Thieme

Controversies in Stereotactic Radiosurgery

Best Evidence Recommendations

Jason P. Sheehan, MD, PhD
Professor
Departments of Neurological Surgery, Radiation Oncology, and Neuroscience
Co-Director
UVa Gamma Knife Center
Riverside-UVa Gamma Knife
University of Virginia School of Medicine
Charlottesville, Virginia

Peter C. Gerszten, MD, MPH
Peter E. Sheptak Professor
Departments of Neurological Surgery and Radiation Oncology
Director
Percutaneous Spine Service
University of Pittsburgh Medical Center
Pittsburgh, Pennsylvania

Thieme
New York • Stuttgart • Delhi • Rio

Thieme Medical Publishers, Inc.
333 Seventh Ave.
New York, NY 10001

Executive Editor: Kay Conerly
Managing Editor: Judith Tomat
Senior Vice President, Editorial and E-Product Development: Cornelia Schulze
Production Editor: Sean Woznicki
International Production Director: Andreas Schabert
Senior Vice President and Chief Operating Officer: Sarah Vanderbilt
President: Brian D. Scanlan
Printer: Sheridan Books

Library of Congress Cataloging-in-Publication Data

Controversies in stereotactic radiosurgery: best evidence recommendations / [edited by] Jason P. Sheehan, MD, PhD, FACS, alumni professor and vice Chair, Department of Neurological Surgery, University of Virginia, Charlottesville, Virginia, USA, Peter Gerszten, MD, MPH, FACS, Peter E. Sheptak, professor of Neurological Surgery and Radiation Oncology, University of Pittsburgh Medical Center, Pittsburgh, Pennsylvania, USA.

pages cm
Includes bibliographical references.
ISBN 978-1-60406-841-2 (hardback) –
ISBN 978-1-60404-842-9 (eISBN)

1. Radiosurgery. 2. Stereoencephalotomy. 3. Evidence-based medicine. I. Sheehan, Jason P., editor of compilation. II. Gerszten, Peter C., editor of compilation. III. Sheptak, Peter E., editor of compilation.
RD594.15.C668 2014
617.4'81059–dc23 2013034350

Thieme Publishers New York 333 Seventh Avenue, New York, NY 10001 USA, 1-800-782-3488, customerservice@thieme.com

Thieme Publishers Stuttgart
Rüdigerstrasse 14, 70469 Stuttgart, Germany, +49 [0]711 8931 421, customerservice@thieme.de

Thieme Publishers Delhi
A-12, Second Floor, Sector-2, NOIDA-201301, Uttar Pradesh, India +91 120 45 566 00, customerservice@thieme.in

Thieme Publishers Rio, Thieme Publicações Ltda.
Argentina Building 16th floor, Ala A, 228 Praia do Botafogo Rio de Janeiro 22250-040 Brazil, +55 21 3736-3631

Printed in the United States of America

5 4 3 2 1

ISBN 978-1-60406–841–2

Also available as an e-book:
eISBN 978-1-60406-842-9

I acknowledge the tremendous support that my family has given me throughout this project. Diane, Kimball, and Darrah were a constant source of encouragement.

Jason P. Sheehan

To my parents, teachers, colleagues, wife, and children. Without their unwavering support and encouragement, this work would not have been possible

Peter C. Gerszten

Contents

Foreword

The field of radiosurgery is now being advanced by arguably a third generation of neurosurgeons and radiation oncologists. Over this period of time, technology has progressed immensely, and a largely empirical-based understanding of how radiosurgery works has evolved considerably. Perhaps most excitingly of all, truly new clinical applications have emerged, especially outside the cranium, which are far removed from the earliest practice of radiosurgery. After so much dramatic change, it is time to take stock of what is known and what is still conjecture within the field. Into that void steps the current treatise.

Controversies in Stereotactic Radiosurgery represents the thinking of some of the leading neurosurgical and radiation oncologic practitioners of radiosurgery in the world today. After reviewing in the opening chapters some recent technological and conceptual advances within radiosurgery, the many coauthors in this book wade into disputed clinical waters. Many chapters are not devoted to radiosurgery itself but represent descriptions of alternative state-of-the-art treatments, such as advanced spinal surgery, microsurgery, and whole-brain radiation therapy; understanding the cost–benefit ratio of radiosurgery necessarily requires a thorough understanding of these alternatives. Despite the absence of level 1 evidence, a few of the "controversies" covered by this book are not entirely "controversial." For example, even the most zealous of microsurgical zealots has finally come to acknowledge some role for using radiosurgery to manage acoustic neuroma in certain clinical situations; in this case, the book provides the reader with an appreciation for what may soon be an emerging consensus. In contrast, for some pathology, it is not clear that we as a discipline are any wiser after the passage of time and experience. For example, one debate that is almost as old as the field of radiosurgery itself is whether or not radiosurgery has any role in treating cavernous malformations of the brain. Without compelling new studies one way or the other, I am not sure we are any closer to definitive answers. Nevertheless, for the radiosurgical neophyte, it is useful to become familiar with the arguments on either side of such issues. For those of us who have been immersed in radiosurgery for the past several decades, revisiting the debate is like spending time with an old friend, or, alternatively, a wound that simply refuses to heal.

Although successive chapters make persuasive arguments on both sides of the many controversies, more often than not the facts unfortunately remain inconclusive. Of course, more rigorous studies would and probably eventually will provide unambiguous answers to some of the uncertainties that currently exist. When a radiosurgical technique has been around for a while, and the condition in question is not rare, prospective and ideally randomized trials can accomplish the goal, especially for brain and spine metastases and glioblastomas. However, some diseases are rarer, the pathology so varied, and the natural history so long that it is unlikely that we will ever see optimal studies conducted, with benign spinal cord tumors and cerebral arteriovenous malformations being cases in point. In these situations, the experience of experts, anecdotal or not, may be as good as our understanding is likely to ever get. With some very new clinical applications that are in many ways still being refined, it is simply not realistic that we as a field are yet able to run rigid definitive head-to-head trials. The ongoing investigation of medial temporal lesioning for temporal lobe epilepsy with radiosurgery provides such an example. I for one believe it is still premature to expect a definitive answer when comparing the radiosurgical approach, which has been explored in only a few dozen patients, with an open surgical resection that has been refined over 60 years and in perhaps as many as 100,000 patients. To elaborate on this, the very recent availability of bevacizumab for treating radiation injury could make it possible to ameliorate the single biggest drawback to radiosurgery and thereby totally transform the risk–benefit ratio.

In a domain of medicine where it is so difficult to successfully perform randomized, controlled clinical trials, the expert guidance in *Controversies in Stereotactic Radiosurgery*, even if perhaps biased, will prove powerful information for any physician whose practice is touched by radiosurgery of the brain or spine. Given the impact of radiosurgery on neurosurgery, I can argue that nearly all neurosurgeons and most radiation oncologists will benefit from a book like this. This is the only book that provides the interested reader with a concise location to explore many of the core controversies within stereotactic radiosurgery. Such a topic can be of considerable interest to those who care for patients with brain and spinal lesions, whether radiosurgeons or not.

Progress is never a straight path, and this book illustrates this point nicely. Much of radiosurgery has progressed merely through the collective will of its enthusiasts, but only to be later beaten back by equally essential doubters. However, with changes in technology and on the back of ever better imaging, as well as opportunities to reframe the underlying thinking about certain diseases themselves, we have been able to witness the radiosurgical frontier being advanced a second or, in some instances, even a third time. This stuttering course of progress inevitably collects controversy, but the reader who approaches this book with an open mind will surely come away the wiser.

John R. Adler, Jr., MD
Dorothy and Thye King Chan Professor of Neurosurgery
Stanford University School of Medicine
Stanford, California

Foreword

From its inception, stereotactic radiosurgery has found itself amid controversy. The field of radiotherapy was already a half century old at the onset of stereotactically guided radiation delivery. For decades, radiotherapists had understood that oligofractionated, or one-stage, dose delivery was associated with toxic late side effects that had previously discredited the field and led to the near decimation of the specialty. No wonder there was such strong and emotional negative reaction to physicians more accustomed to doing surgery now conducting hypofractionated, single-session treatments in, of all places, the central nervous system (CNS). The brain and spinal cord were known to be among the least radiation-tolerant tissue types in the body, not to mention late toxicity could be catastrophically debilitating. The basic controversy about whether these treatments should or should not be done smolders to this day.

Fortunately for our patients, the pioneers of radiosurgery kept their resolve to explore the new therapy. The fundamental hypothesis, understood from the beginning, was that stereotactic radiosurgery must be accurate with precisely localized high-dose potency. In contrast, conventional radiotherapy had evolved to be the opposite, much more encompassing of target and nontarget tissues, yet being forgiven by normal tissue response biology. In the end, they are both clearly useful but different. Radiosurgery uses potent hypofractionation to affect localized, targeted tissue control. The localization is afforded by advanced technology to effectively exclude the sensitive neural tissue surrounding the target. With less need for advanced guidance, conventional radiotherapy "bathes" tissue at risk for tumor infiltration with a more tolerant fractionated dose, facilitating an adjuvant intent. To the credit of the pioneers of stereotactic radiosurgery, the clinical experience over the subsequent half century has shown their hypothesis to be mostly correct. Radiosurgery is clearly beneficial and established in and around the CNS. Furthermore, its guiding principles are being adopted for use in all parts of the body for similarly effective treatment of a large variety of local tumor deposits.

In *Controversies in Stereotactic Radiosurgery*, editors Jason Sheehan and Peter Gerszten bravely face ongoing controversies of CNS radiosurgery. Numerous practical and pertinent issues toward managing these patients are addressed in a fair and balanced forum. While camps of opinion clearly exist, the goal of all should be, simply, to end the controversy. If the controversy is fairly characterized as in this text, appropriate types and amounts of higher level evidence can be gathered that would realign the thinking of any reasonable clinical scientist. Yet we all should recognize that one of the biggest obstacles toward improvement in oncology and neurosurgery has been tradition. If practitioners are satisfied with their time-honored approach, even if outcomes are poor, they frequently will resist change. Change may require new training, new investment, loss of credibility, loss of referrals, or loss of reimbursement. Altruism overcomes these obstacles, and the altruistic route is easier to follow if the pathway is not muddied by poor-quality data and low-level ad hoc experiences. As is made obviously clear in the chapters in this book, many radiosurgery controversies could have been put to rest by cooperation among sites to conduct valid clinical trials. Admittedly, though, other controversies will take more creativity to put to rest. For example, the optic pathway tolerance cannot ethically be determined in a human phase I trial. However, although expensive, tissue tolerance can be appreciated from large animal experimentation. As a pertinent example, the experience described in the text for spinal cord irradiation of pigs has been extremely relevant to radiosurgery, affording both more effective and safer treatments. Similar experiences for a variety of tissues could be conducted to end controversy by finding more accurate boundaries of radiosurgical therapy.

Although several controversies in radiosurgery have been put to rest, including the early basic debate of whether technology can facilitate oligofractionation, many important controversies remain. These controversies and the research that should logically follow constitute opportunities to improve outcomes. *Controversies in Stereotactic Radiosurgery* represents both a balanced summary of differing opinions and, importantly, a practical approach to management decision making both for now and the future. Readers should find it an indispensable resource for evaluations, educating patients, consenting, and applying the stereotactic radiosurgery option most prudently.

Robert Timmerman, MD
Professor of Radiation Oncology and Neurosurgery
University of Texas Southwestern Medical Center
Dallas, TX

Contributors

David W. Andrews, MD
Vice-Chairman of Clinical Services
Department of Neurological Surgery
Thomas Jefferson University
Chief, Division of Neuro-Oncology
Philadelphia, Pennsylvania, USA

Ali A. Baaj, MD
Assistant Professor
Director, Spine Surgery Program
Division of Neurosurgery
University of Arizona
Tucson, Arizona, USA

Igor J. Barani, MD
Assistant Professor In-Residence
Department of Radiation Oncology
University of California, San Francisco
San Francisco, California, USA

Nicholas M. Barbaro, MD
Professor of Neurological Surgery
Department of Neurological Surgery
Indiana University Health
Goodman Campbell Brain and Spine
Indianapolis, Indiana, USA

Mark H. Bilsky, MD
Attending
Department of Neurosurgery
Memorial Sloan-Kettering Cancer Center
Professor
Department of Neurosurgery
Weill Medical College of Cornell University
New York, New York, USA

Seth Blacksburg, MD, MBA
Assistant Professor
Department of Radiation Oncology
Icahn School of Medicine at Mount Sinai
New York, New York, USA

Frank J. Bova, PhD
Professor
Department of Neurosurgery
University of Florida
Gainesville, Florida, USA

Paul D. Brown, MD
Professor
Department of Radiation Oncology
The University of Texas MD Anderson Cancer Center
Houston, Texas, USA

Marc Bussière, MSc
Head Physicist, Stereotactic Service
Department of Radiation Oncology
Massachusetts General Hospital
Boston, Massachusetts, USA

Romain Carron, MD
Neurosurgeon
Department of Functional and Stereotactic Neurosurgery
Gammaknife Radiosurgery Unit
La Timone Univeristy Hospital
Aix-Marseille University
Marseille, France

Eric L. Chang, MD
Professor and Chairman
Department of Radiation Oncology
Keck School of Medicine of USC
Los Angeles, California, USA

Steven D. Chang, MD
Robert C. and Jeannette Powell Professor
Department of Neurosurgery
Stanford University School of Medicine
Stanford, California, USA

Samuel Chao, MD
Assistant Professor
Cleveland Clinic Lerner College of Medicine
Department of Radiation Oncology
Rose Ella Burkhardt Brain Tumor and Neuro-oncology Center
Cleveland Clinic
Cleveland, Ohio, USA

Ephraim W. Church, MD
Neurosurgery Resident
Department of Neurosurgery
Penn State Milton S. Hershey Medical Center
Hershey, Pennsylvania, USA

John Cuaron, MD
Resident
Department of Radiation Oncology
Memorial Sloan-Kettering Cancer Center
New York, New York, USA

Antonio A.F. De Salles, MD, PhD
Professor of Neurosurgery and Radiation Oncology
Departments of Neurosurgery and Radiation Oncology
University of California Los Angeles (UCLA)
HCor Neurosicence
Los Angeles, California
Sao Paulo, Brazil

Anne Donnet, MD
Chief of Chronic Pain Department
Center for Evaluation and Treatment of Pain
Timone Hospital
Marseille, France

Aaron S. Dumont, MD
Charles B. Wilson Professor & Chairman
Department of Neurological Surgery
Tulane University
New Orleans, Louisiana, USA

Christopher J. Farrell, MD
Assistant Professor
Department of Neurological Surgery
Thomas Jefferson University
Philadelphia, Pennsylvania, USA

John C. Flickinger, MD, FACR
Professor
Department of Radiation Oncology
University of Pittsburgh Medical Center – Presbyterian Hospital
Pittsburgh, Pennsylvania, USA

Ryan Foster, PhD
Assistant Professor and Director of Clinical Medical Physics
Department of Radiation Oncology
UT Southwestern Medical Center
Dallas, Texas, USA

William A. Friedman, MD
Professor and Chairman
Department of Neurosurgery
University of Florida
Gainesville, Florida, USA

Kyle S. Gabrick
BS, Medical Student
College of Medicine
University of Tennessee Health Science Center
Semmes Murphey Neurologic and Spine Institute
Memphis, Tennessee, USA

Peter C. Gerszten, MD, MPH
Peter E. Sheptak Professor
Department of Neurological Surgery and Radiation Oncology
Director
Percutaneous Spine Service
University of Pittsburgh Medical Center
Presbyterian University Hospital
Pittsburgh, Pennsylvania, USA

Ziya L. Gokaslan, MD, FACS
Donlin M. Long Professor
Professor of Neurosurgery, Oncology and Orthopaedic Surgery
Director, Neurosurgical Spine Program
Vice Chair
Department of Neurosurgery
Johns Hopkins University School of Medicine
Baltimore, Maryland, USA

John G. Golfinos, MD
Associate Professor and Chairman
Department of Neurosurgery
New York University School of Medicine
New York, New York, USA

Alessandra Gorgulho, MD, MSc
Adjunct Professor of Neurosurgery
Department of Neurosurgery
University of California Los Angeles (UCLA)
HCor Neurosicence - Sao Paulo, Brazil
Los Angeles, California, USA

Ramesh Grandhi, MD
Chief Resident
Department of Neurological Surgery
University of Pittsburgh Medical Center
Pittsburgh, Pennsylvania, USA

Mari L. Groves, MD
Neurosurgery Resident
Department of Neurosurgery
Johns Hopkins University
Baltimore, Maryland, USA

Matthias Guckenberger, MD
Associate Professor
Department of Radiation Oncology
University of Würzburg
Würzburg, Germany

Selena E. Heman-Ackah, MD, MBA
Medical Director of Otology, Neurotology and Audiology
Department of Surgery, Division of Otolaryngology
Beth Israel Deaconess Medical Center, Harvard Medical School
Boston, Massachusetts, USA

Zain A. Husain, MD
Assistant Professor
Department of Therapeutic Radiology
Yale School of Medicine
New Haven, Connecticut, USA

Lee Hwang, MD
Resident Physician
The Cleveland Clinic Department of Neurological Surgery
Cleveland, Ohio, USA

Hideyuki Kano, MD, PhD
Research Assistant Professor
Department of Neurological Surgery
University of Pittsburgh
Pittsburgh, Pennsylvania, USA

Douglas Kondziolka, MD, MSc, FRCSC, FACS
Professor of Neurosurgery and Radiation Oncology
Vice-Chair, Clinical Research (Neurosurgery)
Director, Center for Advanced Radiosurgery
NYU Langone Medical Center
New York University
New York, New York, USA

Ryan M. Kretzer, MD
Neurosurgeon
Department of Neurosurgery
Western Neurosurgery, Ltd.
St. Joseph's Hospital
Tucson, Arizona, USA

Young Kwok, MD
Associate Professor
Department of Radiation Oncology
University of Maryland School of Medicine
Baltimore, Maryland, USA

David A. Larson, MD, PhD
Professor
Departments of Radiation Oncology and Neurosurgery
University of California San Francisco
San Francisco, California, USA

Ilya Laufer, MD
Assistant Attending Neurosurgeon
Department of Neurosurgery
Institution Memorial Sloan-Kettering Cancer Center
New York, New York, USA

Ian Lee, MD
Staff Neurosurgeon
Department of Neurosurgery
Henry Ford Health System
Detroit, Michigan, USA

Daniel Létourneau, PhD
Medical Physicist and Assistant Professor
Radiation Medicine Program
Princess Margaret Cancer Center
University of Toronto
Toronto, Ontario, Canada

Jason Liauw, MD
Resident
Department of Neurosurgery
The Johns Hopkins Hospital
Baltimore, Maryland, USA

Mark E. Linskey, MD, FAANS
Professor of Neurological Surgery
Department of Surgery
University of California, Irvine
Orange, California, USA

Eric Lis, MD
Associate Attending Neuroradiologist
Department of Radiology
Memorial Sloan-Kettering Cancer Center
New York, New York, USA

Sheng-fu Larry Lo, MD, MHS
Assistant Resident
Department of Neurosurgery
Johns Hopkins University
Baltimore, Maryland, USA

Simon S. Lo, MD
Associate Professor of Radiation Oncology and Director of Radiosurgery Services and Neurologic Radiation Oncology
Department of Radiation Oncology
University Hospitals Seidman Cancer Center
Case Comprehensive Cancer Center
Cleveland, Ohio, USA

Jay S. Loeffler, MD, FACR
Professor and Chair
Chief, Department of Radiation Oncology
Herman and Joan Suit Professor of Radiation Oncology
Department of Radiation Oncology
Massachusetts General Hospital
Boston, Massachusetts, USA

L. Dade Lunsford, MD, FACS
Lars Leksell Professor and Distinguished Professor
Department of Neurological Surgery
The University of Pittsburgh
Director, Center for Image Guided Neurosurgery
Director, Neurosurgery Residency Program
Chair, Technology and Innovative Practice Committee
UPMC Presbyterian
Pittsburgh, Pennsylvania, USA

Lijun Ma, PhD
Professor
Department of Radiation Oncology
University of California San Francisco
San Francisco, California, USA

Mitchell Machtay, MD
Professor
Department of Radiation Oncology
University Hospitals Seidman Cancer Center
Case Comprehensive Cancer Center
Case Western Reserve University
Cleveland, Ohio, USA

Usama Mahmood, MD
Assistant Professor
Department of Radiation Oncology
University of Texas MD Anderson Cancer Center
Houston, Texas, USA

Nina A. Mayr, MD, FASTRO, FAAAS
Professor and Chair
Department of Radiation Oncology
UW Medicine, University of Washington
Seattle, Washington, USA

Robert A. McGovern, MD
Resident
Department of Neurological Surgery
Columbia University Medical Center
New York, New York, USA

Guy M. McKhann, MD
Associate Professor of Neurological Surgery
Department of Neurological Surgery
Columbia University Medical Center
New York Presbyterian Hospital
New York, New York, USA

Paul M. Medin, PhD
Associate Professor
Department of Radiation Oncology
University of Texas Southwestern Medical Center
Dallas, Texas, USA

Alireza M. Mohammadi, MD
Clinical Associate of Neurosurgery
Rose Ella Burkhardt Brain Tumor and Neuro-Oncology Center
Cleveland Clinic
Cleveland, Ohio, USA

Edward A. Monaco III, MD, PhD
Assistant Professor
Department of Neurological Surgery
Center for Image-Guided Neurosurgery
University of Pittsburgh Medical Center
Pittsburgh, Pennsylvania, USA

Judith A. Murovic, MD
Clinical Assistant Professor
Department of Neurosurgery
Stanford University Medical Center
Stanford, California, USA

Ajay Niranjan, MD, MBA
Associate Professor of Neurosurgery,
Department of Neurological Surgery
University of Pittsburgh
Pittsburgh, Pennsylvania, USA

Paula L. Petti, PhD
Director of Gamma Knife Physics
Washington Hospital Healthcare System
Fremont, California, USA

Patrick Pezeshkian, MD
Neurosurgery Chief Resident
Department of Neurosurgery
University of California Los Angeles (UCLA)
Los Angeles, California, USA

Gabriel H. Phillips, MD
Neurosurgeon Department of Neurosurgery
New Lexington Clinic
Lexington, Kentucky, USA

Mubina A. Quader, PhD
Clinical Associate Professor
Department of Radiation Oncology
University of Pittsburgh Medical Center
Pittsburgh, Pennsylvania, USA

Mark Quigg, MD, MSc
Professor
Department of Neurology
University of Virginia
Charlottesville, Virginia, USA

Maryam Rahman, MD, MS
Assistant Professor
Department of Neurosurgery
University of Florida
Gainesville, Florida, USA

Pablo F. Recinos, MD
Section Head, Minimally Invasive Skull Base Neurosurgery
Rose Ella Burhardt Brain Tumor and Neuro-Oncology Center
Cleveland Clinic
Cleveland, Ohio, USA

William F. Regine, MD
Isadore and Fannie Schneider Foxman Chair and Professor
Department of Radiation Oncology
University of Maryland
Baltimore, Maryland, USA

Jean Régis, MD
Professor
Department of Functional Neurosurgery & Radiosurgery
Aix Marseille University
Marseille, France

Laurence D. Rhines, MD
Professor of Neurosurgery
Department of Neurosurgery
University of Texas M.D. Anderson Cancer Center
Houston, Texas, USA

Elias B Rizk, MD, MSc
Assistant Professor
Department of Neurosurgery
Penn State Milton S. Hershey Medical Center
Hershey, Pennsylvania, USA

Jack P. Rock, MD
Senior Staff
Department of Neurosurgery
Henry Ford Hospital
Detroit, Michigan, USA

Shaun D. Rodgers, MD
Neurosurgery Chief Resident
Department of Neurosurgery
NYU Langone Medical Center
New York, New York, USA

J. Thomas Roland Jr., MD
Mendik Foundation Chairman Professor of Otolaryngology and Neurosurgery
Department of Otolaryngology-Head and Neck Surgery
NYU Langone Medical Center
New York, New York, USA

Mark Ruschin, PhD, MCCPM
Assistant Professor
Department of Radiation Oncology
University of Toronto
Toronto, Ontario, Canada

Samuel Ryu, MD
Professor
Director of Radiosurgery
Departments of Radiation Oncology and Neurosurgery
Henry Ford Health System
Detroit, Michigan, USA

Arjun Sahgal, MD
Associate Professor of Radiation Oncology and Surgery
Department of Radiation Oncology
Sunnybrook Odette Cancer Centre, University of Toronto
Toronto, Ontario, Canada

David J. Schlesinger, PhD
Associate Professor
Departments of Radiation Oncology and Neurological Surgery
University of Virginia
Charlottesville, Virginia, USA

Daniel M. Sciubba, MD
Assistant Professor of Neurosurgery, Oncology and Orthopaedic Surgery
Department of Neurosurgery
Johns Hopkins University
Baltimore, Maryland, USA

Stephen H. Settle, MD, PhD
Assistant Professor
Department of Radiation Oncology
University of Texas M.D. Anderson Cancer Center
Houston, Texas, USA

Jason P. Sheehan, MD, PhD
Professor
Departments of Neurological Surgery, Radiation Oncology, and Neuroscience
Co-Director
UVa Gamma Knife Center
Riverside-UVa Gamma Knife
University of Virginia School of Medicine
Charlottesville, Virginia, USA

Jonas M. Sheehan, MD, FAANS, FACS
Associate Professor
Department of Neurosurgery
Penn State Milton S. Hershey Medical Center
Hershey, Pennsylvania, USA

Helen A. Shih, MD
Chief, Central Nervous System & Eye Tumor Services
Department of Radiation Oncology
Massachusetts General Hospital
Boston, Massachusetts, USA

Jason W. Sohn, PhD
Associate Professor
Radiation Oncology
Case Western Reserve University
Cleveland, Ohio, USA

Timothy D. Solberg, PhD
Professor and Vice Chair, Director of Medical Physics
Department of Radiation Oncology
University of Pennsylvania
Philadelphia, Pennsylvania, USA

Robert M. Starke, MD, MSc
Neurosurgery Resident
Department of Neurological Surgery
University of Virginia
Charlottesville, Virginia, USA

John H. Suh, MD
Professor and Chairman
Department of Radiation Oncology
Cleveland Clinic
Cleveland, Ohio, USA

Reinhart A. Sweeney, MD, BSc
Director
Department Of Radiation Oncology
MVZ at Leopoldina Hospital
Schweinfurt, Germany

Randa Tao, MD
Resident
Department of Radiation Oncology
The University of Texas M. D. Anderson Cancer Center
Houston, Texas, USA

Constantin Tuleasca, MD; MD-PhD student
Resident
Department of Neurosurgery Service and Gamma Knife Center
Institution Lausanne University Hospital and University of Lausanne
Lausanne, Switzerland
Functional and Stereotactic Neurosurgery Unit and Gamma Knife Unit
Centre Hospitalier Universitaire "La Timone"
Assistance Publique- Hopitaux de Marseille, Aix-Marseille University
Marseille, France
Lausanne, Switzerland

Matthew VanLandingham, MD
Resident
Department of Neurosurgery
University of Tennessee
Semmes-Murphey Clinic
Memphis, Tennessee, USA

Michael A. Vogelbaum, MD, PhD, FAANS, FACS
Professor of Surgery (Neurosurgery)
The Robert W. And Kathryn B. Lamborn Chair for Neuro-Oncology
Rose Ella Burkhardt Brain Tumor and NeuroOncology Center
Cleveland Clinic
Cleveland, Ohio, USA

Jason A. Weaver, MD, FACS
Assistant Professor
Department of Neurosurgery
University of Tennessee
Semmes Murphey Clinic
Memphis, Tennessee, USA

Timothy F. Witham, MD, FACS
Associate Professor of Neurosurgery and Orthopaedic Surgery
Department of Neurosurgery
Johns Hopkins University School of Medicine
Baltimore, Maryland, USA

Jean-Paul Wolinsky, MD
Associate Professor
Departments of Neurosurgery and Oncology
Clinical Director
Johns Hopkins Spine Program
Johns Hopkins Hospital
Baltimore, Maryland, USA

Zhiyuan Xu, MD
Clinical Instructor
Gamma Knife Center
Department of Neurosurgery
University of Virginia
Charlottesville, Virginia, USA

Yoshiya (Josh) Yamada, MD, FRCPC
Associate Attending Radiation Oncologist
Department of Radiation Oncology
Memorial Sloan Kettering Cancer Center
New York, New York, USA

T. Jonathan Yang, MD
Radiation Oncology Resident
Department of Radiation Oncology
Memorial Sloan-Kettering Cancer Center
New York, New York, USA

Kevin C. Yao, MD
Assistant Clinical Professor
Department of Neurosurgery
Mount Sinai Medical Center
New York, New York, USA

Chun-Po Yen, MD
Resident
Department of Neurological Surgery
University of Virginia
Charlottesville, Virginia, USA

1 Introduction

Jason P. Sheehan and Peter C. Gerszten

The field of stereotactic neurosurgery has evolved substantially since the pioneering work of Clarke and Horsley, who developed the first stereotactic system, and Spiegel and Wycis, who applied this methodology clinically.[1,2] Lars Leksell employed the principles of stereotaxis and coupled it with ionizing beams of radiation to devise the concept of "radiosurgery" in 1951.[3] His goal was to develop a technique for destroying localized structures deep within the brain without the degree of collateral brain tissue damage often associated with open neurosurgical procedures. To achieve this goal, he devised the concept of multiple beams of ionizing radiation converging at one stereotactically defined point. An innocuous dose is delivered to the paths of each incident beam. However, at the point of intersection of the various beams, a dose directly proportional to the number of individual beams is delivered. Furthermore, this approach allows for a sharp drop-off of delivered radiation at the edge of the intersection point.

Since its clinical introduction over 60 years ago, stereotactic radiosurgery has revolutionized the clinical approaches of both neurosurgery and radiation oncology. Radiosurgery has altered treatment paradigms for patients with benign and malignant tumors of the brain and spine and vascular malformations, as well as pain and movement disorders. The number of radiosurgical devices and the techniques employed are nearly as diverse as the indications for radiosurgery itself.

Radiosurgery has often been held to a higher standard than other approaches in neurosurgery or radiation oncology. Demand for comprehensive, long-term follow-up of radiosurgical patients has been met with numerous publications detailing the successes and limitations of this approach.[4,5] Also, dose-planning techniques have been carefully refined over the years to ensure improvements in clinical outcomes while maintaining favorable radiologic outcomes.[6]

There are, however, several concepts within the field of radiosurgery for cranial and spinal disorders that remain the subject of much debate. These areas represent controversial subjects for experts in the field and yield continued discussions at scientific meetings and in the printed pages of peer-reviewed journals. In this textbook, we have attempted to cover these important and relevant clinical issues comprehensively while avoiding the dogmatic stances sometimes taken by zealous advocates. At the very least, we hope to facilitate a critical review of the evidence supporting each position that will be

Table 1.1 Classification Scheme for Levels of Evidence

Level of Evidence	Type of Study
I	1. Randomized, controlled trial
	2. Systematic review of randomized, controlled trials
II	1. Prospective cohort study
	2. Randomized trial with low (< 80%) follow-up
	3. Systematic review of level II studies
III	1. Case-control study
	2. Retrospective, cohort study
	3. Systematic review of level III studies
IV	Case series
V	Expert opinion

Table 1.2 Grades of Recommendations

Recommendation Grade	Risk-to-Benefit Clarity	Strength of Supporting Evidence	Clinical Implications
1A	Clear	Randomized trials without appreciable limitations	Strong recommendations that can be applied to most patients
1B	Clear	Randomized trials with important limitations (e.g., methodological flaws)	Strong recommendations that can likely be applied to many patients
1C +	Clear	No randomized trials	Strong recommendations that can be applied to many patients under most circumstances
		Results are based on overwhelming evidence from observational studies	
1C	Clear	Observational studies	Intermediate-strength recommendations
2A	Unclear	Randomized trial without important limitations	Intermediate-strength recommendations; best actions may differ depending on the circumstances of the patient
2B	Unclear	Randomized trials with important limitations (e.g. methodological flaws)	Weak recommendations; alternative approaches may be considered
2C	Unclear	Observational studies	Fairly weak recommendations; other approaches may be equally reasonable

Adapted from Fischer CG, Wood KB. Introduction to and techniques of evidence-based medicine. Spine 2007;32:S66–72.

beneficial for the practitioners of radiosurgery. The evidence will be interspersed with the opinions and practical experience of experts in the field. The reader can then decide the merits of each approach and make an informed decision on how to incorporate this information into his or her clinical practice.

In each case, we have asked the contributing authors to clearly define the controversy that exists, search and critically review the literature with an assessment of the level of evidence each report affords (▶ Table 1.1), and assess outcomes from their particular approach. In addition, they have been asked to make recommendations that they deem fit based on the available literature and their own personal and in many instances vast experience. The recommendations are to follow the grades (▶ Table 1.2) outlined by Fisher and Wood.[7] In some instances, the specific area of controversy itself may not be simply black or white. Shades of gray often encompass clinical situations. The level of evidence currently available may not allow firm, unequivocal recommendations to be drawn. Neurosurgeons and radiation oncologists therefore must make clinical decisions based on the evidence currently available and not the evidence that they wish they had or may have in the future. We hope that this textbook sheds new light on the controversies and adds clarity to challenging clinical situations within the exciting field of stereotactic radiosurgery.

References

[1] Clarke R, Horsley V. THE CLASSIC: on a method of investigating the deep ganglia and tracts of the central nervous system (cerebellum). Br Med J 1906:1799-1800. Clin Orthop Relat Res 2007; 463: 3–6

[2] Spiegel EA, Wycis HT, Marks M, Lee AJ. Stereotaxic apparatus for operations on the human brain. Science 1947; 106: 349–350

[3] Leksell L. The stereotaxic method and radiosurgery of the brain. Acta Chir Scand 1951; 102: 316–319

[4] Gopalan R, Schlesinger D, Vance ML, Laws E, Sheehan J. Long-term outcomes after Gamma Knife radiosurgery for patients with a nonfunctioning pituitary adenoma. Neurosurgery 2011; 69: 284–293

[5] Kondziolka D, Mathieu D, Lunsford LD, et al. Radiosurgery as definitive management of intracranial meningiomas. Neurosurgery 2008; 62: 53–58, discussion 58–60

[6] Niranjan A, Lunsford LD, Flickinger JC, Maitz A, Kondziolka D. Dose reduction improves hearing preservation rates after intracanalicular acoustic tumor radiosurgery. Neurosurgery 1999; 45: 753–762, discussion 762–765

[7] Fisher CG, Wood KB. Introduction to and techniques of evidence-based medicine. Spine 2007; 32 Suppl: S66–S72

Technologies for Intracranial Radiosurgery

2 Frame-based Stereotactic Radiosurgery

Maryam Rahman, Frank J. Bova, and William A. Friedman

Introduction

Stereotactic radiosurgery (SRS) has a rich history, beginning with the first stereotactic frame described by Horsley and Clarke in 1908.[1] In a seminal article published in *Brain*, they described lesioning targets in a monkey brain using an apparatus with an electrode guide based on the three-dimensional Cartesian coordinate system. Many years later Lars Leksell, prior to his description of radiosurgery, developed a stereotactic frame with skull pin fixation for rigid frame immobilization.[1–3] Unlike the orthogonal system of Horsley and Clarke, the electrode advanced along a radius of an arc to which the electrode carrier was attached. The position of the arc was adjustable, and the electrode pointed to the target, regardless of the angle of insertion.[4] He called this the "arc radius" and said, "I was born under the sign of the 'archer' and look forward to sharpshoot into the brain."[5] The arc-radius system subsequently became the Todd-Wells stereotactic system (developed by American neurosurgeon Edwin Todd and engineer Trent Wells). The Cosman-Roberts-Wells (CRW) frame, also in common use today, is arc radius based (▶ Fig. 2.1).

The stereotactic head frame was the crux of radiosurgery, initially described by Leksell in 1951. Radiosurgery, defined as one to five fractions of stereotactically targeted radiation therapy, proposed a paradigm shift in the art of radiation delivery. This approach delivers a high dose of radiation exclusively to the tumor cells, instead of depending on the differential between normal cell and cancer cell repair of sublethal radiation damage. To achieve this high dose of radiation, arcs of noncoplanar beams of radiation or separate cobalt sources are used to converge on the lesion. The stereotactic head frame ensures delivery accuracy necessary for radiosurgery.

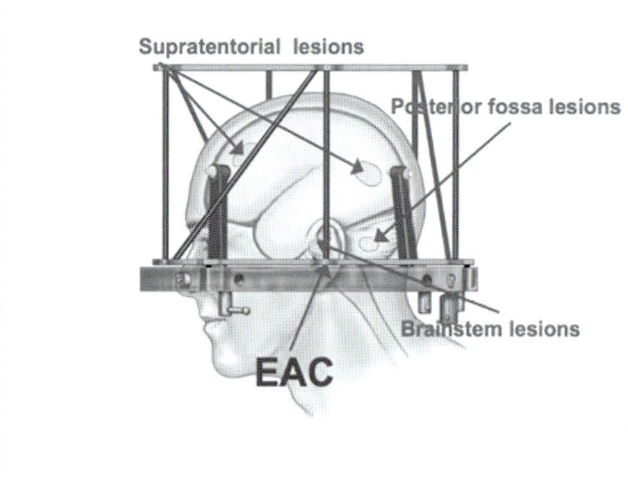

Fig. 2.1 CRW frame with attached localizer used during computed tomography imaging. Note the top of the ring is below the level of the external auditory canal. This ensures that the scan will capture low targets in the middle fossa, brainstem, and posterior fossa.

As imaging techniques have improved, a number of frameless radiosurgery systems have been developed that depend on optical image guidance or stereoscopic X-ray imaging.[6,7] Proponents of frameless radiosurgery note that placement of frames requires premedication, is associated with pain, may slip, causing patient harm, and are less feasible for multiple treatments.[8,9] However, frameless systems are associated with less accuracy and limited immobilization during treatment.[10–12] At the University of Florida, we have developed and continue to improve a frame-based approach to radiosurgery. In this chapter we review the current evidence in the literature and our approach to frame-based radiosurgery.

Literature Review

The goal of SRS is to mimic surgical resection; therefore, the coverage of the planning target volume is set equal to the imaging target volume. The planning process ensures that the full imaged target is covered. Hence, omission of any portion of the target volume is analogous to a subtotal surgical resection due to the steep dose gradient.

The imaging and highly conformal planning with steep dose gradients requires an exquisitely accurate delivery system. The stereotactic target must be aligned with the delivery system, and the system must be able to deliver multiple noncoplanar beams while maintaining alignment.

These criteria were first described with the early Gamma Knife units. The rigid source alignment with the stereotactic reference provided a target to isocenter alignment of 0.3 mm.[13] Initially, linear accelerator (LINAC) systems were unable to maintain such accuracy.

Within 10 years of LINAC development, reports appeared of the use of external beam radiation for radiosurgery.[14] In 1983 Oswaldo Betti and Victor Derechinsky reported the development of a multibeam LINAC coupled with a Talairach stereotactic localization system in Buenos Aires.[14,15] They used circular collimators that could be oriented in multiple coronal planes of a patient sitting in a moveable chair while attached to a rotating head frame.[15,17] Their system uniquely had the patient in a sitting position.[18]

In 1984, a standard LINAC with small modifications was used by Heifetz et al (with Marilyn Wexler's physics contributions) to deliver high-dose radiation to small targets sparing normal brain, similar to Leksell's Gamma Knife.[19] Simultaneously, a neurosurgeon, Federico Colombo, and a group of physicists led by Renzo Avanzo in Vicenza, Italy, reported their stereotactic LINAC radiosurgery system.[20] They wrote about radiosurgical dose schemes of 40 to 50 Gy over two fractions separated by 8 to 10 days for various intracranial targets of 2 to 4 cm in diameter.[21,22] The dose gradient achieved compared well with Gamma Knife data.[22,23] Hartmann et al in Heidelberg, Germany, followed these achievements with the description of a modified stereotactic localization and positioning system to deliver multiple arc radiosurgery treatments.[24] They modified a Riechert-Mundinger stereotactic device, using laser lights to position the frame within the isocenter.

The first published work on LINAC radiosurgery in the United States came from the University of Miami in 1985.[25] However, this system relied on the jaws of the treatment machine for beam collimation instead of the secondary collimation system described by Larsson et al.[26] The technique was regarded as fractionated, rather than single fraction.

One of the first solutions for the requirement to spread out the radiation entrance path and minimize treatment delivery time was described by Ervin Podgorsak at McGill University.[27] He and his colleagues modified a LINAC using extra collimators to define small circular fields and simultaneous gantry and couch rotations. Additionally, the couch and gantry were monitored from the control area, eliminating the need to enter the room during treatment.[28] Due to increased error rates with simultaneous gantry and couch rotation, most institutions have not adopted this system. Concerned with error and quality control, Winston and Lutz published their work on multiple-arc LINAC stereotactic radiosurgery in 1988.[29] Their system included a phantom target device that could easily be used to check the accuracy of each patient treatment as well as evaluate sources of error. Wilson and Lutz found a mechanical accuracy of their system of 0.5 ± 0.2 mm. They suggested that the major error in any radiosurgery system was the error of localization and not mechanical error.[18] In 1989 Friedman and Bova reported on the LINAC radiosurgery system at the University of Florida.[30] A portable add-on stereotactic device was coupled to the LINAC, and high-precision bearings in the device controlled all patient and gantry movements. As a result, the radiation beam accuracy was improved to 0.2 ± 0.1 mm. The accuracy of treatment delivery was further increased with imaging software improvements and the ability to fuse computed tomography (CT) and magnetic resonance (MR) images.[31] More recently, frame-based stereotactic localization with an onboard CT (instead of the UF floor stand) also demonstrated excellent precision (0.3 mm) with localization error of 0.45 mm ± 0.17 mm.[31] Redesigned linear accelerators introduced in the mid-1990s are capable of maintaining submillimeter delivery alignments. These advances have allowed for accurate localization and targeting of intracranial lesions, thereby delivering the appropriate dose to the entire lesion while preserving normal structures.

Accuracy with Frame-based SRS

Accuracy and precision in radiosurgery are limited by several factors, including (1) incorrect mapping of stereotactic coordinates during image analysis or accuracy of imaging (voxel size), (2) accuracy of image fusion if used, (3) planning that does not provide sufficient conformality or gradient, and (4) delivery systems that do not maintain sufficient rigidity precision during noncoplanar beam delivery.

The first limitation has to do with imaging and image manipulation. Imaging includes the stereotactic mapping of the patient's anatomy, as well as the visualization of the target volume. Many targets require magnetic resonance imaging (MRI) to provide sufficient differentiation of the target tissues from the patient's normal anatomy. Unfortunately, MRI is susceptible to distortions from stereotactic hardware and the patient's own anatomy. Therefore, image fusion software is often used to combine the superior contract resolution of MRI with the superior spatial resolution of CT imaging. The overall accuracy is therefore dependent not only on the resolution of the scanned images but also on the accuracy of the fusion of the two image matrixes.

In frame-based procedures, the stereotactic frame, rigidly fixed to the patient's skull, provides a platform for both image acquisition and treatment delivery. The accuracy of the stereotactic mapping is dependent upon not only the in-plane resolution but also the slice thickness and slice spacing. A typical stereotactic frame is on the order of 350 mm in diameter. When a CT scan is displayed on a typical 512 × 512 pixel format, the in-plane resolution is on the order of 0.67 mm/pixel (350 mm/512 pixels). The target resolution is also dependent upon the slice thickness and slice spacing. Typically, contiguous slices of 1 mm provide an end CT resolution of 0.67 mm × 0.67 mm × 1 mm. This voxel size provides the basis for the entire image-planning treatment chain accuracy.

Due to the potential for spatial perturbations, MRI is usually conducted prior to stereotactic ring fixation. This protocol provides for a more spatially uniform image and the ability to limit the scanning volume because the stereotactic ring and fiducial system do not need to be inside the MRI volume. Our typical MRI diameter is on the order of 25 cm with slice thicknesses no greater than 1.0 mm (voxel sizes of 0.5 mm × 0.5 mm × 1.0 mm).

After the nonstereotactic MR image is fused to the stereotactic CT scan, an inspection of the anatomical alignment in the area of the target(s) is carried out by the clinician performing radiosurgery. The overall accuracy is dependent upon the CT pixel resolution, the MR pixel resolution, and the accuracy of the image fusion process.

Images acquired with the ring in place define a virtual patient with a virtual target in the computer. The virtual patient and target serve as a template for designing the trajectory and character of the multiple noncoplanar beam of radiation. The head ring localization defines a coordinate matrix in the computer that is directly transferable to the actual patient and stereotactic subsystem where radiosurgery is delivered. Thus, the patient is treated with specifications assigned by the computer on the basis of the virtual patient in stereotactic space, and the actual treatment in the true treatment room is identical within 0.2 ± 0.1 mm.[32]

The stereotactic frame plays an integral part in ensuring rigidity of the system. Moreover, the rigidity of the stereotactic frame allows accuracy even for extremely small lesions. The frame helps immobilize patients during radiosurgery, especially for plans that are complex and take significant time to deliver. Patients have difficulty holding completely still for radiation treatment. They may cough, itch, or twitch. The frame prevents any movement of the target. In a study of face mask or bite block localization for several SRS treatment sessions, the authors noted that the largest localization deviations took place in the first 2 weeks of therapy due to patient anxiety and movement.[33] The alternative is to monitor the patient's position during treatment, with optical systems. However, these systems add complexity to quality assurance (QA), treatment time, and determining accuracy.

Using the frame and a floor stand greatly simplifies the QA required for radiosurgery. A frameless system requires the use of some other external system, onboard imaging, or lasers. The patient position in relationship to the device can be determined with imaging such as stereoscopic X-ray (Novalis Circle, Brainlab Inc., IL, USA, Brainlab AG, Munich, Germany, and Accuray CyberKnife, Accuray Inc., Sunnyvale, CA) or onboard cone CT (Varian Trilogy, Varian Medical Systems, Inc., Palo Alto, CA; Elekta Synergy, Elekta AB, Stockholm, Sweden; and Siemens ONCOR, Siemens AG, Munich, Germany).[34] However, these systems add to treatment and QA time, potentially precluding the ability to treat multiple patients in 1 day. At the University of Florida, with a rapid QA process, on average 10 patients are treated with a single device per treatment day.

Consensus statements have been made about the controversy between frameless and frame-based stereotaxy. Many believe that frame-based stereotaxy remains the gold standard for accurate targeting and that frameless systems should be used only for lesions > 10 mm in size due to inaccuracies.[35] According to the American Institute of Physics, the stereotactic localization technique should be capable of localizing with on overall uncertainty of no more than 2 mm.[36] Moreover, the mechanical precision of aligning the patient-based or frame-based coordinate system with the treatment machine coordinate system should be < 1 mm.[31]

Even in a surgical setting, frameless neuronavigation systems have demonstrated localization errors between 1.59 and 3.86 mm,[37–39] compared with submillimeter accuracy for frame-based systems.[40] For fractionated radiosurgery, noninvasive fixation systems have been reported with accuracies between 0.5 and 2.0 mm.[32,33] The overall poorer accuracy of frameless systems limits their use for larger lesions or for malignant lesions where a deliberate margin or expansion is placed upon the intracranial target.

Interpretation of the Evidence and Recommended Practice

The evidence for the accuracy of frame-based radiosurgery systems includes single-institution studies and does not include class I data. Moreover, direct prospective studies comparing frameless and frame-based radiosurgery in terms of outcomes have not been performed. Thus, the evidence supporting frame-based radiosurgery over that of frameless radiosurgery is largely based on class III or lower evidence.

At the University of Florida, all radiosurgery patients undergo a pretreatment MRI the morning of their scheduled radiosurgery, then undergo head ring placement after a "time-out" procedure, with local anesthetic after premedication with oral diazepam. The patients subsequently undergo a CT (or computed tomography angiography for vascular lesions) with the addition of a CT localizer on their head frame. The CT and MR images are fused, and dose planning is performed. The patient's head ring is used for immobilization during dose delivery, and the LINAC unit's accuracy is verified prior to each treatment with a step-by-step procedure that verifies the stereotactic coordinate, the cone and collimator settings, and the monitor unit setting for each treatment segment. We recommend frame-based radiosurgery for all cases unless fractionation requires multiple treatments.

References

[1] Leksell L. The stereotaxic method and radiosurgery of the brain. Acta Chir Scand 1951; 102: 316–319

[2] Leksell L. Sterotaxic radiosurgery in trigeminal neuralgia. Acta Chir Scand 1971; 137: 311–314

[3] Rahman M, Murad GJ, Mocco J. Early history of the stereotactic apparatus in neurosurgery. Neurosurg Focus 2009; 27: E12

[4] Gildenberg P. The history of stereotactic neurosurgery. In: Friedman WA, Winn HR, Mayberg MR, eds. Neurosurgery Clinics of North America: Stereotactic Neurosurgery. Vol 1. Philadelphia: W.B. Saunders; 1990:765–780

[5] Lee NIS, Schiff PB, Sisti MB, Germano IM. Historical perspective and basic principles of radiation physics and biology. In: IM G, ed. LINAC and Gamma Knife Radiosurgery. Rolling Meadows, IL: American Association of Neurological Surgeons; 1999:3–10

[6] Ryken TC, Meeks SL, Pennington EC, et al. Initial clinical experience with frameless stereotactic radiosurgery: analysis of accuracy and feasibility. Int J Radiat Oncol Biol Phys 2001; 51: 1152–1158

[7] Verellen D, Soete G, Linthout N, et al. Quality assurance of a system for improved target localization and patient set-up that combines real-time infrared tracking and stereoscopic X-ray imaging. Radiother Oncol 2003; 67: 129–141

[8] Otto K, Fallone BG. Frame slippage verification in stereotactic radiosurgery. Int J Radiat Oncol Biol Phys 1998; 41: 199–205

[9] Ramakrishna N, Rosca F, Friesen S, Tezcanli E, Zygmanszki P, Hacker F. A clinical comparison of patient setup and intra-fraction motion using frame-based radiosurgery versus a frameless image-guided radiosurgery system for intracranial lesions. Radiother Oncol 2010; 95: 109–115

[10] Kooy HM, Dunbar SF, Tarbell NJ, et al. Adaptation and verification of the relocatable Gill-Thomas-Cosman frame in stereotactic radiotherapy. Int J Radiat Oncol Biol Phys 1994; 30: 685–691

[11] Gilbeau L, Octave-Prignot M, Loncol T, Renard L, Scalliet P, Grégoire V. Comparison of setup accuracy of three different thermoplastic masks for the treatment of brain and head and neck tumors. Radiother Oncol 2001; 58: 155–162

[12] Gill SS, Thomas DG, Warrington AP, Brada M. Relocatable frame for stereotactic external beam radiotherapy. Int J Radiat Oncol Biol Phys 1991; 20: 599–603

[13] Lindquist C. Gamma Knife radiosurgery. Semin Radiat Oncol 1995; 5: 197–202

[14] Benedict SH, Bova FJ, Clark B, et al. Anniversary Paper: the role of medical physicists in developing stereotactic radiosurgery. Med Phys 2008; 35: 4262–4277

[15] Betti O, Derechinsky V. Multiple-beam stereotaxic irradiation [in French]. Neurochirurgie 1983; 29: 295–298

[16] Betti OO. Treatment of arteriovenous malformations with the linear accelerator. Appl Neurophysiol 1987; 50: 262

[17] Betti OO, Galmarini D, Derechinsky V. Radiosurgery with a linear accelerator: methodological aspects. Stereotact Funct Neurosurg 1991; 57: 87–98

[18] Friedman WA. Linear accelerator radiosurgery. Clin Neurosurg 1992; 38: 445–471

[19] Heifetz MD, Wexler M, Thompson R. Single-beam radiotherapy knife: a practical theoretical model. J Neurosurg 1984; 60: 814–818

[20] Avanzo RC, Chierego G, Marchetti C, et al. Stereotaxic irradiation with a linear accelerator [in Italian]. Radiol Med (Torino) 1984; 70: 124–129

[21] Colombo F, Benedetti A, Pozza F, et al. Radiosurgery using a 4MV linear accelerator: technique and radiobiologic implications. Acta Radiol Suppl 1986; 369: 603–607

[22] Colombo F, Benedetti A, Pozza F, et al. External stereotactic irradiation by linear accelerator. Neurosurgery 1985; 16: 154–160

[23] Colombo F, Benedetti A, Zanardo A, et al. New technique for three-dimensional linear accelerator radiosurgery. Acta Neurochir Suppl (Wien) 1987; 39: 38–40

[24] Hartmann GH, Schlegel W, Sturm V, Kober B, Pastyr O, Lorenz WJ. Cerebral radiation surgery using moving field irradiation at a linear accelerator facility. Int J Radiat Oncol Biol Phys 1985; 11: 1185–1192

[25] Houdek PV, Fayos JV, Van Buren JM, Ginsberg MS. Stereotaxic radiotherapy technique for small intracranial lesions. Med Phys 1985; 12: 469–472

[26] Larsson B, Lidén K, Sarby B. Irradiation of small structures through the intact skull. Acta Radiol Ther Phys Biol 1974; 13: 512–534

[27] Podgorsak EB, Olivier A, Pla M, Hazel J, de Lotbinière A, Pike B. Physical aspects of dynamic stereotactic radiosurgery. Appl Neurophysiol 1987; 50: 263–268

[28] Podgorsak EB, Olivier A, Pla M, Lefebvre PY, Hazel J. Dynamic stereotactic radiosurgery. Int J Radiat Oncol Biol Phys 1988; 14: 115–126

[29] Winston KR, Lutz W. Linear accelerator as a neurosurgical tool for stereotactic radiosurgery. Neurosurgery 1988; 22: 454–464

[30] Friedman WA, Bova FJ. The University of Florida radiosurgery system. Surg Neurol 1989; 32: 334–342

[31] Soisson ET, Hardcastle N, Tomé WA. Quality assurance of an image guided intracranial stereotactic positioning system for radiosurgery treatment with helical tomotherapy. J Neurooncol 2010; 98: 277–285

[32] Bova FJ, Buatti JM, Friedman WA, Mendenhall WM, Yang CC, Liu C. The University of Florida frameless high-precision stereotactic radiotherapy system. Int J Radiat Oncol Biol Phys 1997; 38: 875–882

[33] Theelen A, Martens J, Bosmans G, et al. Relocatable fixation systems in intracranial stereotactic radiotherapy. Accuracy of serial CT scans and patient acceptance in a randomized design. Strahlenther Onkol 2012; 188: 84–90

[34] Chen JC, Rahimian J, Girvigian MR, Miller MJ. Contemporary methods of radiosurgery treatment with the Novalis linear accelerator system. Neurosurg Focus 2007; 23: E4

[35] Raabe A, Krishnan R, Zimmermann M, Seifert V. Frame-less and frame-based stereotaxy? How to choose the appropriate procedure [in German]. Zentralbl Neurochir 2003; 64: 1–5

[36] Schell MC, Bova FJ, Larson DA, Leavitt DD, Lutz WR, Podgorsak EB, Wu A. Report of Task Group 42 Radiation Therapy Committee. In: Stereotactic Radiosurgery. College Park, Maryland: American Association of Physicists in Medicine; 1995: pp. i–88

[37] Steinmeier R, Rachinger J, Kaus M, Ganslandt O, Huk W, Fahlbusch R. Factors influencing the application accuracy of neuronavigation systems. Stereotact Funct Neurosurg 2000; 75: 188–202

[38] Benardete EA, Leonard MA, Weiner HL. Comparison of frameless stereotactic systems: accuracy, precision, and applications. Neurosurgery 2001; 49: 1409–1415, discussion 1415–1416

[39] Horsley V, Clarke RH. The structure and functions of the cerebellum examined by a new method. Brain 1908; 31: 45–124

[40] Grunert P, Charalampaki K, Kassem M, Boecher-Schwarz H, Filippi R, Grunert P. Frame-based and frameless stereotaxy in the localization of cavernous angiomas. Neurosurg Rev 2003; 26: 53–61

3 Frameless Stereotactic Radiosurgery

Patrick Pezeshkian, Alessandra Gorgulho, and Antonio A. F. De Salles

Introduction

Radiosurgery has a fundamental role in the treatment of such pathologies as primary brain tumors, metastases, and functional disorders. Radiosurgery treatment, when effective, minimizes normal tissue injury by using sharp dose gradients that must be placed accurately at the margins of the target volume. The accuracy and precision of stereotactic treatments depend on a constellation of factors, including factors related to imaging, fiducialization, patient immobilization, patient positioning, device isocentricity, dose-planning algorithms, and device dose output. Patient immobilization and target localization using an invasive head frame have been the cornerstones of radiosurgery.[1,2] Although a variety of noninvasive relocatable frame systems have been used for radiosurgery and fractionated stereotactic treatment,[3–5] there exists ample controversy about their immobilization capability and overall target localization accuracy.[6,7]

To date, there have been no head-to-head comparison studies of frame versus frameless stereotactic intracranial radiosurgery. The ***levels of evidence*** for frameless stereotactic radiosurgery include phantom studies in the medical physics literature and retrospective clinical studies of frameless radiosurgery for various indications, such as brain metastases. In this chapter, we review the evidence as well as the advantages and limitations of frameless intracranial radiosurgery.

Frame-based Radiosurgery

The immobilization reliability and target localization accuracy of invasive frame-based radiosurgery have led to the technique being established as a gold standard. Frame-based radiosurgery using skeletal fixation has the advantage of a mechanical linkage between the target within the patient's head and the radiosurgery device via the stereotactic frame. Therefore, the patient displacement within the fraction is kept to a minimum. However, under some circumstances, patient displacement termed "application error" can occur, which may not be detected at the time of treatment, and is generally ~ 1 mm regardless of the design of the stereotactic frame.[8] Gamma Knife unit devices have been shown to have clinically relevant accuracy in the millimeter range.[9]

Potential Disadvantages of Frame-based Radiosurgery

The use of an invasive head frame is associated with substantial disadvantages. Head frame placement is considered to be a traumatic experience by many patients. Frame placement, although mostly shown to be reliable with low procedural morbidity, is nonetheless associated with a risk of bleeding and infection and requires premedication to sedate the patient, thus requiring close monitoring by anesthesia or by an experienced physician in a setting appropriate for sedation. Moreover, a dedicated nursing and physician support staff is oftentimes necessary to care for patients wearing head frames, thus creating a clinical resource burden on the day of the procedure. Frame-based treatment makes it less feasible to incorporate advanced dose-planning techniques, such as intensity-modulated radiation therapy (IMRT), because it requires treatment planning to be completed following frame placement on the day of treatment. Furthermore, head frames have the potential of slipping, compromising treatment accuracy, and potentially resulting in injury to the patient.[10]

As more patients undergo radiosurgery, and more are being treated on multiple occasions, the potential disadvantages associated with invasive head frames become highlighted. There has been a marked increase in the use of radiosurgery for the treatment of brain metastases, with evidence in the literature suggesting that radiosurgery may improve survival when used with whole-brain radiotherapy for patients with one brain metastasis,[11] and that radiosurgery may be used instead of whole-brain radiotherapy for patients with up to four brain metastases with no decrease in overall survival.[12] Retrospective evidence also suggests that stereotactic radiosurgery is as effective as surgery for local control of brain metastases < 3 cm in size.[13] With improved systemic therapies, as patients with systemic malignancies live longer, the brain becomes a more important potential site of failure, and it becomes increasingly more common to re-treat patients multiple times over several years and leads to a greater number of metastatic lesions.[14] With this in mind, optimizing patient comfort without compromising treatment efficacy becomes even more paramount. Moreover the number of patients being treated per day in units dependent on the stereotactic frame fixation is limited, compared with modern frameless techniques.

Frameless Image-guided Radiosurgery

In an attempt to facilitate fractionated stereotactic radiotherapy and frameless radiosurgery, a variety of relocatable stereotactic immobilization devices such as the Gill-Thomas-Cosman frame were developed;[15] however, the potential weakness of these devices is that the patient may shift relative to the stereotactic immobilization during treatment, making relocation unreliable in subsequent fractions of radiation. Most importantly, the localization may be hampered by patient movement between simulation and treatment.[16]

Over the years, a variety of image-guided frameless radiosurgery systems have been developed for clinical use that rely on optical image guidance, [17,18] X-ray image guidance,[19] or a combination of these for patient localization.[20,21] The difference between X-ray image-guided radiosurgery and frame-based radiosurgery or non-X-ray image-guided frameless radiosurgery is that the relationship between the immobilization device and the skull anatomy need not be preserved from treatment planning to actual treatment. Instead, imaging at the time of treatment is used to directly determine the position of the patient in stereotactic space. Although end-to-end phantom testing supports the technical capability of these systems to accurately localize and deliver the dose to the treatment isocenter under idealized conditions,[19,22] clinical application presents a more complex challenge to the use of these systems. The introduction of frameless image-guided radiosurgery allows for a fully noninvasive treatment with no anesthesia being required for these treatments, thus eliminating the need for close patient monitoring. In addition, no sterile processing is required. Bench testing has provided evidence that frameless image-guided radiosurgery can result in accuracy in treatment similar to frame-based methods.[23–25]

The development of image-guided stereotactic localization methods in the operating room, by virtue of optical image guidance,[17] or stereoscopic X-ray imaging for linear accelerator radiosurgery[20] has provided a foundation for frameless radiosurgical treatment. One such system, the Novalis Body ExacTrac (Brainlab AG, Munich, Germany), utilizes dual floor-mounted kV X-ray tubes that project onto ceiling-mounted amorphous silicon detectors and generate stereoscopic oblique images through machine isocenter.[20] The system creates an image fusion of the kV X-ray images with a digital reconstructed radiograph (DRR) library generated at the time of simulation and generates a predicted position shift to place the patient such that the target is coincident with the planning isocenter (▶ Fig. 3.1). An infrared tracking system is used to verify relative shifts and to provide initial patient position (▶ Fig. 3.2). Phantom-based end-to-end tests have demonstrated overall system accuracy within tolerances appropriate for radiosurgery.[26] Although end-to-end phantom testing provides support for the potential clinical utility of this system, clinical implementation requires careful assessment in patients of system performance relative to the gold standard of invasive frame-based radiosurgery. This allows for stringent evaluation of performance of the image-guided system for various patient anatomies, isocenter localizations, and immobilization systems. Variations in patient anatomy and their interaction with the immobilization and image guidance systems may in theory reduce overall accuracy compared with idealized phantom testing results.

Potential Disadvantages of Frameless Stereotactic Radiosurgery

Although image-guided techniques can correct for any intrafraction positioning error, the lack of rigid skeletal fixation can potentially lead to positioning errors between cycles of imaging. Such positioning errors may be exacerbated in instances of patients with unfavorable body habitus (e.g., morbid obesity) or agitation accompanied with uncontrolled body movements. The amount of intrafraction error also depends in part on the quality of the mask immobilization. Conventional univalve masks used for radiotherapy treatment (e.g., Aquaplast, QFix Systems, Avondale, PA) are flexible and can allow significant motion within the fraction. By using a rigid bivalve mask, intrafraction motion can be minimized. Typically, intrafraction motion can be constrained to < 0.5 mm for cranial radiosurgery under careful monitoring. Monitoring should be especially carefully practiced when treating spinal targets.[27–29]

Despite the availability of frameless radiosurgery methods for more than a decade, few reports exist on the use of this method for indications demanding high geometric precision. True real-time fluoroscopic imaging generally is not used because of excessive patient exposure to orthovoltage-level ionizing radiation. The addition of onboard cone beam computed tomographic imaging during treatment allows for checking on patient positioning independently of optical image guidance[17,18] and X-ray image guidance[19] used in traditional systems such as Novalis[20] and CyberKnife,[19] thereby allowing for advancement in the use of frameless technology to treat challenging and highly precision-demanding targets, as is the case in functional neurosurgery.[30]

Conclusion

Frame-based radiosurgery has wide clinical acceptance as being reliable in all applications of radiosurgery; however, it has limited use when fractions of radiation become necessary. It limits

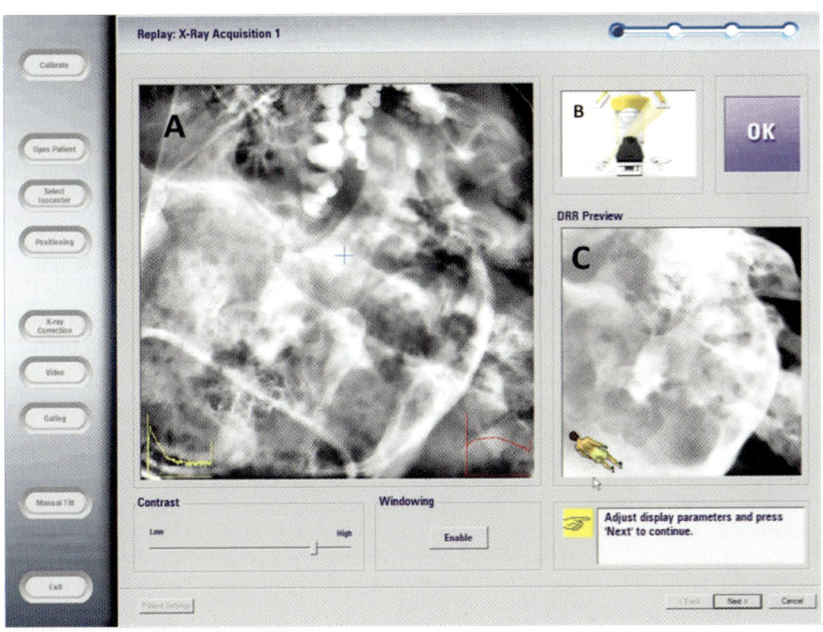

Fig. 3.1 (a) Demonstration of fusion of oblique digital reconstructed radiograph (DRR) obtained during treatment to ascertain position of the target in relation to the linear accelerator isocenter. (b) Direction of the DRR obtained during treatment. (c) Orientation of the DRR in relation to the patient's head position.

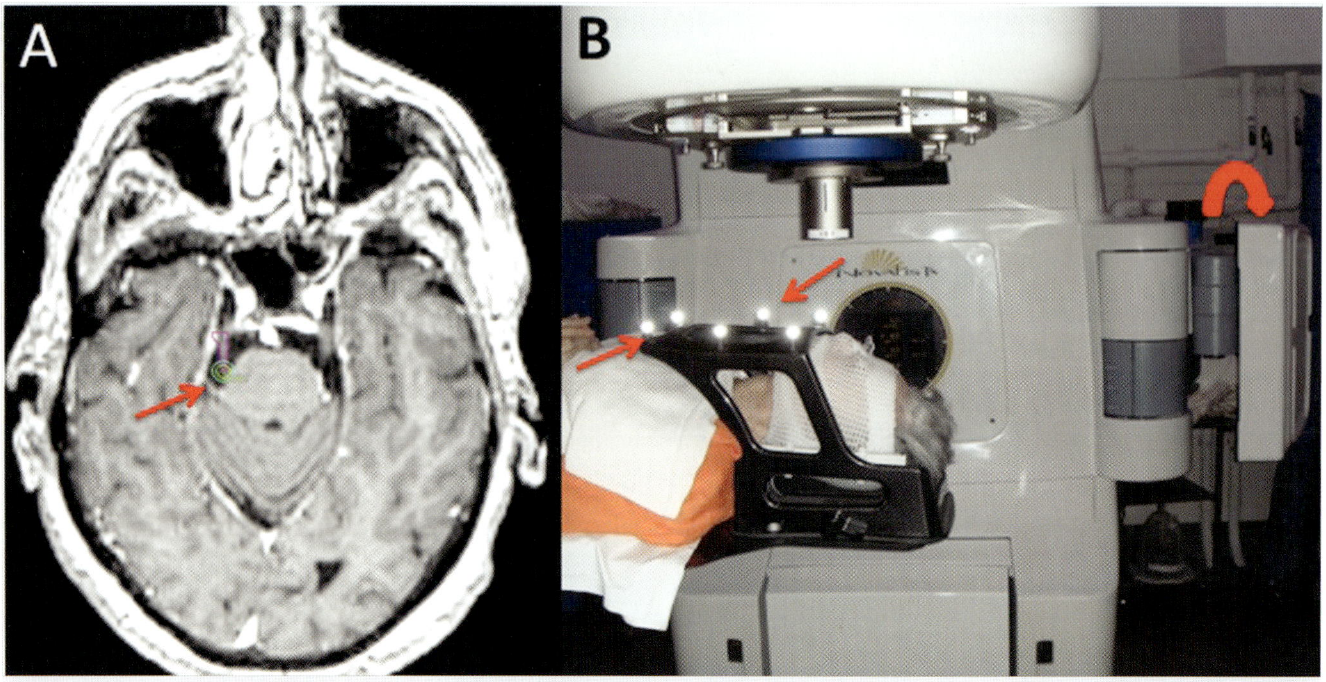

Fig. 3.2 (a) T1-weighted magnetic resonance image with contrast demonstrating the trigeminal nerve segmented and the target in the root entry zone (*arrow*). (b) Patient prepared to receive 90 Gy to the target. Notice the reflective markers (*arrows*) attached to the localizing box for patient positioning and monitoring, as well as the restraining mask. The independent target check is made with cone beam computed tomography (*curved arrow* on the right side of the picture).

the number of patients that can be treated in a day in radiosurgery services, although properly managed radiosurgery programs can treat large numbers of patients daily using multiple stereotactic frames. Frameless radiosurgery techniques are lacking wide clinical acceptance even though reliable data support its use for all applications of radiosurgery. The future will reveal the fate of the stereotactic frame in radiation treatment as the convenience of frameless techniques entice stereotactic surgeons to its use and as the improvement of imaging techniques lead to progressively higher precision and to the acceptance of frameless techniques. As stereotactic radiosurgery invades general oncology, precision is becoming second nature in a medical community that simply does not accept devices that do not ensure submillimeter accuracy of delivery and localization that does not match that of stereotactic frames. The progress of stereotactic radiosurgery demands better comfort for the patients beyond that which the stereotactic frame can sometimes offer.

References

[1] Leksell L. The stereotaxic method and radiosurgery of the brain. Acta Chir Scand 1951; 102: 316–319

[2] Lutz W, Winston KR, Maleki N. A system for stereotactic radiosurgery with a linear accelerator. Int J Radiat Oncol Biol Phys 1988; 14: 373–381

[3] Kooy HM, Dunbar SF, Tarbell NJ, et al. Adaptation and verification of the relocatable Gill-Thomas-Cosman frame in stereotactic radiotherapy. Int J Radiat Oncol Biol Phys 1994; 30: 685–691

[4] Gilbeau L, Octave-Prignot M, Loncol T, Renard L, Scalliet P, Grégoire V. Comparison of setup accuracy of three different thermoplastic masks for the treatment of brain and head and neck tumors. Radiother Oncol 2001; 58: 155–162

[5] Gill SS, Thomas DG, Warrington AP, Brada M. Relocatable frame for stereotactic external beam radiotherapy. Int J Radiat Oncol Biol Phys 1991; 20: 599–603

[6] Rosenberg I, Alheit H, Beardmore C, Lee KS, Warrington AP, Brada M. Patient position reproducibility in fractionated stereotactic radiotherapy: an update after changing dental impression material. Radiother Oncol 1999; 50: 239–240

[7] Kumar S, Burke K, Nalder C, et al. Treatment accuracy of fractionated stereotactic radiotherapy. Radiother Oncol 2005; 74: 53–59

[8] Maciunas RJ, Galloway RL, Latimer JW. The application accuracy of stereotactic frames. Neurosurgery 1994; 35: 682–694, discussion 694–695

[9] Yu C, Apuzzo ML, Zee CS, Petrovich Z. A phantom study of the geometric accuracy of computed tomographic and magnetic resonance imaging stereotactic localization with the Leksell stereotactic system. Neurosurgery 2001; 48: 1092–1098, discussion 1098–1099

[10] Otto K, Fallone BG. Frame slippage verification in stereotactic radiosurgery. Int J Radiat Oncol Biol Phys 1998; 41: 199–205

[11] Andrews DW, Scott CB, Sperduto PW, et al. Whole brain radiation therapy with or without stereotactic radiosurgery boost for patients with one to three brain metastases: phase III results of the RTOG 9508 randomised trial. Lancet 2004; 363: 1665–1672

[12] Aoyama H, Shirato H, Tago M, et al. Stereotactic radiosurgery plus whole-brain radiation therapy vs stereotactic radiosurgery alone for treatment of brain metastases: a randomized controlled trial. JAMA 2006; 295: 2483–2491

[13] Pollock BE. An evidence-based medicine review of stereotactic radiosurgery. Prog Neurol Surg 2006; 19: 152–170

[14] Bhatnagar AK, Flickinger JC, Kondziolka D, Lunsford LD. Stereotactic radiosurgery for four or more intracranial metastases. Int J Radiat Oncol Biol Phys 2006; 64: 898–903

[15] Pollock BE, Phuong LK, Gorman DA, Foote RL, Stafford SL. Stereotactic radiosurgery for idiopathic trigeminal neuralgia. J Neurosurg 2002; 97: 347–353

[16] Dhople AA, Adams JR, Maggio WW, Naqvi SA, Regine WF, Kwok Y. Long-term outcomes of Gamma Knife radiosurgery for classic trigeminal neuralgia: implications of treatment and critical review of the literature. Clinical article. J Neurosurg 2009; 111: 351–358

[17] Ryken TC, Meeks SL, Pennington EC, et al. Initial clinical experience with frameless stereotactic radiosurgery: analysis of accuracy and feasibility. Int J Radiat Oncol Biol Phys 2001; 51: 1152–1158

[18] Keshavarzi S, Meltzer H, Ben-Haim S, et al. Initial clinical experience with frameless optically guided stereotactic radiosurgery/radiotherapy in pediatric patients. Childs Nerv Syst 2009; 25: 837–844

[19] Chang SD, Main W, Martin DP, Gibbs IC, Heilbrun MP. An analysis of the accuracy of the CyberKnife: a robotic frameless stereotactic radiosurgical system. Neurosurgery 2003; 52: 140–146, discussion 146–147

[20] Verellen D, Soete G, Linthout N, et al. Quality assurance of a system for improved target localization and patient set-up that combines real-time infrared tracking and stereoscopic X-ray imaging. Radiother Oncol 2003; 67: 129–141

[21] Calcerrada Díaz-Santos N, Blasco Amaro JA, Cardiel GA, Andradas Aragonés E. The safety and efficacy of robotic image-guided radiosurgery system treatment for intra- and extracranial lesions: a systematic review of the literature. Radiother Oncol 2008; 89: 245–253

[22] Yan H, Yin FF, Kim JH. A phantom study on the positioning accuracy of the Novalis Body system. Med Phys 2003; 30: 3052–3060

[23] Chang SD, Main W, Martin DP, Gibbs IC, Heilbrun MP. An analysis of the accuracy of the CyberKnife: a robotic frameless stereotactic radiosurgical system. Neurosurgery 2003; 52: 140–146, discussion 146–147

[24] Solberg TD, Medin PM, Mullins J, Li S. Quality assurance of immobilization and target localization systems for frameless stereotactic cranial and extracranial hypofractionated radiotherapy. Int J Radiat Oncol Biol Phys 2008; 71 Suppl: S131–S135

[25] Wurm RE, Erbel S, Schwenkert I, et al. Novalis frameless image-guided noninvasive radiosurgery: initial experience. Neurosurgery 2008; 62 Suppl: A11–A17, discussion A17–A18

[26] Lee SW, Jin JY, Guan H, Martin F, Kim JH, Yin FF. Clinical assessment and characterization of a dual tube kilovoltage X-ray localization system in the radiotherapy treatment room. J Appl Clin Med Phys 2008; 9: 2318

[27] Selch MT, Tenn S, Agazaryan N, Lee SP, Gorgulho A, De Salles AA. Image-guided linear accelerator-based spinal radiosurgery for hemangioblastoma. Surg Neurol Int 2012; 3: 73

[28] De Salles AA, Gorgulho AA, Selch M, De Marco J, Agazaryan N. Radiosurgery from the brain to the spine: 20 years' experience. Acta Neurochir Suppl (Wien) 2008; 101: 163–168

[29] Agazaryan N, Tenn SE, Desalles AA, Selch MT. Image-guided radiosurgery for spinal tumors: methods, accuracy and patient intrafraction motion. Phys Med Biol 2008; 53: 1715–1727

[30] Rahimian J, Chen JC, Rao AA, Girvigian MR, Miller MJ, Greathouse HE. Geometrical accuracy of the Novalis stereotactic radiosurgery system for trigeminal neuralgia. J Neurosurg 2004; 101 Suppl 3: 351–355

4 Proton-based Radiosurgery

Marc R. Bussière, Helen A. Shih, and Jay S. Loeffler

Introduction

Protons provide an alternative radiosurgical tool to the more conventional photon approaches. This was the original modality used to pioneer the field of radiosurgery by Lawrence in 1954[1] and Larsson et al in 1957.[2] The Gamma Knife unit was subsequently introduced in 1968, but it was not until 1985 that a linear accelerator (LINAC) was configured and used for radiosurgery.[3] Despite the early implementation of proton radiosurgery programs, the use of this modality was quickly surpassed by the more compact photon units that could be readily obtained from commercial vendors. Therefore, most radiosurgery procedures are delivered using high-energy photons in the form of X-rays generated from a LINAC or γ-rays (gamma rays) emitted from multiple sealed sources contained in a device called a Gamma Knife.[4] Rooms used to house this equipment can be as small as 20 ft × 20 ft but must be designed to incorporate radiation safety shielding.

It took more than 35 years from the initial application of proton radiosurgery until a hospital-based proton center was opened and another 10 years until the radiation oncology community was able to convince commercial vendors of the potential benefits of protons. Despite the more recent proliferation of proton centers, the original challenges remain. These include the initial capital investment for the real-estate infrastructure and equipment, the ongoing operational costs, and the specialized technical expertise required to maintain and operate the facility and ancillary services.

In 2012 there were fewer than 40 proton centers operational worldwide, and very few have been able or willing to further specialize in proton stereotactic radiosurgery (sometimes abbreviated as PSRS). The high demand on proton centers forces them to establish priorities, such as the pediatric population, where the potential clinical benefit is greatest, and generally fractionated cases where larger targets are incompatible with radiosurgical approaches. The increased number of cancer centers with the capability to offer both protons and photons has also improved the feasibility to implement clinical trials to better assess the benefits of proton radiotherapy compared with more conventional photon approaches. Nonetheless, there are a handful of proton centers that have active radiosurgery programs. The largest of these programs is at the Massachusetts General Hospital (MGH) in Boston with over 5,000 proton stereotactic radiosurgery cases treated to date.

Despite the growth in the number of proton centers and in the clinical applications of protons, ***level I evidence*** is limited and is confined to fractionated treatments. These few studies have focused on the question of appropriate dose and incorporating proton therapy as a treatment modality. These include two randomized prostate cancer studies establishing the role for dose escalation in early-stage disease and a less clear role for advanced prostate cancer.[5,6] Neither study specifically evaluated protons as a potential treatment modality superior to conventional photons. There is a recently opened MGH-led multicenter randomized trial of proton versus photon therapy for prostate cancer that may begin to address the true value of protons, but there are disease-specific limitations of daily organ motion and variable immobilization that are not inherent challenges when targeting within the cranium. Other published randomized trials also address questions of dose rather than that of proton therapy as modality. In a study of uveal melanoma patients receiving between 50 and 70 Gy radiobiological effectiveness factor (RBE) delivered in five fractions, patients did not demonstrate a difference in local control or toxicity, presumptively because the lower dose arm still exceeded normal tissue tolerances.[7] Currently, there is a study of non–small cell lung cancer randomizing proton versus photon radiation that will address this issue of use of protons in part. Thoracic irradiation is also unique to cranial radiation because of the inherently large tissue density heterogeneity and organ motion that limit the degree of precision that can be achieved. Dosimetric advantages of protons appear logical, but benefits have not been demonstrated beyond ***level III evidence***. Clinical results referenced in this chapter provide evidence of comparable outcomes for proton and photon radiosurgery. Because many patients are handpicked for proton radiosurgery, any perceived advantage must be considered anecdotal.

Dosimetric Differences between Protons and Photons

The expected clinical advantage of protons lies in their dosimetric properties.

Absorbed energy resulting from ionization processes causes molecular changes that result in cell damage. Tissue responses vary with cell type and radiation. The RBE is used to describe the equivalence between different radiation types.[8] Despite many variables, a generic RBE of 1.1 is used for protons as compared to photons.[9–13] Thus, delivering a physical dose of 18.0 Gy with protons would be considered equivalent to delivering 19.8 Gy with photons, and the proton biologically equivalent dose would be denoted as 19.8 Gy (RBE).[14]

There are significant differences in photon and proton dose distributions. X-rays and γ-rays (gamma rays) are types of photon beams. When these beams travel into matter, they are absorbed, resulting in a smaller number of photons and an exponential reduction in dose as they penetrate deeper into tissues. For a given photon beam, the superficial skin dose can be as low as 20% of the maximal dose delivered due to the tissue dose resulting from radiation interactions dominated by forward scattering. As protons pass through material, they interact and lose energy, resulting in a slowly increasing dose as they penetrate deeper into the body. The bulk of the beam's protons reach the maximum depth determined by their initial energy, at which point the kinetic energy approaches zero. Protons have a higher interaction probability as they decelerate, resulting in a concentrated energy deposition called the Bragg peak just before the particle beam stops. Unlike the photon dose, which is reduced exponentially with depth but always remains nonzero, the dose from protons stops at the Bragg peak. This property of protons is a major advantage over photons due to

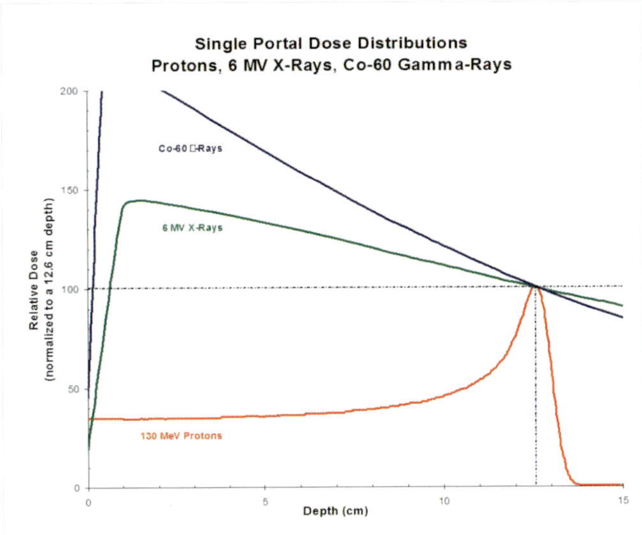

Fig. 4.1 Dose distributions for single proton, 6 MV photon, and cobalt 60 beams. Proton dose is mostly concentrated at the Bragg peak, whereas the photon dose is much higher at shallow depths and continues beyond the target.

the elimination of the dose to the patient beyond the target. The overall nontarget dose known as the integral dose is significantly lower for protons compared with photons regardless of the delivery techniques used. Integral dose contributes only to potential side effects and radiation-induced second malignancies[15–17] (▶ Fig. 4.1).

Practical Aspects of Proton Radiosurgery

The basic principles of proton radiosurgery are the same as those for the more conventional X- and γ-ray approaches, where high-energy ionizing radiation is focused onto a desired small target within the body. The radiation dose focus is achieved by converging radiation beams of multiple incident directions on a common overlap region encompassing the desired treatment volume.

When proton radiosurgery was first used, there was limited ability to determine the placement of the Bragg peak. This was before the era of computed tomography (CT), and patient-specific tissue attenuation characteristics were not available. Therefore, as much as the current main benefit of proton therapy is described as resulting from the Bragg peak effect, the original proton radiosurgery approach used a cross-fire technique that positioned the Bragg peak beyond the exit point of the patient and took advantage of the sharp lateral penumbra offered by the high-energy proton beams. A 1- and 2-mm 80 to 20% dose fall-off was achieved with 340 and 185 MeV protons, respectively.[2,18] This technique was best suited for midline intracranial targets, such as the pituitary.

The use of the Bragg peak for proton radiosurgery was introduced in 1961.[19–23] Most targets, even radiosurgery targets, would be too wide to be fully covered by the narrow Bragg peak. Therefore, individual beams incorporate multiple Bragg peak layers. These are combined to generate a uniform dose spread-out Bragg peak (SOBP). The length of the SOBP is called the modulation. The use of wax or Lucite range compensators allows the depth of the Bragg peak to be adjusted at different points across a field. This has important benefits for larger and more irregular lesions where there is an increased volume of normal tissue adjacent to a desired high-dose region.

Two to six beams are commonly used to generate a proton radiosurgery plan. Beam directions are selected to minimize integral dose overlap with other beams and avoid normal tissue irradiation while maximizing target conformality. Dose shaping is achieved for individual beams using custom brass collimators and Lucite range compensators to conform the Bragg peak fall-off to the geometric shape of the target. The required range along any path is determined by converting CT numbers to proton stopping power. Therefore, special precautions need to be implemented to ensure these accurately reflect the treatment conditions.

Residual rotations or an offset of the immobilization equipment with respect to the patient has little impact for photons due to the shallow depth dose gradient. In contrast, these misalignments can significantly affect proton range. Therefore, beam directions must also be selected to minimize dose gradients within the patient or the immobilization equipment. Immobilization equipment must be designed with small-density gradients. When gradients are unavoidable, the range and modulation of the affected beam must be increased to ensure coverage.

Until recently irregular targets were treated with photons by dividing the volume into multiple segments, but this resulted in heterogeneity of the dose distribution with some areas slightly overdosed and others underdosed. This approach is essential for Gamma Knife techniques and is sometimes still used with LINAC-based procedures. More sophisticated LINAC techniques, such as dynamic conformal arcs, intensity-modulated radiation surgery, and volumetric modulated arc therapy, allow for improved conformality of irregular targets and have reduced, although not eliminated, the proton advantage. Unfortunately, the more conformal photon techniques result in larger low-dose integral dose baths.

Clinical Indications

The clinical applications of photon and proton radiosurgery are the same, with doses of 8 to 24 Gy being administered in one or a few sessions to treat benign or malignant lesions or malformations. Proton radiosurgery is also considered ideal for the treatment of choroidal hemangiomas and uveal melanomas.[24] It has been used to perform thalamotomies for Parkinson disease but has yet to be applied toward the treatment of nerve disorders such as trigeminal neuralgia. The motivation for radiosurgery as an alternative and/or complement to other procedures such as surgery is not presented in this chapter. Rather, we focus on the use of proton radiosurgery itself.

Proton and photon radiosurgery are benefiting from advances in imaging and motion tracking, which has enabled the use of noninvasive fixation for patients and has made the treatment of extracranial sites such as the spine and lung more feasible than in the past.

The first step in the patient selection process is to determine the appropriateness of using radiosurgery regardless of modality. Large centers that offer proton radiosurgery may also benefit from having a parallel conventional radiosurgery program. This allows for an ideal patient selection based on the anticipated dosimetric benefits of one modality over the other. Pediatric patients with expectant long-term survival may benefit the most from the use of protons due to the anticipated normal tissue sparing and potential reduction of late-term complications. Larger targets are considered to benefit most from proton radiosurgery because of the ability to obtain very good conformality and normal tissue sparing. Appropriate applications include treatment of benign meningiomas, pituitary adenomas, vestibular schwannomas, and arteriovenous malformations (AVMs). Patients presenting with atypical meningiomas often require multiple radiosurgery procedures over the slow course of disease progression and often require treatment of long and irregular targets or superficial nodules. These patients may benefit most from normal brain sparing. Metastatic disease in close proximity to critical structures or other lesions can also benefit from the ability to shape proton dose distributions.

Arteriovenous Malformations

AVMs often present with very irregular shapes that lend themselves well to treatment with proton radiosurgery. The first radiosurgical treatment of AVMs was performed with protons in 1965, but it was not until 1972 that a second patient was treated due to a lack of adequate beam-shaping capabilities. An early study of 74 patients treated by the MGH group with proton stereotactic radiosurgery from 1972 to 1978 with follow-up of 2 to 16 years reported a 20% complete obliteration rate, 56% size reduction in half or more, and 13% with no radiographic change.[25] Single-fraction doses of 10 to 50 Gy (RBE) were selected based on AVM diameter, which ranged from 7 to 50 mm. Four of the first 27 patients from this series had large AVMs associated with corticospinal pathways and developed abrupt or progressive hemiparesis after treatment. Dosing was subsequently adjusted following these observations. The same article describes complications for the subsequent 205 patients treated from 1978 to 1980 as having similar complication rates. A series of 95 patients with cavernous malformations treated by the same group reported an annual hemorrhage rate reduction from 17 to 9%, but this series was associated with significant complications, including 16% with permanent neurologic deficit.[26] A study of 63 patients treated from 1980 to 1990 reported clinical improvements in 76% of cases with AVM diameters < 3 cm but symptom progression in 12% of cases. The majority (86%) of patients with Spetzler-Martin grades I and II had improvement of clinical symptoms compared to only 54% of the patients with grade III and 24% with grade IV AVMs.[27] A small study with 26 patients with AVMs ranging in volume from 0.3 to 102 cm^3 treated with two to four fractions to a total of 20 to 25 Gy (RBE) is in agreement with previous studies with an obliteration rate of 70% for AVMs < 25 cm^3 and 30% otherwise.[28] A 2003 retrospective analysis of 1,250 patients treated at MGH between 1965 and 1993 has been used to revise complication risk models for "stereotactic Bragg peak proton therapy."[29,30] In this study, the median AVM volume was 33.7 cm^3 (21% < 10 cm^3 but as large as 927 cm^3), with median follow-up 6.5 years and median dose 10.5 Gy (RBE); 0.5% of patients treated with doses < 12 Gy (RBE) suffered complications. It was found that a 1, 3, and 5% complication rate occurred with malformations receiving doses > 14.8, 19.5, and 22.4 Gy (RBE), respectively, with volumes of 1 cm^3. Larger malformations with volumes of 10 cm^3 had 1, 3, and 5% complication rates when receiving doses of 10.3, 13.6, and 15.6 Gy (RBE), respectively. A study of 64 patients treated with one to three proton stereotactic radiosurgery fractions to a total dose of 16 to 38 Gy (RBE) reported a 67% total obliteration rate in 26 AVMs < 14 cm^3 and 43% for 38 AVMs > 14 cm^3.[31] A recent study reporting on two conservative 7- to 8-Gy (RBE) fractions used to treat small AVMs in critical locations or larger AVMs with volumes > 14 cm^3 included 59 patients with median nidus volume of 23 cm^3 treated between 1991 and 2009, with many patients having had prior surgery or embolization.[32] At a median follow-up of 4.5 years, 15% and 34% had complete or partial obliterations, respectively. Complications included 14% acute and 12% long-term grade I headaches, 2% generalized seizures, and 5% mild neurologic deficits. A companion report of outcomes following single-fraction proton stereotactic radiosurgery included 242 patients treated in the same period, with a median nidus volume of 3.5 cm^3 (0.1 to 28.1).[33] Median follow-up was 4.5 years, and the most common prescription dose was 15 Gy (RBE). In this study, the 5- and 10-year obliteration rates were 68% and 88%, respectively. Complications included 7% acute and 9% long-term seizures controlled with medication. Some of these complications may have been attributable to the AVMs rather than the radiation; thus, true treatment toxicity risks may be lower (▶ Fig. 4.2).

Pituitary Adenomas

Radiation is considered when surgery and pharmacological options have been unable to control symptoms or disease progression. Radiation therapy achieves excellent local control rates of > 95% for nonsecreting tumors and 65 to 85% biochemical control for secretory tumors.[34–37] Fractionated radiotherapy is preferred to radiosurgery for larger tumors where extrasellar disease is present or when there is disease in close proximity to the optic chiasm. Otherwise radiosurgery provides a viable alternative to radiotherapy and has a faster biochemical control response in secretory tumors. Proton radiosurgery is well suited to minimize dose to nearby critical structures, with ideal dose constraints of optic pathways < 8 Gy (RBE), hypothalamus < 12 Gy (RBE), brainstem < 12 Gy (RBE), and minimization of dose to the temporal lobes.

Proton radiosurgery for pituitary ablation was first reported in 1958.[38] Twenty-six patients with breast carcinoma were treated with 340 MeV cross-fire protons delivering doses of 140 to 320 Gy in multiple sessions spanning 9 to 63 days. Results showed clinical improvements in a few patients; the most common changes included depression of I^{131} thyroid uptake and a decrease of 24-hour urinary gonadotropins. An early review of 14 of 22 patients treated with proton radiosurgery using the benefit of the Bragg peak and delivering peak doses of 100 to 120 Gy for the treatment of acromegaly was published in 1968.[39] Twelve lateral fields were used, converging on the sella to minimize the dose to the temporal lobes and avoid the optic

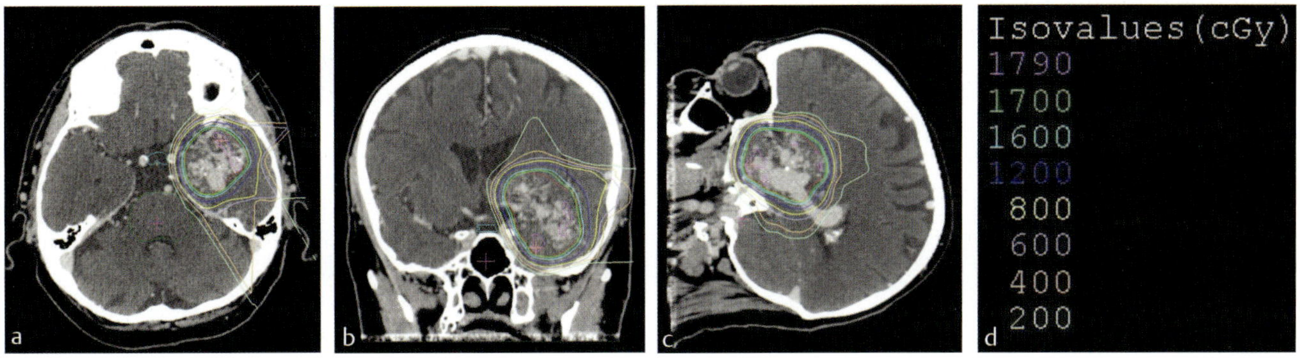

Fig. 4.2 Study of a patient with a 20-year history of minor seizures who presented 1 month after suffering a hemorrhage. A 46-cm^3 left temporal nonoperable arteriovenous malformation (AVM) with intraventricular blood was targeted with a six-field, two-stage proton radiosurgery procedure delivering 8 Gy (RBE) × 2 fractions = 16 Gy (RBE) normalized to the 90% isodose line. (a) Axial, (b) coronal, and (c) sagittal views through the center of the AVM show the proton dose distribution. (d) Isodoses in Gy (RBE). The plan demonstrates the normal brain dose sparing achievable with protons while maintaining a uniform dose distribution within the AVM.

structures. Levels of growth hormone decreased significantly in eight patients. One patient developed unilateral visual loss, and another had anterior pituitary insufficiency; other complications were headaches and diplopia. The technique had results that were considered comparable in both outcome and complications to other procedures at the time. As experience was gained, the peak doses were lowered to 70 Gy, as described in a follow-up summary of 571 patients treated through 1974 with proton radiosurgery for pituitary-related disease.[40] Treatment disorders included 45% acromegaly, 10% Cushing disease, and 8% chromophobe adenoma, while some had the normal pituitary gland irradiated for 32% diabetic retinopathy and 2% breast and prostate carcinoma. The most common complications included temporary oculomotor disturbances in 6% of the first 50 cases; < 1% had temporary field deficits but no blindness. Of the patients with acromegaly, 56% had a complete response, and 29% had a partial response. Patients with Cushing disease had 89% response with lower complication rates. By 1979 over 1,200 patients with pituitary-related disease had been treated with proton radiosurgery by the MGH group.[41]

Despite the potential benefit of proton radiosurgery, there are only two recent studies describing clinical outcomes for pituitary treatments.[42,43] Between 1992 and 2003, 22 patients who had previously failed surgery were treated for persistent acromegaly with median doses of 20 Gy (RBE). Treatments resulted in biochemical improvement in 95% of patients at 6 years, and half reached normal insulinlike growth factor 1 (IGF-1) levels without the need for additional medication. A third of patients developed new pituitary deficits over 1 to 9 years. In the same treatment period, 38 patients who failed surgery were treated with proton radiosurgery for refractory Cushing disease.[43,44] Sustained normalization of urinary-free cortisol was achieved in 50% of patients with a median of 14 months. Partial response was observed in 29% of patients. Approximately one third of patients developed new pituitary deficits within a median time of 2 years. The risk increases with time from radiation, but symptoms can often be managed with medication.

Proton radiosurgery has been comparable to other modalities in demonstrating fast biochemical response and low morbidity for the treatment of pituitary disorders. Macroadenoma with extrasellar disease may benefit from the improved dose homogeneity and conformality offered from protons. Proton radiosurgery can be a viable and convenient alternative to fractionated therapy for patients who present with microadenomas that have sufficient spacing from the chiasm.

Meningiomas

Surgical resection is often the preferred procedure for the treatment of benign meningiomas.[45] Radiotherapy or radiosurgery has demonstrated 5-year control rates of 90 to 95% with 2 to 5% complication rates for patients who have exhausted surgical options.[46–49]

It is very common for meningiomas to have irregular shapes, and the use of radiosurgery as an alternative to radiotherapy is usually determined by volume, shape, and location to avoid complications. Protons offer dosimetric benefits of good conformality and homogeneous dose distributions that are ideally suited for larger targets that require fractionation. Smaller, irregular targets still benefit from the same properties offered by proton radiosurgery.[50] Very little is written on proton radiosurgery, as the focus has been on the fractionated approach.[51–55] A 2001 study reports on 18 patients with lesions ranging in volume from 3 to 63 cm^3 who received three fractions for a total dose of 17 to 24 Gy (RBE).[56] Mean follow-up was 40 months, at which time 89% of patients remained stable, and 11% had developed permanent neurologic deficits. A single retrospective study exists for the treatment of benign meningiomas with proton radiosurgery.[57] Between 1996 and 2007, 50 patients with tumor diameters < 4 cm and no closer than 2 mm to the optic nerves and chiasm received a single treatment dose of 10.0 to 15.5 Gy (RBE) normalized at 90%. At a median radiographic follow-up time of 3 years, 66% had stabilized, 26% had decreased in size, and 10% had grown. Symptoms were improved in 47%, unchanged in 44%, and worsened in 9% of cases. The rate of potential permanent adverse effects was 6%. Despite the short follow-up, these results are consistent with other SRS modalities, having 5-year control rates of 87% and symptom improvements of 81 to 96%.[46,47,58–75]

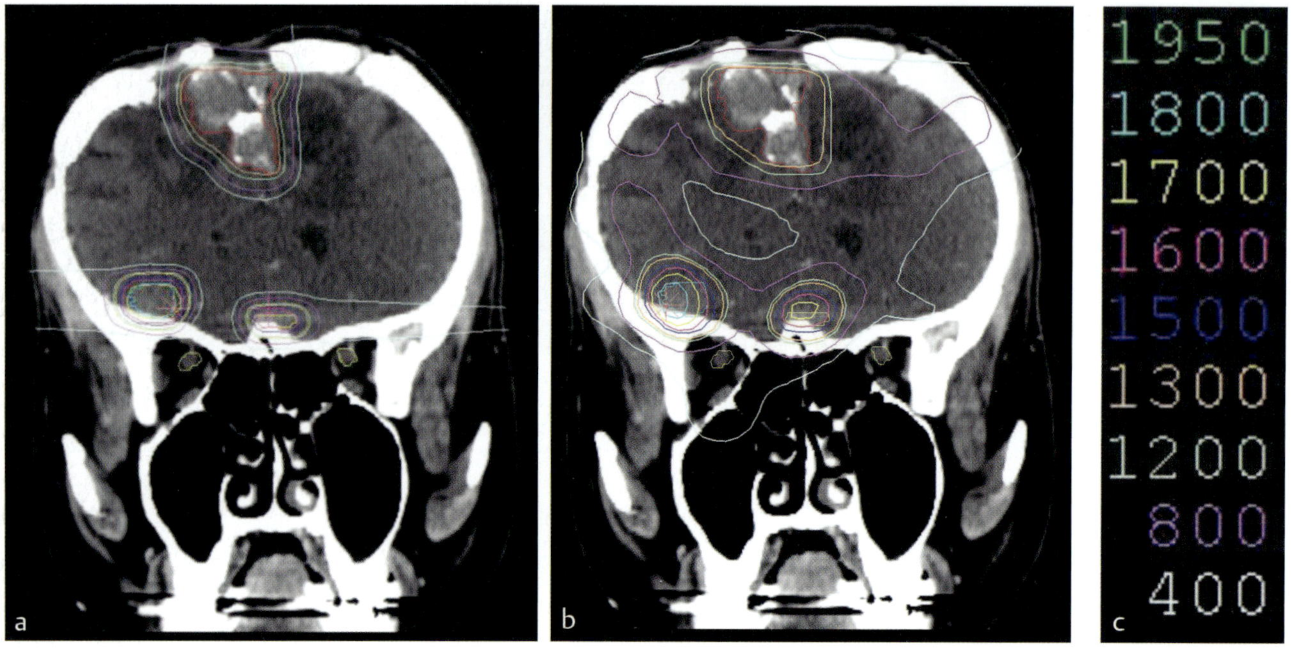

Fig. 4.3 Study of a patient with atypical meningiomas and an extensive history involving multiple craniotomies, stereotactic radiotherapy, and radiosurgery procedures. Five lesions of various sizes, some in close proximity to the optic apparatus, were treated with single doses ranging from 12 to 18 Gy (RBE) as palliative focal radiosurgery in an attempt to alleviate symptoms. Normal brain sparing offered from protons (a) was considered an important benefit as compared with what would have been achievable with photons (b). (c) Isodoses in Gy (RBE).

The reported use of protons for the treatment of atypical and malignant meningiomas is limited to fractioned schemes.[76,77] No reports are available for these treatments with proton radiosurgery. However, small, superficial nodules or long, irregular lesions with moderate volumes have been safely treated with proton radiosurgery while sparing normal brain due to the Bragg peak of protons, which results in no dose beyond the target (▶ Fig. 4.3).

Vestibular Schwannomas

The goal of SRS is to stop tumor growth. In some cases, partial hearing preservation is possible. Five-year control rates of 95% have been obtained regardless of modality.[78–81] Patients with little or no hearing loss are typically treated with fractionated therapy in an attempt to retain auditory capacity. Larger tumors > 2 cm in diameter are also commonly treated using a fractionated scheme in order to minimize facial and trigeminal neuropathy complications, which occur in 1 to 5% of cases.[80] A report of 88 patients treated with proton radiosurgery between 1992 and 2000 to nominal tumor doses of 15 Gy (RBE) had 5-year local control rates of 94% but only 22% hearing preservation and 10% risk of either facial or trigeminal neuropathy.[79] Similar photon radiosurgery studies have shown equal success with doses of 12 to 13 Gy, which is now considered the standard.[82] Not surprisingly, dosimetric comparison shows that protons provide better overall normal tissue sparing than photon techniques; however, no clinical data have substantiated a clinical benefit.[83] Proton radiosurgery is considered equivalent to its photon counterpart with the potential for reducing the already low risk of secondary radiation-induced malignancies.

Uveal Melanomas

The treatment of anterior choroidal melanomas and hemangiomas has been most readily achievable using brachytherapy plaques sutured onto the sclera over the tumor.[84] Enucleation is considered in cases of large tumors. When located near the optic disk, plaques are physically more challenging. Single-fraction Gamma Knife radiosurgery has been used in such cases,[85,86] but most of the clinical experience is with using hypofractionated schedules of four or five fractions. LINAC-based delivery has been successfully used in such cases,[87,88] but proton stereotactic therapy using single en face fields has long been considered the gold standard.[89–96] A surgical procedure precedes the radiation treatment whereby tantalum clips are sutured to the sclera to define the borders of the tumor as observed with the aid of transillumination intraoperatively. These clips are then used as a basis for radiographic treatment alignment. Conventional proton treatments employ five 10- to 14-Gy (RBE) fractions delivered on consecutive days. In 2,069 patients treated at MGH in collaboration with the Massachusetts Eye and Ear Infirmary, 2% of tumors grew between 0.5 and 11.0 years after irradiation. Common complications include cataracts as posterior subcapsular opacities in approximately 19%, 25%, and 38% at 3, 5, and 10 years, respectively, after irradiation. Visual loss can arise from retinal detachment, cataracts, and radiation retinopathy.

Metastatic Disease and Others

Proton therapy is generally allocated to patients perceived as having the greatest clinical gain from the superior dosimetry and who are generally expected to be long-term survivors. Because of limited resources, metastatic disease typically is not treated with protons. However, some intracranial metastastic lesions may be advantageously treated with protons, again because of superior dosimetry. This includes relatively large and particularly irregularly shaped lesions and when treating multiple small lesions in close proximity to each other or to critical structures. There are other, rarer entities that are often managed with proton stereotactic radiosurgery that share the principles of intended clinical benefit from limiting the unnecessary dose to the normal tissues.

References

[1] Lawrence JH. Proton irradiation of the pituitary. Cancer 1957; 10: 795–798

[2] Larsson B, Leksell L, Rexed B, Sourander P, Mair W, Andersson B. The high-energy proton beam as a neurosurgical tool. Nature 1958; 182: 1222–1223

[3] Colombo F, Benedetti A, Pozza F, et al. External stereotactic irradiation by linear accelerator. Neurosurgery 1985; 16: 154–160

[4] Elekta Inc. Manufacturer of the Gamma Knife. US office: Norcross, GA

[5] Zietman AL, Bae K, Slater JD, et al. Randomized trial comparing conventional-dose with high-dose conformal radiation therapy in early-stage adenocarcinoma of the prostate: long-term results from Proton Radiation Oncology Group/American College of Radiology 95-09. J Clin Oncol 2010; 28: 1106–1111

[6] Shipley WU, Verhey LJ, Munzenrider JE, et al. Advanced prostate cancer: the results of a randomized comparative trial of high dose irradiation boosting with conformal protons compared with conventional dose irradiation using photons alone. Int J Radiat Oncol Biol Phys 1995; 32: 3–12

[7] Gragoudas ES, Lane AM, Regan S, et al. A randomized controlled trial of varying radiation doses in the treatment of choroidal melanoma. Arch Ophthalmol 2000; 118: 773–778

[8] Sinclair WK. Relative biological wffectiveness (RBE), quality factor (Q) and radiation weighting factor (Wr). Ann ICRP 2003; 92.

[9] Paganetti H, Niemierko A, Ancukiewicz M, et al. Relative biological effectiveness (RBE) values for proton beam therapy. Int J Radiat Oncol Biol Phys 2002; 53: 407–421

[10] Robertson JB, Williams JR, Schmidt RA, Little JB, Flynn DF, Suit HD. Radiobiological studies of a high-energy modulated proton beam utilizing cultured mammalian cells. Cancer 1975; 35: 1664–1677

[11] Tepper J, Verhey L, Goitein M, Suit HD. In vivo determinations of RBE in a high energy modulated proton beam using normal tissue reactions and fractionated dose schedules. Int J Radiat Oncol Biol Phys 1977; 2: 1115–1122

[12] Urano M, Verhey LJ, Goitein M, et al. Relative biological effectiveness of modulated proton beams in various murine tissues. Int J Radiat Oncol Biol Phys 1984; 10: 509–514

[13] Gerweck L, Paganetti H. Radiobiology of charged particles in proton and charged particle radiotherapy. In: DeLaney TF, Kooy HM, eds. Philadelphia, PA: Lippincott Williams & Wilkins; 2008

[14] International Commission on Radiation Units and Measurements (ICRU). Stopping powers for protons and alpha particles. Report No. 49. Bethesda, MD: ICRU; 1993

[15] Miralbell R, Lomax A, Cella L, Schneider U. Potential reduction of the incidence of radiation-induced second cancers by using proton beams in the treatment of pediatric tumors. Int J Radiat Oncol Biol Phys 2002; 54: 824–829

[16] Schneider U, Lomax A, Pemler P, et al. The impact of IMRT and proton radiotherapy on secondary cancer incidence. Strahlenther Onkol 2006; 182: 11

[17] Winkfield KM, Niemierko A, Bussière MR, et al. Modeling intracranial second tumor risk and estimates of clinical toxicity with various radiation therapy techniques for patients with pituitary adenoma. Technol Cancer Res Treat 2011; 10: 243–251

[18] Tobias CA, Roberts JE, Lawrence JH, et al. Irradiation hypophysectomy and related sudies using 340 MeV deutorons. In: Peaceful Uses Atomic Energy. Geneva: 1955; 10: 95–106

[19] Kjellberg RN, Preston WM. The Bragg peak of a proton beam forIntracerebral lesions. Proc Sec Intl Cong Neurosurg Surg 1961: E103

[20] Kjellberg RN, Sweet WH, Preston WM, Koehler AM. The Bragg peak of a proton beam in intracranial therapy of tumors. Trans Am Neurol Assoc 1962; 87: 216–218

[21] Kjellberg RN, Koehler AM, Preston WM, Sweet WH. Stereotaxic instrument for use with the Bragg peak of a proton beam. Confin Neurol 1962; 22: 183–189

[22] Koehler AM, Dickinson JG, Preston WM. The range of protons in human skull-bone. Radiat Res 1965; 26: 334–342

[23] Preston WM, Koehler AM. Proton beam dosimetry. Harvard Cyclotron Laboratory Technical Note. 1965: 49

[24] Gragoudas ES, Lane AM, Collier JM. Charged particle irradiation of uveal melanomas. In: Adkinson NF, Busse WW, Bochner BS, et al, eds. Albert and Jakobiec's Principles and Practice of Ophthalmology. 3rd ed. Philadelphia, PA: Saunders Elsevier; 2008

[25] Kjellberg RN, Hanamura T, Davis KR, Lyons SL, Adams RD. Bragg peak proton-beam therapy for arteriovenous malformations of the brain. N Engl J Med 1983; 309: 269–274

[26] Amin-Hanjani S, Ogilvy CS, Guillermo JC, et al. Stereotactic radiosurgery for cavernous malformations: Kjellberg's experience with proton beam therapy in 98 cases at the Harvard cyclotron. Neurosurgery 1998; 42: 6

[27] Seifert V, Stolke D, Mehdorn HM, Hoffmann B. Clinical and radiological evaluation of long-term results of stereotactic proton beam radiosurgery in patients with cerebral arteriovenous malformation. J Neurosurg 1994; 81: 683–689

[28] Silander H, Pellettieri L, Enblad P, et al. Fractionated, stereotactic proton beam treatment of cerebral arteriovenous malformations. Acta Neurol Scand 2004; 109: 85–90

[29] Barker FG, Butler WE, Lyons S, et al. Dose-volume prediction of radiation-related complications after proton beam radiosurgery for cerebral arteriovenous malformations. J Neurosurg 2003; 99: 254–263

[30] Lunsford LD. Proton beam for arteriovenous malformations. J Neurosurg 2003; 99: 222–223, discussion 223–224

[31] Vernimmen FJ, Slabbert JP, Wilson JA, Fredericks S, Melvill R. Stereotactic proton beam therapy for intracranial arteriovenous malformations. Int J Radiat Oncol Biol Phys 2005; 62(1): 44: 52

[32] Hattangadi JA, Chapman PH, Bussière MR, et al. Planned two-fraction proton beam stereotactic radiosurgery for high-risk inoperable cerebral arteriovenous malformations. Int J Radiat Oncol Biol Phys 2012; 83: 533–541

[33] Hattangadi JA, Chapman PH, Kim D, et al. Single fraction proton beam stereotactic radiosurgery (PSRS) for inoperable cerebral arteriovenous malformations (AVMs). Int J Radiat Oncol Biol Phys 2012; 84: S38

[34] Estrada J, Boronat M, Mielgo M, et al. The long-term outcome of pituitary irradiation after unsuccessful transsphenoidal surgery in Cushing's disease. N Engl J Med 1997; 336: 172–177

[35] Mitsumori M, Shrieve DC, Alexander E, et al. Initial clinical results of LINAC-based stereotactic radiosurgery and stereotactic radiotherapy for pituitary adenomas. Int J Radiat Oncol Biol Phys 1998; 42: 3

[36] Sasaki R, Murakami M, Okamoto Y, et al. The efficacy of conventional radiation therapy in the management of pituitary adenoma. Int J Radiat Oncol Biol Phys 2000; 47: 1337–1345

[37] Petrovich Z, Yu C, Giannotta SL, et al. Gamma Knife radiosurgery for pituitary adenoma: early results. Neurosurgery 2003; 53: 51: 59

[38] Lawrence JH, Tobias CA, Born JL, et al. Pituitary irradiation with high-energy proton beams: a preliminary report. Cancer Res 1958; 18: 121–134

[39] Kjellberg RN, Shintani A, Frantz AG, Kliman B. Proton-beam therapy in acromegaly. N Engl J Med 1968; 278: 689–695

[40] Kjellberg RN, Kliman B. Bragg peak proton treatment for pituitary-related conditions. Proc R Soc Med 1974; 67: 32–33

[41] Welbourn RB, Friesen SR, Johnston IDA, Sellwood RA. The History of Endocrine Surgery. Westport, CT: Praeger; 1990

[42] Petit JH, Biller BM, Coen JJ, et al. Proton stereotactic radiosurgery in management of persistent acromegaly. Endocr Pract 2007; 13: 726–734

[43] Petit JH, Biller BM, Yock TI, et al. Proton stereotactic radiotherapy for persistent ACTH-producing adenomas. J Clin Endocrinol Metab 2008; 93: 393–399

[44] Aghi MK, Petit J, Chapman P, et al. Management of recurrent and refractory Cushing's disease with reoperation and/or proton beam radiosurgery. In: Clinical Neurosurgery. 2008(5): 141–144

[45] Goldsmith BJ, Wara WM, Wilson CB, Larson DA. Postoperative irradiation for subtotally resected meningiomas: a retrospective analysis of 140 patients treated from 1967 to 1990. J Neurosurg 1994; 80: 195–201

[46] Friedman WA, Murad GJ, Bradshaw P, et al. Linear accelerator surgery for meningiomas. J Neurosurg 2005; 103: 206–209
[47] Hakim R, Alexander E, 3rd, Loeffler JS, et al. Results of linear acceleratorbased radiosurgery for intracranial meningiomas. Neurosurgery 1998; 42: 446–453
[48] Flickinger JC, Kondziolka D, Maitz AH, et al. Gamma Knife radiosurgery of imaging-diagnosed intracranial meningioma. Int J Radiat Oncol Biol Phys 2003; 56: 801–806
[49] Debus J, Wuendrich M, Pirzkall A, et al. High efficacy of fractionated stereotactic radiotherapy of large base-of-skull meningiomas: long-term results. J Clin Oncol 2001; 19: 3547–3553
[50] Verhey LJ, Smith V, Serago CF. Comparison of radiosurgery treatment modalities based on physical dose distributions. Int J Radiat Oncol Biol Phys 1998; 40: 497–505
[51] Gudjonsson O, Blomquist E, Nyberg G, et al. Stereotactic irradiation of skull base meningiomas with high energy protons. Acta Neurochir (Wien) 1999; 141: 933–940
[52] Wenkel E, Thornton AF, Finkelstein D, et al. Benign meningioma: partially resected, biopsied, and recurrent intracranial tumors treated with combined proton and photon radiotherapy. Int J Radiat Oncol Biol Phys 2000; 48: 1363–1370
[53] Weber DC, Lomax AJ, Rutz HP, et al. Spot-scanning proton radiation therapy for recurrent, residual or untreated intracranial meningiomas. Radiother Oncol 2004; 71: 251–258
[54] Noël G, Bollet MA, Calugaru V, et al. Functional outcome of patients with benign meningioma treated by 3D conformal irradiation with a combination of photons and protons. Int J Radiat Oncol Biol Phys 2005; 62: 1412–1422
[55] Arvold ND, Niemierko A, Broussard GP, et al. Projected second tumor risk and dose to neurocognitive structures after proton versus photon radiotherapy for benign meningioma. Int J Radiat Oncol Biol Phys 2012; 83: e495–e500
[56] Vernimmen FJ, Harris JK, Wilson JA, et al. Stereotactic proton beam therapy of skull base meningiomas. Int J Radiat Oncol Biol Phys 2001; 49: 99–105
[57] Halasz LM, Bussière MR, Dennis ER, et al. Proton stereotactic radiosurgery for the treatment of benign meningiomas. Int J Radiat Oncol Biol Phys 2011; 81: 1428–1435
[58] Pollock BE, Stafford SL, Link MJ, Brown PD, Garces Y, Foote RL. Single-Fraction Radiosurgery of Benign Intracranial Meningiomas. Neurosurgery 2012; 71: 604–12
[59] Miralbell R, Linggood RM, de la Monte S, et al. The role of radiotherapy in the treatment of subtotally resected benign meningiomas. J Neurooncol 1992; 13: 157–64
[60] Mendenhall WM, Morris CG, Amdur RJ, et al. Radiotherapy alone or after subtotal resection for benign skull base meningiomas. Cancer 2003; 98: 1473–82
[61] Chang SD, Adler JR, Jr. Treatment of cranial base meningiomas with linear accelerator radiosurgery. Neurosurgery 1997; 41: 1019–1025
[62] DiBiase SJ, Kwok Y, Yovino S, et al. Factors predicting local tumor control after gamma knife stereotactic radiosurgery for benign intracranial meningiomas. Int J Radiat Oncol Biol Phys 2004; 60: 1515–9
[63] Han JH, Kim DG, Chung HT, et al. Gamma knife radiosurgery for skull base meningiomas: long-term radiologic and clinical outcome. Int J Radiat Oncol Biol Phys 2008; 72: 1324–1332
[64] Kreil W, Luggin J, Fuchs I, et al. Long term experience of gamma knife radiosurgery for benign skull base meningiomas. J Neurol Neurosurg Psychiatry 2005; 76: 1425–30
[65] Kimball MM, Friedman WA, Foote KD, et al. Linear accelerator radiosurgery for cavernous sinus meningiomas. Stereotact Funct Neurosurg 2009; 87: 120–127
[66] Kollová A, Liscák R, Novotný J Jr, et al. Gamma Knife surgery for benign meningioma. J Neurosurg 2007; 107: 325–36
[67] Kondziolka D, Mathieu D, Lunsford LD, et al. Radiosurgery as definitive management of intracranial meningiomas. Neurosurg 2008; 62: 53–60
[68] Lee JY, Niranjan A, McInerney J, Kondziolka D, et al. Stereotactic radiosurgery providing long-term tumor control of cavernous sinus meningiomas. J Neurosurg 2002; 97: 65–72
[69] Malik I, Rowe JG, Walton L, et al. The use of stereotactic radiosurgery in the management of meningiomas. Br J Neurosurg 2005; 19: 13–20
[70] Nicolato A, Foroni R, Alessandrini F, et al. The role of Gamma Knife radiosurgery in the management of cavernous sinus meningiomas. Int J Radiat Oncol Biol Phys 2002; 53: 992–1000
[71] Pollock BE, Stafford SL, Utter A, et al. Stereotactic radiosurgery provides equivalent tumor con trol to Simpson Grade 1 resection for patients with small- to medium-size meningiomas. Int J Radiat Oncol Biol Phys 2003; 55: 1000–5
[72] Spiegelmann R, Nissim O, Menhel J, et al. Linear accelerator radiosurgery for meningiomas in and around the cavernous sinus. Neurosurgery 2002; 51: 1373–1379
[73] Stafford SL, Pollock BE, Foote RL, et al. Meningioma radiosurgery: tumor control, outcomes, and complications among 190 consecutive patients. Neurosurgery 2001; 49: 1029–37
[74] Torres RC, Frighetto L, De Salles AA, et al. Radiosurgery and stereotactic radiotherapy for intracranial meningiomas. Neurosurg Focus 2003; 14: e5
[75] Villavicencio AT, Black PM, Shrieve DC, et al. Linac radiosurgery for skull base meningiomas. Acta Neurochir (Wien) 2001; 143: 1141–1152
[76] Boskos C, Feuvret L, Noel G, et al. Combined proton and photon conformal radiotherapy for intracranial atypical and malignant meningioma. Int J Radiat Oncol Biol Phys 2009; 75: 399–406
[77] Hug EB, Devries A, Thornton AF, et al. Management of atypical and malignant meningiomas: role of high-dose, 3D-conformal radiation therapy. J Neurooncol 2000; 48: 151–160
[78] Harsh GR, Thornton AF, Chapman PH, Bussiere MR, Rabinov JD, Loeffler JS. Proton beam stereotactic radiosurgery of vestibular schwannomas. Int J Radiat Oncol Biol Phys 2002; 54: 35–44
[79] Weber DC, Chan AW, Bussiere MR, et al. Proton beam radiosurgery for vestibular schwannoma: tumor control and cranial nerve toxicity. Neurosurgery 2003; 53: 577–586, discussion 586–588
[80] Chan AW, Black P, Ojemann RG, et al. Stereotactic radiotherapy for vestibular schwannomas: favorable outcome with minimal toxicity. Neurosurgery 2005; 57: 1
[81] Lunsford LD, Niranjan A, Flickinger JC, et al. Radiosurgery of vestibular schwannomas: summary of experience in 829 cases. J Neurosurg 2005; 102: 195–199
[82] Miller RC, Foote RL, Coffey RJ, et al. Decrease in cranial nerve complications after radiosurgery for acoustic neuromas: a prospective study of dose and volume. Int J Radiat Oncol Biol Phys 1999; 43: 305–311
[83] Bolsi A, Fogliata A, Cozzi L. Radiotherapy of small intracranial tumours with different advanced techniques using photon and proton beams: a treatment planning study. Radiother Oncol 2003; 68: 1–14
[84] Finger PT, Berson A, Ng T, Szechter A. Palladium-103 plaque radiotherapy for choroidal melanoma: an 11-year study. Int J Radiat Oncol Biol Phys 2002; 54: 5
[85] Kim YT, Kang SW, Lee JI. Gamma Knife radiosurgery for choroidal hemangioma. Int J Radiat Oncol Biol Phys 2011; 81: 1399–1404
[86] Schirmer CM, Chan M, Mignano J, et al. Dose de-escalation with Gamma Knife radiosurgery in the treatment of choroidal melanoma. Int J Radiat Oncol Biol Phys 2009; 75: 170–176
[87] Dunavoelgyi R, Dieckmann K, Gleiss A, et al. Local tumor control, visual acuity, and survival after hypofractionated stereotactic photon radiotherapy of choroidal melanoma in 212 patients treated between 1997 and 2007. Int J Radiat Oncol Biol Phys 2011; 81: 199
[88] Dunavoelgyi R, Dieckmann K, Gleiss A, et al. Radiogenic side effects after hypofractionated stereotactic photon radiotherapy of choroidal melanoma in 212 patients treated between 1997 and 2007. Int J Radiat Oncol Biol Phys 2012; 83: 121–128
[89] Courdi A, Caujolle JP, Grange JD, et al. Results of proton therapy of uveal melanomas treated in Nice. Int J Radiat Oncol Biol Phys 1999; 45: 5–11
[90] Damato B, Kacperek A, Chopra M, Campbell IR, Errington RD. Proton beam radiotherapy of choroidal melanoma: the Liverpool-Clatterbridge experience. Int J Radiat Oncol Biol Phys 2005; 62: 1405–1411
[91] Dendale R, Lumbroso-Le Rouic L, Noel G, et al. Proton beam radiotherapy for uveal melanoma: results of Curie Institut-Orsay Proton Therapy Center (ICPO). Int J Radiat Oncol Biol Phys 2006; 65: 780–787
[92] Egger E, Schalenbourg A, Zografos L, et al. Maximizing local tumor control and survival after proton beam radiotherapy of uveal melanoma. Int J Radiat Oncol Biol Phys 2001; 51: 138–147
[93] Höcht S, Bechrakis NE, Nausner M, et al. Proton therapy of uveal melanomas in Berlin. 5 years of experience at the Hahn-Meitner Institute. Strahlenther Onkol 2004; 180: 419–424
[94] Gragoudas E, Li W, Goitein M, Lane AM, Munzenrider JE, Egan KM. Evidence-based estimates of outcome in patients irradiated for intraocular melanoma. Arch Ophthalmol 2002; 120: 1665–1671
[95] Gragoudas ES, Marie Lane A. Uveal melanoma: proton beam irradiation. Ophthalmol Clin North Am 2005; 18: 111–118
[96] Gragoudas ES. Proton beam irradiation of uveal melanomas: the first 30 years. The Weisenfeld Lecture. Invest Ophthalmol Vis Sci 2006; 47: 4666–4673

5 Gamma Knife versus CyberKnife versus Multileaf Collimator Nonrobotic LINAC-based Radiosurgery

Arjun Sahgal, Lijun Ma, Mark Ruschin, Simon S. Lo, Paula Petti, Daniel Letourneau, David A. Larson, and Eric L. Chang

Introduction

There have been dramatic advances in radiation oncology technologies over the past 10 years, specifically in the application of brain stereotactic radiosurgery (SRS). In the beginning of SRS, the main technologies were the Leksell Gamma Knife (Elekta AB, Stockholm, Sweden) and linear accelerators (LINACs) that were retrofitted to perform SRS using circular collimators and noncoplanar arc-based radiation delivery.[1]

Both technical platforms have undergone major changes, and in this chapter we review these changes, including the development of a nonisocentric robotic delivery unit and the potential benefits of one platform over another specific to SRS for brain metastases. Current SRS technologies allow multiple brain metastases to be treated in a single session,[2–4] and we provide details on the various technologies in the context of the radiosurgical treatment of such metastases. The clinical details of the treatment of multiple metastases with SRS are discussed elsewhere.

Stereotactic Radiosurgery Platforms

Leksell Gamma Knife Perfexion

The Leksell Gamma Knife (LGK) Perfexion unit shown in ▶ Fig. 5.1 features 192 cobalt 60 sources arranged in a cone section configuration.[1,5] During fabrication of the collimator system, multiple rings of collimating holes are drilled directly into one tungsten piece, creating three beam sizes of 16, 8, and 4 mm in diameter at the isocenter. Just beyond the tungsten collimator assembly are eight sliding source sectors, each of which contains 24 sources. When individual sectors slide along the outside surface of the tungsten collimator to align with different rings of predrilled holes, 192 16-mm-diameter beams, 192 8-mm-diameter beams, and 192 4-mm-diameter beams are possible. Individual sectors can also be blocked to conform the isodose distribution at the target by placing them between predrilled holes, creating 0-mm-diameter beams, for an overall combination of beam apertures at each isocenter of 65,535. Intermediate collimator sizes can also be created within any sector by serially superimposing different collimator sizes on different relative weights, that is, the beam-on time. Therefore, the independently moving sector design allows for significantly enhanced flexibility in the number and diameter of beams intersecting at the isocenters, as compared with previous generations of LGK models.

For multiple metastatic lesion treatments, automatic sector selection and automatic patient positioning via full couch positioning significantly improve the overall treatment delivery efficiency. Compared with earlier models of LGK delivery, where the overall treatment time may last 100 to 200% longer than the actual beam-on time for a multiple-lesion treatment session (due to repeat repositioning of the patient to reach different targets), the overall treatment time with LGK Perfexion is nearly identical to the overall beam-on time, as each isocenter shift can now be accomplished within a few seconds. In addition, the accessible coordinate range for the LGK Perfexion has also nearly doubled compared with earlier models, making all intracranial lesions readily treatable in a single frame placement.

Besides new hardware designs, several advancements in the Leksell Gamma Plan (LGP) software have facilitated multiple metastatic brain lesions to be addressed in a single treatment. For example, automatic image registration and fusion in the latest LGP now allow both pre- and postplanning management of multiple metastatic lesions. The preplanning feature allows the user to design the treatment plan of a known number of lesions before the treatment day without a frame in place. In particular, the latest LGP system enables automatic mapping of a treatment plan based on multiple imaging modalities to any treatment coordinate system as defined by the LGK frame on the day of patient treatment. The postplanning feature enables the user to map previously treated lesions on prior treatment planning magnetic resonance imaging (MRI) to new follow-up imaging studies (with superimposed previously treated isodose lines) to differentiate new lesions requiring treatment from those previously treated. In addition to the improved planning features, there are software-based developments, including a more accurate dose calculation based on the convolution method, as well as an inverse planning module that is designed to optimize conformity index.

In the past, LGK SRS of multiple brain lesions was limited to single-fraction treatments. This was primarily because of the need for an invasive frame, making it impractical and potentially unreliable for a patient to remain immobilized in a frame over multiple days. However, the LGK Extend system[6] allows frameless LGK SRS and hypofractionated SRS. In particular, for large tumors > 3 cm in diameter, hypofractionation allows for high-dose delivery as opposed to the dose reductions required with single-fraction SRS based on size. For multiple brain metastases, it may also allow the treatment to extend over a few days, as treatment times can still be excessively long. For example, in a patient with 32 brain metastases and a surgical cavity treated with single-fraction LGK Perfexion SRS, the treatment time was 421.3 min (dose rate 2.1 Gy/min), with 54 shots used (▶ Fig. 5.2).

CyberKnife

The Accuray CyberKnife (Accuray Inc., Sunnyvale, CA) is a nonisocentric compact LINAC mounted on a highly flexible, multijointed robotic arm[7–9] (▶ Fig. 5.3). Fundamentally, it is a paradigm shift in radiation delivery such that the LINAC itself is repositioned in near-real time in all six degrees of freedom to compensate for patient/tumor motion. The radiation beam is collimated by circular collimators of fixed diameters ranging

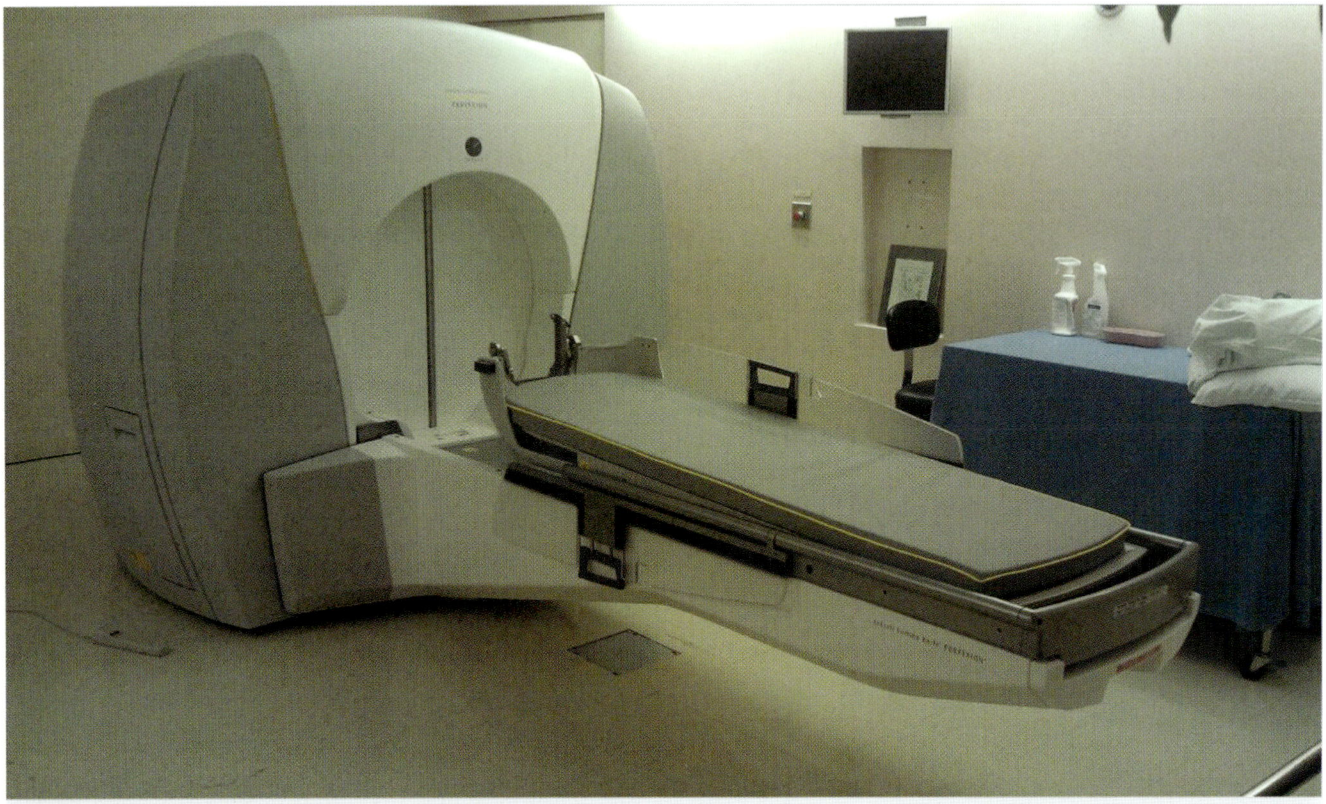

Fig. 5.1 The Leksell Gamma Knife Perfexion unit installed at the University Hospitals Seidman Cancer Center, Cleveland, Ohio.

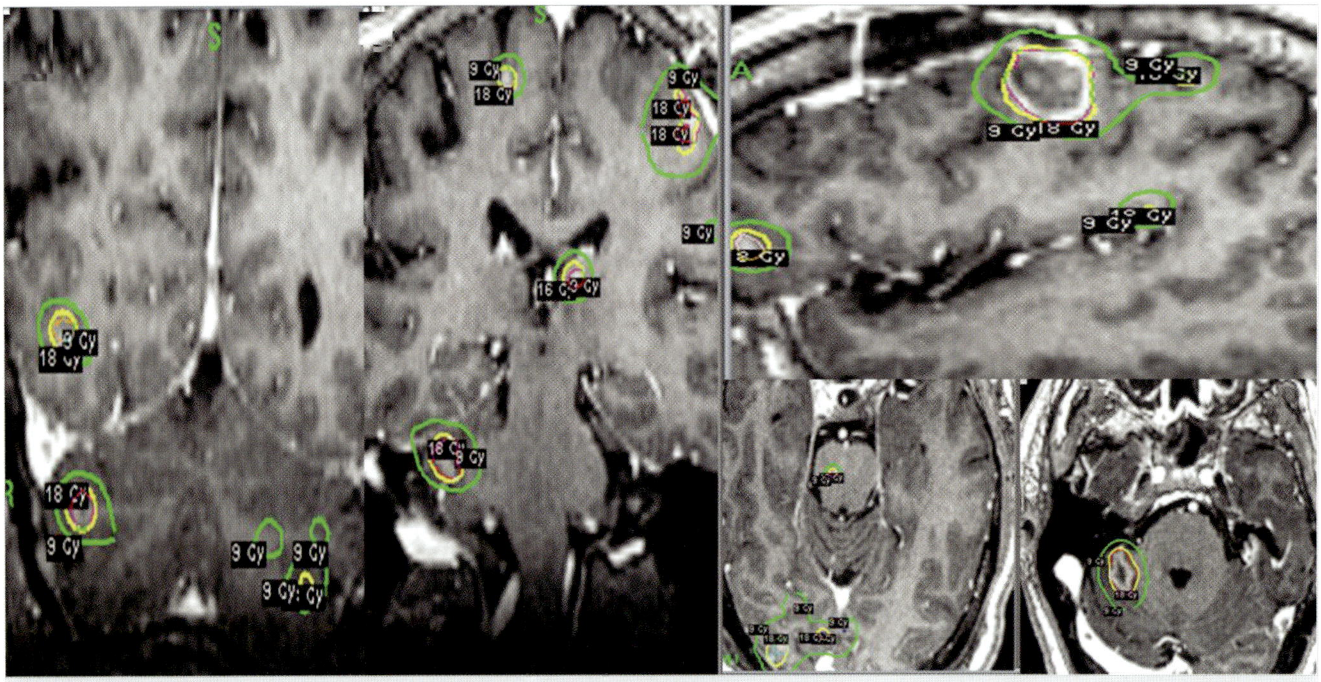

Fig. 5.2 A patient with 32 brain metastases and a surgical cavity treated with the Leksell Gamma Knife Perfexion unit in a single session. The treatment time was 421.3 min (dose rate 2.1 Gy/min), and we used 54 shots.

from 0.5 to 6.0 cm. It relies on a set of noncoplanar beams cross-firing at various angles from a large number of points (nodes) on the surface of a sphere or ellipsoid surrounding the patient (~ 100–200 beams). Treatment planning is achieved with an inverse planning algorithm for the optimization of the beams' number and orientation. The additive effect of the

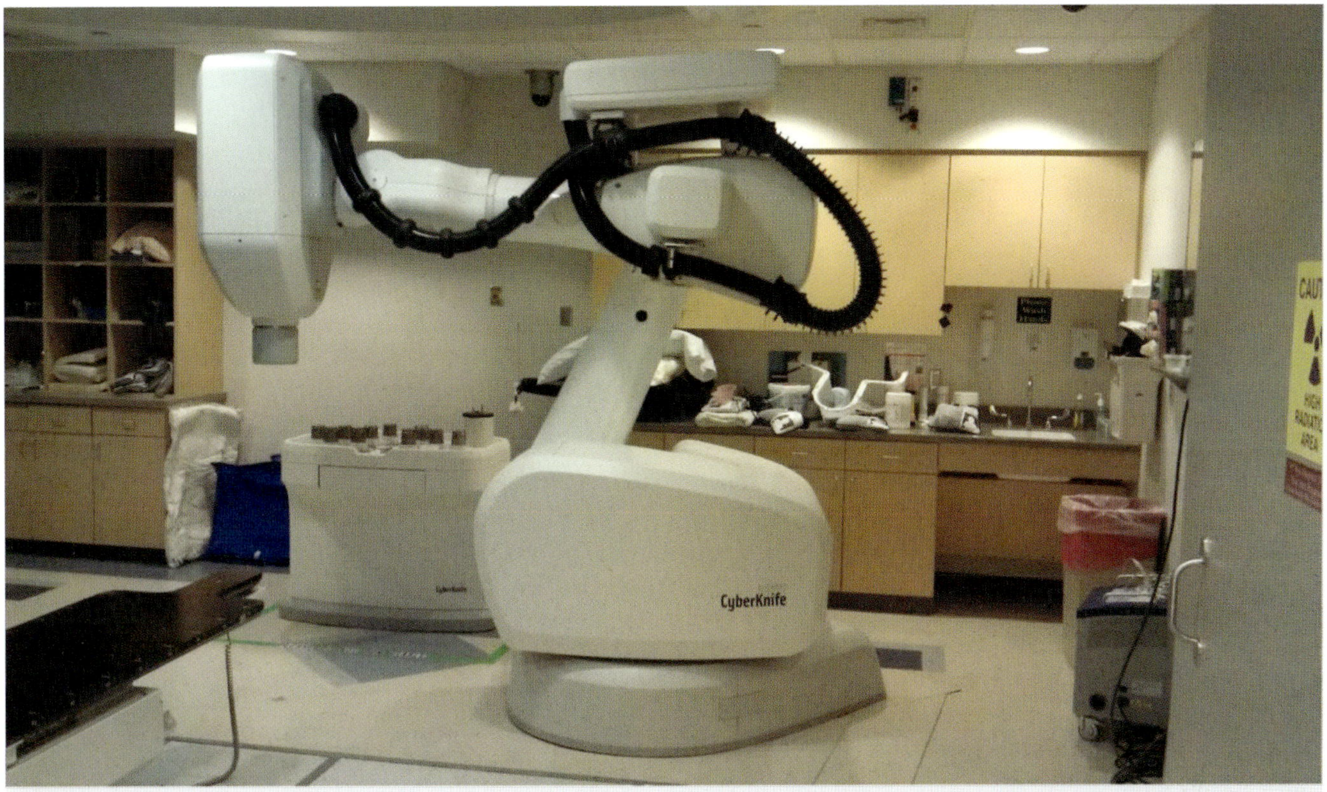

Fig. 5.3 The CyberKnife robotic unit currently installed at the University Hospitals Seidman Cancer Center, Cleveland, Ohio.

individual beam-on times results in conformal dose distribution. Highly conformal plans with steep dose gradients are typically achieved within the target.[10–12] Recent advances in the CyberKnife include a treatment planning system that allows for a sequential optimization routine, as opposed to the prior iterative process,[13] and Monte Carlo–based dose calculations. Benefits of the new treatment planning system include the potential for better sparing of organs at risk.[12] The self-contained collimator unit allows the aperture to independently and automatically vary the beam diameter (range 0.5–6.0 cm); however, it does not adjust dynamically while the beam is on to modulate the radiation. There has been promising exploratory work in intensity-modulated CyberKnife delivery using multileaf collimators (MLCs), but no commercial device is currently available.[14]

With respect to treatment planning for multiple brain metastases, research done by Ma et al concentrated on improving the optimization for multiple targets to be treated in a single session.[13] The two-step optimization method addressed in that study resulted in significantly lower volumes of normal brain receiving relatively low doses. For example, the study demonstrated that the normal brain volume receiving 12 Gy was reduced by an average of 42% (range 34–47%). Furthermore, the gains observed typically increased with an increasing number of targets treated regardless of size. It should be noted that this new optimization is not yet commercially available. Importantly, this study also reports the nonlinear dependence of the normal brain dose with increasing number of targets. A nonlinear dependency (i.e., the rate of change in isodose volumes varies as N increases) suggested that simple extrapolation of normal brain tolerance from $N = 1$, or a small number of targets treated, is likely invalid.

LINAC-based Stereotactic Radiosurgery

LINAC-based SRS systems initially consisted of retrofitted conventional S-band LINACs with modifications that included the addition of tertiary circular collimator cones of varying diameter (minimum diameter ~ 5 mm at the isocenter), additional monitoring devices for couch motion to ensure precise motions, and a couch attachment to dock a stereotactic head frame.[1] As SRS practice grew, dedicated high-output LINACs with improved mechanical accuracy were developed with dedicated treatment planning systems (or planning system modules) to support LINAC-based SRS using noncoplanar arc therapy with cones. Recent developments of high-definition MLCs, forward or inverse treatment planning allowing for intensity-modulated radiation therapy (IMRT), and onboard image guidance systems (computed tomographic [CT], stereoscopic, or both) have allowed the practice of MLC-based intensity-modulated radiosurgery (IMRS) with mechanical accuracy in the range of 1 to 2 mm.[1] However, using this technology does not circumvent the use of proper immobilization, as a thermoplastic mass is generally insufficient to provide the appropriate precision according to SRS standards.[15] A more sophisticated mask equipped with a bite block system with image guidance is suggested for single-fraction frameless SRS, and several are on the market.[16] An evaluation by Memorial Sloan-Kettering for the Aktina system (Aktina Medical Corp., Congers, NY) has shown positioning to be equivalent to an invasive frame.[16]

With a high-definition MLC (leaf width 2.5–5 mm), the requirement for circular collimators is questionable except for very small lesions (< 0.5 to 1.0 cm). The primary concern is the beam penumbra, which is wider with an MLC than that achievable with a cone. The distance between the beam-shaping device and the patient is smaller for cones than for MLCs, which explains the difference in penumbra width. As a result, for the same degree of conformity, more normal brain tissue may be exposed with MLC-based SRS, especially for very small tumors. However, for larger tumors or tumors that are nonspherical, IMRT-based systems often achieve greater conformity than cones, as cone-based treatment planning is limited by the number of isocenters.

MLC-based LINAC delivery has undergone another evolution with the advent of volumetric modulated arc therapy (VMAT). In this system, radiation is delivered along a gantry arc motion, with the beam aperture changing dynamically as a function of the gantry motion (the MLC moves simultaneously with gantry rotation) during delivery. The beam dose rate and the gantry speed are also allowed to vary during delivery, providing additional degrees of freedom to generate a conformal dose distribution. The treatment is delivered with continuous gantry rotation. Fundamentally, VMAT delivers the same treatment quality as IMRT but uses beam angles more efficiently. The rotational delivery also affords greater degrees of freedom in terms of delivery parameters such as beam direction, dose rate, and gantry speed. These allow greater flexibility in the treatment planning optimization parameter space, which may translate to better treatment planning solutions. An example of a VMAT multiple brain metastases plan is shown in ▶ Fig. 5.4, as planned using Pinnacle treatment planning software version 9.0 (Philips Radiation Oncology Systems, Fitchburg, WI), and delivered using the Elekta Axesse equipped with a 4-mm high-definition MLC, cone beam CT for image guidance, and a Hexapod couch.

A practical advantage of IMRT/VMAT over cone-based solutions in the treatment of multiple brain metastases is that it uses only a few or even a single isocenter setup.[2] This means that the composite dose distribution for all lesions can be generated using an inverse treatment planning algorithm that takes into account both the dose objectives for each target and the dose limits for the organs at risk.[2] Coupled with VMAT, treatment time can be substantially shortened, thereby allowing multiple brain metastases to be treated with high efficiency and making SRS a more convenient and more tolerable experience for the patient.

The latest major advance in LINAC-based MLC radiation delivery involves flattening filter-free beam delivery. Essentially, the dose rate output has been markedly increased from the typical 400 to 600 monitor units per minute (MU/min) to as high as 2,400 MU/min. The flattening filter is normally used to make the beam profile flat at a given depth in tissue. By physically removing the flattening filter from the beam path, the resulting elimination of beam attenuation substantially increases the dose rate and gives the beam profile a cone shape centered on the beam axis. The use of IMRT, MLC, and inverse treatment planning algorithms can take into account the nonuniform nature of these beams while taking advantage of the high dose rate for delivery efficiency. The Varian TrueBeam (Varian Medical Systems, Inc., Palo Alto, CA) is one such unit (▶ Fig. 5.5). The unit can couple RapidArc volumetric modulated arc technology with flattening filter-free technology, and the net result is improved delivery efficiency. A recent investigation by Reggiori et al reported a delivery of 75 Gy in three fractions in 2.2 min per fraction and 8.2 min in flattening filter-free delivery and conventional delivery, respectively.[17]

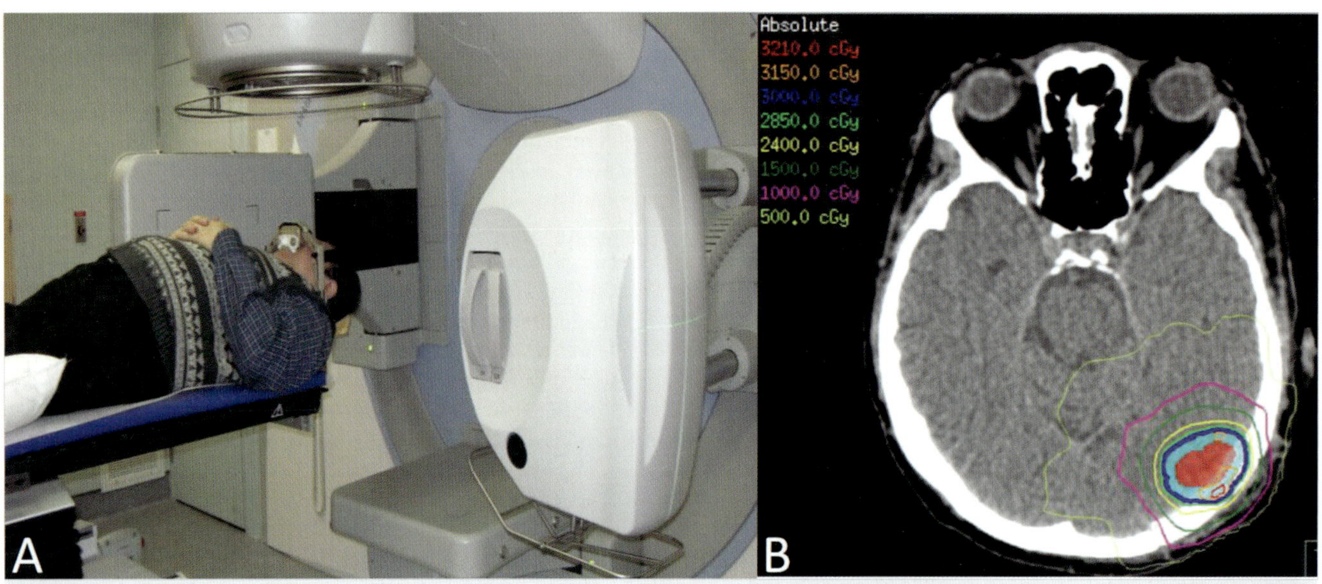

Fig. 5.4 (a) The Elekta Axesse equipped with a 4-mm high-definition multileaf collimator and cone beam computed tomography scanner for image guidance. (b) A typical volumetric modulated arc therapy plan treating a 4.3-cm^3 brain metastasis (*red*) with a planning target volume (*cyan*) to 30 Gy in five fractions.

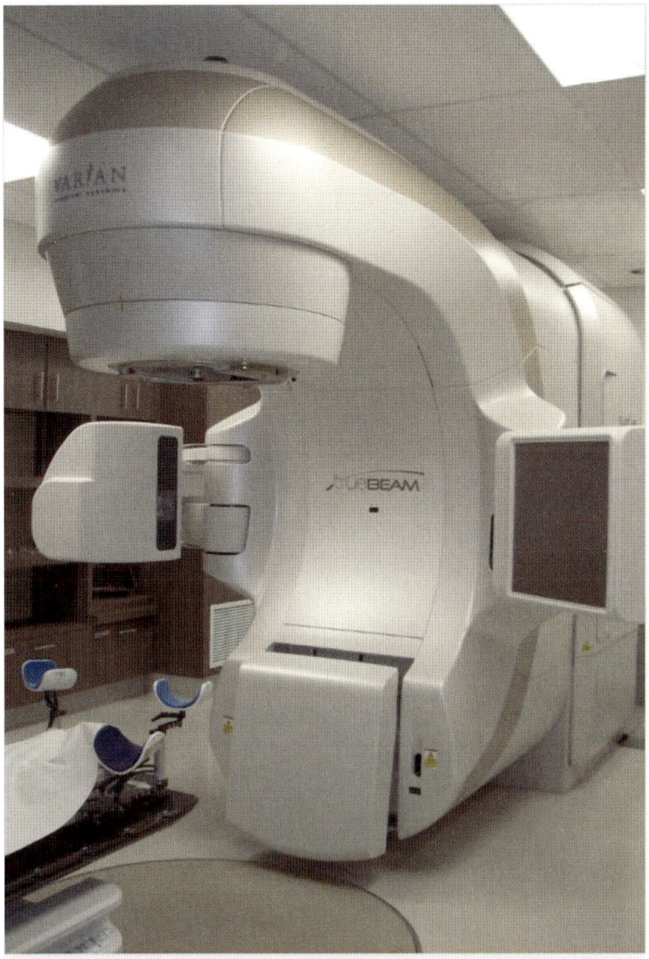

Fig. 5.5 The Varian TrueBeam currently installed at the Princess Margaret Hospital, University of Toronto.

Comparing the Technologies

There are inherent differences in target central-dose distribution according to each category of SRS technology that are fundamentally linked to the prescription practice. With LGK SRS, we commonly prescribe the dose to the 50% isodose line; that is, the maximum dose in the target is twice the prescribed dose. LINAC-based SRS using a single isocenter and a tertiary circular collimator (i.e., a cone) is typically prescribed to the 80 to 90% isodose line. With MLC-based IMRS, treatment planning is most often designed to produce homogeneous plans in the order of plus or minus 10 to 20%, but it can also be designed to emulate cone-based or LGK plans if the physician wishes to emphasize a steep dose gradient. With CyberKnife technology, we typically prescribe at an intermediate isodose line between that of LGK and traditional LINAC-based SRS practice.

In terms of *evidence-based medicine,* there have never been any clinical data to support one technology as being superior to another with regard to local control. With respect to survival rates, in a randomized trial of whole-brain radiation plus or minus boost SRS (***level I evidence***), no difference in overall survival was reported between Gamma Knife and LINAC-based SRS in the subset analysis.[18] Moreover, looking at ***level II and level III evidence***, survival after radiosurgical treatment for either malignant or benign tumors appears comparable regardless of the radiosurgical device used.

One area where there may be differences in SRS technologies is the peripheral dose distribution. Differences in peripheral dose distribution could equate to a difference in the risk of radiation necrosis. For the radiosurgical treatment of arteriovenous malformations (AVMs), it is well known that the risk of radiation necrosis increases as the volume encompassed by the 10- and 12-Gy isodose increases.[19] Differences in 12-Gy volumes have been the focus of several investigations led by the University of California, San Francisco, and the University of Toronto.[10,11,20] However, from an evidence-based medicine standpoint, the differences in peripheral dose distribution among devices have not yet been rigorously studied in a case-controlled or prospective fashion, and they have not been causally linked to differences in outcome or safety among the various radiosurgical platforms. Nevertheless, these theoretical differences warrant some discussion.

The Impact of Each Platform on a Single Target

Ma et al examined the peripheral dose fall-off for individual lesions treated with LGK Perfexion, CyberKnife, and the Novalis MLC-based stereotactic unit (Brainlab AG, Munich, Germany).[11] The investigators observed that the peripheral dose fall-off was nearly identical among technologies, but the heterogeneity within the target volume was greatest for LGK Perfexion plans. The importance of this observation lies in the application of V10 and V12 (i.e., the volume of normal brain tissue receiving 10 Gy and 12 Gy, respectively) as predictors of necrosis being applicable across technologic platforms. Based on radiobiologic modeling of the normal tissue doses, some interesting observations were made. First, for fast-growing tumors, such as brain metastases, a hypofractionated course may be biologically better than single-fraction delivery. The movement toward hypofractionated SRS is growing, and some clinical data are starting to emerge supporting better outcomes. Second, for slow-growing targets, such as AVMs, single-fraction SRS may in fact be the preferred therapeutic approach. This conclusion is supported by clinical data reporting suboptimal obliteration rates achieved using fractionated SRS.[21]

The Impact of Each Platform on Multiple Targets

In a study reported by Ma et al, the peripheral dose fall-off was given for 3, 6, 9, and 12 targets treated in a single session.[10] This study accounted for the effects of dose spillage beyond the target on the peripheral dose fall-off characteristics and whole-brain dose.

The authors observed a nonlinear trend of increase in the volume of normal brain tissue receiving a peripheral dose of 4 to 20 Gy among the three modalities. The LGK Perfexion plans resulted in the least normal brain volumes receiving any particular dose. This discrepancy was typically on the order of a factor of 2 or 3 in favor of LGK Perfexion. The clinical significance with respect to normal brain tissue functioning is not known.

However, the impact on the dose prescribed is an issue and is explained in the following section.

The Impact of Multiple Metastases Treated in a Single Session on the Prescription

Sahgal et al investigated the impact on the treatment of multiple brain metastases of the prescription practice according to guidelines based on the Radiation Therapy Oncology Group (RTOG) 9005 study.[20] The authors observed that the peripheral isodose volume was dependent on an increasing number of targets, but not on the total intracranial target volume. This suggests that as the number of targets increases, the near 12-Gy peripheral isodose line volume increases for each individual target, and hence the risk of radiation necrosis. Based on a simulation of 1 to 60 targets to be treated randomly within the brain, the average increase in the total 12-Gy volume was 0.87%, 1.9%, and 4.4% per each additional target treated at the 15-, 18-, and 24-Gy dose prescription level, respectively. The increase was approximately linear in nature over this dose prescription range. The authors concluded that to maintain a constant 12-Gy isodose volume surrounding each target, with a single target treated as the reference, a dose reduction by 1 Gy at the 24-Gy prescription practice level would yield an additional 4 targets to be treated, an additional 9 targets at the 18-Gy prescription dose level, and an additional 23 targets at the 15-Gy prescription dose level. Based on these results, users must be knowledgeable and adapt the prescription practice when multiple brain metastases are being treated in a single radiosurgical session.

Authors' Practice

The authors' practice is to use single-fraction SRS for targets < 2-3 cm with either a cone-based LINAC system or LGK Perfexion technology. The choice is based entirely on the site at which the patient is being treated, as well as on whether an invasive head frame is being used. For metastases > 2-3 cm, or if patients refuse the invasive head frame and the tumors are > 1 cm, the authors currently use image-guided IMRT on a LINAC with the patient immobilized in a sturdy thermoplastic mask or non-invasive re-locatable frame with a bite block and vacuum suction, and the typical dose is 30 Gy in five fractions. We are in the process of implementing VMAT to deliver the dose faster. With the planned acquisition of a frameless non-invasive head immobilization system at the Sunnybrook Health Sciences Center, Toronto, our aim is to deliver frameless single-fraction IMRS for tumors < 3 cm using the Elekta Axesse.

Future Directions

Frameless SRS for LGK Perfexion is in use with the release of the Extend system, and frameless SRS will continue to grow in practice, as patients do not enjoy the application of the invasive frame. Frameless LGK Perfexion also permits hypofractionated SRS, and the recent development of a mounted cone beam CT unit onto the LGK Perfexion will improve the day-to-day reliability of the patient's position.[22]

LINAC-based systems will likely discard the invasive frame and be solely frameless. Treatment times will become extremely fast as flattening filter-free units emerge into mainstream centers and mature. This will also increase the availability of SRS for patients and permit the move toward multiple metastases treated with SRS alone and reserve whole-brain radiation as a salvage therapy. Hypofractionated SRS should also continue to grow in practice, in particular in the treatment of large metastases.

Conclusion

At present, there are no clinical data to support one SRS technology over others with respect to treatment efficacy or safety. SRS using the LGK Perfexion has been reported to yield the lowest integral brain dose, as well as an asymptotic peripheral dose within the brain, when multiple metastases are treated. This may allow for optimal dosing to the targets and a lower risk of radiation necrosis; however, treatment times can be prohibitively long. New flattening filter-free, high-output MLC-based LINACs with VMAT capacity may yield SRS treatment times in the order of minutes and a new paradigm in LINAC SRS delivery. What is needed are head-to-head trials as part of randomized studies comparing the technologies, but there are significant barriers to such studies. There is no doubt that SRS technologies are evolving at a rapid pace, and the challenge is for users to become highly proficient in the technologies' capabilities and limitations in order to perform treatment safely.

References

[1] Sahgal A, Ma L, Chang E, et al. Advances in technology for intracranial stereotactic radiosurgery. Technol Cancer Res Treat 2009; 8: 271–280

[2] Nath SK, Lawson JD, Simpson DR, et al. Single-isocenter frameless intensity-modulated stereotactic radiosurgery for simultaneous treatment of multiple brain metastases: clinical experience. Int J Radiat Oncol Biol Phys 2010; 78: 91–97

[3] Yamamoto M, Ide M, Nishio Si, Urakawa Y. Gamma Knife radiosurgery for numerous brain metastases: is this a safe treatment? Int J Radiat Oncol Biol Phys 2002; 53: 1279–1283

[4] Serizawa T, Hirai T, Nagano O, et al. Gamma Knife surgery for 110 brain metastases without prophylactic whole-brain radiation therapy: analysis of cases meeting the Japanese prospective multi-institute study (JLGK0901) inclusion criteria. J Neurooncol 2010; 98: 163–167

[5] Sahgal A, Ma L, Tsao M, et al. Gamma Knife radiosurgery. In: Vaezy S, Zderic V, eds. Image-Guided Therapy Systems. ARTECH HOUSE; 2009: 161–175

[6] Ruschin M, Nayebi N, Carlsson P, et al. Performance of a novel repositioning head frame for gamma knife perfexion and image-guided linac-based intracranial stereotactic radiotherapy. Int J Radiat Oncol Biol Phys 2010; 78: 306–313

[7] Antypas C, Pantelis E. Performance evaluation of a CyberKnife G4 image-guided robotic stereotactic radiosurgery system. Phys Med Biol 2008; 53: 4697–4718

[8] Sahgal A, Chou D, Ames C, et al. Image-guided robotic stereotactic body radiotherapy for benign spinal tumors: the University of California San Francisco preliminary experience. Technol Cancer Res Treat 2007; 6: 595–604

[9] Adler JR, Chang SD, Murphy MJ, Doty J, Geis P, Hancock SL. The CyberKnife: a frameless robotic system for radiosurgery. Stereotact Funct Neurosurg 1997; 69: 124–128

[10] Ma L, Petti P, Wang B, et al. Apparatus dependence of normal brain tissue dose in stereotactic radiosurgery for multiple brain metastases. J Neurosurg 2011; 114: 1580–1584

[11] Ma L, Sahgal A, Descovich M, et al. Equivalence in dose fall-off for isocentric and nonisocentric intracranial treatment modalities and its impact on dose fractionation schemes. Int J Radiat Oncol Biol Phys 2010; 76: 943–948
[12] Ma L, Sahgal A, Cozzi L, et al. Apparatus-dependent dosimetric differences in spine stereotactic body radiotherapy. Technol Cancer Res Treat 2010; 9: 563–574
[13] Ma L, Sahgal A, Hwang A, et al. A two-step optimization method for improving multiple brain lesion treatments with robotic radiosurgery. Technol Cancer Res Treat 2011; 10: 331–338
[14] van de Water S, Hoogeman MS, Breedveld S, Nuyttens JJ, Schaart DR, Heijmen BJ. Variable circular collimator in robotic radiosurgery: a time-efficient alternative to a mini-multileaf collimator? Int J Radiat Oncol Biol Phys 2011; 81: 863–870
[15] Lightstone AW, Tsao M, Baran PS, et al. Cone beam CT (CBCT) evaluation of inter- and intra-fraction motion for patients undergoing brain radiotherapy immobilized using a commercial thermoplastic mask on a robotic couch. Technol Cancer Res Treat 2012; 11: 203–209
[16] Li G, Ballangrud A, Kuo LC, et al. Motion monitoring for cranial frameless stereotactic radiosurgery using video-based three-dimensional optical surface imaging. Med Phys 2011; 38: 3981–3994
[17] Reggiori G, Mancosu P, Castiglioni S, et al. Can volumetric modulated arc therapy with flattening filter free beams play a role in stereotactic body radiotherapy for liver lesions? A volume-based analysis. Med Phys 2012; 39: 1112–1118
[18] Andrews DW, Scott CB, Sperduto PW, et al. Whole brain radiation therapy with or without stereotactic radiosurgery boost for patients with one to three brain metastases: phase III results of the RTOG 9508 randomised trial. Lancet 2004; 363: 1665–1672
[19] Korytko T, Radivoyevitch T, Colussi V, et al. 12 Gy Gamma Knife radiosurgical volume is a predictor for radiation necrosis in non-AVM intracranial tumors. Int J Radiat Oncol Biol Phys 2006; 64: 419–424
[20] Sahgal A, Barani IJ, Novotny J, et al. Prescription dose guideline based on physical criterion for multiple metastatic brain tumors treated with stereotactic radiosurgery. Int J Radiat Oncol Biol Phys 2010; 78: 605–608
[21] Laing RW, Childs J, Brada M. Failure of conventionally fractionated radiotherapy to decrease the risk of hemorrhage in inoperable arteriovenous malformations. Neurosurgery 1992; 30: 872–875, discussion 875–876
[22] Ruschin M, Komljenovic PT, Ansell M, et al. Cone beam computed tomography image guidance system for a dedicated intracranial radiosurgery treatment unit. Int J Radiat Oncol Biol Phys 2013; 85: 243–250

Benign Intracranial Tumors

6 Single-Session Radiosurgery for Acoustic Neuromas

Ajay Niranjan, Douglas Kondziolka, John C. Flickinger, and L. Dade Lunsford

Introduction

Patients with acoustic neuromas can choose among different therapeutic approaches, including observation with further imaging, microsurgery, radiosurgery, and fractionated radiation therapy. To make an informed decision, patients need to be presented with up-to-date information regarding clinical outcomes and complications of different management techniques. Over the past 15 years, stereotactic radiosurgery (SRS) has emerged as an effective and well-studied alternative to surgical removal of small to moderate-sized vestibular schwannomas. The evolution of single-session radiosurgery has influenced the management algorithm for the treatment of these tumors.[1] Advanced dose-planning software, intraoperative magnetic resonance imaging (MRI) for targeting, and dose optimization reflect the evolution of this technology. Long-term results from multiple international sites have established Gamma Knife (Elekta AB, Stockholm, Sweden) radiosurgery as an important minimally invasive alternative to microsurgery. The goals of acoustic neuroma Gamma Knife radiosurgery are to prevent further tumor growth, preserve cochlear and facial nerve function, and maintain or improve the patient's neurologic status.

Single-Session Radiosurgery: Clinical Results

Tumor Growth Control

Long-term results of Gamma Knife radiosurgery for vestibular schwannomas have been documented.[2–7] Recent reports suggest a tumor control rate of 93 to 100% after radiosurgery.[2–24] Kondziolka et al studied 5- to 10-year outcomes in 162 patients with vestibular schwannomas who had radiosurgery at the University of Pittsburgh.[17] In this long-term study, a 98% tumor control rate was reported (▶ Fig. 6.1). Sixty-two percent of tumors became smaller, 33% remained unchanged, and 6% became slightly larger. Some tumors initially enlarged 1 to 2 mm during the first 6 to 12 months after radiosurgery as they lost their central contrast enhancement. Such tumors generally regressed in volume compared to their preradiosurgery size. Less than 2% of patients required additional management, such as tumor resection after radiosurgery. Norén, in his 28-year experience with vestibular schwannoma radiosurgery, reported a 95% long-term tumor control rate.[22] Litvack et al reported a 98% tumor control rate at a mean follow-up of 31 months after radiosurgery using a 12-Gy margin dose.[25] Niranjan et al analyzed the outcome of intracanalicular tumor radiosurgery performed at the University of Pittsburgh.[26] All patients had imaging-documented tumor growth control. Flickinger et al performed an outcome analysis of patients with acoustic neuromas who were treated between August 1992 and August 1997 at the University of Pittsburgh. The actuarial 5-year clinical tumor control rate (no requirement for surgical intervention) was 99.4 ± 0.6%.[3,9]

In a long-term (10- to 15-year) outcome study that included 157 patients with vestibular schwannomas, the median follow-up for patients still living at the time of the study ($n = 136$) was 10.2 years. Serial imaging studies after radiosurgery ($n = 157$) showed a decrease in tumor size in 114 patients (73%), no change in 40 patients (25.5%), and an increase in 3 patients who later had resection (1.9%).[6] No patient developed a radiation-associated malignant or benign tumor (defined as a histologically confirmed and distinct neoplasm arising in the initial radiation field after at least 2 years have passed).

Hearing Preservation

Preradiosurgery hearing can now be preserved in 60 to 70% of patients, with higher preservation rates found for smaller tumors. In a long-term (5- to 10-year follow-up) study conducted at the University of Pittsburgh, 51% of patients had no change in

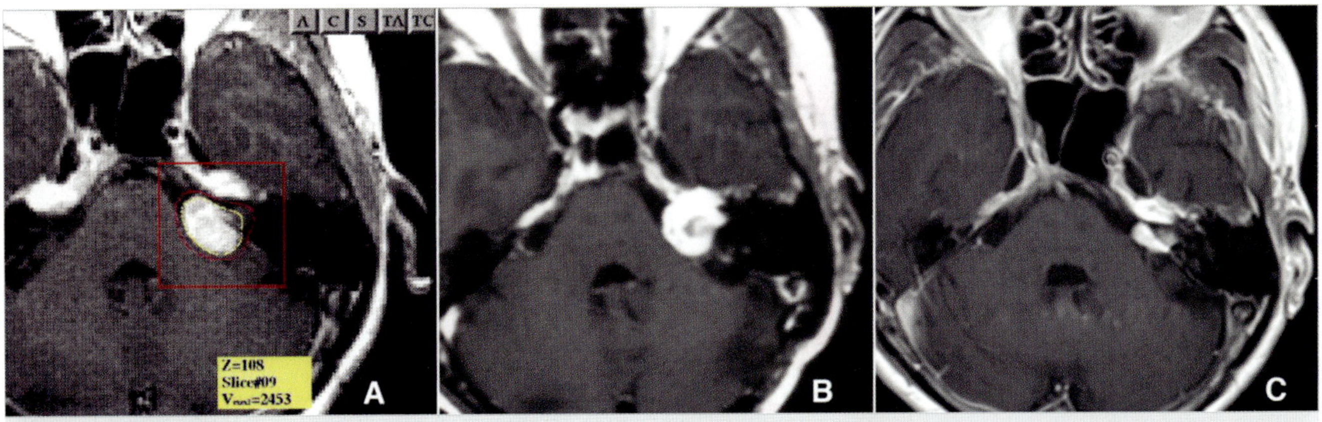

Fig. 6.1 (a) Contrast-enhanced axial magnetic resonance imaging (MRI) of a 59-year-old woman showing the Gamma Knife radiosurgery dose plan for a residual acoustic neuroma. (b) A 5-year follow-up MRI showing the unchanged tumor. (c) Follow-up MRI obtained 19 years after radiosurgery shows a significantly regressed tumor.

hearing ability.[9,17] All patients who were treated with a margin dose ≤ 14 Gy maintained a serviceable level of hearing after intracanalicular tumor radiosurgery.[26] Among patients treated after 1992, the 5-year actuarial rates of hearing level and speech preservation were 75.2% and 89.2%, respectively, for patients ($n = 89$) treated with a 13-Gy tumor margin dose. The 5-year actuarial rates of hearing level and speech preservation were 68.8% and 86.3%, respectively, for patients ($n = 103$) treated with > 14 Gy as the tumor margin dose.[3]

In an SRS study, Kano et al evaluated factors related to hearing preservation in 77 patients with acoustic neuromas.[27] The median tumor volume was 0.75 cm, and the median radiation dose to the tumor margin was 12.5 Gy. At a median of 20 months after SRS, serviceable hearing was preserved in 71% of all patients and in 89% of those with GR class I hearing. Significant prognostic factors for serviceable hearing preservation were Gardner-Robertson (GR) class I hearing, a patient age < 60 years, an intracanalicular tumor location, and a tumor volume < 0.75 cm. Patients who received a radiation dose < 4.2 Gy to the central cochlea had significantly better hearing preservation of the same GR class.

Facial and Trigeminal Nerve Preservation

Facial and trigeminal nerve function can now be preserved in almost all patients. In the early experience at the University of Pittsburgh, normal facial function was preserved in 79% of patients after 5 years, and normal trigeminal nerve function was preserved in 73%. These facial and trigeminal nerve preservation rates reflected the higher tumor margin dose of 18 to 20 Gy used during the computed tomography (CT)–based planning era (before 1991). In a recent study using MRI-based dose planning, a 13-Gy tumor margin dose was associated with 0% risk of new facial weakness and 3.1% risk of facial numbness (5-year actuarial rates). A margin dose > 14 Gy was associated with a 2.5% risk of new-onset facial weakness and a 3.9% risk of facial numbness (5-year actuarial rates).[3] None of the patients who had radiosurgery for intracanalicular tumors developed new facial or trigeminal neuropathies.

Single-Session Radiosurgery for Younger Patients

Despite robust long-term outcome data on radiosurgery, many surgeons continue to offer microsurgery to younger patients. Our experience indicates that Gamma Knife SRS is an effective management strategy for younger patients with vestibular schwannomas. Lobato-Polo et al reviewed long-term outcomes in 55 younger patients with acoustic neuromas.[28] The 5-year rate of freedom from additional management was 96%. Serviceable hearing was maintained in 100%, 93%, and 93% of patients at 3, 5, and 10 years, respectively. Hearing preservation was related to a margin dose < 13 Gy ($p = 0.017$). None of the patients treated with doses < 13 Gy experienced facial or trigeminal neuropathy. All patients continued their previous level of activity or employment after Gamma Knife SRS. No patient developed a secondary radiation-related tumor.

Single-Session Radiosurgery for Larger Tumors

SRS is an important management option for patients with small- and medium-sized vestibular schwannomas. Several investigators have started assessing its potential role for larger tumors as well. In one recent study, Milligan et al evaluated long-term results of Gamma Knife surgery in patients with larger tumors. The median maximum posterior fossa diameter was 2.8 cm (range 2.5–3.8 cm) in this group of 22 patients.[29] The median tumor margin dose was 12 Gy (range 12–14 Gy). The 3-year actuarial rates of tumor control, freedom from new facial neuropathy, and preservation of functional hearing were 86%, 92%, and 47%, respectively. At the most recent follow-up, 91% of tumors were smaller. Yang et al studied 65 patients with larger acoustic neuromas (3–4 cm in diameter, median tumor volume 9 mL) who underwent radiosurgery.[30] At 6 months, 2 patients needed resections; of the remaining patients, 89% had stable or smaller-volume tumors. Eleven percent had slightly enlarged acoustic neuromas (one had repeat SRS). Serviceable hearing was preserved in 82% of patients. For smaller tumors, the long-term outcome data are clear and consistent. The value of radiosurgery in selected patients with large tumors is encouraging but must be individualized after taking into consideration the surgeon's experience and the patient's expectations and desires.

Gamma Knife Radiosurgery Technique for Acoustic Neuromas

Preradiosurgery Evaluation

Patients with vestibular schwannomas are evaluated with high-resolution MRI and audiological tests that include pure tone average (PTA) and speech discrimination score (SDS) measurements. Hearing is graded using the GR classification. "Serviceable" hearing (class I and II) is defined as a PTA or speech reception threshold < 50 dB and SDS score > 50%. The Committee on Hearing and Equilibrium of the American Academy of Otolaryngology–Head and Neck Surgery (AAO-HNS) has established guidelines for reporting vestibular schwannoma results. In this classification, hearing loss at a higher frequency (3,000 Hz) is included in calculating the PTA. Serviceable hearing (class A and B) is similar to GR class I and II. Facial nerve function is assessed according to the House-Brackmann grading system.

Radiosurgery Technique

In Gamma Knife radiosurgery, the procedure begins with rigid fixation of an MRI-compatible Leksell stereotactic frame (model G, Elekta) to the patient's head. High-resolution images are acquired with a fiducial system attached to the stereotactic frame. For acoustic neuroma radiosurgery, a three-dimensional (3D) volume acquisition MRI using a gradient pulse sequence (divided into 1-mm-thick axial slices) is performed. A T2-weighted 3D volume sequence is performed to visualize cranial nerves and delineate inner ear structures (cochlea and semicircular canals). Dose planning is performed on narrow-slice thickness axial MR images with coronal and sagittal reconstructions.

Radiosurgical Dose Planning

Dose planning is a critical aspect of radiosurgery. Complete 3D conformal coverage of the tumor and preservation of facial, cochlear, and trigeminal nerve function are given priority during dose planning. For large tumors, preservation of brainstem function is also a consideration. A conformal radiosurgery plan is necessary for hearing and facial nerve preservation. Highlights of Gamma Knife acoustic neuroma radiosurgery planning include use of multiple isocenters, beam weighting, and use of plug patterns to optimize both conformality (i.e., 3D fit) and selectivity (sharp dose fall-off outside the tumor volume). Precise 3D conformality between treatment and tumor volumes is needed to avoid radiation-related complications.[18] This degree of conformality can be achieved through complex multi-isocenter planning using composite isocenters. Acoustic neuroma dose planning is usually performed using a combination of small beam diameter (4- and 8-mm) collimators. For large tumors, few sectors of 16-mm collimators are also used. A series of 4-mm isocenters are used to create a tapered isodose plan to conform to the intracanalicular portion of the tumor. Sector blocking can be used to create sharp fall-off toward the cochlea. The success of vestibular schwannoma radiosurgery depends on high conformality to the tumor margin. Because the facial and cochlear nerve complex generally courses along the anterior margin and anteroinferior side of the tumor, the dose plan should be highly conformal in this region. Although with current imaging techniques the cochlear nerve cannot be well visualized, efforts should be made to achieve high conformality at the anterior and inferior margins of the tumor. Conformal dose planning using 4-mm collimators for the intracanalicular portion of the tumor may prevent further injury to the cochlear nerve. It is likewise important to minimize radiation of the cochlea.[31]

Dose Prescription

The margin dose to the tumor is determined after considering the goal of radiosurgery in an individual patient and the tolerance of the surrounding structures. Dose prescription for acoustic neuroma has changed significantly over the past 15 years. In Gamma Knife radiosurgery, a dose of 12 to 13 Gy is typically prescribed to the 50% (or other) isodose line that conforms to the tumor margin. A margin dose of 12 to 13 Gy is associated with a low complication rate, yet maintains a high rate of tumor control. After prescribing the margin dose, the fall-off rates on the cochlea, semicircular canal, and brainstem are checked to keep them below the tolerance level.

Dose Delivery

Gamma Knife radiosurgery is performed with a 201-source, cobalt 60 unit (model C or 4C) or a 192-source Leksell Gamma Knife (LGK) Perfexion model. Dose delivery is accomplished in a single session by positioning the head serially for each subsequent isocenter until a fully conformal field encompasses the tumor volume.

Postoperative Care and Evaluations

There is no consensus on the use of corticosteroids on the day of radiosurgery. Some practitioners do not use steroids at all before, during, or after radiosurgery. At our centers, patients receive an intravenous dose of 40 mg of methylprednisolone at the onset or conclusion of the procedure. The stereotactic frame is removed immediately after radiosurgery. Patients are observed for a few hours in the same-day-surgery unit and are usually discharged within 24 hours. After radiosurgery, all patients are followed up with serial gadolinium-enhanced MRI scans, which are generally requested following a schedule such as 6 months, 12 months, and 2, 4, 8, and 16 years. All patients who have some preserved hearing are advised to obtain audiological tests (PTA and SDS) near the time of their MRI follow-ups.

Stereotactic Radiotherapy: Clinical Results

Stereotactic radiotherapy (SRT) or fractionated stereotactic radiotherapy (FSRT) refers to the delivery of a standard fractionation scheme of radiation using relocatable stereotactic guiding devices. To reduce complication rates, some linear accelerator (LINAC)-based radiosurgery centers have shifted to FSRT for vestibular schwannomas.[15,32–38]

Ishihara et al reported a 94% tumor control rate at a median follow-up of 31.9 months in a series of 38 patients who had CyberKnife (Accuray Inc., Sunnyvale, CA) SRT for vestibular schwannoma. One patient developed transient facial paresis (2.6%), and one developed trigeminal nerve neuropathy (2.6%).[15] Fuss et al described 51 patients with vestibular schwannomas who were treated with SRT.[39] Mean follow-up was 42 months, and the actuarial 5-year tumor control rate was 95%. One patient developed transient facial nerve paresis, and two noted new trigeminal dysesthesias. Chung et al, using SRT for 25 patients with useful hearing, reported 57% hearing preservation at 2 years.[40] The mean pre- and post-SRT speech recognition threshold was 20 and 38 dB, respectively. The mean proportion of pre- and post-SRT speech discrimination was 91% and 59%, respectively. Sawamura et al treated 101 patients with vestibular schwannomas using FSRT at a radiation level of 40 to 50 Gy, administered in 20 to 25 fractions over a 5- to 6-week period.[35] The median follow-up period was 45 months, and the actuarial 5-year rate of tumor control was 91.4%. The actuarial 5-year rate of useful hearing preservation (GR class I or II) was 71%. The complications of FSRT included transient facial nerve palsy (4%), trigeminal neuropathy (14%), and balance disturbance (17%). Eleven patients (11%) who had progressive communicating hydrocephalus after FSRT required a shunt.

Sakanaka et al evaluated their 8 years of experience with hypofractionated stereotactic radiotherapy (hypo-FSRT) for acoustic neuromas using two types of treatment schedules.[41] Thirteen patients received a margin dose of 30 to 39 Gy using 10 to 13 fractions (regimen A), whereas 12 patients received 20 to 24 Gy in 5 or 6 fractions (regimen B). These treatments were scheduled to be delivered in three fractions per week. Local control rates achieved in 100% with regimen A and in 92% with regimen B. Serviceable hearing was preserved in 57% (4 of 5 patients in regimen B but no patients in regimen A). Kapoor et al studied 385 patients to assess long-term tumor control after FSRT for unilateral acoustic neuromas.[42] In 11 patients (3%) required salvage (microsurgical) treatment. Radiologic progression was observed in 116 patients (30.0%), including 35 patients (9%) in whom the treatment volume more than doubled during the follow-up period, although none required surgical resection. Treatment-induced neurologic morbidity included 8 patients (1.6%) with new facial weakness, 12 patients (2.8%) with new trigeminal paresthesias, 4 patients (0.9%) with hydrocephalus (1 communicating and 3 obstructive), and 2 patients (0.5%) with possibly radiation-induced neoplasia. Hearing preservation was not assessed.

Hansasuta et al examined tumor control and complication rates after multisession SRS in a study of 383 patients, the majority of whom (90%) were treated with 18 Gy in three sessions with a median tumor volume of 1.1 cm^3.[43] The 5-year tumor control rate was 98% for tumors < 3.4 cm^3. The crude rate of serviceable hearing was preserved in 76%. Eight patients (2%) developed trigeminal dysfunction, half of which was transient. Powell et al evaluated 72 patients with acoustic neuromas treated with FSRT (45–50 Gy in 25 to 30 fractions over 5 to 6 weeks) and reported an 11% rate of hydrocephalus within 19 months of radiotherapy.[44]

In a recent study, Andrews et al evaluated hearing preservation in 89 patients treated with SRT.[45] The high-dose cohort (HDC) had 43 patients (treated to 50.4 Gy), and the low-dose cohort (LDC) had 46 patients (treated to 46.8 Gy). The median audiometric follow-up in HDC and LDC was 13 months and 16 months, respectively. The authors concluded that the actuarial hearing preservation rate was significantly longer for the LDC than for the HDC. However, their Kaplan-Meier plots showed that all patients who had preradiosurgery GR grade II hearing and were treated with HDC lost hearing within 7 months of SRT. Eventually, all patients in the LDC group lost serviceable hearing by the end of 42 months.

Comparison of LINAC Single-Session Radiosurgery with Stereotactic Radiotherapy

Meijer et al performed a single-institution trial to study whether FSRT is superior to single-session LINAC-based radiosurgery with respect to treatment-related toxicity and local control in patients with vestibular schwannomas.[46] These authors analyzed 129 patients with vestibular schwannomas who were treated at a LINAC-based radiosurgery facility. SRT was performed on 80 patients with a relocatable guidance device using either 5 × 4 or 5 × 5 Gy at the 80% isodose. Forty-nine patients had SRS using 10 or 12.5 Gy at the 80% isodose using a stereotactic frame. There was no statistically significant difference between the single-fraction group and the fractionated group with respect to mean tumor diameter (2.6 vs 2.5 cm) or mean follow-up time (both 33 months). Outcome differences between the single-session group and the fractionated treatment group with respect to 5-year local control probability (100% vs 94%), 5-year facial nerve preservation probability (93% vs 97%), and 5-year hearing preservation probability (75% vs 61%) were not statistically significant.

Collen et al evaluated and compared outcomes for patients with acoustic neuromas treated with LINAC-based SRS or FSRT.[47] Of 119 patients, 78 received SRS, 41 patients, with 42 VSs, received SRT. A median single dose of 12.5 Gy (range 11–14 Gy) was prescribed to the 80% isodose line encompassing the target. Of the 42 tumors in the FSRT group, 32 had 10 fractions of 3 to 4 Gy, and 10 patients received 25 sessions of 2 Gy, prescribed to the 100%, with the 95% isodose line encompassing the planning target volume. Mean largest tumor diameter was 16.6 mm in the SRS and 24.6 mm in the FSRT group. Median follow-up was 62 months; 5 patients progressed, resulting in an overall 5-year local tumor control of 95%. The overall 5-year facial nerve preservation probability was 88%, and facial nerve neuropathy was statistically significantly higher after SRS, after prior surgery, for larger tumors, and in Koos grade ≥ 3. The overall 5-year trigeminal nerve preservation probability was 96%. The overall 4-year probability of preservation of useful hearing (GR score 1 or 2) was 68%, not significantly different between SRS and FSRT. Combs et al evaluated the outcomes of 200 patients with vestibular schwannomas treated with FSRT and compared them to patients treated with SRS.[48] For patients receiving FSRT, a median total dose of 57.6 Gy was prescribed, with a median fractionation of 5 × 1.8 Gy per week. For patients who underwent SRS, a median single dose of 13 Gy was prescribed to the 80% isodose. Local control was not statistically different for both groups. The probability of maintaining the pretreatment hearing level after SRS with doses ≤ 13 Gy was comparable to that for FSRT. In the group of patients treated with SRS (doses ≤ 13 Gy), cranial nerve toxicity was comparable to that of the FSRT group. Kopp et al studied 115 consecutive cases of acoustic neuromas treated with SRS or FSRT.[49] The FSRT group (47 patients), including those with larger tumors, received a total dose of 54 Gy at 1.8 Gy per fraction. The SRS group received a total dose of 12 Gy at the 100% isodose. The tumor control rate was 97.9% in the FSRT group, for a mean follow-up time of 32.1 months, and 98.5% in the SRS group, for a mean follow-up time of 30.1 months. Hearing function was preserved after SRS in 85% of the patients and after FSRT in 79%.

The studies based on FSRT have not shown better outcome in comparison to single-session radiosurgery. However, there is no ***level I evidence*** comparing both modalities. Given the entrenched philosophies as well as logistical challenges and financial costs, there will probably not be a prospective, randomized trial of FSRT versus SRS for patients with acoustic neuromas. The available data on SRT or FSRT is sparse and heterogeneous in terms of dose and number of fractions. The outcome data on single-session radiosurgery are robust and homogeneous. In a recent meta-analysis, Yang et al performed an analytical review of the published literature on Gamma Knife radiosurgery for patients with acoustic neuromas in order to mitigate institutional and practitioner bias.[50] These authors evaluated 45 articles that met the authors' inclusion criteria and represented 4,234 patients. At a median follow-up of 35 months, an overall hearing preservation rate was 51%, irrespective of radiation dose, patient age, or tumor volume. With margin doses ≤ 13-Gy higher hearing preservation rate (60.5%) was noted. Patients with smaller tumors (average tumor volume 1.5 cm^3) had a higher hearing preservation rate (62%), comparable to patients harboring larger tumors (61%) ($p = 0.8968$). This type of objective analysis provides a less biased assessment of a hearing preservation with Gamma Knife radiosurgery for acoustic neuromas. There is no such meta-analysis for patients treated with FSRT. Currently, there are limited data on SRT for vestibular schwannomas. For some centers, SRT may be an option for vestibular schwannomas if they have a higher complication rate using LINAC radiosurgery.

Reasons to Select Single-Session Radiosurgery for Acoustic Neuroma

Reasons to select single-session radiosurgery for acoustic neuroma include the following:

- There are no compelling radiobiological principles supporting the use of SRT over radiosurgery for achieving an optimal therapeutic response for the slowly proliferating, late-responding tissue of a schwannoma.
- Excellent long-term outcome data are available for single-session radiosurgery.
- Single-session radiosurgery is convenient for patients and their families.
- Highly conformal plans are feasible because of rigid, frame-based head fixation.
- FSRT is less accurate and has a lower biological tumor dose.
- Available data do not show any benefit to FSRT in comparison to single-session radiosurgery.
- No consensus exists on dose and fraction regimen for FSRT.
- FSRT appears to be associated with a reduced rate of tumor regression at 4 to 5 years' follow-up.
- Higher rates of hydrocephalus are reported in SRT series (may be due to larger tumors or to regional irradiation).
- No meta-analysis of FSRT is available.

Radiosurgery has become a well-documented management option for patients with acoustic neuromas or vestibular schwannomas. It is an effective option but one that requires very high conformality and selectivity of dose delivery, as with Gamma Knife technology. As a minimally invasive strategy, we now know the expected success rate and risks. Not all radiosurgery technologies are the same. The evolution of radiosurgery has led to enhanced outcomes for patients diagnosed with such tumors. There are currently no randomized, prospective clinical trials comparing single-session radiosurgery with SRT. Obtaining clinical equipoise in such a proposed trial would be impossible. We therefore rely on the analysis of information from the retrospective case series from different centers. Although the dose range, planning technique, and dose delivery in single-session radiosurgery using the Gamma Knife are performed in a homogeneous manner across the world, the literature on FSRT or multisession radiosurgery in the management of acoustic neuromas suffers from a lack of homogeneity in terms of number of fractions, total dose, and dose prefraction, as well as the technique of dose delivery. This makes it difficult to compare outcomes of single-session radiosurgery and FSRT. Before a meaningful and rigorous scientific comparison can be made, a uniform SRT technique and standardized reporting are necessary.

References

[1] Niranjan A, Madhavan R, Gerszten PC, Lunsford LD. Intracranial radiosurgery: an effective and disruptive innovation in neurosurgery. Stereotact Funct Neurosurg 2012; 90: 1–7

[2] Chung WY, Liu KD, Shiau CY, et al. Gamma knife surgery for vestibular schwannoma: 10-year experience of 195 cases. J Neurosurg 2005; 102 Suppl: 87–96

[3] Flickinger JC, Kondziolka D, Niranjan A, Maitz A, Voynov G, Lunsford LD. Acoustic neuroma radiosurgery with marginal tumor doses of 12 to 13 Gy. Int J Radiat Oncol Biol Phys 2004; 60: 225–230

[4] Hasegawa T, Kida Y, Kobayashi T, Yoshimoto M, Mori Y, Yoshida J. Long-term outcomes in patients with vestibular schwannomas treated using gamma knife surgery: 10-year follow up. J Neurosurg 2005; 102: 10–16

[5] Kondziolka D, Lunsford LD, Flickinger JC. Acoustic neuroma radiosurgery: origins, contemporary use and future expectations. Neurochirurgie 2004; 50: 427–435

[6] Kondziolka D, Nathoo N, Flickinger JC, Niranjan A, Maitz AH, Lunsford LD. Long-term results after radiosurgery for benign intracranial tumors. Neurosurgery 2003; 53: 815–821, discussion 821–822

[7] Lunsford LD, Niranjan A, Flickinger JC, Maitz A, Kondziolka D. Radiosurgery of vestibular schwannomas: summary of experience in 829 cases. J Neurosurg 2005; 102 (Suppl): 195–199

[8] Delbrouck C, Hassid S, Massager N, et al. Preservation of hearing in vestibular schwannomas treated by radiosurgery using Leksell Gamma Knife: preliminary report of a prospective Belgian clinical study. Acta Otorhinolaryngol Belg 2003; 57: 197–204

[9] Flickinger JC, Kondziolka D, Niranjan A, Lunsford LD. Results of acoustic neuroma radiosurgery: an analysis of 5 years' experience using current methods. J Neurosurg 2001; 94: 1–6

[10] Flickinger JC, Kondziolka D, Pollock BE, Lunsford LD. Evolution in technique for vestibular schwannoma radiosurgery and effect on outcome. Int J Radiat Oncol Biol Phys 1996; 36: 275–280

[11] Foote KD, Friedman WA, Buatti JM, Meeks SL, Bova FJ, Kubilis PS. Analysis of risk factors associated with radiosurgery for vestibular schwannoma. J Neurosurg 2001; 95: 440–449

[12] Harsh GR, Thornton AF, Chapman PH, Bussiere MR, Rabinov JD, Loeffler JS. Proton beam stereotactic radiosurgery of vestibular schwannomas. Int J Radiat Oncol Biol Phys 2002; 54: 35–44

[13] Horstmann GA, Van Eck AT. Gamma Knife model C with the automatic positioning system and its impact on the treatment of vestibular schwannomas. J Neurosurg 2002; 97 Suppl: 450–455

[14] Inoue HK. Low-dose radiosurgery for large vestibular schwannomas: long-term results of functional preservation. J Neurosurg 2005; 102 Suppl: 111–113

[15] Ishihara H, Saito K, Nishizaki T, et al. CyberKnife radiosurgery for vestibular schwannoma. Minim Invasive Neurosurg 2004; 47: 290–293

[16] Kondziolka D, Lunsford LD, Flickinger JC. Gamma Knife radiosurgery for vestibular schwannomas. Neurosurg Clin N Am 2000; 11: 651–658

[17] Kondziolka D, Lunsford LD, McLaughlin MR, Flickinger JC. Long-term outcomes after radiosurgery for acoustic neuromas. N Engl J Med 1998; 339: 1426–1433

[18] Linskey ME. Stereotactic radiosurgery versus stereotactic radiotherapy for patients with vestibular schwannoma: a Leksell Gamma Knife Society 2000 debate. J Neurosurg 2000; 93 (Suppl 3): 90–95

[19] Linskey ME, Johnstone PA. Radiation tolerance of normal temporal bone structures: implications for Gamma Knife stereotactic radiosurgery. Int J Radiat Oncol Biol Phys 2003; 57: 196–200

[20] Linskey ME, Lunsford LD, Flickinger JC. Tumor control after stereotactic radiosurgery in neurofibromatosis patients with bilateral acoustic tumors. Neurosurgery 1992; 31: 829–838, discussion 838–839

[21] Lunsford LD. Vestibular schwannomas. Neurochirurgie 2004; 50: 151–152

[22] Norén G. Long-term complications following Gamma Knife radiosurgery of vestibular schwannomas. Stereotact Funct Neurosurg 1998; 70 (Suppl 1): 65–73

[23] Meijer OW, Wolbers JG, Vandertop WP, Slotman BJ. Stereotaxic irradiation of vestibular schwannoma (acoustic neuroma). Ned Tijdschr Geneeskd 2000; 144: 2088–2093

[24] Petit JH, Hudes RS, Chen TT, Eisenberg HM, Simard JM, Chin LS. Reduced-dose radiosurgery for vestibular schwannomas. Neurosurgery 2001; 49: 1299–1306, discussion 1306–1307

[25] Litvack ZN, Norén G, Chougule PB, Zheng Z. Preservation of functional hearing after Gamma Knife surgery for vestibular schwannoma. Neurosurg Focus 2003; 14: e3

[26] Niranjan A, Lunsford LD, Flickinger JC, Maitz A, Kondziolka D. Dose reduction improves hearing preservation rates after intracanalicular acoustic tumor radiosurgery. Neurosurgery 1999; 45: 753–762, discussion -762–765

[27] Kano H, Kondziolka D, Khan A, Flickinger JC, Lunsford LD. Predictors of hearing preservation after stereotactic radiosurgery for acoustic neuroma. J Neurosurg 2009; 111: 863–873

[28] Lobato-Polo J, Kondziolka D, Zorro O, Kano H, Flickinger JC, Lunsford LD. Gamma knife radiosurgery in younger patients with vestibular schwannomas. Neurosurgery 2009; 65: 294–300, discussion 300–301

[29] Milligan BD, Pollock BE, Foote RL, Link MJ. Long-term tumor control and cranial nerve outcomes following Gamma Knife surgery for larger-volume vestibular schwannomas. J Neurosurg 2012; 116: 598–604

[30] Yang HC, Kano H, Awan NR, et al. Gamma Knife radiosurgery for larger-volume vestibular schwannomas: clinical article. J Neurosurg 2011; 114: 801–807

[31] Wackym PA, Runge-Samuelson CL, Nash JJ, et al. Gamma Knife surgery of vestibular schwannomas: volumetric dosimetry correlations to hearing loss suggest stria vascularis devascularization as the mechanism of early hearing loss. Otol Neurotol 2010; 31: 1480–1487

[32] Szumacher E, Schwartz ML, Tsao M, et al. Fractionated stereotactic radiotherapy for the treatment of vestibular schwannomas: combined experience of the Toronto-Sunnybrook Regional Cancer Centre and the Princess Margaret Hospital. Int J Radiat Oncol Biol Phys 2002; 53: 987–991

[33] Suh JH, Barnett GH, Sohn JW, Kupelian PA, Cohen BH. Results of linear accelerator-based stereotactic radiosurgery for recurrent and newly diagnosed acoustic neuromas. Int J Cancer 2000; 90: 145–151

[34] Shirato H, Sakamoto T, Takeichi N, et al. Fractionated stereotactic radiotherapy for vestibular schwannoma (VS): comparison between cystic-type and solid-type VS. Int J Radiat Oncol Biol Phys 2000; 48: 1395–1401

[35] Sawamura Y, Shirato H, Sakamoto T, et al. Management of vestibular schwannoma by fractionated stereotactic radiotherapy and associated cerebrospinal fluid malabsorption. J Neurosurg 2003; 99: 685–692

[36] Sakamoto T, Shirato H, Takeichi N, Aoyama H, Fukuda S, Miyasaka K. Annual rate of hearing loss falls after fractionated stereotactic irradiation for vestibular schwannoma. Radiother Oncol 2001; 60: 45–48

[37] Poen JC, Golby AJ, Forster KM, et al. Fractionated stereotactic radiosurgery and preservation of hearing in patients with vestibular schwannoma: a preliminary report. Neurosurgery 1999; 45: 1299–1305, discussion 1305–1307

[38] Meijer OW, Wolbers JG, Baayen JC, Slotman BJ. Fractionated stereotactic radiation therapy and single high-dose radiosurgery for acoustic neuroma: early results of a prospective clinical study. Int J Radiat Oncol Biol Phys 2000; 46: 45–49

[39] Fuss M, Debus J, Lohr F, et al. Conventionally fractionated stereotactic radiotherapy (FSRT) for acoustic neuromas. Int J Radiat Oncol Biol Phys 2000; 48: 1381–1387

[40] Chung HT, Ma R, Toyota B, Clark B, Robar J, McKenzie M. Audiologic and treatment outcomes after linear accelerator-based stereotactic irradiation for acoustic neuroma. Int J Radiat Oncol Biol Phys 2004; 59: 1116–1121

[41] Sakanaka K, Mizowaki T, Arakawa Y, et al. Hypofractionated stereotactic radiotherapy for acoustic neuromas: safety and effectiveness over 8 years of experience. Int J Clin Oncol 2011; 16: 27–32

[42] Kapoor S, Batra S, Carson K, et al. Long-term outcomes of vestibular schwannomas treated with fractionated stereotactic radiotherapy: an institutional experience. Int J Radiat Oncol Biol Phys 2011; 81: 647–653

[43] Hansasuta A, Choi CY, Gibbs IC, et al. Multisession stereotactic radiosurgery for vestibular schwannomas: single-institution experience with 383 cases. Neurosurgery 2011; 69: 1200–1209

[44] Powell C, Micallef C, Gonsalves A, Wharram B, Ashley S, Brada M. Fractionated stereotactic radiotherapy in the treatment of vestibular schwannoma (acoustic neuroma): predicting the risk of hydrocephalus. Int J Radiat Oncol Biol Phys 2011; 80: 1143–1150

[45] Andrews DW, Werner-Wasik M, Den RB, et al. Toward dose optimization for fractionated stereotactic radiotherapy for acoustic neuromas: comparison of two dose cohorts. Int J Radiat Oncol Biol Phys 2009; 74: 419–426

[46] Meijer OW, Vandertop WP, Baayen JC, Slotman BJ. Single-fraction vs. fractionated linac-based stereotactic radiosurgery for vestibular schwannoma: a single-institution study [see comment] Int J Radiat Oncol Biol Phys 2003; 56: 1390–1396

[47] Collen C, Ampe B, Gevaert T, et al. Single fraction versus fractionated linac-based stereotactic radiotherapy for vestibular schwannoma: a single-institution experience. Int J Radiat Oncol Biol Phys 2011; 81: e503–e509

[48] Combs SE, Welzel T, Schulz-Ertner D, Huber PE, Debus J. Differences in clinical results after LINAC-based single-dose radiosurgery versus fractionated stereotactic radiotherapy for patients with vestibular schwannomas. Int J Radiat Oncol Biol Phys 2010; 76: 193–200

[49] Kopp C, Fauser C, Müller A, et al. Stereotactic fractionated radiotherapy and LINAC radiosurgery in the treatment of vestibular schwannoma-report about both stereotactic methods from a single institution. Int J Radiat Oncol Biol Phys 2011; 80: 1485–1491

[50] Yang I, Sughrue ME, Han SJ, et al. A comprehensive analysis of hearing preservation after radiosurgery for vestibular schwannoma. J Neurosurg 2010; 112: 851–859

7 Fractionated Stereotactic Radiotherapy for Acoustic Neuromas

Christopher J. Farrell and David W. Andrews

Introduction

Since 1969, when Lars Leksell treated the first patient with an acoustic neuroma with stereotactic radiosurgery (SRS), the relative merits of surgery and radiation therapy for these benign, slow-growing tumors have been contentiously debated.[1] With the apparent incidence of acoustic neuromas on the rise and patients increasingly diagnosed earlier in their clinical course, the need for high-quality data to guide both patients and clinicians through the treatment decision-making process has become paramount.[2,3] Unfortunately, the early literature describing radiation therapy for acoustic neuromas was limited by its retrospective nature with short-term follow-up periods and incomplete or inconsistent data collection. In 2002 Nikolopoulos and O'Donoghue used evidence-based methods to evaluate the existing scientific literature and determined that no significant evidence favored one treatment modality over the other.[4] Since that time, however, several prospective cohort studies have been published demonstrating improved or equivalent treatment outcomes, including cranial nerve morbidity and quality of life (QOL) assessment using radiation therapy for the treatment of acoustic neuromas compared with microsurgical resection.[5–7] These findings, along with the emergence of reports consistently documenting effective long-term tumor control following radiation therapy, have led to a prevailing role for radiation therapy in the management of small- and medium-sized tumors. From the patients' perspective, this migration away from surgery to radiosurgery is evident in the 2007–2008 patient survey conducted by the Acoustic Neuroma Association (ANA; http://anausa.org/index.php/patient-surveys). ▶ Table 7.1 illustrates the treatment choices made by respondents in each of the three surveys conducted by the ANA to date. ANA members have shifted from surgical patients seeking interventions for chronic postoperative morbidities to newly diagnosed patients seeking treatment options.

Table 7.1 Results of the ANA surveys over 3 decades

Treatment reported by respondents	2007–2008	1998	1983
Translabyrinthine approach	33%	51%	72%
Retrosigmoid approach	17%	28%	11%
Middle fossa approach	10%	6%	3%
Don't know approach	0%	0%	14%
Total, microsurgical resection	60%	85%	100%
Stereotactic radiosurgery (SRS)	12%	NA	NA
Fractionated stereotactic radiotherapy (FSRT)	8%	NA	NA
Total SRS/FSRT	20%	5%	0%
Watch and wait	20%	4%	0%
Don't know what type of treatment	NA	6%	0%
Total	100%	100%	100%

Abbreviations: ANA, Acoustic Neuroma Association; NA, not available

In this chapter, we examine the benefits of fractionated stereotactic radiotherapy (FSRT) over other radiation therapy strategies that have emerged for the treatment of acoustic neuromas.

Natural History

Despite the significant advances made in the treatment of acoustic neuromas, a period of observation remains a reasonable option for many patients. Several meta-analyses have been performed demonstrating that only 43 to 54% of tumors will grow over an observational period of ~ 3 years and that a small percentage (4–6%) of tumors will regress in size without intervention.[8,9] numerous studies have attempted to better predict the natural history of untreated acoustic neuromas, growth pattern remains incompletely understood, and no resolute clinical or radiographic indicators of tumor growth or symptom progression have been identified. Haioff et al identified extracanalicular tumors as more likely to grow and fail conservative management, and other studies have suggested that younger age and growth within the first year of radiographic surveillance may be predictive of subsequent progression.[10–12]Unfortunately, these studies and others have consistently shown that hearing may irrevocably deteriorate even in the absence of radiographic tumor growth, contributing to the fear that a conservative "wait and scan" approach may lead to missed opportunities for hearing preservation.[12,13] In a review of 34 published studies containing hearing outcome data for patients who underwent observation management for small- and medium-sized acoustic neuromas, Sughrue et al found that tumors exhibiting a growth rate > 2.5 mm/year were significantly (75% vs 32%) less likely to retain serviceable hearing compared to those with slower growing tumors.[14] In a large series of patients from Denmark managed conservatively, Stangerup et al identified initial speech discrimination score as predictive of long-term hearing retention. Among patients with a speech discrimination score of 100% at the time of tumor diagnosis, 69% maintained good hearing after more than 10 years of observation compared to only 38% of patients with a slight discrimination loss at the time of initial diagnosis.[15] The results of any radiation or surgical intervention aimed at hearing preservation must be carefully balanced against the anticipated rate of hearing maintenance during a period of observation based on the individual clinical, radiographic, and audiometric data. We and others[16] have found that early detection of any sensorineural hearing loss (SNHL) associated with acoustic neuroma warrants early intervention with the highest likelihood of improved hearing outcomes.

Stereotactic Radiosurgery

Since the initial report from the Karolinska Institute describing the use of SRS for the treatment of acoustic neuromas, a steady increase in the utilization of radiation therapy as either primary therapy or for residual disease following microsurgical resection has been observed, with the results of modern radiosurgical series consistently demonstrating its efficacy and safety.[1,7,17–22] Stereotactic techniques currently employed include SRS and FSRT, with SRS most commonly delivered using either a Gamma Knife (Elekta AB, Stockholm, Sweden) or linear accelerator (LINAC). Early experience with SRS delivered prescription doses ranging from 16 to 20 Gy and achieved excellent rates of local tumor control (89–100%). However, the observed rate of facial and trigeminal neuropathy was 29 to 67% and 33 to 59%, respectively, with multivariate analysis revealing that tumor size and prescription dose correlated with the development of cranial neuropathy.[23–25] In 1996 Flickinger et al reviewed the University of Pittsburgh experience and found that following introduction of magnetic resonance imaging (MRI)–based treatment planning and reduction of the prescription dose to 14 Gy, facial and trigeminal nerve morbidity was significantly decreased without any change in the tumor control rate.[26]

Currently, most institutions perform SRS using a marginal dose of 12 to 14 Gy. Although the published literature for SRS using this reduced prescription dose has been fairly consistent in terms of treatment outcomes, the available data are beset by inadequate follow-up periods, varied treatment protocols, and nonuniform criteria for assessing tumor control and morbidity, making comparative analyses between the available treatment modalities for acoustic neuromas difficult.[27,28] To facilitate more reliable comparisons across institutions, the Consensus Meeting on Systems for Reporting Results in Acoustic Neuroma was convened in 2003.[29] Although these guidelines have led to improved reporting of tumor size, facial nerve function, hearing preservation, and other treatment-related complications, the inconsistent reporting of important dosimetry variables, including target volume, prescription dose, prescription isodose line, and fractionation scheme, continues to limit the data interpretation.[30]

Tumor Control

One of the major inconsistencies in the radiosurgical literature is the definition of tumor control, which has been variably assessed as an increase in tumor diameter > 1 to 2 mm, progressive enlargement on serial imaging, and the need for further surgical or radiation salvage treatment.[31] Bassim et al found that in more than one third of the cases in the radiosurgical literature, no definition of tumor control was specified.[28] This is an important consideration, given that transient tumor expansion has been observed in up to 24 to 54% of patients following SRS with radiographic enlargement typically noted between 6 and 30 months after treatment.[31–33] Chopra et al reported their experience in treating 216 patients with a median marginal tumor dose of 13 Gy.[17] They observed a 10-year actuarial control rate of 98.3% when defined as the need for subsequent surgical resection. Using an alternative definition of tumor control based on any radiographic enlargement, their control rate diminished to 90%. Despite the inconsistencies in data reporting, the overall results for SRS treatment of acoustic neuromas are excellent. Multiple large SRS series with at least 5-year median follow-up periods have yielded local tumor control rates of 89 to 100% using prescription doses of 12 to 14 Gy. Attempts at further SRS dose reduction, however, have met with unacceptable levels of tumor recurrence.[34] Despite differences in dose conformality and homogeneity, the results of LINAC-based SRS are highly comparable to those of Gamma Knife in terms of both tumor control and associated morbidity.[21,35–39]

Facial Nerve Preservation and Trigeminal Neuropathy

Preservation of facial nerve function represents a principal consideration for patients undergoing acoustic neuroma treatment and a major source of contention in the debate between radiation therapy and microsurgical resection. Facial nerve outcomes are typically reported using the House-Brackmann (HB) classification. Yang et al performed a meta-analysis assessing facial nerve outcomes after Gamma Knife SRS and found an overall facial nerve preservation rate of 96.2%.[40] Patients receiving ≤ 13 Gy of radiation at the marginal dose had significantly better facial nerve outcomes than those receiving a higher dose. Additional factors associated with improved outcome were tumor volume ≤ 1.5 cm^3 and age ≤ 60 years. Similarly, Friedman et al observed a direct correlation between tumor volume and facial nerve outcome with the risk of facial weakness increasing by 17% with each cubic centimeter increase in tumor volume.[41] In a prospective cohort analysis of patients with unilateral acoustic neuromas < 3 cm comparing microsurgical resection and SRS, Pollock et al reported improved rates of normal facial function in the SRS group at 3 months (100% vs 61%), at 1 year (100% vs 69%), and at last follow-up (100% vs 75%), providing ***level II evidence*** in favor of radiosurgery for small- to medium-sized tumors with regard to facial nerve preservation.[7]

Similar to facial nerve injury, the incidence of trigeminal neuropathy, characterized by facial paresthesias, or pain, is clearly dose dependent. As mentioned previously, initial experience with SRS for acoustic neuromas using prescription doses up to 20 Gy reported rates of trigeminal neuropathy as high as 59%.[24] With dose reduction, the rate has been reduced to 2.3% overall and 1.6% when doses < 13 Gy are administered.[24,42]

Hearing Preservation

In a prospective study assessing QOL measures in patients undergoing observational, surgical, and radiation therapy for acoustic neuromas, nearly one third of patients cited hearing as the single most important factor affecting their QOL.[6] With the widespread availability of MRI, patients are increasingly being diagnosed with acoustic neuromas and preserved functional hearing, defined as Gardner-Robertson (GR) classification I or II[43] or American Association of Otolaryngology–Head and Neck Surgery (AAO-HNS) class A or B. As discussed in the Natural History section of this chapter, hearing loss may be unpredictable during the course of an observational period. In a meta-analysis performed by Smouha et al, 51% of patients with functional hearing at the time of diagnosis lost hearing over an average observational period of ~ 3 years.[8] Similar to the natural history of hearing loss with these tumors, hearing loss associated with SRS treatment has also shown great variability, with the overall results remaining inconclusive in terms of their superiority relative to conservative management. In a systematic analysis of the literature, Yang et al reported a hearing preservation rate following SRS of 57% with an average follow-up period of 41.2 months.[44] The only significant variable found to correlate positively with hearing preservation was marginal treatment dose ≤ 12.5 Gy. Hearing loss may occur as early as 3 months following SRS with the potential to decline many years after treatment.[37,45] Chopra et al reported that after 3 years of follow-up, the hearing preservation rate was 74%, but it had declined to 44% at 10 years.[17,25] Similarly, Roos et al reported 5- and 10-year hearing preservation rates of 57% and 24%, respectively.[37]

Radiation therapy is believed to induce SNHL via injury to the cochlea, cochlear nerve, or brainstem auditory nuclei, and many recent studies have focused on identifying patient-related and dosimetry variables that may allow for improved preservation of functional hearing. Several studies have demonstrated that patients with GR class I were more likely to retain functional hearing compared to GR class II patients, suggesting that interventions aimed at hearing preservation should be considered as early as possible, particularly for younger patients.[46–48] In our practice, we have incorporated the findings from Denmark demonstrating excellent long-term natural hearing preservation rates for patients with 100% speech discrimination scores and recommend treatment for this subset of patients only at the time of hearing decline based on serial audiogram assessment.[15] Several studies have also suggested that radiation dose to the cochlea may be a critical determinant of preserved hearing function. Kano et al reported the results of 77 patients treated with a marginal dose of 12.5 Gy and found that after controlling for GR class, patients who received a central cochlear dose < 4.2 Gy were more likely to retain serviceable hearing.[48] Additional studies have confirmed the influence of cochlear dose on hearing preservation. Unfortunately, it is not always possible to limit the cochlear dose to a safe level while still prescribing an effective dose necessary to achieve tumor control.[49–53]

Quality of Life

With the excellent long-term tumor control achieved with SRS for small- and medium-sized tumors and the significant reduction in cranial neuropathy associated with current dosing regimens, a shift in focus toward QOL measures is necessary to better guide treatment recommendations. In particular, the effect of SRS on dizziness, balance, and tinnitus remains to be fully elucidated. Using static stabilometry and caloric testing, Fukuoka et al demonstrated that 90% of patients with acoustic neuromas have evidence of vestibular dysfunction at the time of diagnosis.[54] Several retrospective studies have suggested that surgical intervention with sectioning of the vestibular nerve may be associated with improved vestibular outcomes. However, the prospective study of Pollack et al comparing SRS to microsurgical resection failed to confirm this conventional perception.[7,55,56] In addition to greater imbalance, the surgical resection group reported worsened outcomes at 1 year in terms of other QOL measures, including physical functioning and bodily pain. Conversely, the prospective cohort analysis performed by Di Maio and Akagami revealed no QOL differences in observation, radiation treatment, and surgical resection, including assessments of dizziness and tinnitus.[6] Both of these prospective studies were limited by short-term follow-up periods, but they demonstrate the need for more detailed attention to these important QOL measures.

Fractionated Stereotactic Radiotherapy

As summarized above, SRS represents the pioneering intervention that broadened the treatment alternatives for patients with acoustic neuromas. Originally practiced with the Gamma Knife, radiosurgery techniques were soon adapted to retrofitted LINAC systems[57] and subsequently to LINACs designed for and dedicated to radiosurgery.[58] It was this development that enabled the design of fractionated stereotactic techniques with noninvasive relocatable frames and marked the beginning of modern stereotactic techniques, as described below. The following sections discuss the radiobiological rationale and advantages of FSRT, as well as published outcomes as they relate to acoustic tumors.

Radiobiological Principles of Fractionation for Selected Late-Responding Tissues

We previously reviewed the advantages of FSRT and derived a hearing radiation effect therapy (RET) formula to guide dose-fractionation strategies,[59] as discussed below. SRS has made the treatment of skull base tumors far more precise with modern imaging and versatile three-dimensional (3D) treatment planning software that, through dose volume histograms maximizes dose to target with high conformality and minimizes dose to contiguous normal structures. Two exceptions are optic nerve sheath meningiomas and acoustic neuromas, where these cranial nerves are intrinsic to the target volume. With special sensory cranial nerves, injury to sensory function occurs much more frequently than either sensory or motor function in mixed cranial nerves, reflecting a lower threshold for injury. To make matters even more complicated when considering acoustic neuromas, recent literature has focused on the cochlea itself, which may have a different radiobiological tolerance.[48] We will advance arguments based on published data that tumors involving or near special sensory cranial nerves should be treated with FSRT using daily low conventional fraction sizes.

Optic Nerve Sheath Meningiomas

Single doses of 15 or 54 Gy in 30 daily fractions result in excellent control of meningiomas.[60] The SRS dose of 15 Gy, however, exceeds the generally accepted single-dose tolerance of the optic nerves (8–10 Gy) and may be associated with a risk of optic neuropathy approaching 78%.[61] For fractionated radiotherapy, decades of experience have led to guidelines for normal tissue tolerance. For the optic nerve and chiasm, guidelines have evolved that have proven to be extremely safe and are generally based on the optic RET dose recommended by Goldsmith et al,[62] later corroborated by a large retrospective analysis by Parsons et al.[63] We adopted the observations set forth by Parsons and colleagues and dropped the daily dose to the optic nerve to 1.8 Gy and the total dose to 54 Gy—both below the threshold for injury established by the optic RET formula and corroborated by Parsons et al. Our results yielded excellent tumor control and a compelling preservation of or improvement in vision in these patients.[64] These were the first data supporting FSRT as a means of controlling a benign tumor while simultaneously preserving or restoring the function of a special sensory cranial nerve.

The Biologically Effective Dose for Acoustic Neuromas

We noted that reports of hearing preservation are not uniform, ranging from subjective hearing outcomes to standard audiometric outcomes scales. The most widely cited scale is the Gardner-Robertson;[43] despite this scale, there still exist disparities in reported outcomes due to differences, for example, in the derivation of pure tone average. We reviewed published literature and selected only those studies that featured audiometric outcomes using the GR scale as confirmed by audiometric data.[59] Other scales or outcomes based on subjective hearing results were excluded. The most informative reports included the actual audiometric data, but most reports did not. As we noted, radiosurgery doses that reflected excellent tumor control rates also showed that Gamma Knife dose deescalations over time improved rates of cranial neuropathy. Other than our recent publication,[47] literature does not reflect dose iterations for FSRT. From past literature, high rates of tumor control have been achieved for both a single dose of 12 to 13 Gy and 45 to 50 Gy in1.8- to 2-Gy daily fractions, suggesting a dose equivalence for treatment of acoustic neuromas. Unlike the optic apparatus, however, acceptably low rates of hearing loss have not yet been generally agreed upon. In our single institution experience of dose deescalation for FSRT, we have found the lower dose cohort of 46.8 Gy achieves an excellent tumor control rate while improving hearing preservation.[47] It remains unclear, however, if further dose reductions improve hearing deficits even more while maintaining high rates of tumor control.

To guide and optimize future treatments, we need to understand the radiobiological rationale for fractionation for acoustic neuromas. We must first acknowledge that the target is a late-responding tissue radiographically inseparable from a special sensory cranial nerve that could be compromised by radiation treatment. Fractionation allows time between fractions for normal tissues (i.e., the cochlear nerve) to repair sublethal damage (tumor tissue is less efficient at repair due to faulty repair mechanisms). This leads to the separation of tumor and normal tissue cell survival curves, thereby minimizing normal tissue toxicity while maximizing tumor cell kill. This is depicted in ▶ Fig. 7.1.

The radiobiology of high-dose single fraction involves more than sublethal damage, and the major effects have been documented to involve both lethal DNA damage and endothelial damage. Though favorable for tumor cell kill, these dual effects may have adverse effects on the normal neurophil and vasculature of the cochlear nerve.

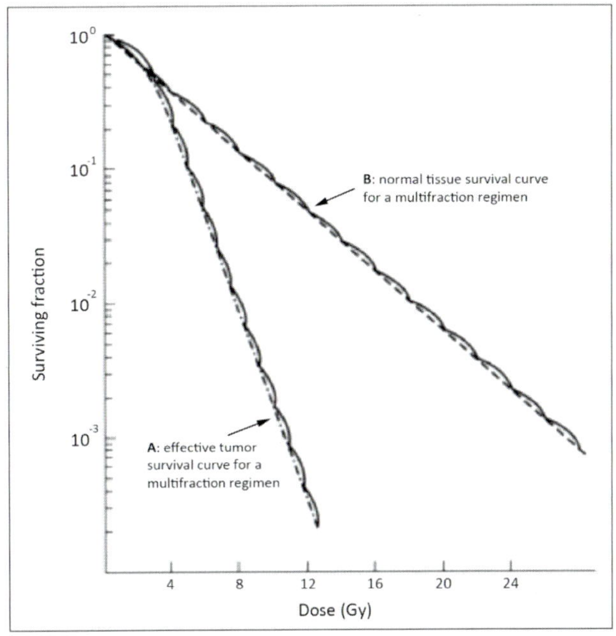

Fig. 7.1 Graph illustrating the effects of fractionation on the survival of tumor (line A) and normal (line B) cells. Because normal cells have intact repair mechanisms, whereas tumor cells do not, fractionation effectively separates the survival curves for tumor cells and normal cells, thereby sparing normal cells while killing tumor cells. (With permission from Balagamwala EH, Chao ST, Suh JH (2012) Principles of radiobiology of stereotactic radiosurgery and clinical applications in the central nervous system. Technology in cancer research & treatment 11:3-13)

To better understand an optimal dose regimen for the treatment of acoustic neuromas, it is important to review the concept of a biologically effective dose (BED), which is useful for quantifying treatment expectations[65] and is an inherent part of the linear quadratic formula for radiation effect. For a review of the derivation and significance of α/β ratios and the linear quadratic equation, the reader is referred to an excellent review by Balagamwala et al.[66] The radiation cell kill (or effect E) can be expressed as

$$\text{Cell kill } E = n\left(\alpha d + \beta d^2\right) \quad (1)$$

Where α and β are the radiosensitivity coefficients, n is the number of fractions, and d is the dose per fraction such that the total dose $(D) = nd$.

Historically, radiosurgical dose reductions for acoustic tumors have been performed empirically to improve hearing outcomes. Consistent with this exercise, consider a progressive reduction in d approaching but not reaching zero. Although the number of fractions n will then need to be increased to maintain the same effect, βd^2 will be very small in comparison to αd, and when d is very small, the above equation can be simplified to

$$E = n\alpha d = \alpha D \quad (2)$$

This demonstrates that the total dose D of radiotherapy given at a very low dose per fraction represents the highest total dose required to obtain a specific effect, in this case simultaneously high rates of tumor control and hearing preservation. This total dose represents the BED in situations where neoplastic cellular repopulation can be ignored, which is the case for acoustic neuromas. Equation 2 can be redefined as

$$BED = D = E/\alpha \tag{3}$$

With this assumption, BED for any practical radiotherapy application can be derived by first dividing both sides of equation 1 by α such that

$$BED = \frac{E}{\alpha} = \frac{n(\alpha\, d + \beta d^2)}{\alpha} = nd\left[1 + \frac{d}{\alpha/\beta}\right] \tag{4}$$

It is perhaps difficult to understand that one BED can be obtained by different dose/fractionation schedules. Drawing from an analogy by Jones et al,[65] the height of a mountain could be viewed as a BED. BED represents the absolute height using the longest route (i.e., the lowest dose) to the summit, but it is possible to climb to the summit by a steeper and hence shorter route. Carrying the analogy forward, the steeper route represents a shorter distance, or in biological terms, the use of larger fractions results in a shorter time course with a smaller total dose.

Currently, disparate focused radiation dose-fractionation schedules are practiced worldwide for acoustic tumors, including single-fraction SRS, FSRT, and hypofractionated FSRT or fractionated SRS. Doses of 12 Gy in a single fraction, 46.8 Gy in 1.8-Gy daily fractions, or 18 Gy in three fractions all achieve excellent tumor control rates with serviceable hearing preservation rates that vary roughly from 60 to 80%. One might argue that these dose-fractionation schedules are not biologically equivalent because of variable outcomes in hearing preservation, but for purposes of this model, we will assume they are. We can correspondingly assign values of BED1, BED2, and BED3, respectively, to these dose-fraction schemes.

Assuming BED1 = BED2 for tissue of an unknown α/β, or in terms of total dose D and fraction dose d,

$$D1\left[1 + \frac{d1}{\left(\frac{\alpha}{\beta}\right)}\right] = D2\left[1 + \frac{d2}{\left(\frac{\alpha}{\beta}\right)}\right], \text{ or} \tag{5}$$

$$\frac{\alpha}{\beta} = \frac{D1 \times d1 - D2 \times d2}{D2 - D1}$$

For acoustic neuromas using the assumption of equivalent BED for 12 Gy in a single fraction ($d1$ = 12 Gy) and 46.8 Gy in 26 fractions ($d2$ = 1.8 Gy),

$$\frac{\alpha}{\beta} = \frac{(12 \times 12) - (46.8 \times 1.8)}{46.8 - 12} = 1.72 \tag{6}$$

and the corresponding BED based on this α/β ratio is calculated as

$$BED = 12\left(1 + \frac{12}{1.72}\right) = 46.8\left(1 + \frac{1.8}{1.72}\right) = 95.7Gy_{1.72} \tag{7}$$

Having derived an isoeffective BED for acoustic tumors, we can now test an alternate dose fractionation schedule by substituting actual values from equation 4 above for BED3, an actual dose fractionation schedule recently reported,[67] to see if our derived α/β ratio actually yields the same dose per fraction solving for d as the unknown:

$$3d\left[1 + \frac{d}{1.72}\right] = 95.7Gy_{1.72} \tag{8}$$

which is rearranged as

$$3d + 1.74d^2 - 95.7 = 0 \tag{9}$$

For a general quadratic equation such as $ad^2 + bd + c = 0$, the positive solution for d is given as

$$d = \frac{-b + \sqrt{a^2 - 4ac}}{2a} \tag{10}$$

where $a = 1.74$, $b = 3$, and $c = 95.7$. The solution for d above is 6.6 Gy, which is within a 10% error of 6 Gy. As a working model, therefore, an α/β ratio of 1.72 yielding an isoeffective BED of 95.7 $Gy_{1.72}$ is a reasonable derivation from current literature regarding focused radiation for acoustic neuromas.

Although an α/β ratio of 1.72 is low and consistent with late-responding normal central nervous system tissues,[68] this model has potential pitfalls, including an oversimplification of single Gamma Knife radiosurgery, which necessarily involves multiple isocenter hot spots, and a two-target model (DNA damage and endothelial cell apoptosis), especially at high doses per fraction. In the former case, a single one-point calculation will not be representative of the biological effect throughout a larger acoustic tumor with multiple hot spots, and multiple BED evaluations would be necessary.[65] In the latter case, a modification of the linear quadratic equation, such as a generalized linear quadratic[69] or universal survival curve,[70] might be more appropriate. As a starting point, we felt this model would be useful for dose-fractionation schedules designed for treating acoustic tumors. Its utility as a predictive model of serviceable hearing loss, however, remains unclear due to the significant variations in hearing outcomes mentioned above.

Derivation of a Hearing RET Formula for Acoustic Neuromas

We felt that a more systematic approach to serviceable hearing preservation would be the derivation and application of a hearing RET formula.[59] A prospective trial by Pan et al[71]documented that for almost all cases in which significant hearing loss occurred in the affected ear receiving radiation, the dose was ≥ 45 Gy. Among published data available, we were able to plot the log of dose versus the log of the number of fractions drawing from Goldsmith's model[3] for reports with hearing preservation rates of at least 70% based on GR criteria. The linear regression gave us a formula for dose/fraction size regimens with a high correlation coefficient (R^2 = 0.9705). Drawing from

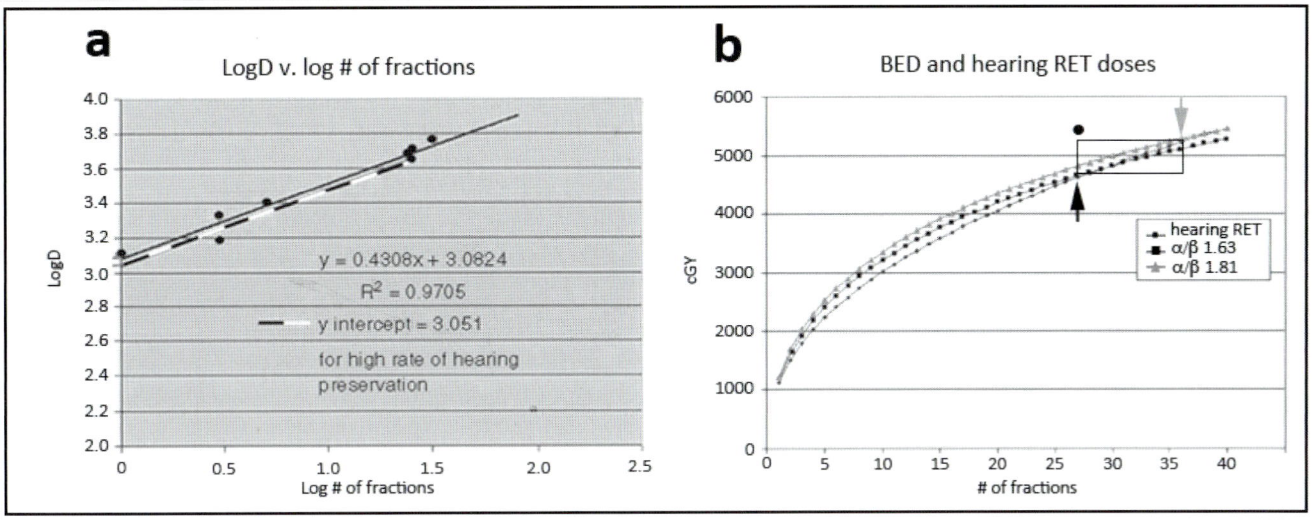

Fig. 7.2 (a) Logarithmic plot of total dose versus number of fractions for cases reporting preservation of serviceable hearing. (b) Plots of biologically equivalent doses (BEDs) using the linear quadratic formula with α/β ratios as ± 10% of the calculated α/β value, with comparison to the hearing resolution enhancement technology (RET) plot. The dose prescription schemes predicting the highest yield of hearing preservation fall within the box at or below the hearing RET curve, depending on which α/β ratio is used. The *black arrow* represents the point beyond which dose-fractionation schemes predict a higher likelihood of hearing preservation for a lower α/β ratio; the *gray arrow*, a higher α/β ratio. The *black point* represents a recent study[72] that documented a high rate of hearing loss and falls above the hearing RET range.

Goldsmith's optic RET derivation, we postulated that dose-fractionation schemes with very high hearing preservation rates could be represented by a parallel line on the same plot, intersecting at a point corresponding to the dose-fractionation scheme documented as safe. Data from Pan et al[71] suggest that 45 Gy in 25 × 1.8 Gy fractions (or less) is such a point. By adding this value in the linear regression equation,

$$\text{intercept} = \log(4500) - 0.4308 \times \log(25) \text{ with an intercept at } 3.051 \quad (11)$$

So the line equation is

$$\log D = 0.431 \times \log N + 3.051 \quad (12)$$

where *N* is the number of fractions. This can be folded into Equation 13

$$D = 1120 \times N^{0.43} \quad (13)$$

or 1,120 hearing $\text{RET} = D \times N^{0.43}$ for dose-fractionation schemes with high hearing preservation rates.

For one fraction, $D = 11.2$ Gy. This implies that the radiosurgical dose should not exceed a threshold ~ 11.2 Gy to obtain high rates of hearing preservation. Based on this hearing RET formula, single-fraction doses > 11.2 Gy or a cumulative FSRT dose > 45 Gy in a 25-fraction regimen could result in higher rates of hearing loss. For SRS, any dose < 13 Gy results in loss of tumor control,[39] so even with an ~ 60% hearing preservation rate, 13 Gy may represent the most optimal dose achievable with SRS. Based on our earlier literature review, a median value of 13 Gy has, in fact, resulted in reported serviceable hearing losses ranging from 17 to 67%.[59] A median FSRT dose of 47.5 Gy, while maintaining excellent tumor control, has resulted in reported serviceable hearing losses ranging from 29 to 43%.[59] As noted in ▶ Fig. 7.2, the dose prescription schemes with the highest yield of hearing preservation fall within the box that includes the 10% variance of the α/β ratio we derived. The single point represents a recently published paper that describes a high probability of hearing loss with a dose-fractionation scheme for acoustic neuromas described as a total dose of 54 Gy in 27 fractions.[72] Applying an α/β ratio of 1.63 for tumor control and the hearing RET formula as a guide for hearing preservation, the total dose should not exceed 46.2 Gy for 27 fractions to maximize the chance of hearing preservation while maintaining excellent tumor control.

Further Radiobiological Advantages: Large Tumors

With the progressive shift in treatment patterns toward use of radiation therapies for acoustic neuromas, some authors have suggested that relative indications for microsurgical resection include the presence of medically refractory trigeminal neuralgia; hydrocephalus; symptomatic mass effect, including disabling ataxia or hemiparesis; intractable headache; and large tumor size. Although the definition of large tumor size remains somewhat arbitrary, maximal tumor diameter > 3 cm has conventionally been used as a cutoff for SRS treatment based on studies demonstrating rates of effective tumor control as low as 57% and increased risk of complication compared to SRS treatment of small- and medium-sized tumors.[73] Milligan et al described their experience using SRS for tumors with volumes more than one standard deviation above the mean during a

9-year period and demonstrated a 5-year actuarial tumor control rate of 83%.[74] Impairment of facial nerve function was observed in 14% of patients, and 15% required prolonged corticosteroid administration for symptomatic radiation-induced brainstem or cerebellum edema. Based on their results, the authors recommended consideration of surgical resection for tumors > 2.7 cm in the posterior fossa. A group from the Netherlands recently reported primary SRS treatment of 33 patients with large tumors defined as tumor volume > 6 cm^3 with indentation of the brainstem (Koos grades III and IV). Patients with neurofibromatosis 2 (NF2), symptomatic mass effect, or maximum extracanalicular dimension ≥ 4 cm were excluded from primary SRS treatment. A radiographic tumor control rate of 88% was reported over a median follow-up time of 30 months, although 7 of 33 patients required further microsurgical or SRS treatment for development of either progressive neurologic symptoms or radiographic enlargement. Transient facial and trigeminal neuropathy occurred in 9% and 14% of patients, respectively, with good facial nerve function (HB grades I and II) preserved in all patients at 1 year posttreatment. Interestingly, of the 12 patients included in the study who reported pretreatment symptoms of trigeminal hypesthesia, 11 (92%) experienced resolution of their condition following SRS likely related to the 67% incidence of tumor volume shrinkage observed on radiographic follow-up.

FSRT has been recommended as an alternative radiation modality for the treatment of larger tumors adjacent to the brainstem, although few data exist to suggest improved outcome relative to SRS for this population of tumors. Mandl et al reported a cohort of patients with tumors > 3 cm in diameter treated primarily with multisession SRS using a maximum dose of 25 Gy delivered in 5-Gy fractions.[75] The actuarial 5-year tumor control and facial nerve function rates were 82% and 80%, respectively. We have updated our review of FSRT treatment for acoustic neuromas, and of 154 tumors treated in the 46.8-Gy cohort, 15 were > 6 cm^3 in size. In this subgroup, we have documented no treatment failures, and of six patients with serviceable hearing, three have maintained hearing in a serviceable range at a median follow-up of 35 months. At conventional fraction sizes, we have also noted no other cranial neuropathies in this subgroup of patients. See ▶ Fig. 7.3 as an example.

The theoretical advantage of fractionation for large tumors is depicted in ▶ Fig. 7.4. For larger treatment volumes, the penumbra affecting contiguous normal tissues is often judged to be prohibitive for single-fraction SRS. In a review of 149 patients with posterior fossa tumors treated with SRS, factors that

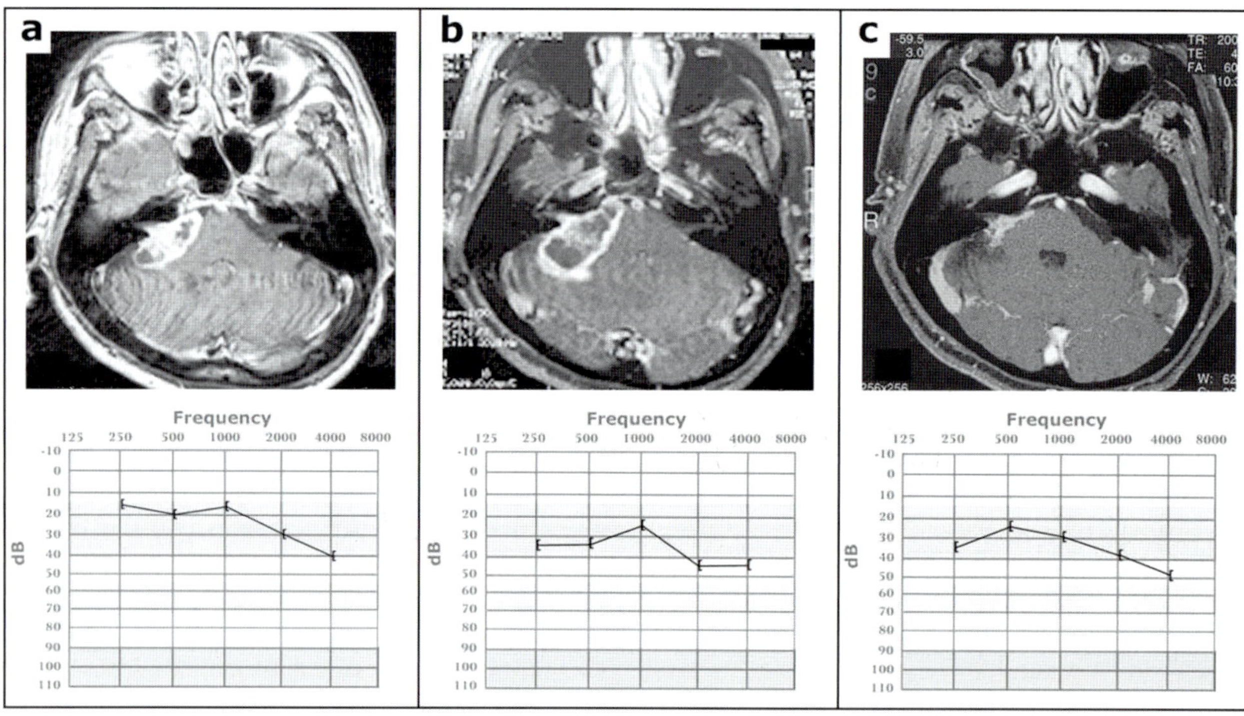

Fig. 7.3 Serial magnetic resonance imaging scans with associated audiograms obtained at the same time in a patient treated with fractionated stereotactic radiotherapy to 46.8 Gy. **(a)** Pretreatment T1-weighted gadolinium-enhanced axial image featuring a right acoustic neuroma. Audiogram reflects pure tone average (PTA) of 22 and speech discrimination score (SDS) of 95%, representing Gardner-Robertson (GR) level I pretreatment serviceable hearing. **(b)** Posttreatment T1-weighted gadolinium-enhanced axial image at 6 months featuring some enlargement and extensive central necrosis of the tumor. Audiogram at 6 months after treatment reflects some audiometric decay with PTA of 35 and SDS of 100%, representing a decrease to GR level II serviceable hearing. **(c)** Posttreatment T1-weighted gadolinium-enhanced axial image at 42 months featuring marked diminution in tumor size. Audiogram at 42 months after treatment reflects stable audiogram with PTA of 30 and SDS of 92%, back to the lowest range of GR level I serviceable hearing. (With permission from Andrews DW, Werner-Wasik M, Den RB, et al. Toward dose optimization for fractionated stereotactic radiotherapy for acoustic neuromas: comparison of two dose cohorts. Int J Radiat Oncol Biol Phys 2009;74(2):419–426.)

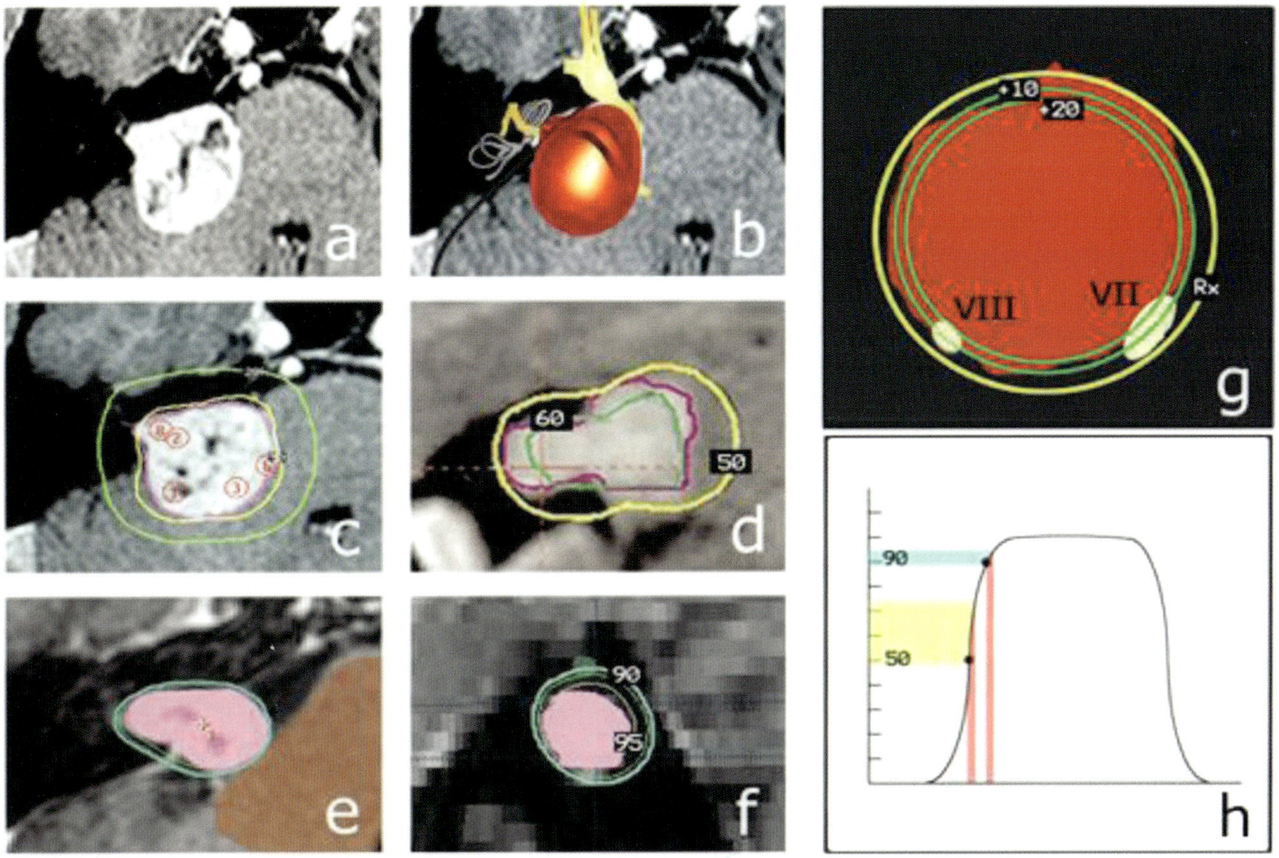

Fig. 7.4 Comparison of dose distribution to the cochlear nerve with Gamma Knife and fractionated stereotactic radiotherapy (FSRT) treatments. (a) Axial T1 gadolinium-enhanced magnetic resonance imaging (MRI) scan of a right acoustic neuroma. (b) Artist's rendering of a translucent acoustic tumor with cranial nerves (CN) VII and VIII adherent to the anterior and caudal surface of the tumor, coursing to the internal auditory canal. (c) Eight-shot Gamma Knife radiosurgery treatment plan with a 12-Gy prescription to the 50% isodose line (*yellow*) for a right acoustic neuroma. (d) Magnified sagittal view of an actual treatment plan in the distal porus acusticus [outer line (*yellow*) is 50% isodose prescription line; middle line (*magenta*) is tumor surface; inner line (*green*) is 60% isodose line]. Assuming the cochlear nerve is around the 7 o'clock position, the nerve is within a 10% dose gradient above the isodose prescription. (e) Single-shot Novalis FSRT treatment plan with a 1.8-Gy prescription to the 90% isodose line for a right acoustic neuroma (tumor is shaded; outer line is 90% isodose prescription line). (f) Magnified sagittal view of an actual treatment plan in the distal porus acusticus (tumor is shaded; outer line is 90% isodose prescription line; inner line is 95% isodose line). Assuming the cochlear nerve is around the 7 o'clock position, the nerve is within a 5% dose gradient above the isodose prescription. (g) Artist's rendering of panel d (magnified sagittal cross section of the intracanalicular portion of a tumor treated with the Gamma Knife). CN VIII at the 7 o'clock position is within the prescribed isodose line and exposed to higher dose gradients. (h) Profile of a focused radiation beam with typical isodose prescriptions at 50% (Gamma Knife) and 90% (FSRT). Vertical columns in either scenario could represent the narrow location range of the cochlear nerve relative to the tumor (e.g., within 1 mm of the tumor surface). The broad inferior horizontal bar represents the potential actual dose range delivered to the cochlear nerve with 50% isodose prescription; the narrow superior horizontal bar represents the potential actual dose range delivered to the cochlear nerve with 90% isodose prescription. The potential dose gradient at a 50% isodose prescription is more than 3 times greater than the 90% prescription at the same distance.

predicted cranial nerve palsy included maximum dose of ≥ 17.5 Gy, a prescribed isosurface dose ≥ 12.5 Gy, length of cranial nerve > 16 mm, and tumor volume of 1.7 cm^3.[76]

More specifically, dose inhomogeneity within that penumbra is less favorable than a fractionation technique that delivers a homogeneous dose of radiation with high conformality within the hearing RET formula. Homogeneity promises to minimize injury to the cochlear nerve, and high conformality promises to minimize injury to the cochlea, a structure too small for reliable dose-volume histograms. Our analysis, limited to the cochlear nerve, is based on an actual comparison of a multishot/high-conformality Gamma Knife SRS treatment to a single-isocenter dynamic arc FSRT treatment on a Novalis Classic (Brainlab AG, Munich, Germany). The dose distribution penumbra is a depiction of a circular collimator instead of a dynamic arc penumbra to allow a uniform comparison of dose prescription conventions with both techniques. Particularly for larger acoustic tumors, both the dose prescription convention and the design of multiple isocenters to achieve conformality increase the likelihood of overdosing the cochlear nerve. The comparison is different for the cochlea. We have since learned that the dose fall-off outside the prescription to tumor volume (PTV) isosurface prescription is important when considering the cochlear dose, and an 80 to 85% isosurface prescription for LINAC can achieve the best dose distribution for both the cochlea and the cochlear nerve.

History and Progress in Clinical Outcomes Using Fractionated Stereotactic Radiotherapy

In 1987 Wallner et al described the use of FSRT for the treatment of acoustic neuromas following subtotal resection. They demonstrated that when doses ≥ 45 Gy were administered, the tumor recurrence rate could be significantly decreased. Several years later, a group from France described their experience using FSRT as primary therapy for acoustic neuromas, including a small subset of patients with NF2 and preexisting unilateral deafness secondary to previous surgical resection of a contralateral tumor. At an average follow-up of 70 months, hearing was preserved in three of the five patients with no evidence of tumor progression. Based on these encouraging early results, a number of groups posited that combining the radiobiological advantages of dose fractionation with the precision of stereotactic techniques may enable effective treatment of acoustic neuromas with reduced cranial neuropathy and improved hearing preservation.

Studies reporting outcomes using FSRT have consistently demonstrated excellent tumor control rates comparable to those achieved with SRS and low risk of cranial nerve morbidity. The optimal dose-fractionation scheme for FSRT remains uncertain, with the widespread variation in treatment practices at different institutions precluding definitive comparisons of FSRT and SRS. Several recent studies have described outcomes using FSRT with maximum doses ranging from 46.8 to 57.6 Gy, typically administered in conventional 1.8- to 2.0-Gy fractions. Overall, functional hearing preservation was observed in 61 to 94% of patients over an average follow-up time of ~ 50 months.[77–84] In 2001 our group at Thomas Jefferson University performed a nonrandomized prospective cohort analysis comparing outcomes after SRS and FSRT using a maximum dose of 50.4 Gy for 122 patients. Tumor control, facial nerve preservation, and trigeminal neuropathy rates were equivalent among the two cohorts; however, hearing preservation rates were 2.5 times higher in the FSRT group, with a crude hearing preservation rate of 81% compared to 33% in the SRS cohort.[77] Limitations of this prospective study included short-term length of audiometry data and an SRS hearing preservation rate toward the low range of reported outcomes. Subsequently, Combs et al reported their single-institution prospective experience comparing SRS to FSRT using a marginal dose of 57.6 Gy. Their study revealed no overall difference in terms of hearing preservation between the two modalities when the SRS prescription dose was ≤ 13 Gy.[85] The FSRT group in this study, however, represented only 10 patients.

As in the early stages of SRS, the optimal FSRT prescription dose necessary to achieve long-term tumor control while minimizing damage to normal structures, such as the cochlea and cochlear nerve, remains to be established. We previously demonstrated that FSRT dose reduction from 50.4 to 46.8 Gy enabled improved hearing outcomes without sacrificing tumor control. These results are consistent with data using FSRT for nasopharyngeal cancer, revealing that hearing loss is significantly increased when the mean cochlear dose is > 48 Gy.[47,86] Conversely, in the same patient population, hearing is preserved for a mean cochlear dose < 45 Gy.[71] Importantly, hearing impairment after FSRT appears to have a delayed time to onset relative to SRS, and longer-term data will be necessary to fully evaluate this treatment modality.[45]

Several groups have reported their experience using a multisession SRS scheme in an effort to balance the advantages of fractionation with the convenience of SRS. Hansasuta et al described the extensive experience of the Stanford group delivering 18 Gy over three treatment sessions using the CyberKnife (Accuray Inc., Sunnyvale, CA).[67] During a median follow-up period of 3 years, they found a 98% tumor control rate and accompanying 76% hearing preservation rate. Meijer et al, however, reported the results of a prospective cohort study comparing single versus multisession LINAC-based SRS and observed no differences in either tumor control or hearing preservation rates between the two cohorts, which were 75% and 61%, respectively, for serviceable hearing.[84] A slight but statistically significant reduction in trigeminal neuropathy incidence was noted with multisession SRS.

As mentioned above, we have modeled the radiobiology of fractionation for acoustic neuromas, including a hearing RET formula, as a guideline for treatment. Summarizing the above literature, there remains no systematic application of radiobiological principles to the treatment of acoustic neuromas. In fact, none of the FSRT or SRS studies we previously analyzed provided uniform treatment planning data such as maximum dose to prescribed dose (MDPD) ratios or PTV ratios as measures, respectively, of dose homogeneity and dose conformality. For circular collimation, a uniform reporting mechanism should include mean number of isocenters stratified by tumor sizes, and these data might build a relationship between such variables as tumor size, serviceable hearing loss, and mean number of isodose centers as a measure of conformality. Newer techniques, such as mini-multileaf collimation with dynamic arc or intensity modulation (Novalis TrueBeam, Brainlab) and nonisocentric smearing with pencil beams (CyberKnife),[87]promise to maintain conformality and increase dose homogeneity and should also include MDPD and PTV values.

Despite a broad variety of dose-fractionation schedules without a clear rationale, recent systematic literature review by Arthurs et al favors FSRT when assessing hearing preservation[83] (▶ Table 7.1). These data are remarkably similar to those we previously compiled from published series.[59]

Drawing from the patients' perspective, we once again refer to the ANA's 2007–2008 patient survey, recognizing that all data collected were self-reported by patients and reported as is. ▶ Table 7.2 indicates the self-reported GR class 1 and 2 results of respondents who underwent either SRS or FSRT. If this survey is any indication, FSRT provides a more favorable outcome when assessing serviceable hearing preservation.

■ Future Directions

Future treatment possibilities for acoustic neuromas remain both challenging and hopeful. The challenge will remain the

Table 7.1 Summary of treatment outcomes for SRS and FSRT, 2004–2009

Treatment	N	Tumor volume (cc)	Dose (Gy)	Follow-(months)	Tumor control rate (%)	Hearing preservation rate (%)
SRS	1,850	2.3	12.6	71	89	60
FSR	404	4.1	52.4	53	95.8	79

With permission from Arthurs BJ, Fairbanks RK, Demakas JJ, et al. A review of treatment modalities for vestibular schwannoma. Neurosurg Rev 2011;34 (3):265–277

Table 7.2 Summary of serviceable hearing outcomes from the 2007–2008 ANA survey

Treatment	Hearing status (*N*) before treatment	Hearing status (*N*) after treatment	Rate of serviceable hearing preservation
SRS	108	22	20%
FSR	84	41	49%

design of appropriate prospective trials that guide practitioners with useful ***level 1*** data. Although radiosurgery and FSRT have become common, physicians seem wedded to the commercial platform they use, which makes prospective, randomized comparisons of different treatment techniques on different platforms extremely difficult. Also, further refinements in our understanding of the radiobiological tolerances of the cochlea and the cochlear nerve, including the hearing RET formula, will be important new information critical to the design of new radiation treatment strategies. Uniform analyses of reliable audiometric data immediately before and at routine intervals after treatment will yield better outcome data. Associating pure tone averages with cochlear doses and speech discrimination scores with cochlear nerve doses may provide further insight into the radiobiology of these structures and guide future treatment plans. Although there remains solid evidence to support the use of FSRT for patients with acoustic neuromas, the evidence remains at ***level III*** There are no randomized or nonrandomized prospective studies (i.e., ***level I evidence***) that permit rigorous comparison of radiotherapeutic modalities in terms of the ideal hearing preservation therapy.[88]

The optimal treatment outcome will include the excellent tumor control rates already achieved with better hearing preservation and possibly recovery of hearing. The latter achievement may include a combination of targeted chemotherapy and radiation. In one recent application of chemotherapy, vascular endothelial growth factor (VEGF) blockade with bevacizumab improved hearing in some, but not all, patients with NF2 and was associated with a reduction in the volume of most growing acoustic neuromas.[89] The impact bevacizumab may have on sporadic tumors remains unknown. The molecular mechanisms at play in sporadic tumors, as reviewed by Neff et al, notably merlin's interactions with other proteins and regulation of the NF2 gene,[90]could spawn new targeted molecular therapies that may complement existing focused radiation strategies or supersede them altogether.

Acknowledgments

We thank our colleagues from the Department of Radiation Oncology, Drs. Wenyin Shi and Haisong Liu, for their helpful comments during the preparation of this chapter.

References

[1] Leksell L. A note on the treatment of acoustic tumours. Acta Chir Scand 1971; 137: 763–765

[2] Stangerup SE, Tos M, Caye-Thomasen P, Tos T, Klokker M, Thomsen J. Increasing annual incidence of vestibular schwannoma and age at diagnosis. J Laryngol Otol 2004; 118: 622–627

[3] Propp JM, McCarthy BJ, Davis FG, Preston-Martin S. Descriptive epidemiology of vestibular schwannomas. Neuro-oncol 2006; 8: 1–11

[4] Nikolopoulos TP, O'Donoghue GM. Acoustic neuroma management: an evidence-based medicine approach. Otol Neurotol 2002; 23: 534–541

[5] Myrseth E, Moller P, Pedersen PH, Lund-Johansen M. Vestibular schwannoma: surgery or gamma knife radiosurgery? A prospective, nonrandomized study. Neurosurgery 2009; 64: 654–661, discussion 661–663

[6] Di Maio S, Akagami R. Prospective comparison of quality of life before and after observation, radiation, or surgery for vestibular schwannomas. J Neurosurg 2009; 111: 855–862

[7] Pollock BE, Driscoll CL, Foote RL, et al. Patient outcomes after vestibular schwannoma management: a prospective comparison of microsurgical resection and stereotactic radiosurgery. Neurosurgery 2006; 59: 77–85, discussion 77–85

[8] Smouha EE, Yoo M, Mohr K, Davis RP. Conservative management of acoustic neuroma: a meta-analysis and proposed treatment algorithm. Laryngoscope 2005; 115: 450–454

[9] Selesnick SH, Johnson G. Radiologic surveillance of acoustic neuromas. Am J Otol 1998; 19: 846–849

[10] Hajioff D, Raut VV, Walsh RM, et al. Conservative management of vestibular schwannomas: third review of a 10-year prospective study. Clin Otolaryngol 2008; 33: 255–259

[11] Matthies C, Samii M. Management of 1000 vestibular schwannomas (acoustic neuromas): clinical presentation. Neurosurgery 1997; 40: 1–9, discussion 9–10

[12] Flint D, Fagan P, Panarese A. Conservative management of sporadic unilateral acoustic neuromas. J Laryngol Otol 2005; 119: 424–428

[13] Bakkouri WE, Kania RE, Guichard JP, Lot G, Herman P, Huy PT. Conservative management of 386 cases of unilateral vestibular schwannoma: tumor growth and consequences for treatment. J Neurosurg 2009; 110: 662–669

[14] Sughrue ME, Yang I, Aranda D, et al. The natural history of untreated sporadic vestibular schwannomas: a comprehensive review of hearing outcomes. J Neurosurg 2010; 112: 163–167

[15] Stangerup SE, Thomsen J, Tos M, Cayé-Thomasen P. Long-term hearing preservation in vestibular schwannoma. Otol Neurotol 2010; 31: 271–275

[16] Roos DE, Potter AE, Zacest AC. Hearing preservation after low dose linac radiosurgery for acoustic neuroma depends on initial hearing and time. Radiother Oncol 2011; 101: 420–424

[17] Chopra R, Kondziolka D, Niranjan A, Lunsford LD, Flickinger JC. Long-term follow-up of acoustic schwannoma radiosurgery with marginal tumor doses of 12 to 13 Gy. Int J Radiat Oncol Biol Phys 2007; 68: 845–851

[18] Chen DA. Acoustic neuroma in a private neurotology practice: trends in demographics and practice patterns. Laryngoscope 2007; 117: 2003–2012

[19] Flickinger JC, Kondziolka D, Niranjan A, Maitz A, Voynov G, Lunsford LD. Acoustic neuroma radiosurgery with marginal tumor doses of 12 to 13 Gy. Int J Radiat Oncol Biol Phys 2004; 60: 225–230

[20] Kalogeridi MA, Georgolopoulou P, Kouloulias V, Kouvaris J, Pissakas G. Long-term results of LINAC-based stereotactic radiosurgery for acoustic neuroma: the Greek experience. J Cancer Res Ther 2009; 5: 8–13

[21] Hasegawa T, Fujitani S, Katsumata S, Kida Y, Yoshimoto M, Koike J. Stereotactic radiosurgery for vestibular schwannomas: analysis of 317 patients followed more than 5 years. Neurosurgery 2005; 57: 257–265, discussion 257–265

[22] Murphy ES, Barnett GH, Vogelbaum MA, et al. Long-term outcomes of Gamma Knife radiosurgery in patients with vestibular schwannomas. J Neurosurg 2011; 114: 432–440

[23] Flickinger JC, Lunsford LD, Linskey ME, Duma CM, Kondziolka D. Gamma Knife radiosurgery for acoustic tumors: multivariate analysis of four year results. Radiother Oncol 1993; 27: 91–98

[24] Foote RL, Coffey RJ, Swanson JW, et al. Stereotactic radiosurgery using the Gamma Knife for acoustic neuromas. Int J Radiat Oncol Biol Phys 1995; 32: 1153–1160

[25] Murphy ES, Suh JH. Radiotherapy for vestibular schwannomas: a critical review. Int J Radiat Oncol Biol Phys 2011; 79: 985–997

[26] Flickinger JC, Kondziolka D, Lunsford LD. Dose and diameter relationships for facial, trigeminal, and acoustic neuropathies following acoustic neuroma radiosurgery. Radiother Oncol 1996; 41: 215–219

[27] Conley GS, Hirsch BE. Stereotactic radiation treatment of vestibular schwannoma: indications, limitations, and outcomes. Curr Opin Otolaryngol Head Neck Surg 2010; 18: 351–356

[28] Bassim MK, Berliner KI, Fisher LM, Brackmann DE, Friedman RA. Radiation therapy for the treatment of vestibular schwannoma: a critical evaluation of the state of the literature. Otol Neurotol 2010; 31: 567–573

[29] Kanzaki J, Tos M, Sanna M, Moffat DA, Monsell EM, Berliner KI. New and modified reporting systems from the consensus meeting on systems for reporting results in vestibular schwannoma. Otol Neurotol 2003; 24: 642–648, discussion 648–649

[30] Han SJ, Oh MC, Sughrue ME, Rutkowski MJ, Aranda D, Barani IJ, Parsa AT. The effect of the 2003 Consensus Reporting Standards on publications describing patients with vestibular schwannoma treated with stereotactic radiosurgery. J Clin Neurosci; 19: 1144–1147

[31] Hayhurst C, Zadeh G. Tumor pseudoprogression following radiosurgery for vestibular schwannoma. Neuro-oncol 2012; 14: 87–92

[32] Kim KM, Park CK, Chung HT, Paek SH, Jung HW, Kim DG. Long-term outcomes of Gamma Knife stereotactic radiosurgery of vestibular Schwannomas. J Korean Neurosurg Soc 2007; 42: 286–292

[33] Farrell CJ, Plotkin SR. Genetic causes of brain tumors: neurofibromatosis, tuberous sclerosis, von Hippel-Lindau, and other syndromes. Neurol Clin 2007; 25: 925–946, viii

[34] Mendenhall WM, Friedman WA, Buatti JM, Bova FJ. Preliminary results of linear accelerator radiosurgery for acoustic schwannomas. J Neurosurg 1996; 85: 1013–1019

[35] Andrews DW, Bednarz G, Evans JJ, Downes B. A review of 3 current radiosurgery systems. Surg Neurol 2006; 66: 559–564

[36] Likhterov I, Allbright RM, Selesnick SH. LINAC radiosurgery and radiotherapy treatment of acoustic neuromas. Otolaryngol Clin North Am 2007; 40: 541–570, ixix

[37] Roos DE, Potter AE, Brophy BP. Stereotactic radiosurgery for acoustic neuromas: what happens long term? Int J Radiat Oncol Biol Phys 2012; 82: 1352–1355

[38] Hsu PW, Chang CN, Lee ST, et al. Outcomes of 75 patients over 12 years treated for acoustic neuromas with linear accelerator-based radiosurgery. J Clin Neurosci 2010; 17: 556–560

[39] Pollock BE, Link MJ, Foote RL. Failure rate of contemporary low-dose radiosurgical technique for vestibular schwannoma. J Neurosurg 2009; 111: 840–844

[40] Yang I, Sughrue ME, Han SJ, et al. Facial nerve preservation after vestibular schwannoma Gamma Knife radiosurgery. J Neurooncol 2009; 93: 41–48

[41] Friedman WA, Bradshaw P, Myers A, Bova FJ. Linear accelerator radiosurgery for vestibular schwannomas. J Neurosurg 2006; 105: 657–661

[42] Sughrue ME, Yang I, Han SJ, et al. Non-audiofacial morbidity after Gamma Knife surgery for vestibular schwannoma. Neurosurg Focus 2009; 27: E4

[43] Gardner G, Robertson JH. Hearing preservation in unilateral acoustic neuroma surgery. Ann Otol Rhinol Laryngol 1988; 97: 55–66

[44] Yang I, Aranda D, Han SJ, et al. Hearing preservation after stereotactic radiosurgery for vestibular schwannoma: a systematic review. J Clin Neurosci 2009; 16: 742–747

[45] Bhandare N, Jackson A, Eisbruch A, et al. Radiation therapy and hearing loss. Int J Radiat Oncol Biol Phys 2010; 76 (Suppl): S50–S57

[46] Hasegawa T, Kida Y, Kato T, Iizuka H, Yamamoto T. Factors associated with hearing preservation after Gamma Knife surgery for vestibular schwannomas in patients who retain serviceable hearing. J Neurosurg 2011; 115: 1078–1086

[47] Andrews DW, Werner-Wasik M, Den RB, et al. Toward dose optimization for fractionated stereotactic radiotherapy for acoustic neuromas: comparison of two dose cohorts. Int J Radiat Oncol Biol Phys 2009; 74: 419–426

[48] Kano H, Kondziolka D, Khan A, Flickinger JC, Lunsford LD. Predictors of hearing preservation after stereotactic radiosurgery for acoustic neuroma. J Neurosurg 2009; 111: 863–873

[49] Massager N, Nissim O, Delbrouck C, et al. Irradiation of cochlear structures during vestibular schwannoma radiosurgery and associated hearing outcome. J Neurosurg 2007; 107: 733–739

[50] Paek SH, Chung HT, Jeong SS, et al. Hearing preservation after Gamma Knife stereotactic radiosurgery of vestibular schwannoma. Cancer 2005; 104: 580–590

[51] Brown M, Ruckenstein M, Bigelow D, Judy K, Wilson V, Alonso-Basanta M, Lee JY. Predictors of hearing loss after gamma knife radiosurgery for vestibular schwannomas: age, cochlear dose, and tumor coverage. Neurosurgery; 69: 605–613, discussion 613–614

[52] Linskey ME, Johnstone PA, O'Leary M, Goetsch S. Radiation exposure of normal temporal bone structures during stereotactically guided Gamma Knife surgery for vestibular schwannomas. J Neurosurg 2003; 98: 800–806

[53] Tamura M, Carron R, Yomo S, et al. Hearing preservation after Gamma Knife radiosurgery for vestibular schwannomas presenting with high-level hearing. Neurosurgery 2009; 64: 289–296, discussion 296

[54] Fukuoka S, Takanashi M, Hojyo A, Konishi M, Tanaka C, Nakamura H. Gamma Knife radiosurgery for vestibular schwannomas. Prog Neurol Surg 2009; 22: 45–62

[55] Coelho DH, Roland JT, Rush SA, et al. Small vestibular schwannomas with no hearing: comparison of functional outcomes in stereotactic radiosurgery and microsurgery. Laryngoscope 2008; 118: 1909–1916

[56] Humphriss RL, Baguley DM, Moffat DA. Change in dizziness handicap after vestibular schwannoma excision. Otol Neurotol 2003; 24: 661–665

[57] Winston KR, Lutz W. Linear accelerator as a neurosurgical tool for stereotactic radiosurgery. Neurosurgery 1988; 22: 454–464

[58] Das IJ, Downes MB, Corn BW, Curran WJ, Werner-Wasik M, Andrews DW. Characteristics of a dedicated linear accelerator-based stereotactic radiosurgery-radiotherapy unit. Radiother Oncol 1996; 38: 61–68

[59] Andrews DW, Bednarz G, Werner-Wasik M, Downes-Phillips B. Fractionated stereotactic radiotherapy: rationale, indications, and treatment technique. In: Chin L, Regine W, eds. Principles and Practice of Stereotactic Radiosurgery. New York: Springer; 2008:289–298

[60] Shrieve DC, Hazard L, Boucher K, Jensen RL. Dose fractionation in stereotactic radiotherapy for parasellar meningiomas: radiobiological considerations of efficacy and optic nerve tolerance. J Neurosurg 2004; 101 (Suppl 3): 390–395

[61] Leber KA, Berglöff J, Pendl G. Dose-response tolerance of the visual pathways and cranial nerves of the cavernous sinus to stereotactic radiosurgery. J Neurosurg 1998; 88: 43–50

[62] Goldsmith BJ, Rosenthal SA, Wara WM, Larson DA. Optic neuropathy after irradiation of meningioma. Radiology 1992; 185: 71–76

[63] Parsons JT, Bova FJ, Fitzgerald CR, Mendenhall WM, Million RR. Radiation optic neuropathy after megavoltage external-beam irradiation: analysis of time-dose factors. Int J Radiat Oncol Biol Phys 1994; 30: 755–763

[64] Andrews DW, Faroozan R, Yang BP, et al. Fractionated stereotactic radiotherapy for the treatment of optic nerve sheath meningiomas: preliminary observations of 33 optic nerves in 30 patients with historical comparison to observation with or without prior surgery. Neurosurgery 2002; 51: 890–902, discussion 903–904

[65] Jones B, Dale RG, Deehan C, Hopkins KI, Morgan DA. The role of biologically effective dose (BED) in clinical oncology. Clin Oncol (R Coll Radiol) 2001; 13: 71–81

[66] Balagamwala EH, Chao ST, Suh JH. Principles of radiobiology of stereotactic radiosurgery and clinical applications in the central nervous system. Technol Cancer Res Treat 2012; 11: 3–13

[67] Hansasuta A, Choi CY, Gibbs IC, et al. Multisession stereotactic radiosurgery for vestibular schwannomas: single-institution experience with 383 cases. Neurosurgery 2011; 69: 1200–1209

[68] Jones B, Dale RG. Mathematical models of tumour and normal tissue response. Acta Oncol 1999; 38: 883–893

[69] Wang JZ, Huang Z, Lo SS, Yuh WT, Mayr NA. A generalized linear-quadratic model for radiosurgery, stereotactic body radiation therapy, and high-dose rate brachytherapy. Sci Transl Med 2010; 2: 39ra48

[70] Park C, Papiez L, Zhang S, Story M, Timmerman RD. Universal survival curve and single fraction equivalent dose: useful tools in understanding potency of ablative radiotherapy. Int J Radiat Oncol Biol Phys 2008; 70: 847–852

[71] Pan CC, Eisbruch A, Lee JS, Snorrason RM, Ten Haken RK, Kileny PR. Prospective study of inner ear radiation dose and hearing loss in head-and-neck cancer patients. Int J Radiat Oncol Biol Phys 2005; 61: 1393–1402

[72] Rasmussen R, Claesson M, Stangerup SE, et al. Fractionated stereotactic radiotherapy of vestibular schwannomas accelerates hearing loss. Int J Radiat Oncol Biol Phys 2012; 83: e607–e611

[73] van de Langenberg R, Hanssens PE, Verheul JB, et al. Management of large vestibular schwannoma: II. Primary Gamma Knife surgery: radiological and clinical aspects. J Neurosurg 2011; 115: 885–893
[74] Milligan BD, Pollock BE, Foote RL, Link MJ. Long-term tumor control and cranial nerve outcomes following γ knife surgery for larger-volume vestibular schwannomas. J Neurosurg 2012; 116: 598–604
[75] Mandl ES, Meijer OW, Slotman BJ, Vandertop WP, Peerdeman SM. Stereotactic radiation therapy for large vestibular schwannomas. Radiother Oncol 2010; 95: 94–98
[76] Foote KD, Friedman WA, Buatti JM, Meeks SL, Bova FJ, Kubilis PS. Analysis of risk factors associated with radiosurgery for vestibular schwannoma. J Neurosurg 2001; 95: 440–449
[77] Andrews DW, Suarez O, Goldman HW, et al. Stereotactic radiosurgery and fractionated stereotactic radiotherapy for the treatment of acoustic schwannomas: comparative observations of 125 patients treated at one institution. Int J Radiat Oncol Biol Phys 2001; 50: 1265–1278
[78] Chan AW, Black P, Ojemann RG, et al. Stereotactic radiotherapy for vestibular schwannomas: favorable outcome with minimal toxicity. Neurosurgery 2005; 57: 60–70, discussion 60–70
[79] Combs SE, Volk S, Schulz-Ertner D, Huber PE, Thilmann C, Debus J. Management of acoustic neuromas with fractionated stereotactic radiotherapy (FSRT): long-term results in 106 patients treated in a single institution. Int J Radiat Oncol Biol Phys 2005; 63: 75–81
[80] Koh ES, Millar BA, Ménard C, et al. Fractionated stereotactic radiotherapy for acoustic neuroma: single-institution experience at the Princess Margaret Hospital. Cancer 2007; 109: 1203–1210
[81] Maire JP, Huchet A, Milbeo Y, et al. Twenty years' experience in the treatment of acoustic neuromas with fractionated radiotherapy: a review of 45 cases. Int J Radiat Oncol Biol Phys 2006; 66: 170–178
[82] Thomas C, Di Maio S, Ma R, et al. Hearing preservation following fractionated stereotactic radiotherapy for vestibular schwannomas: prognostic implications of cochlear dose. J Neurosurg 2007; 107: 917–926
[83] Arthurs BJ, Fairbanks RK, Demakas JJ, et al. A review of treatment modalities for vestibular schwannoma. Neurosurg Rev 2011; 34: 265–277, discussion 277–279
[84] Meijer OW, Vandertop WP, Baayen JC, Slotman BJ. Single-fraction vs. fractionated linac-based stereotactic radiosurgery for vestibular schwannoma: a single-institution study. Int J Radiat Oncol Biol Phys 2003; 56: 1390–1396
[85] Combs SE, Burkholder I, Edler L, et al. Randomised phase I/II study to evaluate carbon ion radiotherapy versus fractionated stereotactic radiotherapy in patients with recurrent or progressive gliomas: the CINDERELLA trial. BMC Cancer 2010; 10: 533
[86] Chen WC, Jackson A, Budnick AS, et al. Sensorineural hearing loss in combined modality treatment of nasopharyngeal carcinoma. Cancer 2006; 106: 820–829
[87] Gevaert T, Levivier M, Lacornerie T, et al. Dosimetric comparison of different treatment modalities for stereotactic radiosurgery of arteriovenous malformations and acoustic neuromas. Radiother Oncol 2013 Feb; 106: 192–7
[88] Murphy ES, Suh JH. Radiotherapy for vestibular schwannomas: a critical review. Int J Radiat Oncol Biol Phys 2011; 79: 985–997
[89] Plotkin SR, Stemmer-Rachamimov AO, Barker FG, et al. Hearing improvement after bevacizumab in patients with neurofibromatosis type 2. N Engl J Med 2009; 361: 358–367
[90] Neff BA, Welling DB, Akhmametyeva E, Chang LS. The molecular biology of vestibular schwannomas: dissecting the pathogenic process at the molecular level. Otol Neurotol 2006; 27: 197–208

8 Microsurgery for Acoustic Neuromas

Shaun D. Rodgers, Selena Heman-Ackah, J. Thomas Roland Jr., and John G. Golfinos

Introduction

Microsurgery for the treatment of acoustic neuromas remained the gold standard until the late 20th century. Radiosurgery then emerged as an alternative management strategy for this slow-growing, benign tumor. The treatment of a benign disease process with radiation was fairly counterintuitive to the understanding of radiation biology (i.e., induced DNA damage). Ample historical and retrospective data are present in the literature for both treatment modalities. However, ***level I and II evidence*** remains scant. In this chapter we present data supporting the continued use of microsurgery and radiosurgery as a multimodality approach to the management of acoustic neuromas.[1–5]

Microsurgery Versus Radiosurgery

Which patients or tumors are appropriate for microsurgery versus radiosurgery? Which patient should just be observed with imaging? A multidisciplinary approach to the management of each patient is advocated, with individualization of the patient's treatment paradigm dependent upon specific factors. These factors include age, size of tumor, comorbidity, presence of neurofibromatosis, serviceable hearing, and individual patient risk strategy. The treatment modality of choice for an elderly patient with significant comorbidities will differ significantly from that for a child with neurofibromatosis 2 (NF2), for example. The middle-aged adult with a 1.5-cm acoustic neuroma in the classic "ice cream cone" shape represents a controversy, as the tumor is amenable to either treatment modality. Many groups have attempted to decipher which patients will fare better with microsurgery or radiosurgery.[6–16] Using current treatment paradigms supported by evidence within the literature, microsurgery remains the treatment of choice for the following clinical scenarios: small tumors < 1 cm with serviceable hearing, especially tumors impacted near the fundus and hence the cochlea; large tumors > 3 cm; intracanalicular acoustic neuromas with no serviceable hearing; patients with NF2; individuals presenting with severe vertigo, especially elderly individuals; and any patient in which the surgical risk compares favorably to the radiosurgery risk at high-volume centers with good outcomes. Given the number of variables and the permutations of their combinations, therapy should be individually tailored.

Literature Review

There remains no ***level I evidence*** for microsurgery or radiosurgery in the treatment of acoustic neuromas. The majority of available literature is ***levels III, IV,*** and ***V***, which includes cohort studies, retrospective reviews, descriptive studies, and case reports. There are only three ***level II*** studies in the literature.[7,10,13] There is no consensus regarding the optimal treatment for acoustic neuromas. In particular circumstances, microsurgery and radiosurgery each have specific advantages, so that a practitioner versed in both can recommend the optimal treatment.

The general outcomes and morbidities associated with microsurgery have been very well elucidated over many years of follow-up. A meta-analysis by Sughrue et al found an overall mortality rate of 0.2% with a cerebrospinal fluid (CSF) leak rate of 8.5%. Only 1% of patients had a vascular complication and an overall neurologic complication rate of 8.6%, with a decreasing trend for small tumors. Infections occurred in 3.8% of cases and was usually meningitis.[17] On review of surgical outcomes in patients younger than 21 years, complication rates were comparable.[18] For the translabyrinthine approach, the CSF leak rate has declined significantly from the historical rate of 17% to a rate much closer to 6.6%.[19] Samii et al presented a robust retrospective review providing some of the most definitive surgical data in acoustic neuroma microsurgery. Gross total resection by retrosigmoid approach was achieved in 979 of 1,000 tumors, with 21 being planned partial resections. The facial nerve preservation rate was 93%, and cochlear nerve rate, 68%. Lower cranial nerve palsy occurred in 5.5% of patients. Other morbidities in this series were CSF leak (9.2%), hydrocephalus (2.3%), meningitis (1.2%), and wound revision (1.1%). The series had a 1.1% mortality rate.[20] In 200 cases, with serviceable hearing, a preservation rate of 47% was achieved in a very diverse cohort.[21]

The outcome and morbidity profiles for radiosurgery continue to approach the microsurgery data. Park et al prospectively followed 59 patients who underwent stereotactic radiosurgery (SRS) with a serviceable hearing rate of 47% at 12 months; no decline in quality of life was reported. However, this study was plagued with poor follow-up.[22] In a meta-analysis by Sughrue et al, a dose > 13 Gy was found to increase trigeminal neuropathy with no correlation for hydrocephalus. The low-dose group had worse vertigo and tinnitus.[23] A fractionated cochlear dose and viewing the cochlea as an organ at risk may help to reduce radiosurgery morbidity.[24] A prospective trial of 25 patients with serviceable hearing by Paek et al reported a control rate of 92%, with 13 patients (52%) retaining serviceable hearing and no facial palsies. It was concluded that the dose to the cochlear nucleus was the sole prognostic factor.[25] Additionally, data for linear accelerator (LINAC) radiosurgery identified the best margin dose to be 12.5 Gy with a corresponding tumor control rate of 93%, with 59% of tumors regressing and 7.5% remaining stable. The 5-year tumor control rate was 87%.[26]

Park et al retrospectively examined 46 patients with acoustic neuromas with serviceable hearing comparing retrosigmoid approach to SRS. The retrosigmoid approach was found to have a 7% preservation rate, while 45% was observed following Gamma Knife (Elekta AB, Stockholm, Sweden) surgery.[6] Coelho et al retrospectively compared 22 patients with small tumors < 1.5 cm and significant preoperative dizziness. Twelve patients who had undergone radiosurgery and 10 patients who had undergone microsurgical resection via the translabyrinthine approach were included in this study. Both groups experienced tumor control.[9] However, patients in the radiosurgery cohort experienced worse long-term imbalance.[9] Some authors advocate for microsurgery as a best first option in the management of acoustic neuromas except in elderly patients or poor surgical candidates.[11] Still other authors contend that the data on radiosurgery remain too mixed, given the different protocols with unclear secondary tumor rates, to draw accurate conclusions.[12]

To address the radiosurgery versus microsurgery controversy more effectively, a prospective cohort was needed. Three prospective trials have been performed to date representing the only ***level II evidence*** known.[7,10,13] Myrseth et al prospectively studied a nonrandomized cohort of 91 patients with tumors < 2.5 cm. Twenty-eight patients underwent microsurgery, and 63 underwent Gamma Knife radiosurgery. Follow-up at 2 years favored radiosurgery.[7] Reduced facial function was observed in 13 of 28 patients in the microsurgery group but only 1 of 63 patients in the radiosurgery group. All patients in the microsurgery group lost serviceable hearing, while 68% of patients in the radiosurgery group preserved hearing. This study, however, was limited in terms of follow-up (2 years), which is short for a slow-growing vestibular schwannoma. Additionally, there was no observation arm, as commented on by Teo and Eljamel.[8] The microsurgery arm would likely have a different profile, depending on the center. A prospective study by Pollock et al evaluated 82 patients with tumors < 3 cm in size; 36 patients underwent microsurgery, and 46 underwent radiosurgery. The mean follow-up was only 42 months, but no difference was identified in tumor control. Radiosurgery had a better outcome for facial function and hearing preservation at a limited follow-up of 1 year.[10] The third prospective study, by Régis et al, compared 97 Gamma Knife radiosurgery patients to 110 microsurgery patients in terms of functional outcome and quality of life as determined by a questionnaire. All radiosurgery patients and 63% of microsurgery patients had no new facial motor disturbance. Time away from work was significantly lower and hearing function was better preserved in the radiosurgery patients at 4 years.[13] However, the study was limited by its questionnaire style. Other retrospective studies have attempted comparisons but remain lacking in general application. A meta-analysis by Kaylie et al favored microsurgery for tumor control and better outcome for tumors < 4 cm.[15] However, most results in the short term appear to favor radiosurgery for its obviously gentle upfront morbidity.[14,16] ▶ Fig. 8.1 represents a case very much still in debate based on the literature. Most neurosurgeons would choose a different treatment modality if the patient were 25 years old versus 75 years old.

Recent reviews have singled out the positive attributes of both treatment paradigms. The options of microsurgery, radiosurgery, and observation appear valid in different cases. A recent meta-analysis found that, during observation, tumors grew in 29 to 54% of cases. Although 16 to 26% of patients required additional treatment, 54 to 63% were able to preserve functional hearing. Radiosurgery in these cases was able to preserve hearing in 44 to 55% of patients, with only 2 to 4% requiring additional treatment.[2] Tumor control data for radiosurgery is slowly accumulating with the increasing years of follow-up. The importance of minimizing the cochlear dose to preserve hearing also continues to gain ground. Microsurgery remains the best option for cytoreduction. Large tumors > 3 cm are best treated with microsurgery, but with potential facial and hearing morbidity.[1] A valid option, with less morbidity, may be subtotal resection followed by observation and radiosurgery for documented growth.[27,28] There is too little information available at present to determine the viability of this approach.

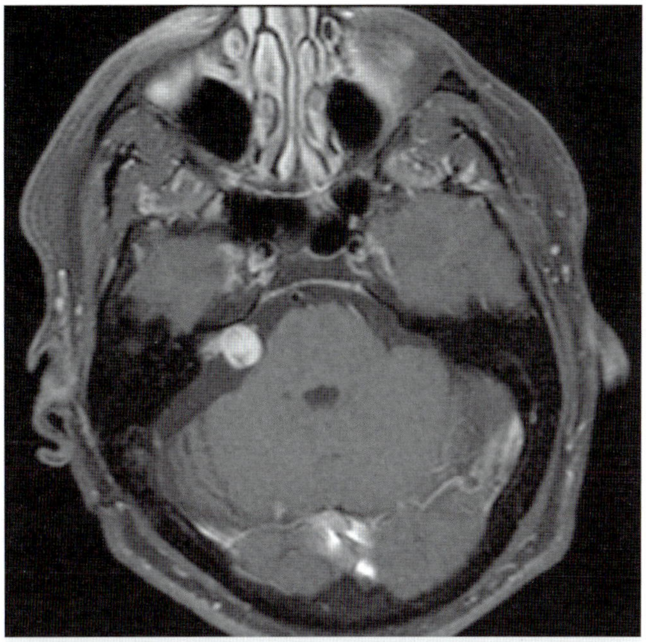

Fig. 8.1 A 1.5-cm acoustic neuroma with serviceable hearing and minimal comorbidities. This tumor would be amenable to both microsurgical resection and stereotactic radiosurgery. The patient underwent total resection via the retrosigmoid approach.

Large tumors remain an obvious target for microsurgery. An example is given in ▶ Fig. 8.2. The morbidity, chiefly facial nerve morbidity, for microsurgery on a large tumor may be significant. Hearing is rarely an issue in large tumors, although in one series, serviceable hearing was preserved in 21.4% of patients.[29] Key observations used in predicting hearing outcome were the quality of preoperative hearing and whether the CSF cleft was near the apex of the internal auditory canal.[29] Another series showed tumors > 4 cm in diameter had facial outcomes described as excellent in 75% of patients, fair in 19%, and poor in 6%.[30] Large tumors treated with microsurgery appear to have outcomes inversely proportional to tumor size.[30,31] In the series by Roland et al of tumors > 3 cm treated mainly via the translabyrinthine approach, a House-Brackmann (HB) grade of 3 or better was obtained in 90% of cases and grade 2 or better in 84% of cases.[32] In a review of patients with tumors > 4 cm in size who underwent microsurgical resection using the translabyrinthine approach, Briggs et al reported HB grades 1 to 4 in 75% of cases and grade 1 or 2 in 42%.[33] Complication rates included 4.8% vascular, 9.6% CSF leaks, and 8.3% meningitis.[33] Microsurgery remains the best option for large tumors > 3 cm.

Subtotal resection is an additional surgical strategy for a certain percentage of large tumors. The data concerning subtotal resection are limited, but with a recent resurgence in the popularity of subtotal resection as a strategy, new evidence is being generated. Van de Langenberg et al presented a cohort of 50 planned subtotal resections followed by radiosurgery.[34] Clinical control was achieved in 92% of patients with radiological control in 90%. An HB grade of 1 or 2 was observed in 94% of patients.[34] Haque et al reported the outcomes of 20 patients with

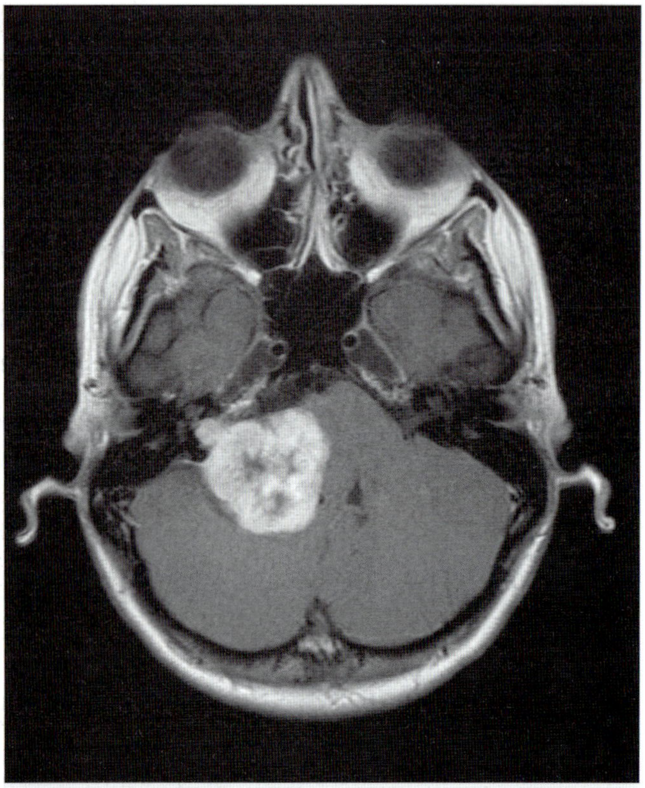

Fig. 8.2 This patient presented with a large 4.5-cm acoustic neuroma with brainstem compression. Note, however, there remains patency of the fourth ventricle. The patient underwent microsurgical resection via the translabyrinthine approach with good facial nerve outcomes.

large tumors who underwent subtotal resections followed by radiosurgery treatment. In this cohort, the facial nerve outcome was described as excellent in 96% of patients.[27] Salvage therapy in some cases may also be warranted.[35] Recurrence rates depending on the amount of resection have been reported as 3.8% for gross total, 9.4% for near total, and 27.6% for subtotal resection. Good facial nerve outcome (HB 1–3) was reported as 15.4% for gross total, 40.6% for near total, and 46.6% for subtotal resection. However, no difference remained at long-term follow-up.[36] If microsurgery is not feasible, fractionated radiosurgery may be an alternative.[37]

Some groups have attempted radiosurgery on large acoustic neuromas. Milligan et al treated 22 patients with acoustic tumors of maximum diameter 2.8 cm with 12 Gy. Four patients went on to fail treatment; tumor control at 3 years was 86%, with no facial palsy in 92% and hearing preservation in 47%. At 5 years, this dropped to a tumor control rate of 82%, with no facial palsy in 85% and hearing preservation in 47%.[38] Although the hearing preservation rates are impressive in tumors this size, the failure rate of 18% is notable and indicates that hearing preservation and facial nerve preservation are achieved at the expense of not treating the tumor definitively. Yang et al presented 65 patients with 3- to 4-cm-diameter tumors treated with radiosurgery. At 5-month follow-up, 8% of tumors expanded, 82% remained stable, and 11% were smaller.[39] Three percent of patients went on to require resection at 6 months. At 2-year follow-up, 25% of tumors showed a reduction in volume by half, and 35% showed $\ll 50\%$ reduction. Twenty-nine percent of tumors remained stable and 11% enlarged; 82% of patients retained serviceable hearing. Five percent of patients developed hydrocephalus, and 6% developed trigeminal neuralgia. Van de Langenberg et al reported the experience with 33 patients with tumors > 6 cm^3 that indented the brainstem. The growth control was 88%, with 79% clinical control. However, two patients required placement of a ventriculoperitoneal shunt. Hearing preservation was noted in 58% of patients, with 91% intact facial function at 30 months.[34] The follow-up data remain small for these cohorts, and significant risk remains for these patients to develop hydrocephalus and brainstem compression, as well as trigeminal dysfunction. More research is necessary to determine whether radiosurgery for large tumors is a viable option or merely forcing the use of a tool for a job for which it was never intended.

Small acoustic neuromas, with or without serviceable hearing, represent another area of controversy. Two examples are shown in ▶ Fig. 8.3 and ▶ Fig. 8.4. Small tumors, without serviceable hearing, represent a great target for the translabyrinthine approach. In a study of 91 patients with gross total resection, Schmerber et al found no recurrences on magnetic resonance imaging (MRI) at 11 years, with minimal morbidity.[40] The small tumor size combined with the excellent internal auditory canal exposure afforded by the translabyrinthine approach resulted in facial nerve functional preservation rates approaching 100%. Radiosurgery represents a valid option as well with increased age and significant comorbidities. The experience with the translabyrinthine approach of the neuro-otologist or neurosurgeon becomes critical in these

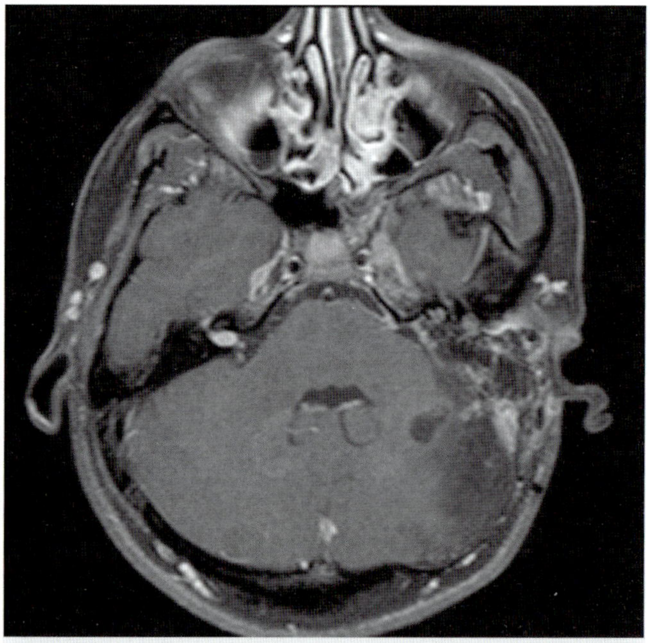

Fig. 8.3 The clinical presentation in patients with neurofibromatosis type 2 (NF2) can pose a challenge. This patient with NF2 previously underwent acoustic neuroma resection via the left translabyrinthine approach. The patient then presented with a right acoustic neuroma < 1 cm and without serviceable hearing. The patient underwent resection via the right translabyrinthine approach with auditory brainstem implantation done concurrently.

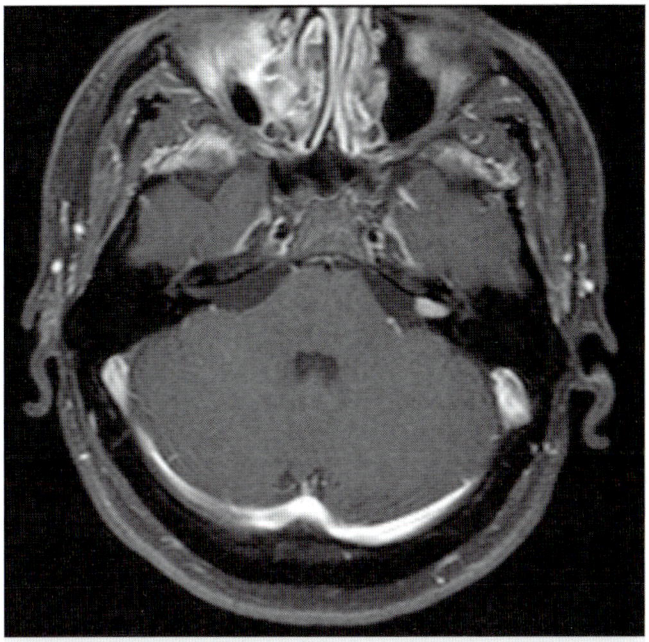

Fig. 8.4 This patient presented with an acoustic neuroma < 1 cm with serviceable hearing and minimal comorbidities. He underwent the middle fossa approach.

cases when a complete mastoid drill-out and skeletonizing of the internal auditory canal can be completed in less than 2½ hours versus the 4 to 5 hours needed by a less experienced surgeon. Because the dissection on a small tumor takes less than 1 hour in most cases, the approach time becomes a significant determinant of the morbidity of the case for an elderly patient or one with comorbidities.

An acoustic neuroma < 1 cm in a young patient with serviceable hearing should remain a microsurgery target using the middle fossa or retrosigmoid approach. The definition of "young" becomes the sticking point. Because patients younger than age 50 have an additional life expectancy of more than 35 years, a definitive management option providing more than 30 years of control is required for their tumors. The middle fossa approach has been shown to preserve serviceable hearing function in 76.7% versus 73.2% for the retrosigmoid approach. However, hearing preservation rates of up to 90% have been reported by a few surgeons with the middle fossa approach.[41] In one study, temporary facial weakness was slightly higher with the middle fossa approach.[42] With a purely intracanalicular acoustic neuroma < 1 cm in size in a young patient with serviceable hearing, the middle fossa approach remains an excellent option. In a review of 162 consecutive patients with unilateral acoustic neuromas with a diameter of 0.2 to 2.5 cm resected via the middle fossa approach, Meyer et al found that both tumor size and preoperative word recognition scores related to postoperative word recognition scores. Normal facial function was preserved in all patients with tumors 1 cm, and hearing was preserved in 72% of patients. Complications were extremely low, with a 5.5% CSF leak rate and 0.6% recurrence rate.[43] A middle fossa approach in this scenario appears easily justified. The controversy arises in older patients, with the age cutoff a fluid number that seems to change more with society's view of what is old rather than with statistical evidence of increased surgical morbidity. Given hearing preservation rates of > 40% at 10 years with radiosurgery, radiation has to be considered a viable option for those patients who prioritize hearing preservation over risk of recurrence.[10] Certainly, patients over the age of 60 become poorer candidates for a middle fossa approach compared to the minimal morbidity of radiosurgery, where hearing preservation is the goal. Finally, in comparing the middle fossa approach to radiosurgery for hearing preservation, the proximity of the lateral end of the tumor to the fundus of the internal auditory canal and, in turn, the cochlea becomes a critical consideration. Although radiosurgery was touted early on as the perfect solution to the difficult problem of intracanalicular tumors, the proliferation of strategies for reducing the cochlear dose testifies to the limits of radiosurgery in hearing preservation. In determining the best strategy for preserving hearing in a young patient with a small tumor at the fundus, the choice is between a middle fossa approach with the possibility of mild facial weakness and noninvasive radiosurgery with a compromised likelihood of hearing preservation and lower long-term tumor control.

The use of radiosurgery, or any radiation, for that matter, in patients with NF2 is still hotly debated. In our institution, we try to avoid the use of radiosurgery in patients with NF2, leaving microsurgery as the best strategy. The goal of management in this chronic disease remains to preserve function and balance quality of life with tumor burden. Samii et al advocated for avoiding radiation in this patient population despite the demonstrated poorer surgical results. In their study of 120 tumors in 82 patients with NF2, complete resection was achieved in 105 cases; 15 cases were planned subtotal resections. Serviceable hearing was preserved in 24% of patients with large tumors (3 cm and greater) and in 57% with small tumors (less than 3 cm). Eighty-five percent of patients had facial nerve preservation.[44] The proliferation of reports of secondary malignancy in patients with NF2 compared to the population of patients with sporadic acoustic neuromas gives pause to any recommendation of radiation in these patients. Moreover, even with radiosurgery, hearing preservation rates are lower and tumor control rates are lower as well. As these patients are now living longer, the long-term morbidities of radiation which were previously unimportant become more significant. Currently, we advocate microsurgery as the treatment modality of choice in cases of NF2. We believe that the competition in the future for surgery will come from targeted chemotherapies rather than radiation.

Salvage therapy after failed radiosurgery warrants the use of microsurgery. Perhaps this is the area of least controversy in the use of microsurgery for acoustic neuromas. Freidman et al presented results from 73 patients treated with radiosurgery that required salvage microsurgery. A gross total resection was achieved in 79.5% of patients, planned subtotal in 5.5%, and intraoperative decision for partial removal in 15.1% of cases. At 1-year postoperative follow-up, 50% of patients in the gross total resection group had an HB grade of 1 or 2 compared to 85.7% in the partial removal group. Interestingly, 21.7% of the gross total resection group had an unsatisfactory facial function outcome (HB grade 5 or 6) versus only 7% in the partial resection group.[45]

The weakness of the literature remains evident in the paucity of ***level II*** and lack of ***level I evidence***. No ***level I*** recommendation may be given for microsurgery versus radiosurgery in the treatment of acoustic neuromas. Microsurgery and radiosurgery are rarely compared in a uniform fashion, while cross-study comparisons and meta-analysis remain inadequate.[2,3,15] What remains is largely ***level III* or lower evidence** to guide clinicians on microsurgery versus radiosurgery for acoustic neuromas.

Authors' Experience at New York University

Microsurgery has been the gold standard of treatment for acoustic neuromas for many years. However, complications and upfront surgical morbidity are not trivial. Radiosurgery represents an excellent option in select cases. Our multidisciplinary approach treats acoustic neuromas with either option as well as observation. Our clinical paradigm takes into account many clinical attributes specific to each patient. We have operated on a large cohort of patients with NF2 where radiosurgery may have posed a significant risk. Likewise, large acoustic neuromas (> 3 cm) have not been a traditional target for radiosurgery. Our strategy for maximal safe tumor resection has remained to afford brainstem decompression and prevent hydrocephalus. Some data have been presented recently for large acoustic neuromas, but long-term data are lacking.[34,38,39] Microsurgery remains a necessary treatment modality in cases of significant brainstem compression. It also offers a significant advantage when vertigo is a major complaint.[9]

Individualized Patient Approach

A multidisciplinary group, working at a high-volume center, must be able to treat acoustic neuromas in an up-to-date fashion. The treatment paradigm should take into account a program tailored to each patient.[4,5] Treatment options for acoustic neuromas today include microsurgery, SRS, conservative observation, and, most recently, chemotherapy. With the exception of chemotherapy, which is currently limited to our patients with NF2, all of these treatment options are offered to each patient in the discussion of disease management. Although some patients arrive at the consultation with ideas of how they want to be treated, we urge all patients to consider all the options in light of their priorities. The responsibility of the surgeon, then, is to match the correct treatment to the correct patient, maximizing the benefits of treatment and minimizing the risks. It is not infrequent to have two patients of the same age with virtually identical tumors choose different treatment options, based on how they tolerate risk and how they prioritize their goals. The mandate for the surgeon treating acoustic neuromas is to have expertise with all of the treatment options so as to be able to speak from personal experience buttressed by the limited objective data available.

Future Studies

The future treatment of acoustic neuromas would benefit greatly from randomized prospective trials comparing microsurgery and radiosurgery. These trials would allow practitioners to better classify outcomes and compare risks in a uniform manner. Currently, ***level II evidence*** is scarce in the literature, and no ***level I*** data exist. We rely heavily on personal experience and ***level III, IV,*** and ***V evidence***. The long-term outcomes for radiosurgery need to be further evaluated for recurrence, quality of life, and secondary malignancy. Patients with NF2 represent a subpopulation requiring further investigation.[44] The treatment paradigm of subtotal resection followed by observation, radiosurgery, or further microsurgery needs to be studied further.[27,28,46,47]

Conclusion

A multidisciplinary team approach must be taken for acoustic neuroma management. A team offering multimodality treatment at a high-volume center will be able to better serve patients. The morbidity of either microsurgery or radiosurgery will be minimized at large centers. We have seen excellent results with microsurgery and radiosurgery, but both treatments are not benign. Individualized treatment should be offered to each patient.

References

[1] Theodosopoulos PV, Pensak ML. Contemporary management of acoustic neuromas. Laryngoscope 2011; 121: 1133–1137

[2] Arthurs BJ, Fairbanks RK, Demakas JJ, et al. A review of treatment modalities for vestibular schwannoma. Neurosurg Rev 2011; 34: 265–277, discussion 277–279

[3] Pollock BE. Vestibular schwannoma management: an evidence-based comparison of stereotactic radiosurgery and microsurgical resection. Prog Neurol Surg 2008; 21: 222–227

[4] Wackym PA. Stereotactic radiosurgery, microsurgery, and expectant management of acoustic neuroma: basis for informed consent. Otolaryngol Clin North Am 2005; 38: 653–670

[5] Briggs RJ, Fabinyi G, Kaye AH. Current management of acoustic neuromas: review of surgical approaches and outcomes. J Clin Neurosci 2000; 7: 521–526

[6] Park CE, Park BJ, Lim YJ, Yeo SG. Functional outcomes in retrosigmoid approach microsurgery and Gamma Knife stereotactic radiosurgery in vestibular schwannoma. EUR Arch Otolaryngol 2011; 268: 955–959

[7] Myrseth E, Møller P, Pedersen PH, Lund-Johansen M. Vestibular schwannoma: surgery or gamma knife radiosurgery? A prospective, nonrandomized study. Neurosurgery 2009; 64: 654–661, discussion 661–663

[8] Teo M, Eljamel MS. Vestibular schwannoma. Neurosurgery 2010; 67: E878

[9] Coelho DH, Roland JT, Rush SA, et al. Small vestibular schwannomas with no hearing: comparison of functional outcomes in stereotactic radiosurgery and microsurgery. Laryngoscope 2008; 118: 1909–1916

[10] Pollock BE, Driscoll CL, Foote RL, et al. Patient outcomes after vestibular schwannoma management: a prospective comparison of microsurgical resection and stereotactic radiosurgery. Neurosurgery 2006; 59: 77–85, discussion 77–85

[11] Kaylie DM, McMenomey SO. Microsurgery vs Gamma Knife radiosurgery for the treatment of vestibular schwannomas. Arch Otolaryngol Head Neck Surg 2003; 129: 903–906

[12] Coker NJ. The radiosurgical option: too many unanswered questions. Arch Otolaryngol Head Neck Surg 2003; 129: 906–907

[13] Régis J, Pellet W, Delsanti C, et al. Functional outcome after Gamma Knife surgery or microsurgery for vestibular schwannomas. J Neurosurg 2002; 97: 1091–1100

[14] Karpinos M, Teh BS, Zeck O, et al. Treatment of acoustic neuroma: stereotactic radiosurgery vs. microsurgery. Int J Radiat Oncol Biol Phys 2002; 54: 1410–1421

[15] Kaylie DM, Horgan MJ, Delashaw JB, McMenomey SO. A meta-analysis comparing outcomes of microsurgery and Gamma Knife radiosurgery. Laryngoscope 2000; 110: 1850–1856

[16] Pollock BE, Lunsford LD, Kondziolka D, et al. Outcome analysis of acoustic neuroma management: a comparison of microsurgery and stereotactic radiosurgery. Neurosurgery 1995; 36: 215–224, discussion 224–229
[17] Sughrue ME, Yang I, Aranda D, et al. Beyond audiofacial morbidity after vestibular schwannoma surgery. J Neurosurg 2011; 114: 367–374
[18] Mirzayan MJ, Gerganov VM, Lüdemann W, Oi S, Samii M, Samii A. Management of vestibular schwannomas in young patients-comparison of clinical features and outcome with adult patients. Childs Nerv Syst 2007; 23: 891–895
[19] Fishman AJ, Marrinan MS, Golfinos JG, Cohen NL, Roland JT. Prevention and management of cerebrospinal fluid leak following vestibular schwannoma surgery. Laryngoscope 2004; 114: 501–505
[20] Samii M, Matthies C. Management of 1000 vestibular schwannomas (acoustic neuromas): surgical management and results with an emphasis on complications and how to avoid them. Neurosurgery 1997; 40: 11–21, discussion 21–23
[21] Samii M, Matthies C. Management of 1000 vestibular schwannomas (acoustic neuromas): hearing function in 1000 tumor resections. Neurosurgery 1997; 40: 248–260, discussion 260–262
[22] Park SS, Grills IS, Bojrab D, et al. Longitudinal assessment of quality of life and audiometric test outcomes in vestibular schwannoma patients treated with gamma knife surgery. Otol Neurotol. 2011; 32: 676–679
[23] Sughrue ME, Yang I, Han SJ, et al. Non-audiofacial morbidity after Gamma Knife surgery for vestibular schwannoma. Neurosurg Focus 2009; 27: E4
[24] Thomas C, Di Maio S, Ma R, et al. Hearing preservation following fractionated stereotactic radiotherapy for vestibular schwannomas: prognostic implications of cochlear dose. J Neurosurg 2007; 107: 917–926
[25] Paek SH, Chung HT, Jeong SS, et al. Hearing preservation after Gamma Knife stereotactic radiosurgery of vestibular schwannoma. Cancer 2005; 104: 580–590
[26] Foote KD, Friedman WA, Buatti JM, Meeks SL, Bova FJ, Kubilis PS. Analysis of risk factors associated with radiosurgery for vestibular schwannoma. J Neurosurg 2001; 95: 440–449
[27] Haque R, Wojtasiewicz TJ, Gigante PR, et al. Efficacy of facial nerve-sparing approach in patients with vestibular schwannomas. J Neurosurg 2011; 115: 917–923
[28] van de Langenberg R, Hanssens PE, van Overbeeke JJ, et al. Management of large vestibular schwannoma: I. Planned subtotal resection followed by Gamma Knife surgery: radiological and clinical aspects. J Neurosurg 2011; 115: 875–884
[29] Di Maio S, Malebranche AD, Westerberg B, Akagami R. Hearing preservation after microsurgical resection of large vestibular schwannomas. Neurosurgery 2011; 68: 632–640, discussion 640
[30] Samii M, Gerganov VM, Samii A. Functional outcome after complete surgical removal of giant vestibular schwannomas. J Neurosurg 2010; 112: 860–867
[31] Park CK, Jung HW, Kim JE, Son YJ, Paek SH, Kim DG. Therapeutic strategy for large vestibular schwannomas. J Neurooncol 2006; 77: 167–171
[32] Roland JT, Fishman AJ, Golfinos JG, Cohen N, Alexiades G, Jackman AH. Cranial nerve preservation in surgery for large acoustic neuromas. Skull Base 2004; 14: 85–90, discussion 90–91
[33] Briggs RJ, Luxford WM, Atkins JS, Hitselberger WE. Translabyrinthine removal of large acoustic neuromas. Neurosurgery 1994; 34: 785–790, discussion 790–791
[34] van de Langenberg R, Hanssens PE, Verheul JB, et al. Management of large vestibular schwannoma, II: Primary Gamma Knife surgery: radiological and clinical aspects. J Neurosurg 2011; 115: 885–893
[35] Prasad D, Steiner M, Steiner L. Gamma surgery for vestibular schwannoma. J Neurosurg 2000; 92: 745–759
[36] Seol HJ, Kim CH, Park CK, et al. Optimal extent of resection in vestibular schwannoma surgery: relationship to recurrence and facial nerve preservation. Neurol Med Chir (Tokyo) 2006; 46: 176–180, discussion 180–181
[37] Bambakidis NC, Lo SS, Selman WR. Large vestibular schwannomas. J Neurosurg 2011; 115: 894–895
[38] Milligan BD, Pollock BE, Foote RL, Link MJ. Long-term tumor control and cranial nerve outcomes following Gama Knife surgery for larger-volume vestibular schwannomas. J Neurosurg 2012; 116: 598–604
[39] Yang HC, Kano H, Awan NR, et al. Gamma Knife radiosurgery for larger-volume vestibular schwannomas: clinical article. J Neurosurg 2011; 114: 801–807
[40] Schmerber S, Palombi O, Boubagra K, Charachon R, Chirossel JP, Gay E. Long-term control of vestibular schwannoma after a translabyrinthine complete removal. Neurosurgery 2005; 57: 693–698, discussion 693–698
[41] Woodson EA, Dempewolf RD, Gubbels SP, et al. Long-term hearing preservation after microsurgical excision of vestibular schwannoma. Otol Neurotol 2010; 31: 1144–1152
[42] Sameshima T, Fukushima T, McElveen JT, Friedman AH. Critical assessment of operative approaches for hearing preservation in small acoustic neuroma surgery: retrosigmoid vs middle fossa approach. Neurosurgery 2010; 67: 640–644, discussion 644–645
[43] Meyer TA, Canty PA, Wilkinson EP, Hansen MR, Rubinstein JT, Gantz BJ. Small acoustic neuromas: surgical outcomes versus observation or radiation. Otol Neurotol. 2006; 27: 380–392
[44] Samii M, Matthies C, Tatagiba M. Management of vestibular schwannomas (acoustic neuromas): auditory and facial nerve function after resection of 120 vestibular schwannomas in patients with neurofibromatosis 2. Neurosurgery 1997; 40: 696–705, discussion 705–706
[45] Friedman RA, Berliner KI, Bassim M, et al. A paradigm shift in salvage surgery for radiated vestibular schwannoma. Otol Neurotol. 2011; 32: 1322–1328
[46] Kondziolka D. Facial nerve and acoustic neuromas. J Neurosurg 2011; 115: 915–916, author reply 916
[47] Kondziolka D. Role of radiosurgery for larger vestibular schwannomas. J Neurosurg 2011; 115: 896–897

9 Treating Cavernomas with Radiosurgery

Douglas Kondziolka, Edward A. Monaco III, Ajay Niranjan, Hideyuki Kano, Ramesh Grandhi, John C. Flickinger, and L. Dade Lunsford[1]

Introduction

Symptomatic cavernous malformations (CMs) of the brain present a challenge. Symptoms are usually due to hemorrhage that can be defined on imaging. In certain cases, imaging does not confirm the presence of acute blood, and regional ischemia, edema, or microhemorrhage may be present. CMs of the brain occur in 0.1 to 4.0% of the population but represent 8 to 15% of all vascular lesions in the brain.[1–4] These angiographically occult vascular malformations can occur anywhere in the brain. Brainstem location is reported to account for 9 to 35% of all CMs.[5–7] CMs may be single and incidental or develop due to genetic, postsurgical, or postradiation effects.[8–10] Up to one third of patients harboring CMs possess associated developmental venous anomalies (DVAs).[11–14]

CMs are a diagnosis of the magnetic resonance imaging (MRI) era. MRI has helped physicians understand the epidemiology and natural history of these lesions.[2,11,15–21] Whereas supratentorial CMs can cause seizures, deficits, or headache, brainstem malformations typically present with focal neurologic deficits due to bleeding. The annual hemorrhage risk has been estimated to be 0.1 to 2.5% per lesion-year and 0.25 to 16.5% per patient-year, but this risk is much higher (up to 34% annual risk) for patients with prior imaging-confirmed hemorrhages.[22,23]

Controversies

Most CMs are managed with surgical resection, and complete removal usually confers cure. When accessible with low risk, clinical outcomes are good.[24–27] However, microsurgery for CMs in the brainstem, thalamus, or basal ganglia carries with it higher rates of morbidity (up to 35%), demands complete resection, and is only reasonably suited for those lesions that present to an ependymal or pial surface.[18,20,28] For this reason, we began to use stereotactic radiosurgery for high-risk symptomatic CMs in 1988, as an alternative to either observation or resection. Radiosurgery is controversial because there is no imaging test to confirm cure or complete obliteration with no further risk of hemorrhage. This can also be true after resection. Another controversy relates to the natural history of CM. Studies, noted below, provide annual hemorrhage rates. However, such rates can vary significantly from year to year, which affects how data are interpreted. Thus, only long-term studies provide any strength to the argument in favor of radiosurgery. Fortunately, such studies are available.

University of Pittsburgh Patient Population

We have performed Gamma Knife (Elekta AB, Stockholm, Sweden) radiosurgery in 130 patients from 1988–2012. This review will focus on those patients with brainstem CMs ($n = 68$). The average patient age was 41 years (range 5–79 years). All patients had previously experienced at least two hemorrhages, and 37% had suffered three or more bleeds (range 3–12 bleeds). Bleeding events were defined as the development of a new neurologic deficit with imaging evidence of new blood products in a newly discovered or previously identified CM. Information pertaining to clinical events was obtained via discussions with patients and/or their treating physicians combined with review of all available imaging studies. The diagnosis of a CM was made by computed tomography (CT) prior to 1990 and by MRI after 1990. Sixty-four patients (94.1%) presented with preexisting neurologic deficits caused by hemorrhage. Nine patients (13.2%) had previously undergone partial surgical resection.

Radiosurgical Technique

CM stereotactic radiosurgery (SRS) has been described in several reports.[29–31] Briefly, the Leksell model G stereotactic frame (Elekta) was applied to the patient's head after the administration of local anesthetic and, as needed, conscious sedation. For the three patients under the age of 12, frame application and SRS were performed under general anesthesia. Before 1990, CT was used for dose planning (17 patients), while stereotactic MRI has been used since 1991. Upon the administration of MR contrast, three-dimensional (3D) volume acquisition using the spoiled gradient recalled (SPGR) in steady-state sequence (1- to 1.5-mm-thick slices) was performed. An additional variable echo multiplanar (3/0 thickness) sequence was obtained to identify the hemosiderin signal surrounding the CM. Images were exported to dose-planning workstations for the U, B, C, or 4C Gamma Knife instruments (Elekta).

Gamma Knife radiosurgery dose plans using single or multiple isocenters (range 1–9) were created to yield highly conformal (to the lesion's 3D geometry) and selective (rapid dose falloff outside the CM margin) dosing (▶ Fig. 9.1). The targeted edge of the CM was considered to be the region characterized by mixed signal change within the T2-defined hemosiderin ring. This margin served as the 50% or greater isodose line. In general, targeting of eccentric accumulated blood products was avoided, as iron breakdown products are potential radiation sensitizers. Following completion of SRS, each patient received a single 40-mg dose of methylprednisolone.

Follow-up

Clinical and follow-up MRI was requested at 6-month intervals during the first 2 years after SRS, after which it was recommended on an annual basis. Sixty-six patients (97.1%) had follow-up of at least 2 years, 40 (58.8%) had follow-up from 2 to 5 years, 17 (25%) had follow-up from 5 to 10 years, and 9 (13.2%) had follow-up for more than 10 years.

Hemorrhage was defined as imaging evidence of a new area of blood signal corresponding to a new neurologic sign or symptom. The annual hemorrhage rate was calculated using the following formula: total number of hemorrhages in all

[1] Disclosure: Drs. Lunsford, Kondziolka, and Niranjan are consultants with Elekta AB. Dr. Lunsford is also a stockholder in Elekta AB.

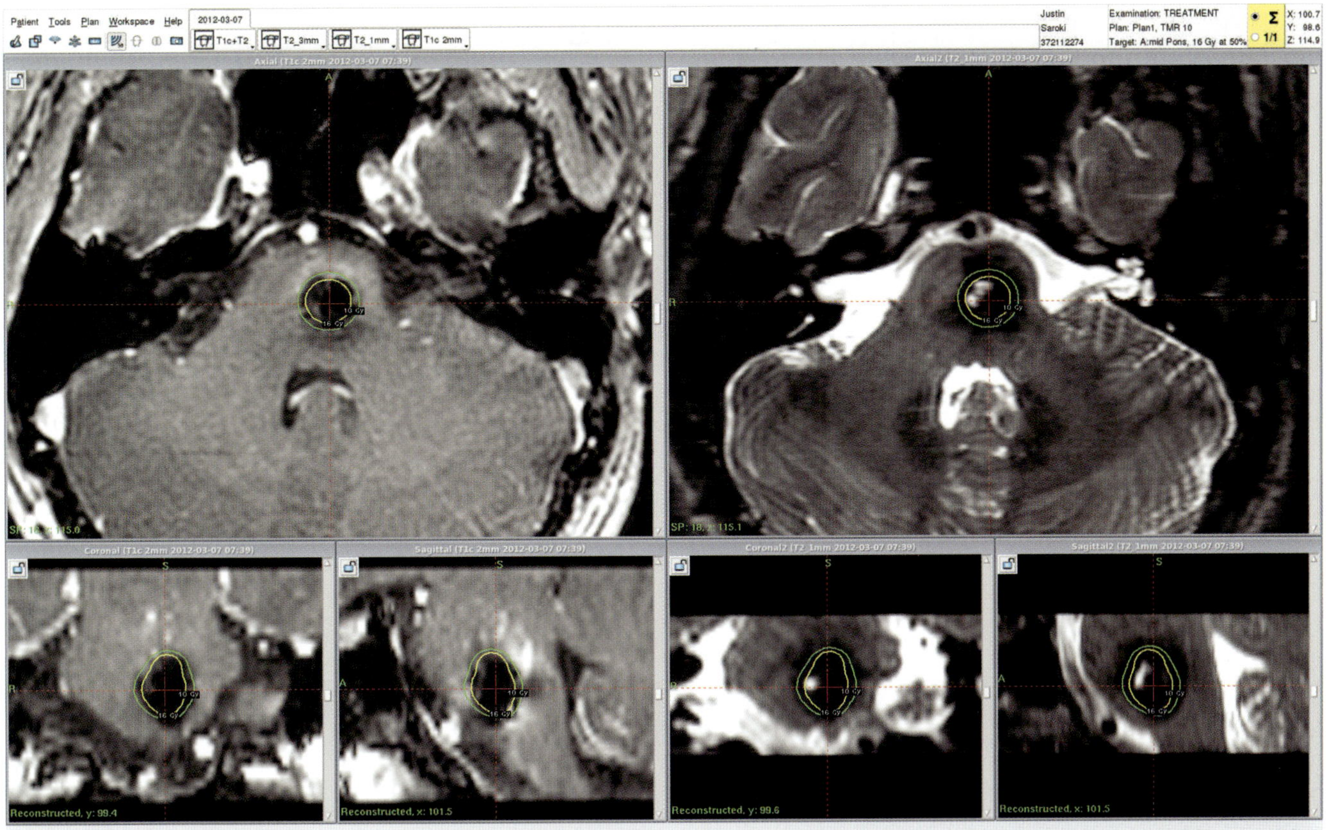

Fig. 9.1 Magnetic resonance imaging–based stereotactic radiosurgery dose plan in a 26-year-old man who had suffered a symptomatic hemorrhage from a cavernous malformation in the brainstem. The dose plan is shown on axial T1- and T2-weighted images (*top*) and coronal and sagittal images (*bottom*). Radiosurgery was performed with a margin dose of 16 Gy, a maximal dose of 32 Gy, to a total volume of 0.48 mL.

patients/total number of patient-years observed. Hemorrhage rates were compared before and after SRS using a paired *t*-test.

Preradiosurgery Hemorrhage Rate

The time of observation was defined as the time from the first symptomatic, image-documented hemorrhage to the time of SRS. Thus, a total of 386 patient-years were observed, with a mean observation period of 5.68 years (range 1–38 years). There were 193 hemorrhages documented during this time (2.84 per patient). All patients had at least two hemorrhages prior to SRS (range 2–12). After exclusion of the first hemorrhage (193 – 68 = 125 hemorrhages), the calculated annual hemorrhage rate was 32.38% (125 hemorrhages in 386 patient-years observed).

Postradiosurgery Hemorrhage Rate

The observation period following radiosurgery was considered to be the time following the procedure until either of the following: most recent clinical follow-up, surgical intervention, or death. Thus, postradiosurgical follow-up averaged 5.2 years per patient (range 0.58–12.41 years), with a total observation period of 353 patient-years. During follow-up after SRS, seven patients died (10.3%). Two patients died in the setting of subsequent microsurgical resection of lesions that rebled; the remaining five died of either unknown causes or causes unrelated to their CMs (one myocardial infarction, three cancer related, and one unknown). There were no deaths directly attributable to SRS.

Fourteen hemorrhages in 13 patients were documented during this period (0.21 hemorrhage per patient). Eleven of these bleeds occurred in 10 patients within a 2-year period after SRS, whereas only three occurred after 2 years. The annual hemorrhage rate during the first 2 years after SRS was 8.2% (11 hemorrhages/133.75 patient-years). The annual hemorrhage rate after the initial 2 years then dropped to 1.4% (3 hemorrhages/219.25 patient-years). This represented a significant reduction ($p < 0.0001$) in the annual hemorrhage rate after SRS (32.38 vs 8.22%), as well as a reduction in the mean number of hemorrhages per patient (2.84 before vs 0.21 after SRS, $p < 0.0001$). Additionally, there was a statistically significant reduction ($p < 0.0447$) in the annual hemorrhage rate after the first 2 years had passed (8.2% vs 1.4%).

Morbidity

Eight patients (11.8%) demonstrated new neurologic symptoms following SRS in the absence of a new hemorrhage. In all but one of these patients, the neurologic worsening was transient and responded fully to a short course of corticosteroids. The remaining patient manifested a permanent new neurologic deficit and went on to microsurgical resection. Two patients (2.94%)

were discovered to have new T2 signal abnormality surrounding their CMs, but they were neurologically asymptomatic. Overall, at the most recent follow-up, 79.4% of patients were either stable or improved in their neurologic condition following SRS.

Determining the Role of Radiosurgery

In contrast to supratentorial CM, brainstem malformation may have a higher rate of rehemorrhage.[10,33,37] This risk has been estimated to be up to 60% annually with corresponding neurologic deficits. As discussed previously, a CM may cause a symptomatic bleeding event below the resolution of current imaging modalities. Interestingly, the literature regarding surgical resection is not large. There are only a few hundred patients reported with multiple hemorrhagic, symptomatic CMs of the brainstem in several retrospective series. As such, management is not clearly defined. Although controversial to some, we and others have shown that in a highly selective group of patients with surgically high-risk symptomatic brainstem CMs, SRS is a reasonable alternative with a safety profile similar to or better than other treatment approaches.

Porter et al[20] reviewed a series of 86 cases of patients who had resection of a brainstem CM. Fifty-two percent of the CMs in this series reached the pial surface. Following surgery, 33% of patients had new cranial nerve deficits, 30% demonstrated cerebellar findings, and 29% had new-onset weakness. The overall rate of temporary and/or permanent morbidity and mortality was 35%. Overall mortality was 8%, and all-cause 30-day mortality was 3.5%. Twelve percent had permanent or severe deficits. Eleven patients required additional surgery to either manage the target lesion or address a complication.

Mathiesen et al[18] reported on a series of patients with deep-seated CMs, including 40 with CMs confined to the brainstem, 17 of whom underwent microsurgical resection. They noted a 69% incidence of transient and an 8% risk of permanent neurologic deterioration. There was a 15% rate of rehemorrhage after surgery, in each case attributed to subtotal resection. From these data, it was concluded that microsurgery for symptomatic lesions was feasible as long as radical resection could be confidently and safely achieved. In a retrospective series of 137 patients with brainstem CMs treated by microsurgery by Wang et al,[28] 4.6% of patients harbored residual CM after surgery, and 27.7% deteriorated after surgery or developed new neurologic deficits. Hauck et al[32] reported 44 microsurgical patients with brainstem CMs, all of whom had symptomatic hemorrhages. Postoperatively, one patient was found to have residual CM and went on to suffer a subsequent hemorrhage. Fourteen percent of the patients experienced increased cranial nerve deficits, 7% had worsened hemiparesis, and 4% had new deafness. In a series of 45 patients with brainstem CMs treated surgically by a supracerebellar infratentorial approach, de Oliveira et al[33] found that 44% of patients had new postoperative deficits, with almost half of these being permanent. Twenty-nine percent of patients experienced treatment-related complications, including hydrocephalus, cerebrospinal leak, meningitis, and pseudomeningocele. Four patients required placement of a tracheostomy and feeding tube. Seven had a recurrence even if initial imaging appeared to show no lesion.

In our most recent report on CM in all brain locations,[31] we showed that for 103 patients with surgically high-risk CMs, the rate of rehemorrhage significantly declined from a pre-SRS annual rate of 32.5% to a rate of 10.8% in the 2 years following treatment and to an annual rate of 1.06% thereafter. Adverse radiation effects (AREs) were observed in 13.5% of patients, with most being transient and occurring early in the experience. In 2010 the Sheffield Gamma Knife experience was published.[34] The authors of that study reported 113 patients with 79 brainstem CMs. The annual rebleeding rate before radiosurgery was 30.5%, which decreased to 15% during the first 2 years after radiosurgery, then to 2.4% thereafter. The Sheffield group found that 7% of patients had a permanent ARE with minor neurologic deficits.[34] They concluded that CM radiosurgery was safe and believed that early use of radiosurgery for patients with a hemorrhagic CM in a deep location was justified.

In 57 patients harboring surgically inaccessible CMs, Chang et al[1] observed a pre-SRS hemorrhage annual rate of 9.4% that declined to 1.6% 36 months after treatment. Only 7% of these patients suffered AREs. Using stereotactic Bragg-peak proton beam therapy, Amin-Hanjani et al[24] treated 95 patients with 98 CMs. They observed a reduction in the hemorrhage rate from a pretreatment annual rate of 17.5% to 4.5% after a 2-year latency period. However, 16% of patients suffered permanent neurologic deficit, and 3% died. Liu et al[17] treated 125 patients with a reduction in the annual hemorrhage rate from 10.3% pretreatment to 3.3% after. Seventeen (13.1%) of these patients experienced AREs. In a smaller study of 22 patients with CMs treated by SRS, Kim et al[35] documented an annual hemorrhage rate reduction of 35.5 to 3.55%, with six patients demonstrating AREs. Finally, García-Muñoz et al[36] reported 15 patients treated with SRS and showed that the annual hemorrhage rate decreased from 34.45% to 7.17%. Other reports have failed to reproduce similar reductions in hemorrhage risk, but they are limited by their size, details of treatment, and/or limited follow-up.[18,20,37]

Although Pollock and colleagues treated 17 patients and showed a reduction in annual hemorrhage rates from 40% prior to SRS to 2.9% after a 2-year latency period, they did not conclude that radiosurgery was protective against hemorrhage.[14] Indeed, 59% of these patients had evidence of AREs, a finding possibly attributable to a high median target dose of 18 Gy causing toxicity in the radiation-sensitized adjacent hemosiderin-containing brain. Some others have expressed concerns related to the high risk of reactive edema around treated CMs.[18,38] However, this may be the result of adverse effects on coexistent DVAs, as many of the patients in these reports harbored DVAs. Far fewer patients in the current series experienced AREs, with only 11.8% of patients being symptomatic. We have hypothesized that the radiobiological effect of SRS on CMs is similar to that for arteriovenous malformations: progressive endothelial cell proliferation and hyalinization yielding luminal closure. Gewirtz et al[16] reviewed the histopathological changes in eight CMs following surgical resection after failed SRS treatment (with 18- to 26-Gy equivalents). These lesions demonstrated fibrinoid necrosis when compared to untreated controls but still possessed patent vascular channels. Nyáry et al[19] identified endothelial cell destruction and marked fibrosis in the connective tissue stroma of a thalamic CM 1 year after 40-Gy irradiation. Taken together with clinical data, these reports suggest that CMs may respond to SRS in a fashion similar to other vascular lesions via delayed luminal closure of vascular channels.

The role of radiosurgery for CM has evolved slowly. We recommend observation more than we recommend resection or radiosurgery because most patients we see have incidental lesions. Slow accrual in clinical series has prevented large data pools. A randomized trial comparing resection to radiosurgery for brainstem CM was begun but later closed due to poor accrual. Thus, no ***level I*** or ***II evidence*** exists. All published series provide ***level III evidence***. In addition, there are no consensus statements on the role of radiosurgery. Thus, selection bias is likely to contribute to the results of current reports. In this instance, only patients with brainstem CMs who had two or more hemorrhages confirmed by the observation of new neurologic findings and new MRI evidence. Importantly, although the natural history of brainstem CMs is better understood than it was 20 years ago, it has not yet been fully defined.

References

[1] Chang SD, Levy RP, Adler JR, Martin DP, Krakovitz PR, Steinberg GK. Stereotactic radiosurgery of angiographically occult vascular malformations: 14-year experience. Neurosurgery 1998; 43: 213–220, discussion 220–221

[2] Larson JJ, Ball WS, Bove KE, Crone KR, Tew JM. Formation of intracerebral cavernous malformations after radiation treatment for central nervous system neoplasia in children. J Neurosurg 1998; 88: 51–56

[3] Maraire JN, Awad IA. Intracranial cavernous malformations: lesion behavior and management strategies. Neurosurgery 1995; 37: 591–605

[4] Zimmerman RS, Spetzler RF, Lee KS, Zabramski JM, Hargraves RW. Cavernous malformations of the brain stem. J Neurosurg 1991; 75: 32–39

[5] Fritschi JA, Reulen HJ, Spetzler RF, Zabramski JM. Cavernous malformations of the brain stem: a review of 139 cases. Acta Neurochir (Wien) 1994; 130: 35–46

[6] Kondziolka D, Lunsford LD, Kestle JRW. The natural history of cerebral cavernous malformations. J Neurosurg 1995; 83: 820–824

[7] Simard JM, Garcia-Bengochea F, Ballinger WE, Mickle JP, Quisling RG. Cavernous angioma: a review of 126 collected and 12 new clinical cases. Neurosurgery 1986; 18: 162–172

[8] Del Curling O, Kelly DL, Elster AD, Craven TE. An analysis of the natural history of cavernous angiomas. J Neurosurg 1991; 75: 702–708

[9] Kida Y, Kobayashi T, Mori Y. Radiosurgery of angiographically occult vascular malformations. Neurosurg Clin N Am 1999; 10: 291–303

[10] Nyáry I, Major O, Hanzély Z, Szeifert GT. Pathological considerations to irradiation of cavernous malformations. Prog Neurol Surg 2007; 20: 231–234

[11] Labauge P, Brunereau L, Lévy C, Laberge S, Houtteville JP. The natural history of familial cerebral cavernomas: a retrospective MRI study of 40 patients. Neuroradiology 2000; 42: 327–332

[12] Liscák R, Vladyka V, Simonová G, Vymazal J, Novotny J. Gamma Knife surgery of brain cavernous hemangiomas. J Neurosurg 2005; 102 (Suppl): 207–213

[13] Mitchell P, Hodgson TJ, Seaman S, Kemeny AA, Forster DM. Stereotactic radiosurgery and the risk of haemorrhage from cavernous malformations. Br J Neurosurg 2000; 14: 96–100

[14] Pollock BE, Garces YI, Stafford SL, Foote RL, Schomberg PJ, Link MJ. Stereotactic radiosurgery for cavernous malformations. J Neurosurg 2000; 93: 987–991

[15] Aiba T, Tanaka R, Koike T, Kameyama S, Takeda N, Komata T. Natural history of intracranial cavernous malformations. J Neurosurg 1995; 83: 56–59

[16] Gewirtz RJ, Steinberg GK, Crowley R, Levy RP. Pathological changes in surgically resected angiographically occult vascular malformations after radiation. Neurosurgery 1998; 42: 738–742, discussion 742–743

[17] Liu KD, Chung WY, Wu HM, et al. Gamma Knife surgery for cavernous hemangiomas: an analysis of 125 patients. J Neurosurg 2005; 102 (Suppl): 81–86

[18] Mathiesen T, Edner G, Kihlström L. Deep and brainstem cavernomas: a consecutive 8-year series. J Neurosurg 2003; 99: 31–37

[19] Nyáry I, Major O, Hanzély Z, Szeifert GT. Histopathological findings in a surgically resected thalamic cavernous hemangioma 1 year after 40-Gy irradiation. J Neurosurg 2005; 102 (Suppl): 56–58

[20] Porter RW, Detwiler PW, Spetzler RF, et al. Cavernous malformations of the brainstem: experience with 100 patients. J Neurosurg 1999; 90: 50–58

[21] Rigamonti D, Drayer BP, Johnson PC, Hadley MN, Zabramski J, Spetzler RF. The MRI appearance of cavernous malformations (angiomas). J Neurosurg 1987; 67: 518–524

[22] Chang SD, Steinberg GK, Levy RP, et al. Microsurgical resection of incompletely obliterated intracranial arteriovenous malformations following stereotactic radiosurgery. Neurol Med Chir (Tokyo) 1998; 38 (Suppl): 200–207

[23] Karlsson B, Kihlström L, Lindquist C, Ericson K, Steiner L. Radiosurgery for cavernous malformations. J Neurosurg 1998; 88: 293–297

[24] Amin-Hanjani S, Ogilvy CS, Candia GJ, Lyons S, Chapman PH. Stereotactic radiosurgery for cavernous malformations: Kjellberg's experience with proton beam therapy in 98 cases at the Harvard Cyclotron. Neurosurgery 1998; 42: 1229–1236, discussion 1236–1238

[25] McLaughlin MR, Kondziolka D, Flickinger JC, Lunsford S, Lunsford LD. The prospective natural history of cerebral venous malformations. Neurosurgery 1998; 43: 195–200, discussion 200–201

[26] Otten P, Pizzolato GP, Rilliet B, Berney J. One hundred thirty-one cases of cavernous angioma (cavernomas) of the CNS, discovered by retrospective analysis of 24,535 autopsies [in French]. Neurochirurgie 1989; 35: 82–83

[27] Porter PJ, Willinsky RA, Harper W, Wallace MC. Cerebral cavernous malformations: natural history and prognosis after clinical deterioration with or without hemorrhage. J Neurosurg 1997; 87: 190–197

[28] Wang CC, Liu A, Zhang JT, Sun B, Zhao YL. Surgical management of brain-stem cavernous malformations: report of 137 cases. Surg Neurol 2003; 59: 444–454, discussion 454

[29] Hasegawa T, McInerney J, Kondziolka D, Lee JY, Flickinger JC, Lunsford LD. Long-term results after stereotactic radiosurgery for patients with cavernous malformations. Neurosurgery 2002; 50: 1190–1197, discussion 1197–1198

[30] Kondziolka D, Lunsford LD, Flickinger JC, Kestle JR. Reduction of hemorrhage risk after stereotactic radiosurgery for cavernous malformations. J Neurosurg 1995; 83: 825–831

[31] Lunsford LD, Khan AA, Niranjan A, Kano H, Flickinger JC, Kondziolka D. Stereotactic radiosurgery for symptomatic solitary cerebral cavernous malformations considered high risk for resection. J Neurosurg 2010; 113: 23–29

[32] Hauck EF, Barnett SL, White JA, Samson D. Symptomatic brainstem cavernomas. Neurosurgery 2009; 64: 61–70, discussion 70–71

[33] de Oliveira JG, Lekovic GP, Safavi-Abbasi S, et al. Supracerebellar infratentorial approach to cavernous malformations of the brainstem: surgical variants and clinical experience with 45 patients. Neurosurgery 2010; 66: 389–399

[34] Nagy G, Razak A, Rowe JG, et al. Stereotactic radiosurgery for deep-seated cavernous malformations: a move toward more active, early intervention. Clinical article. J Neurosurg 2010; 113: 691–699

[35] Kim DG, Choe WJ, Paek SH, Chung HT, Kim IH, Han DH. Radiosurgery of intracranial cavernous malformations. Acta Neurochir (Wien) 2002; 144: 869–878, discussion 878

[36] García-Muñoz L, Velasco-Campos F, Lujan-Castilla P, Enriquez-Barrera M, Cervantes-Martínez A, Carrillo-Ruiz J. [Radiosurgery in the treatment of brain cavernomas: experience with 17 lesions treated in 15 patients [in French] Neurochirurgie 2007; 53: 243–250

[37] Seo Y, Fukuoka S, Takanashi M, et al. Gamma Knife surgery for angiographically occult vascular malformations. Stereotact Funct Neurosurg 1995; 64 (Suppl 1): 98–109

[38] Lindquist C, Guo WY, Karlsson B, Steiner L. Radiosurgery for venous angiomas. J Neurosurg 1993; 78: 531–536

10 The Argument Against Treating Cavernomas with Radiosurgery

Chun-Po Yen, David Schlesinger, and Jason Sheehan

Introduction

Following successful obliteration of a series of cerebral arteriovenous malformations (AVMs) using the Gamma Knife (Elekta AB, Stockholm, Sweden) in the 1970s, Steiner et al tried the same technique for cavernous malformations (CMs). Between 1983 and 1987, they treated 15 cases with unexpected unfavorable outcomes (▶ Fig. 10.1).[1] Karlsson et al in Stockholm and Lindquist in London continued to treat a few patients but again achieved unsatisfactory results.[1,2] Although these early endeavors proved that radiosurgery occasionally resulted in a limited decrease in the hemorrhage rate and reduced frequency of seizure, Steiner et al concluded that the high incidence of radiation-induced complications did not justify the limited protection the treatment could afford.[1] With more natural history studies available,[3,4] there is little doubt that asymptomatic or mildly symptomatic CMs are better treated with observation, given the hemorrhage rate of CMs in general is low. When lesions become symptomatic, especially those present with multiple hemorrhages, interventions may be required, and microsurgery is usually the treatment of choice if the lesions are readily accessible.

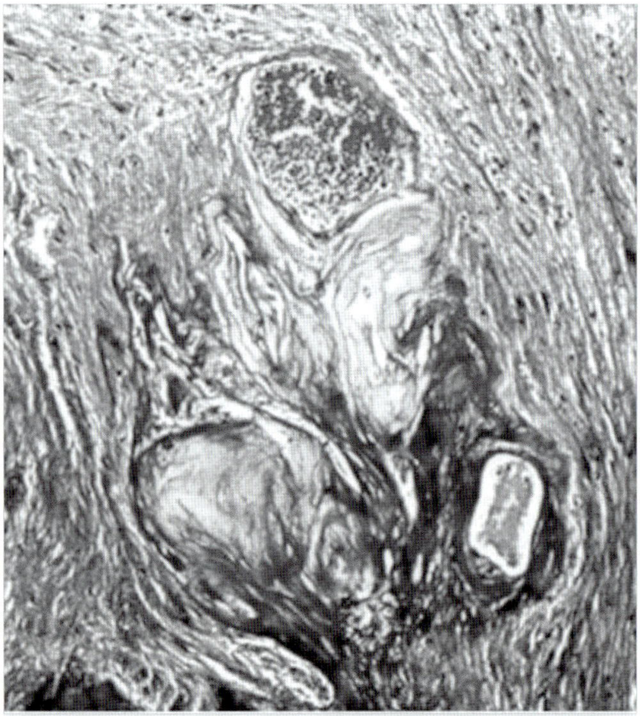

Fig. 10.1 Photograph showing a section of a cavernous malformation (CM) that was treated with Gamma Knife radiosurgery. Imaging did not show any change in the size, and the patient continued to have seizures. The CM was extirpated, and a histology study revealed that part of the CM had been obliterated. (Used with Permission from Steiner L, Karlsson B, Yen CP, Torner JC, Lindquist C, Schlesinger D. Radiosurgery in cavernous malformations: anatomy of a controversy. J Neurosurg 2010;113(1):16–21)

Currently, the radiosurgical literature pertaining to the treatment of CMs is limited to retrospective cohort studies, case series, and expert opinion. Thus, the evidence both for and against treatment is ***level III*** or lower.[1,5–10] The analysis of the relevant literature has resulted in disparate recommendations based in part on biases.

Several researchers, led by the Pittsburgh group, however, have revisited the feasibility of Gamma Knife radiosurgery for CMs since 1988 using magnetic resonance imaging (MRI) (unavailable earlier in Stockholm) for targeting and lower prescription doses. These studies reported favorable outcomes. In 1995 Kondziolka et al published a retrospective study suggesting that radiosurgery protect CMs from rupture.[7] The same group later reported longer-term results emphasizing improvement of the natural history of CMs following radiosurgery and advocating its use in cases of difficult approach for microsurgery.[6,8] An increasing number of neurosurgeons followed the policy of Pittsburgh without any reservation.[11–13] Others did so but with some caveats.[5,10,14] Pollock et al stated that "limitations in our knowledge of the natural history of untreated CMs make it impossible to conclude that radiosurgery protects against the future risk of bleeding. Radiosurgery of CMs does appear to entail a greater risk of radiation-related complications compared with that of AVMs."[10] Hua et al, commenting on the impressive results of Hasegawa et al, emphasized selection bias as well as the difference between hemorrhage and outcomes reported by Hasegawa and colleagues and those previously reported. They also criticized the use of the study group as its own control.[6] Nagy and colleagues advocated for the use of early radiosurgery for deep-seated CMs with more than one symptomatic hemorrhage.[9] However, as we pointed out in an editorial, the rate of hemorrhage was not appreciably different before and after treatment if one excludes the period of temporal clustering of hemorrhages well known to exist.[15]

None of the pathologies treated with Gamma Knife have been as controversial as CMs. Why is there such disagreement over radiosurgery for CMs, given that the radiosurgical techniques are now more available? Because they are angiographically occult vascular malformations, imaging cannot establish if CMs are affected by the radiation thus, the treatment success for a patient cannot be directly assessed. In fact, the changes typically seen are adverse radiological effects from the radiosurgery, resolution of a prior hemorrhage, or a new hemorrhage. Because the radiosurgical effects cannot be fully evaluated by imaging, an alternative to evaluating the outcome of radiosurgery for CMs is to calculate whether the rates of hemorrhage decrease following radiosurgery. This approach opens another area of controversy in using radiosurgery for CMs.[1]

Natural Course of Cavernous Malformations

Optimal management cannot be justified without a thorough understanding of the natural history. Studies analyzing the natural course of CMs are either prospective or retrospective. Retrospective studies can be further divided into two groups, depending on the methodology used. The first group of studies simply divides the number of observed hemorrhages by the number of risk-years (method A). The method assumes that all patients are born with the CMs and that the annual risk of hemorrhage is constant. Initially considered as developmental anomalies, there is now compelling evidence demonstrating that CMs can develop de novo. The second group of retrospective studies excludes the first hemorrhage, as well as the time at risk before the first hemorrhage, the rationale being that one cannot be sure when the patients with CMs will be at risk for hemorrhages. This group also uses the number of observed hemorrhages divided by the number of risk-years, but starting from the day after the first hemorrhage (method B), making the method insensitive for the time of the development of the CMs.

Under both methods, the retrospective studies report on incidence of hemorrhage, which may or may not equal the prospective risk of hemorrhage. A selection bias may result in a significant difference between the calculated incidence and the actual annual risk of a hemorrhage. The likelihood of drawing skewed conclusions is very high if the patient selection is based on those with prior ruptures. The impact of this selection bias is much weaker in prospective studies, making it reasonable to assume that the calculated incidence of hemorrhages equals the actual risk for hemorrhage.

In ▶ Table 10.1, the annual risks of hemorrhage obtained in four published studies analyzing the natural history of CMs are provided.[4,16–18] The incidence of hemorrhage using prospective methods ranged from 0.8 to 3.8%. Recalculating the same group of patients using retrospective method A results in a range of 0.3 to 2.3%.The minimal difference can be explained by the way patient-years at risk are calculated. In method A, we assume that patients were born with CMs, which might not be true because of the de novo CMs in sporadic and familial cases.[19,20]

Because the natural course of CMs is still poorly understood, it is tempting to use the pretreatment incidence of hemorrhage in the treated patient population as an indicator of the pretreatment risk instead of the 0.3 to 3.8% annual risk found in the articles analyzing the natural course of CMs.[3,4,18,21,22] The argument used is that the CMs in the treated patient population represent a higher risk for hemorrhages than other CMs, the proof being that they hemorrhaged frequently before the treatment. This assumption may potentially lead to erroneous conclusions.

In ▶ Table 10.2, we analyze the annual risk of hemorrhage of CM patients from radiosurgical series, which selected only so-called high-risk patients. Using retrospective method A, hemorrhage rates in these high-risk patients ranged from 3.9 to 6.5%, a little higher than the reported rates of 0.3 to 3.8% in studies of natural history. Recalculating with method B, the hemorrhage rates become 17 to 36%.[5,6,10,22–24] Can this difference be explained by a much higher hemorrhage risk among the patients selected for radiosurgery, or is it mainly caused by a methodo-

Table 10.1 Incidence of annual hemorrhage from studies analyzing the natural history of cavernous malformations using retrospective method A before and prospective method after the cases enter the studies

			Prospective			Retrospective method A		
Study	No. of patients	Follow-up	Hemorrhages*	Risk-years	Annual incidence	Hemorrhages*	Risk-years	Annual incidence
Robinson et al[4]	66	66	6	2,284	0.3%*	1	119	0.8%
Kondziolka et al[7]	122	122	61	4,551	1.3%	9	342	2.6%
Kim et al[16]	62	28	57	2,510	2.3%	2	52	3.8%
Porter et al[18]	173	110	44	6,488	0.7%*	7	427	1.6%

* Hemorrhagic rate are calculated by us from the numbers of hemorrhages and risk-years reported by the authors in the publications.

Table 10.2 Incidence of annual hemorrhage from radiosurgical series using retrospective methods A and B

		Method A			Method B		
Study	No. of patients	Hemorrhages	Risk-years	Annual incidences	Hemorrhages	Risk-years	Annual incidences
Amin-Hanjani et al[5]	95	132	2,635	5.0%	59	339	17%
Pollock et al[10]	17	48	748	6.4%	31	125	25%
Tsien et al[24]	21	34	863	3.9%	36	121	30%
Hasegawa et al[6]	82	202	3,091	6.5%	120	354	34%
Kim et al[22]	22	30	750	4.0%	10	28	36%
Liu et al[23]	125	167	NA	NA	55	188	29%

logical flaw? If we agree that the higher risk of subsequent hemorrhages for some period of time (i.e., clustering of hemorrhages) occurs in patients with prior symptomatic hemorrhage, as proposed by Barker et al,[25] the calculation of hemorrhage rate using method B will be problematic. This is because the increased number of hemorrhages at this specific time period and the prematurely terminated follow-up time by radiosurgery result in a skewed high hemorrhage rate.

Increased Hemorrhage Risk for Some Cavernous Malformations

The available evidence suggests that CMs are not static lesions where the risk for a clinically detectable hemorrhage is constant and independent of anatomical and clinical factors. It has been suggested that the risk for hemorrhage is higher in female patients,[3,4] and in centrally located CMs.[17,18] Numerous studies also observed that the risk of CMs having a clinically detectable hemorrhage increases after an earlier one.[6–8] It is unknown, however, how long this increased risk persists. It is reasonable to believe that the increase in risk is temporary. If not, a larger number of CMs would have a higher risk for hemorrhage, as the majority of these lesions show imaging evidence of either acute or subacute hemorrhage. It should also be noted that, although blood degradation products suggest prior hemorrhages, they may occur also from extravasations of small amounts of erythrocytes.

To our knowledge, the length of the increased risk has not been analyzed in any publications. Therefore, we cannot exclude the possibility that the decrease in hemorrhage rate seen after the treatment of recently hemorrhaged CMs is at least to some extent caused by a reset to prehemorrhage bleeding risk rather than caused by the treatment.

Postradiosurgery Hemorrhage Rate and Incidence of Complications

If all patients are summarized in the 15 studies reporting results following CM radiosurgery, 132 (19%) of the patients developed a complication, of which around half were permanent.[1,5,6,10–14,22–24,26–29] Amin-Hanjani et al reported three lethal complications. Thus, the incidence and the severity of complications are not trivial after radiosurgery for CMs.[5]

Risk/Benefit Analysis

Based on the presented facts, one cannot use the pretreatment incidence of hemorrhage to assess if radiosurgery has or has not affected the natural course of disease. Instead, one can use a fundamental principle in radiobiology: the relation between the radiation dose and the risk for complications. There would be a higher risk for complications with the higher the dose given. If CMs respond to radiosurgery, there must be a relation between the dose and the response as well; the higher the dose given, the lower the posttreatment incidence of hemorrhages after 2 years. Thus, by extracting the complications and posttreatment hemorrhage rates from different clinical studies, we can get an idea of how steep the dose-response curve is for CMs in relation to the dose-risk curve. For this, we used 10 publications where the results could be extracted from the information published.[1,5,6,10,14,23,24,26,29] As seen in ▶ Fig. 10.2, there is a big difference in outcome in different centers, the most common being a 2 to 4% risk for hemorrhage and a 10 to 30% risk for symptomatic complications. The trend in the meta-analysis is that the incidence for complications increases with an increasing incidence of hemorrhages 2 years or more after radiosurgery. Given the small number of patients in the studies used, the conclusion is tentative. However, the data suggest that the dose-response relation is weak, which can be interpreted as a very limited response to radiation, or that the maximum radiation response is already reached when a low radiation dose is given.

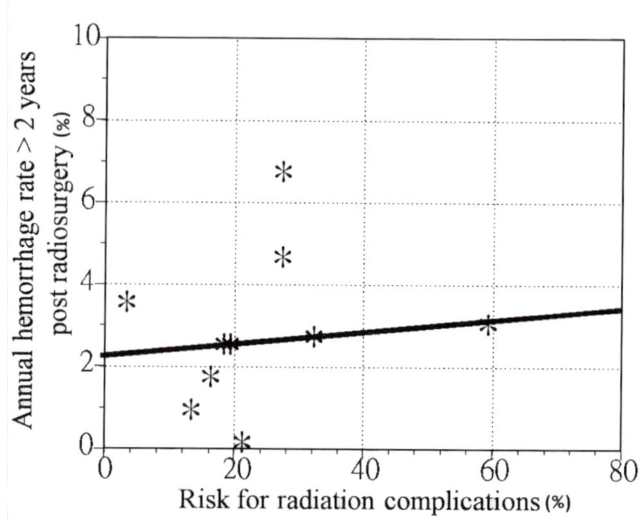

Fig. 10.2 Relation between the incidence of complications and the annual incidence of hemorrhages > 2 years after the treatment. The line represents the linear regression after the highest and lowest annual hemorrhage rates have been excluded. (from Steiner L, Karlsson B, Yen CP, Torner JC, Lindquist C, Schlesinger D. Radiosurgery in cavernous malformations: anatomy of a controversy. J Neurosurg 2010;113(1):16–21, with permission.)

Radiosurgery for Cavernous Malformations Considered High Risk for Surgical Resection

The controversy regarding the use of radiosurgery for CMs boils down to the validity of the methods used to calculate and compare pre- versus postradiosurgery hemorrhage rates. Concerning the feasibility of surgical extirpation with reasonable risks, the opinions of a neurosurgeon high on the learning curve of the management of this kind of lesion should be sought, in addition to the decision of the local multidisciplinary stereotactic radiosurgery conference. Criteria for the inoperability of CMs remain a matter of debate and vary tremendously based on neurosurgical bias and expertise. More frequent use of neurophysiological testing when selecting the appropriate approach to the lesion as well as changing the technique may make microsurgery for CMs at a distance from the pia feasible.

Conclusion

Radiosurgery for CMs, although conceptually attractive, does not fulfill the rigid criteria of minimal risk and beneficial risk/benefit ratio for a lesion with a benign natural history. Patient-year analysis (such as methods A and B) has some flaws, such as the question of constancy or randomness of risk. A prospective, randomized study is needed to establish the role of radiosurgery in the management of CMs. At present, recommendations both for and against treatment have been made in the literature. At most, these should be considered grade 2C recommendations based on studies with significant methodological flaws.

References

[1] Steiner L, Karlsson B, Yen CP, Torner JC, Lindquist C, Schlesinger D. Radiosurgery in cavernous malformations: anatomy of a controversy. J Neurosurg 2010; 113: 16–21, discussion 21–22

[2] Karlsson B, Kihlström L, Lindquist C, Ericson K, Steiner L. Radiosurgery for cavernous malformations. J Neurosurg 1998; 88: 293–297

[3] Moriarity JL, Wetzel M, Clatterbuck RE, et al. The natural history of cavernous malformations: a prospective study of 68 patients. Neurosurgery 1999; 44: 1166–1171, discussion 1172–1173

[4] Robinson JR, Awad IA, Little JR. Natural history of the cavernous angioma. J Neurosurg 1991; 75: 709–714

[5] Amin-Hanjani S, Ogilvy CS, Candia GJ, Lyons S, Chapman PH. Stereotactic radiosurgery for cavernous malformations: Kjellberg's experience with proton beam therapy in 98 cases at the Harvard Cyclotron. Neurosurgery 1998; 42: 1229–1236, discussion 1236–1238

[6] Hasegawa T, McInerney J, Kondziolka D, Lee JY, Flickinger JC, Lunsford LD. Long-term results after stereotactic radiosurgery for patients with cavernous malformations. Neurosurgery 2002; 50: 1190–1197, discussion 1197–1198

[7] Kondziolka D, Lunsford LD, Flickinger JC, Kestle JR. Reduction of hemorrhage risk after stereotactic radiosurgery for cavernous malformations. J Neurosurg 1995; 83: 825–831

[8] Lunsford LD, Khan AA, Niranjan A, Kano H, Flickinger JC, Kondziolka D. Stereotactic radiosurgery for symptomatic solitary cerebral cavernous malformations considered high risk for resection. J Neurosurg 2010; 113: 23–29

[9] Nagy G, Razak A, Rowe JG, et al. Stereotactic radiosurgery for deep-seated cavernous malformations: a move toward more active, early intervention. Clinical article. J Neurosurg 2010; 113: 691–699

[10] Pollock BE, Garces YI, Stafford SL, Foote RL, Schomberg PJ, Link MJ. Stereotactic radiosurgery for cavernous malformations. J Neurosurg 2000; 93: 987–991

[11] Huang YC, Tseng CK, Chang CN, Wei KC, Liao CC, Hsu PW. LINAC radiosurgery for intracranial cavernous malformation: 10-year experience. Clin Neurol Neurosurg 2006; 108: 750–756

[12] Kida Y, Kobayashi T, Tanaka T. Treatment of symptomatic AOVMs with radiosurgery. Acta Neurochir Suppl (Wien) 1995; 63: 68–72

[13] Liscák R, Vladyka V, Simonová G, Vymazal J, Novotny J. Gamma knife surgery of brain cavernous hemangiomas. J Neurosurg 2005; 102 (Suppl): 207–213

[14] Mitchell P, Hodgson TJ, Seaman S, Kemeny AA, Forster DM. Stereotactic radiosurgery and the risk of haemorrhage from cavernous malformations. Br J Neurosurg 2000; 14: 96–100

[15] Sheehan J, Schlesinger D. Editorial. Radiosurgery and cavernous malformations. J Neurosurg 2010; 113: 689–690, discussion 690

[16] Kim DS, Park YG, Choi JU, Chung SS, Lee KC. An analysis of the natural history of cavernous malformations. Surg Neurol 1997; 48: 9–17, discussion 17–18

[17] Kondziolka D, Lunsford LD, Kestle JR. The natural history of cerebral cavernous malformations. J Neurosurg 1995; 83: 820–824

[18] Porter PJ, Willinsky RA, Harper W, Wallace MC. Cerebral cavernous malformations: natural history and prognosis after clinical deterioration with or without hemorrhage. J Neurosurg 1997; 87: 190–197

[19] Brunereau L, Levy C, Laberge S, Houtteville J, Labauge P. De novo lesions in familial form of cerebral cavernous malformations: clinical and MR features in 29 non-Hispanic families. Surg Neurol 2000; 53: 475–482, discussion 482–483

[20] Zabramski JM, Wascher TM, Spetzler RF, et al. The natural history of familial cavernous malformations: results of an ongoing study. J Neurosurg 1994; 80: 422–432

[21] Del Curling O, Kelly DL, Elster AD, Craven TE. An analysis of the natural history of cavernous angiomas. J Neurosurg 1991; 75: 702–708

[22] Kim DG, Choe WJ, Paek SH, Chung HT, Kim IH, Han DH. Radiosurgery of intracranial cavernous malformations. Acta Neurochir (Wien) 2002; 144: 869–878, discussion 878

[23] Liu AL, Wang C, Sun S, Wang M, Liu P. Gamma knife radiosurgery for tumors involving the cavernous sinus. Stereotact Funct Neurosurg 2005; 83: 45–51

[24] Tsien C, Souhami L, Sadikot A, et al. Stereotactic radiosurgery in the management of angiographically occult vascular malformations. Int J Radiat Oncol Biol Phys 2001; 50: 133–138

[25] Barker FG, Amin-Hanjani S, Butler WE, et al. Temporal clustering of hemorrhages from untreated cavernous malformations of the central nervous system. Neurosurgery 2001; 49: 15–24, discussion 24–25

[26] Chang SD, Levy RP, Adler JR, Martin DP, Krakovitz PR, Steinberg GK. Stereotactic radiosurgery of angiographically occult vascular malformations: 14-year experience. Neurosurgery 1998; 43: 213–220, discussion 220–221

[27] Kim MS, Pyo SY, Jeong YG, Lee SI, Jung YT, Sim JH. Gamma knife surgery for intracranial cavernous hemangioma. J Neurosurg 2005; 102 (Suppl): 102–106

[28] Stea RA, Schicker L, King GA, Winfield JA. Stereotactic linear radiosurgery for cavernous angiomas. Stereotact Funct Neurosurg 1994; 63: 255–265

[29] Zhang N, Pan L, Wang BJ, Wang EM, Dai JZ, Cai PW. Gamma knife radiosurgery for cavernous hemangiomas. J Neurosurg 2000; 93 (Suppl 3): 74–77

11 Optic Apparatus Tolerance Up to 8 Gy

Jason P. Sheehan and Zhiyuan Xu

In medicine, the guiding principle of the Hippocratic oath is to do no harm. In the early days of stereotactic radiosurgery (SRS), neurosurgeons and radiation oncologists grappled with dose selection to achieve a favorable rate of tumor control while avoiding harm to critical structures, particularly the optic nerve and chiasm in intracranial radiosurgery. Over the years, 8 Gy has become accepted as the tolerable dose for the optic apparatus in single-session radiosurgery.[1] This 8-Gy tolerance has meant different things to clinicians even at leading centers. Some have advocated 8 Gy as the maximum tolerated dose, whereas others have maintained that 8 Gy can be delivered to a "short" segment of the nerve or to 1% volume of the optic apparatus. The 8-Gy tolerance also led to the concept that 5-mm clearance was required between the planned treatment volume and the optic apparatus for single-session radiosurgery.

The 8-Gy standard appears to have arisen from a few retrospective studies based on patients treated in the 1990s (▶ Table 11.1). All of these reports represent ***level III evidence***. Certainly, the authors of these studies analyzed the optic apparatus tolerance with the best evidence available at the time. In this chapter, we evaluate the scientific foundations that led to the origination of the 8-Gy limit for the optic apparatus.

The Neuroanatomical Features of the Optic Apparatus

The optic nerves begin at the posterior portion of each globe. They pass through the approximate center of each orbit and are encompassed by the rectus muscles and periorbital fat. From each globe, they angle rostrally to pass through the optic canals and exit near the anterior clinoid process. Both nerves meet at the chiasm. Typically, the chiasm lies above the diaphragma sellae and the pituitary gland. However, ~ 30% of patients demonstrate either a pre- or postfixed chiasm. A prefixed chiasm overlies the tuberculum sellae; a postfixed chiasm, above the dorsum sellae.

Nerve fibers within the optic nerves partially divide at the optic chiasm. Medially located fibers cross to the contralateral optic tract, whereas laterally located fibers remain in the ipsilaterally located tract. The optic tracts represent the visual projections just beyond the chiasm. On magnetic resonance imaging (MRI) or computed tomography (CT), the optic tracts are usually visual for 1 to 2 cm beyond the chiasm before the fibers project into the brain parenchyma and become less distinct. Diffusion tensor MRI can be used to track the optic radiations; such information can be co-registered in radiosurgical planning systems.[2]

The optic apparatus comprises the optic nerves, chiasm, and optic tracts; these structures are typically defined on neuroimaging studies and contoured appropriately. Because the diameter of the optic nerve is ~ 2 to 5 mm, careful attention to neuroimaging protocols and tomographic slice orientation is important for accurate contouring. In frame-based radiosurgery, it is useful to angle the base of the frame parallel to the direction of the rostrally projecting optic nerves. Thin-sliced, volume acquisition axial and coronal neuroimaging with and without fat suppression techniques is prudent for delineation of the optic apparatus. Dose-volume histograms can be used to determine the dose given to the optic apparatus.

The Concern for Radiation Injury to the Optic Apparatus

Radiation-induced optic injury has long been a feared complication of external beam radiotherapy (EBRT) and radiosurgery. It is generally believed that there is a 5% risk of developing an optic neuropathy within 5 years when delivering 50 Gy to the chiasm and that there is a 50% risk of blindness when delivering 65 Gy of fractionated radiotherapy to the chiasm.[3] With EBRT, radiation-induced optic neuropathy typically manifested itself at 10 to 20 months posttreatment (range 6 months to 3 + years).[4,5] For EBRT, fractionation, total dose, treatment volume, and dose rate all appear to contribute to the risk of an adverse effect to the visual system.[6–8] For radiosurgery, the issue of fractionation plays less of a role, as most radiosurgery is delivered in a single session, although it can occasionally be delivered in as many as five sessions.

The underlying mechanism for radiation-induced optic neuropathy is not fully understood. Moreover, it is likely multifactorial. It is believed that radiation-induced injury to the microvasculature of the optic apparatus plays a role in visual decline. Endothelial cells are sensitive to radiation. They may be stimulated to proliferate and compromise vital blood flow to the optic pathways. Also, inflammatory processes may be triggered to induce a vasculitis and thereby alter myelin composition of the optic nerves. Optic nerves are myelinated, and radiation could disrupt the normal composition, metabolism, and formation of myelin.[9] Such mechanisms have been supported to a degree by experimental research that indicates radiation effectuates changes through induction of inflammation and changes to the microvasculature and oligodendroglia.[10–12]

Early Reports on Radiosurgical Tolerance of the Optic Apparatus

In 1993 Tishler et al pooled the experience of two leading centers to examine the tolerance of cranial nerves in and around the cavernous sinus.[34] The cohort of patients included 62 patients, of which 42 had meningiomas near the cavernous sinus. Thirty-three of these patients were treated with Gamma Knife (Elekta AB, Stockholm, Sweden) radiosurgery at the University of Pittsburgh, and 29 were treated with a 6-MV linear accelerator (LINAC) at the Joint Center for Radiation Therapy at Harvard. Maximum doses were computed for the optic nerve and chiasm. With a median follow-up of 19 months (range 3–49

Table 11.1 Selected studies of radiosurgical tolerance of the optic apparatus

Study	No. of patients	Prescription dose (range, Gy)	Dose/fraction (range, Gy)	D_{max} to OA (range, Gy)	Visual decline rate (%)	Level of evidence
Tishler et al (1993)[34]	62	10–40	Single session	< 8	0	III
				8–10	50	
				> 10	20	
Leber (1998)[35]	45	14.3 (8.0–25.0)	Single session	< 10	0	III
				10–15	26.7	
				> 15	77.8	
Stafford et al (2003)[14]	215	18 (12–30)	Single session	< 8	1.7	III
				8–10	1.7	
				10–12	0	
				> 12	6.9	
Adler et al (2006)[15]	49	20.3 (15.0–30.0)	2–5 sessions	< 8	6*	III
Lee (2008)[36]	11	25 (18–38)	5 (3.8–6.7)	< 5/fraction	0	III
Pollock (2008)[37]	62	16.3 (11.0–20.0)	Single session	9.5 (5.0–12.6)	0	III
Hasegawa et al (2010)[16]	94	11.4 (10.0–18.0)	Single session	≤ 8	7	III
				9–14	0	
				> 15	38	
Marchetti et al (2011)[17]	17	25	5	25	0	III

* *Two percent radiosurgery-induced.*
Abbreviations: D_{max}, *maximum dose; OA, optic apparatus.*

months), four optic neuropathies developed. In those patients receiving > 8 Gy to any part of the optic apparatus (i.e., optic nerves or chiasm), 24% (4 of 17) developed visual complications. This was in marked distinction to a 0 percent incidence of optic neuropathy in the subgroup (0 of 35 patients) who received < 8 Gy. It is worth noting that the median and minimum follow-up periods in this series were fairly short. Moreover, many of these patients were treated in the early era of SRS. Hence, the contouring of the optic apparatus was performed in some patients with CT alone, and the dosimetry did not rely on current, robust computer-based algorithms. Also, patients in this study did not routinely get neuro-ophthalmologic assessments as part of their follow-up.

Nearly 5 years later, Leber et al published their experience with 50 patients who had undergone Gamma Knife radiosurgery for benign skull base tumors.[35] In this case, the minimum follow-up was 24 months, and the mean was 40 months. Follow-up examinations did include neuro-ophthalmologic assessments. The mean dose to the optic structures was computed for 66 at-risk eyes. Of these, vision was unchanged in 51.5% and improved in 25.8%. Radiation-induced optic neuropathy was identified in 22.7% of the at-risk eyes. In those with a critical dose < 10 Gy, no signs of radiation-induced optic neuropathy were noted. However, the incidence of optic neuropathy for those receiving 10 to 15 Gy was 26.7%; for those receiving a dose ≥ 15 Gy, the incidence was 77.8%. The authors computed a hazard ratio for radiation-induced optic neuropathy of 1.47 per Gy. They concluded that a dose as high as 10 Gy to the optic apparatus is likely to be tolerated without adverse effects. Of note, the analysis did rely at least in part on CT-based imaging and the early KULA 4.3 software for dose calculations.

More Recent Reports on Radiosurgical Tolerance of the Optic Apparatus

Radiosurgery has evolved over the past 40 years. This evolution has involved technological improvements in the radiosurgical device, integration of MRI and more sophisticated neuroimaging, refinement of treatment protocols, and improvements in dose planning. As such, the more recent reports on radiosurgical tolerance to the optic apparatus draw from patients being treated with contemporary radiosurgical techniques. One such report from Ove et al evaluated 18 patients undergoing Gamma Knife radiosurgery for perisellar tumors.[13] Most of these patients had pituitary adenomas, but some harbored a meningioma. Patients underwent both pre- and postoperative neuro-ophthalmologic assessment, including visual field and cranial nerve examinations. Median follow-up in this series was 24 months (range 11–43 months) for visual field testing and 30 months for other clinical testing. With regard to radiation delivered, two of the patients underwent EBRT in addition to Gamma Knife radiosurgery, and two patients were treated twice with Gamma Knife radiosurgery. The volume-averaged dose to the chiasm ranged from 1 to 8.8 Gy (mean 5.2 Gy); the maximum chiasmal dose ranged from 2.5 to 14.1 Gy (mean 9 Gy). In this study, no patients were noted to have worsened function of the optic apparatus. The authors contend that 8 Gy is a conservative estimate for single-fraction radiosurgical tolerance and that 10 Gy may be a more justifiable limit.

In another landmark work published in 2003, Stafford et al detailed the dose to the optic apparatus and the incidence of optic neuropathy in 215 patients with sellar and parasellar tumors.[14] In this patient cohort, 122 had meningiomas, 89 harbored pituitary adenomas, and 7 had craniopharyngiomas. Overall, the median maximum dose to the optic nerve was 10 Gy (range 0.4–16 Gy). The incidence of radiation-induced optic neuropathy was 1.9% ($n = 4$ patients) at a median time of 4 years after radiosurgery. Seventy-five percent of the patients who developed optic neuropathy had EBRT either prior to or after SRS. The authors note that the risk of developing optic neuropathy was 1.1% for those receiving ≤ 12 Gy to their optic apparatus. In this series, those patients with visual complaints had routine testing of visual fields and acuity. However, patients who did not complain of visual decline did not appear to have routine testing. Thus, this study may have underestimated the risk of optic neuropathy. Nevertheless, the authors contend that 12 Gy conferred a low risk of visual decline in patients undergoing single-session radiosurgery. This represented a 50% increase over the traditionally held view of a tolerable 8-Gy maximum dose.

In 2006 Adler et al reported on their experience with multisession SRS with the CyberKnife (Accuray Inc., Sunnyvale, CA).[15] In this study, they reported on a cohort of 49 patients with diverse neuropathologies in and around the optic apparatus. The histologies included meningioma ($n = 27$), pituitary adenoma ($n = 19$), craniopharyngioma ($n = 2$), and mixed germ cell tumor ($n = 1$). A total marginal dose of 20.3 Gy (range 15.0–30.0 Gy) was delivered at a mean isodose line of 80% (range 70–95%). Patients were treated with five ($n = 19$), four ($n = 2$), three ($n = 17$), and two sessions ($n = 11$); sessions were separated by 12 to 24 hours. The authors noted that they tried not to exceed a maximum dose of 8 Gy per session to the anterior visual pathways. In instances where the optic pathways were well demarcated on neuroimaging studies, the optic structures were usually kept to < 5 Gy per session. Ophthalmologic testing was performed at 6-month intervals on all patients for the first 3 years posttreatment and then yearly thereafter. With a mean ophthalmologic follow-up of 49 months (range 6–96 months), visual fields were stable or improved in 94% of patients. Two patients had visual decline in the setting of demonstrable tumor progression. A third patient had visual decline likely related to radiation-induced injury. This particular patient had undergone prior radiotherapy and three separate radiosurgical procedures to treat a progressive pituitary adenoma. Such a finding underscores the diminished radiosurgical tolerance of the optic apparatus when prior radiotherapy has been administered. Limitations of the study include the retrospective nature, the wide range in biological equivalent dose (76.1–220.0 Gy, assuming an α/β ratio of 2), and the imprecise notion of exactly how much dose was given to the optic apparatus. Nevertheless, this study demonstrated that an 8-Gy maximum dose to the optic apparatus per session conferred a low risk of visual decline.

In two more recent publications by Hasegawa et al and Marchetti et al, the tolerance of the optic apparatus to radiosurgery is further assessed under contemporary practice paradigms.[16,17] In particular, dose planning used MRI and generally robust computer-based software. Hasegawa and colleagues evaluated the risk of visual decline in a cohort of 94 patients with craniopharyngiomas followed up for a median period of 68 months. They delivered a median dose of 10 Gy to the optic apparatus (range 2–18 Gy). The overall risk of optic neuropathy in this series was 5%. The authors further analyzed the groups in terms of low (≤ 8 Gy), medium (9–14 Gy), and high (≥ 15 Gy) dose to the optic apparatus; the optic neuropathy rates were 7%, 0%, and 38% in the low, medium, and high groups, respectively. The one patient in the low-dose group who developed optic neuropathy had undergone prior EBRT. A less touted but perhaps more important finding in the study was that 15 patients underwent repeat radiosurgery 6 to 79 months after initial radiosurgery. In those undergoing repeat radiosurgery, a cumulative dose of 14 to 20 Gy was given. At a median follow-up period of 42 months, none of the 15 patients developed optic neuropathy. These rates of optic neuropathy must be considered conservative in that the clinical follow-up was obtained through information from referring doctors, patient questionnaires, or telephone interviews. The authors noted that visual examination data, including visual acuity and field information, was incorporated into the analysis, but they did not specify the precise intervals for neuro-ophthalmologic follow-up in the study.

Marchetti et al reported on their use of multisession radiosurgery for the treatment of optic nerve sheath meningiomas for 17 evaluable patients.[17] The target volume was covered by an isodose line that ranged from 75 to 85%. Patients underwent routine neuro-ophthalmologic evaluations at 3 months after treatment and then at 6-month intervals for 2 years, yearly thereafter. They used a prescription dose of 25 Gy delivered in five fractions on consecutive days. With a median follow-up of 27 months (range 11–68 months), visual fields improved in 35% and remained stable in 65%. Visual acuity improved in 27% and remained stable in 87%. No decline in visual fields or acuity was noted.

In treating more than 800 patients with pituitary adenomas with SRS at our center, we have observed a < 1% risk of optic apparatus injury when limiting to a dose of 8 Gy to < 1% of the optic apparatus volume.[18–21] Even so, we have observed a few patients who have developed radiation-induced neuropathies with < 8 Gy to the optic apparatus (▶ Fig. 11.1). Such patients usually have had nonmalignant systemic comorbidities (e.g., diabetes or multiple sclerosis) or had received prior fractionated radiation therapy to the area. Radiosurgical dose planning requires the meticulous contouring of

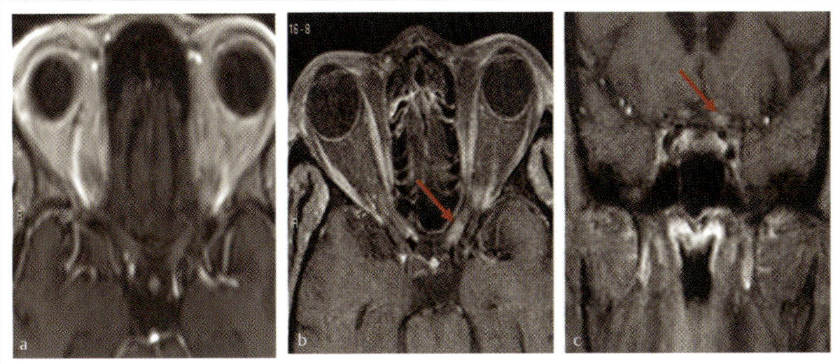

Fig. 11.1 (a) A postcontrast, T1-weighted axial magnetic resonance (MR) image of a patient prior to radiosurgery. The patient had radiation therapy, then underwent stereotactic radiosurgery. A maximum dose of 4 Gy was delivered to the optic apparatus. Several months after radiosurgery, the patient developed visual decline. The postcontrast, T1-weighted axial (b) and coronal (c) MR images show enhancement of the left optic nerve consistent with radiation-induced neuropathy.

the optic nerves, chiasms, and tracts and running dose-volume histograms to assess the optic apparatus. In current SRS systems, extensive shielding generally can be used to achieve delivery of a maximum dose of 8 Gy to the optic apparatus and still deliver 12 to 25 Gy to most sellar and parasellar tumors (▶ Fig. 11.2).

Potential Factors Increasing the Risk of Optic Neuropathy

In the radiosurgical literature, there is little to no accounting for comorbidities that can affect the tolerance of the optic apparatus to radiation. However, it is clear that nonmalignant comorbidities can affect the tolerance of neural structures, including the optic apparatus, to radiation. It is also widely believed, although not well proven from the standpoint of evidence-based medicine, that those patients with preexisting visual deficits may be at greater risk of a radiosurgically induced visual decline.

The risk of optic neuropathy appears to increase with age. For patients undergoing radiation therapy with a dose > 60 Gy, Parsons et al noted the incidence of optic neuropathy was 26% in patients 50 to 70 years old and 56% for patients older than age 70.[7] Bhandare et al noted optic neuropathy rates of 0% (< 20 years old), 4% (20–50 years old), 13% (51–70 years old), and 14% (> 70 years old).[22]

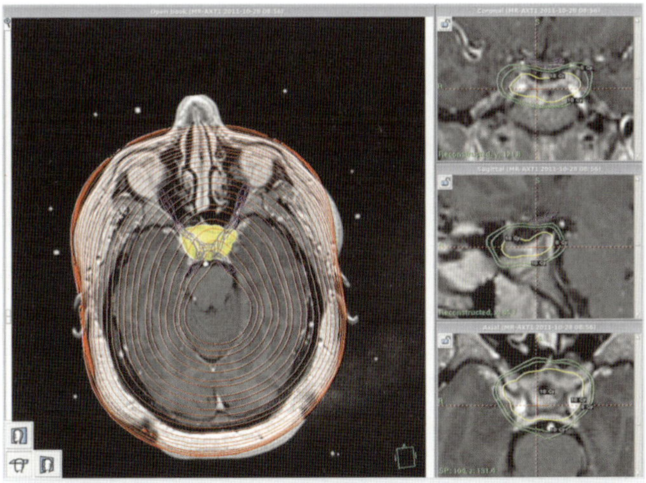

Fig. 11.2 Steep dose gradients can be achieved in dose planning with currently available radiosurgical units. This dose plan depicts a patient with recurrent pituitary adenoma for which the prescription isodose line of 18 Gy (*yellow line*) is surrounded by the 10 Gy (*inner green isodose line*) and 8 Gy (*outer green line*) that bend around the optic apparatus.

Other nonmalignant systemic diseases have been shown to be linked to increased risks after radiation. These include diabetes, hypertension, collagen vascular disease, and inflammatory disease. In an analysis of 15 studies published in the literature, Chon and Loeffler determined that the majority of the studies revealed a lower radiation tolerance for patients with such nonmalignant systemic diseases.[23] Lowell et al noted a significantly increased risk of serious toxicity in six patients with multiple sclerosis who underwent SRS with a median margin dose of 13 Gy (range 12–21 Gy). These toxicities included some permanent cranial nerve injuries.[24] Daniels et al[25] reported a serious case of radiation-induced optic neuritis in a patient with multiple sclerosis who underwent radiosurgery for a pituitary adenoma. Whether controlling these diseases reduces the risk of radiation-induced injury remains to be determined.

Chemotherapy may cause optic apparatus injury and could potentiate the risk of optic neuropathy after radiation therapy or radiosurgery.[26] Also, previous radiation to the optic apparatus likely increases the risk of subsequent radiosurgically induced optic neuropathy.[21] Flickinger et al reported a 10% risk of optic neuropathy in reirradiated patients receiving 46 Gy ~ 7.5 years after an initial 40 Gy.[27] In a series of 90 patients undergoing SRS for persistent Cushing's Disease, JPS team noted that 80% of those experiencing damage to cranial nerves in the sellar region had prior EBRT or radiosurgery.[21] The specific repair and recovery that can occur in the optic apparatus after previous radiation therapy or radiosurgery has not been well studied. None of the available literature examining tolerance of the optic apparatus to radiosurgery sheds enough light on the decreased tolerance related to age, comorbidities, or previous radiation. It does seem intuitively pleasing to deduce that patients in these risk groups may warrant a lower dose than those without such risk factors.

Potential Treatments

Whenever possible, optic neuropathy is to be avoided. However, optic neuropathy will always be a risk of radiosurgery to the sellar and parasellar region. When radiation-induced optic neuropathy occurs, the standard approach is to employ a short course of corticosteroids to treat it.[1] Additional but largely anecdotal reports have indicated therapeutic benefits for treating optic neuropathy with bevacizumab (Avastin), vitamin E, pentoxifylline (Trental), optic nerve sheath fenestration, and hyperbaric oxygen.[4,28–31] Anticoagulants have not been shown to be helpful in preventing or treating radiation-induced optic neuropathy.[32,33]

Conclusion

In a commencement speech at Stanford University, Steve Jobs said, "Don't be trapped by dogma—which is living with the results of other people's thinking." Challenging the 8-Gy standard may be justified based on the literature from which it was derived; however, the evidence leading to the 8-Gy rule appears to be constrained by inherent limitations in study design. Certainly, the practice of SRS has evolved substantially from the era from which the data were derived. A reevaluation of the 8-Gy standard thus appears justified for some cases. A higher tolerance of the optic apparatus in most patients than previously believed could increase the number of patients for whom radiosurgery is indicated. It may also allow delivery of a higher dose to a tumor adjacent to the optic apparatus, thereby permitting a better chance of tumor control and endocrine remission.

Nevertheless, some patients receiving < 8 Gy to the optic apparatus have developed radiosurgically induced optic neuropathy. Based on available literature, then, the safest maximum dose to the optic apparatus is still 8 Gy. The maximum dose to the optic apparatus can be pushed to 12 Gy in select circumstances in which no prior radiation was given and no concerning comorbidities exist.

References

[1] Girkin CA, Comey CH, Lunsford LD, Goodman ML, Kline LB. Radiation optic neuropathy after stereotactic radiosurgery. Ophthalmology 1997; 104: 1634–1643

[2] Maruyama K, Kamada K, Shin M, et al. Optic radiation tractography integrated into simulated treatment planning for Gamma Knife surgery. J Neurosurg 2007; 107: 721–726

[3] Emami B, Lyman J, Brown A, et al. Tolerance of normal tissue to therapeutic irradiation. Int J Radiat Oncol Biol Phys 1991; 21: 109–122

[4] Borruat FX, Schatz NJ, Glaser JS, Matos L, Feuer W. Radiation optic neuropathy: report of cases, role of hyperbaric oxygen therapy, and literature review. Neuroophthalmology 1996; 16: 255–266

[5] Danesh-Meyer HV. Radiation-induced optic neuropathy. J Clin Neurosci 2008; 15: 95–100

[6] Parsons JT, Bova FJ, Mendenhall WM, Million RR, Fitzgerald CR. Response of the normal eye to high dose radiotherapy. Oncology (Williston Park) 1996; 10: 837–847, discussion 847–848, 851–852

[7] Parsons JT, Bova FJ, Fitzgerald CR, Mendenhall WM, Million RR. Radiation optic neuropathy after megavoltage external-beam irradiation: analysis of time-dose factors. Int J Radiat Oncol Biol Phys 1994; 30: 755–763

[8] Mayo C, Martel MK, Marks LB, Flickinger J, Nam J, Kirkpatrick J. Radiation dose-volume effects of optic nerves and chiasm. Int J Radiat Oncol Biol Phys 2010; 76 (Suppl): S28–S35

[9] Crompton MR, Layton DD. Delayed radionecrosis of the brain following therapeutic x-radiation of the pituitary. Brain 1961; 84: 85–101

[10] Rogers M, Myers R, Jenkinson T, Hornsey S. Histology of the irradiated rat brain in the first post-irradiation year. Br J Radiol 1982; 55: 208–212

[11] LeCouteur RA, Gillette EL, Powers BE, Child G, McChesney SL, Ingram JT. Peripheral neuropathies following experimental intraoperative radiation therapy (IORT). Int J Radiat Oncol Biol Phys 1989; 17: 583–590

[12] Szeifert GT, Kondziolka D, Lunsford LD, et al. Introduction: the contribution of pathology to radiosurgery. Prog Neurol Surg 2007; 20: 1–15

[13] Ove R, Kelman S, Amin PP, Chin LS. Preservation of visual fields after peri-sellar Gamma Knife radiosurgery. Int J Cancer 2000; 90: 343–350

[14] Stafford SL, Pollock BE, Leavitt JA, et al. A study on the radiation tolerance of the optic nerves and chiasm after stereotactic radiosurgery. Int J Radiat Oncol Biol Phys 2003; 55: 1177–1181

[15] Adler JR, Gibbs IC, Puataweepong P, Chang SD. Visual field preservation after multisession cyberknife radiosurgery for perioptic lesions. Neurosurgery 2006; 59: 244–254, discussion 244–254

[16] Hasegawa T, Kobayashi T, Kida Y. Tolerance of the optic apparatus in single-fraction irradiation using stereotactic radiosurgery: evaluation in 100 patients with craniopharyngioma. Neurosurgery 2010; 66: 688–694, discussion 694–695

[17] Marchetti M, Bianchi S, Milanesi I, et al. Multisession radiosurgery for optic nerve sheath meningiomas: an effective option: preliminary results from a monoinstitutional experience. Neurosurgery 2011 Nov; 69: 1116–22, discussion 1122–3

[18] Gopalan R, Schlesinger D, Vance ML, Laws E, Sheehan J. Long-term outcomes after Gamma Knife radiosurgery for patients with a nonfunctioning pituitary adenoma. Neurosurgery 2011; 69: 284–293

[19] Jagannathan J, Sheehan JP, Pouratian N, Laws ER, Steiner L, Vance ML. Gamma Knife radiosurgery for acromegaly: outcomes after failed transsphenoidal surgery. Neurosurgery 2008; 62: 1262–1269, discussion 1269–1270

[20] Mauermann WJ, Sheehan JP, Chernavvsky DR, Laws ER, Steiner L, Vance ML. Gamma Knife surgery for adrenocorticotropic hormone-producing pituitary adenomas after bilateral adrenalectomy. J Neurosurg 2007; 106: 988–993

[21] Jagannathan J, Sheehan JP, Pouratian N, Laws ER, Steiner L, Vance ML. Gamma Knife surgery for Cushing's disease. J Neurosurg 2007; 106: 980–987

[22] Bhandare N, Monroe AT, Morris CG, Bhatti MT, Mendenhall WM. Does altered fractionation influence the risk of radiation-induced optic neuropathy? Int J Radiat Oncol Biol Phys 2005; 62: 1070–1077

[23] Chon BH, Loeffler JS. The effect of nonmalignant systemic disease on tolerance to radiation therapy. Oncologist 2002; 7: 136–143

[24] Lowell D, Tatter SB, Bourland JD, et al. Toxicity of Gamma Knife radiosurgery in the treatment of intracranial tumors in patients with collagen vascular diseases or multiple sclerosis. Int J Radiat Oncol Biol Phys 2011; 81: e519–e524

[25] Daniels TB, Pollock BE, Miller RC, Lucchinetti CF, Leavitt JA, Brown PD. Radiation-induced optic neuritis after pituitary adenoma radiosurgery in a patient with multiple sclerosis: case report. J Neurooncol 2009; 93: 263–267

[26] Shurin SB, Rekate HL, Annable W. Optic atrophy induced by vincristine. Pediatrics 1982; 70: 288–291

[27] Flickinger JC, Deutsch M, Lunsford LD. Repeat megavoltage irradiation of pituitary and suprasellar tumors. Int J Radiat Oncol Biol Phys 1989; 17: 171–175

[28] Finger PT. Anti-VEGF bevacizumab (Avastin) for radiation optic neuropathy. Am J Ophthalmol 2007; 143: 335–338

[29] Mohamed IG, Roa W, Fulton D, et al. Optic nerve sheath fenestration for a reversible optic neuropathy in radiation oncology. Am J Clin Oncol 2000; 23: 401–405

[30] Williamson R, Kondziolka D, Kanaan H, Lunsford LD, Flickinger JC. Adverse radiation effects after radiosurgery may benefit from oral vitamin E and pentoxifylline therapy: a pilot study. Stereotact Funct Neurosurg 2008; 86: 359–366

[31] Borruat FX, Schatz NJ, Glaser JS, Feun LG, Matos L. Visual recovery from radiation-induced optic neuropathy: the role of hyperbaric oxygen therapy. J Clin Neuroophthalmol 1993; 13: 98–101

[32] Danesh-Meyer HV, Savino PJ, Sergott RC. Visual loss despite anticoagulation in radiation-induced optic neuropathy. Clin Experiment Ophthalmol 2004; 32: 333–335

[33] Barbosa AP, Carvalho D, Marques L, et al. Inefficiency of the anticoagulant therapy in the regression of the radiation-induced optic neuropathy in Cushing's disease. J Endocrinol Invest 1999; 22: 301–305

[34] Tishler RB, Loeffler JS, Lundsford LD, Duma C, Alexander E 3rd, Kooy HM, Flickinger JC. Tolerance of cranial nerves of the cavernous sinus to radiosurgery. Int J Radiat Oncol Biol Phys 1993 Sep 30; 27: 215–21

[35] Leber KA, Bergloeff J, Pendl G. Dose-response tolerance of the visual pathways and cranial nerves of the cavernous sinus to stereotactic radiosurgery

[36] Lee M, Kalani MY, Cheshier S, Gibbs IC, Adler JR, Chang SD. Radiation therapy and Cyberknife radiosurgery in the management o craniopharyngiomas. Neurosurg Focus 2008; 24: E4

[37] Pollock BE, Cochran J, Nat N, Brown PD, Erickson D, Link MJ, Garces YI, Foote RL, Stafford SL, Schomberg PJ. Gamma knife radiosurgery for patients with nonfunctioning pituitary adenomas: results from a 15-year experinece. Int J Radiat Oncol Biol Phys 2008 Apr 1; 70: 1325–9

12 Optic Apparatus Tolerance Greater than 8 Gy

John C. Flickinger, Douglas Kondziolka, and L. Dade Lunsford

How high a dose can the optic nerves and chiasm, or optic apparatus, take from radiosurgery before there is an unacceptable risk of radiation injury? Is 8 Gy the upper limit that should be set? Radiosurgery dose-response analyses are challenging to interpret because of the steep dose gradients across very small volumes.[1] Unlike conventional large-field fractionated radiotherapy, where injury to the optic system usually results in global loss, the small treatment volumes in radiosurgery are more likely to produce more focal optic injuries that may result in a more tolerable visual field cut. This means that taking a 1 to 3% risk of optic nerve injury may be reasonable for radiosurgery but usually not for large-field fractionated radiotherapy, especially if dose-response data for tumor control may not demand such high doses. Because of the proximity of the optic nerves and chiasm to pituitary adenomas, cavernous sinus and parasellar meningiomas, and craniopharyngiomas, optic nerve tolerance was a key question in early radiosurgery for these tumors and has remained a controversial area.[1,2]

Clearly imaging the entire optic pathway was a problem during the early years of radiosurgery. Prior to 1990, most radiosurgery was planned with computed tomography (CT), alone, and the only optic apparatus doses quoted were usually for the middle of the optic chiasm. Tishler et al reviewed optic nerve injury for 62 radiosurgery patients with no prior radiotherapy from the early experiences of the Harvard Joint Center and the University of Pittsburgh.[2] A limit of 8 Gy for optic tolerance was recommended from that analysis. Four of 17 patients (24%) receiving > 8 Gy to any part of the optic apparatus developed optic neuropathy, whereas none developed it among 35 patients receiving < 8 Gy. The lowest dose for optic neuropathy identified in that study was 9.7 Gy for the middle of the optic chiasm. From those data, setting 8 Gy as the upper limit for optic tolerance made sense. If the whole optic system were carefully delineated on magnetic resonance imaging (MRI), it is quite likely that the maximum dose within the optic apparatus for that patient who suffered optic injury at 9.7 Gy could have been substantially higher. Following 8 Gy as a conservative upper dose limit for radiation injury in an era when the optic nerve doses were difficult to delineate probably prevented cases of optic injury in patients for whom optic doses were underestimated.

This 8-Gy limit for optic tolerance was questioned first by the Mayo Clinic experience.[3] Stafford et al reported that optic neuropathy developed in 4 of 215 Mayo Clinic patients receiving a median maximum dose of 10 Gy to the optic apparatus, with maximum chiasm/optic nerve doses of 0.4 to 16.0 Gy. The risk of radiation-induced optic injury in this series of patients (11 of whom had prior radiotherapy) was estimated at 1.7%, 1.8%, 0%, and 6.9% for maximum optic doses of < 8, 8 to 10, 10 to 12, and > 12 Gy, respectively. Of those four patients who developed optic injury, three had previous external beam radiotherapy with combined (radiotherapy + radiosurgery) doses of (58.8 + 7) Gy, (45 + 9) Gy, and (50.4 + 9 + 12) Gy. The only injury in a previously unirradiated patient occurred after an optic dose of 12.8 Gy. From this report, it appeared that the risks of optic injury without prior radiotherapy above and below 12 Gy were ~ 3% and 0%, respectively. In a later study of nonfunctioning pituitary adenomas, Pollock et al observed no cases of optic injury among 62 patients undergoing Gamma Knife (Elekta AB, Stockholm, Sweden) radiosurgery at the Mayo Clinic, with maximum optic doses < 12 Gy and a median maximum to the optic apparatus of 9.5 ± 1.7 Gy.[4] The same group later reported bilateral visual decline in a patient with multiple sclerosis following Gamma Knife radiosurgery for a prolactin-secreting pituitary adenoma. Maximum doses were 9.5 Gy to the right and 10.5 Gy to the left optic nerves.[5]

Leber et al analyzed optic neuropathy risks in 50 patients 24 to 60 months (median follow-up 40 months) after Gamma Knife radiosurgery for benign skull base tumors. They reported optic neuropathy risks of 0% with < 10 Gy, 27% with 10 to 15 Gy, and 78% with > 15 Gy.[6]

Hasegawa et al evaluated optic nerve tolerance in 100 patients with craniopharyngiomas after a median follow-up period of 68 months following Gamma Knife radiosurgery.[7] Thirteen had prior radiotherapy (range 30–60 Gy; mean 46 Gy). The maximum doses to any part of the optic apparatus varied from 2 to 18 Gy (median 10 Gy). Out of 94 patients with evaluable visual function, 3 developed radiation-induced optic neuropathy, for an overall radiation-induced optic neuropathy rate of 5%. One patient who received a maximum optic dose of 8 Gy had prior radiation therapy with a biologically effective dose of 60 Gy. The other two patients had no prior radiotherapy but received maximum doses of 15 or 18 Gy to the optic system. The authors estimated the actuarial risk of optic neuropathy to be 38%, 0%, and 7% for maximum optic doses of 15 to 18 Gy, 9 to 14 Gy, and < 8 Gy, respectively. The 7% risk for < 8 Gy was confounded by including patients with prior radiotherapy and would have been 0% if previously irradiated patients were excluded.

▸ Table 12.1 summarizes the key findings of these studies of radiosurgery optic tolerance; these represent ***level III evidence***. The variation in risks for doses between 10 and 15 Gy could possibly come from uncertainties in defining the optic pathways, particularly in retrospective studies conducted in the era of lower resolution imaging. The optic system can be very difficult to define in patients with prior surgery or compression of the optic system by tumor. We recommend carefully outlining the optic apparatus on two or more separate high-resolution sequences such as 1-mm contrast-enhanced spoiled gradient recalled images and 1-mm heavily T2-weighted volume acquisition images.

What is a safe upper dose limit for the optic nerves or optic chiasm from radiosurgery? For patients with no prior radiotherapy and no conditions that may predispose to radiation injury, 8 Gy appears to be too low a limit, as radiosurgery doses of 10 to 11 Gy to the optic apparatus appear to represent very low risk. An optic dose of 10 Gy seems to be a more reasonable limit. When prior radiotherapy doses ≥ 55 Gy have been delivered to the optic system, 8 Gy from later radiosurgery may still result in a focal radiation injury. If there is a reasonably high chance that additional radiosurgery or fractionated radiotherapy may be

Table 12.1 Optic neuropathy dose-response analyses for radiosurgery

Study	Dose (Gy)	Risk of optic injury	Limitations/comments
Tishler et al[2]	< 8 Gy > 9 Gy	0% 24%	Limited imaging and dosimetry
Stafford et al[3]	< 8 Gy 8–10 Gy 10–12 Gy with no XRT > 12 Gy	1.7% (0% no XRT) 1.8% (0% no XRT) 0.0% 6.9% (3% no XRT)	Includes patients with prior radiotherapy
Pollock et al[4]	9.5 Gy median, < 12 Gy	0/62 nonfunctional	Augment above series
Daniels et al[5]	9.5 and 10.5 Gy with MS	Bilateral optic injury	
Leber et al[6]	< 10 Gy 10 15 Gy > 15 Gy	0% 27% 78%	Risks seem high > 10 Gy compared to other series
Hasegawa et al[7]	< 8 Gy 8–14 Gy 15–18 Gy	7% (0% for no XRT) 0% 38%	Includes patients with prior radiotherapy

Abbreviations: *MS, multiple sclerosis; XRT, radiotherapy.*

needed in the future, using 8 Gy as the dose limit for the optic apparatus may be prudent.

References

[1] Mayo C, Martel MK, Marks LB, Flickinger J, Nam J, Kirkpatrick J. Radiation dose-volume effects of optic nerves and chiasm. Int J Radiat Oncol Biol Phys 2010; 76 (Suppl): S28–S35

[2] Tishler RB, Loeffler JS, Lunsford LD, et al. Tolerance of cranial nerves of the cavernous sinus to radiosurgery. Int J Radiat Oncol Biol Phys 1993; 27: 215–221

[3] Stafford SL, Pollock BE, Leavitt JA, et al. A study on the radiation tolerance of the optic nerves and chiasm after stereotactic radiosurgery. Int J Radiat Oncol Biol Phys 2003; 55: 1177–1181

[4] Pollock BE, Cochran J, Natt N, et al. Gamma Knife radiosurgery for patients with nonfunctioning pituitary adenomas: results from a 15-year experience. Int J Radiat Oncol Biol Phys 2008; 70: 1325–1329

[5] Daniels TB, Pollock BE, Miller RC, Lucchinetti CF, Leavitt JA, Brown PD. Radiation-induced optic neuritis after pituitary adenoma radiosurgery in a patient with multiple sclerosis: case report. J Neurooncol 2009; 93: 263–267

[6] Leber KA, Berglöff J, Langmann G, Mokry M, Schröttner O, Pendl G. Radiation sensitivity of visual and oculomotor pathways. Stereotact Funct Neurosurg 1995; 64 (Suppl 1): 233–238

[7] Hasegawa T, Kobayashi T, Kida Y. Tolerance of the optic apparatus in single-fraction irradiation using stereotactic radiosurgery: evaluation in 100 patients with craniopharyngioma. Neurosurgery 2010; 66: 688–694, discussion 694–695

13 Radiosurgery of Arteriovenous Malformations without Embolization

Robert M. Starke and Aaron S. Dumont

Introduction

Cerebral arteriovenous malformations (AVMs) are often associated with a significant risk of morbidity and mortality due to intracerebral hemorrhage, seizure, or neurologic deficits secondary to venous hypertension or vascular steal. Intervention may be indicated to eliminate the risk of hemorrhage and to preserve or improve neurologic function. For each patient, a treatment plan must include a complete assessment of the risks of intervention and the clinical history as well as the angioarchitecture of the normal brain and AVM. Treatment should be undertaken only if the risks of the intervention plan are deemed lower than the risks of hemorrhage and complications from the predicted natural history.

Treatment strategies for cerebral AVMs have evolved significantly; currently, there are three major interventions. In patients where the risks of intervention outweigh the risks of expectant monitoring, microsurgery, radiosurgery, and embolization have all been successfully used either alone or in combination. For certain AVMs, combination therapy may decrease the overall risks of aggressive intervention with a single modality. Although multimodality therapy may be a beneficial treatment plan, the risks of each procedure must be taken into account to assess the additive risk and overall therapeutic plan.

Although treatment options of AVMs have been refined over many years, the best therapeutic strategies remain unclear, and there have been no randomized clinical trials. Endovascular therapy is associated with low rates of obliteration as a primary therapy, and associated morbidity and mortality have limited its potential use. Despite these drawbacks, endovascular therapy is a common intervention for AVMs, and complication rates appear to be decreasing. Even though it is commonly used prior to radiosurgery, the additive risks of intervention may outweigh the benefits in some instances. This chapter reviews the outcomes of endovascular therapy for cerebral AVMs and addresses its controversial role as an adjunctive treatment to radiosurgery.

Alterations in Pathophysiology following Embolization and Radiosurgery

Although significant strides have been made in understanding the basic biology underlying cerebral AVMs,[1] alterations following both radiosurgery and endovascular therapy are less clear. Additionally, AVMs are dynamic lesions with significant angiogenic potential that may grow de novo.[2–5] Alterations following treatment are also not static, and final obliteration following radiosurgery may take years.[6,7] Additionally, microarray studies following intervention have demonstrated significant alteration in gene expression.[8,9] It is believed that radiosurgery causes endothelial cell proliferation, progressive vessel wall thickening, and eventually luminal closure.[10,11] Experimental studies have demonstrated that radiosurgery decreases neovascularization following Gamma Knife (Elekta AB, Stockholm, Sweden) radiosurgery as compared to untreated AVMs.[12,13] Additionally, there was a dose-dependent response to inhibition of neovascularization.[12]

Although the response may differ according to embolic agents, endovascular therapy results in an inflammatory process and fibrosis that may lead to vessel occlusion. When the nidus is incompletely embolized, collateral vessels can form, leading to recanalization.[14] Studies have found significant rates of recanalization of embolized specimens on pathological inspection even following the use of permanent embolic agents.[15–17] Experimental studies have also found increased angiogenesis as compared to AVMs treated with Gamma Knife radiosurgery or untreated lesions.[13] These underlying alterations in AVMs treated with embolization may partially explain the low rates of obliteration when endovascular therapy is the only intervention.

Outcomes following Embolization

Currently, embolization may be used as primary curative therapy, adjuvant therapy prior to definitive microsurgery or radiosurgery, or palliative therapy for inoperable or otherwise incurable AVMs. To assess the role of embolization as an adjunctive treatment to radiosurgery, the risks and outcomes of embolization must be assessed, as the morbidity and mortality may be additive.

Overall complication rates following embolization of cerebral AVMs vary considerably, with morbidity rates from 0 to 50% and mortality rates from 0 to 4%.[17–45] Variance is due in part to differences in patient and AVM characteristics, patient selection, embolic agents, experience of the treating team, and treatment goals. In the majority of series, neurologic deficits most commonly occur in 10 to 14% of patients, disabling deficits in 2 to 5%, and death in ~ 1%.[20,21,24,46–57] A recent comparative effectiveness review of the National Inpatient Sample, which covered a total of 33,997 admissions for cerebral AVMs over an 8-year period, found that those patients treated with endovascular therapy as opposed to other therapies had the highest mortality index (1.6% in unruptured and 10.6% in ruptured AVMs).[58] We have found low rates of mortality in well-selected patients, and a majority of patients experiencing deficits due to embolization will improve over time.[59] Key determinants of complications following embolization reported in the literature are the number of embolization procedures, number of arterial feeders embolized, eloquent location, location in the basal ganglia, deep venous drainage, size < 3 cm, size > 6 cm, Spetzler-Martin grade III to V, venous penetration of glue cast, and AVMs with a pure fistula or a nidus with a fistulous component.[46,50,54,57,59] Although AVMs treated with primary embolization tend to be smaller in size with fewer arterial pedicles, rates of complications following either primary or adjuvant embolization have been similar.[50,51,56,60] Further components that play an important role in endovascular-related complications are patient age and medical condition, as well as degree of vessel atherosclerosis.

Rates of complete obliteration following primary embolization are limited, with success rates generally ranging from 5 to 20%, but up to 70% in some patients.[18,23,24,29–31,39,45,50,51,60–64] A review of 1,246 patients treated from 1960 to 1995 found an overall cure rate of 5%.[30] Rates in patients treated more recently were similar to those treated earlier.[30] Curative embolization rates have been similar in patients treated with Onyx (ev3, Inc., Irvine, CA) and *N*-butyl-cyanoacrylate (NBCA; Cordis Microvascular, Inc., New Brunswick, NJ) and range between ~ 15 and 50%,[65–72] but they may be higher in cohorts of select patients.

These patients require long-term follow-up, as a small number of patients will experience recanalization following the use of permanent embolic agents.[15–17] Even with complete angiographic obliteration, delayed recanalization may occur due to formation of collateral channels.[14] Incompletely embolized AVMs may be an increased risk of hemorrhage.[15–17] A study by Heidenreich et al demonstrated that a reduction of > 60% without complete obliteration resulted in a 19-fold increase in risk of hemorrhage.[73] Thus, because of the associated morbidity and mortality, rates of obliteration, and risk of recanalization, embolization as a primary treatment option is reserved for only select patients.[74]

Treatment of Small Arteriovenous Malformations

For small AVMs, or Spetzler-Martin grade I and II lesions, microsurgery is the preferred treatment option. Favorable outcome can be achieved in 92 to 100% and 94 to 95% of patients, respectively.[22,75–77] Although studies have demonstrated that preoperative embolization leads to decreased operative time, blood loss, and morbidity and mortality in cerebral AVM surgery,[32,47,78] embolization is often unnecessary because of the additive risk of multiple procedures (▶ Fig. 13.1 and ▶ Fig. 13.2). For the majority of patients with small AVMs, the lesion can be removed without embolization (▶ Fig. 13.3 and ▶ Fig. 13.4).

Radiosurgery has been shown to be an effective treatment option for AVMs, especially for those < 3 cm in diameter.[6,7,79–89] For patients with Spetzler-Martin grade I and II lesions, radiosurgery may be a less invasive option for those medically unsuitable or unwilling to be treated with surgical therapy.[82] In patients with small AVMs, obliteration rates are ~ 80 to 90% and are associated with low rates of radiation-induced complications.[90] Because of the high rates of obliteration and low rates of complications following radiosurgery of small AVMs, embolization as an adjuvant therapy is rarely indicated.

Therapeutic Options for Large Arteriovenous Malformations

In certain AVMs, the risks of surgery alone may be associated with unacceptably high rates of morbidity and mortality. In select AVMs, excellent or good outcomes range from 68 to 96% in Spetzler-Martin grade III lesions[22,75] and 71 to 75% in grade IV lesions.[22,76,91] In grade V lesions, the reported good/excellent rate is 50 to 70%, with a 14 to 25% rate of poor outcome and a 0 to 5% mortality rate at long-term follow-up.[22,75,91,92] Because of higher rates of morbidity and mortality in these patients, multimodality treatment is often indicated.

For large lesions located in deep locations, the risk following surgery alone may be considerable. In the study by Morgan et al,[93] five of six patients (86%) with grade III AVMs fed by lenticulostriate arteries suffered a new neurologic deficit. For this reason, the modified Spetzler-Martin (mSM) grading scale was created to address differences in outcome in grade III AVMs.[92,94] The mSM has two subgroups under grade III: grade IIIA (size > 6 cm) and grade IIIB (venous drainage and/or eloquence). De Oliveira et al found that 2 of 44 patients (4%) with grade IIIa AVMs had new neurologic deficits versus 29 of 97 (30%) of patients with grade IIIB lesions.[94] Others have found similar outcomes, with surgical risks (new deficit or death) in Spetzler-Martin grade III AVMs of 2.9% for small AVMs (S1V1E1), 7.1% for medium/deep AVMs (S2V1E0), and 14.8% for medium/eloquent AVMs (S2V0E1).[95] Thus, a recommended treatment plan for large grade III lesions without eloquent location may be microsurgery with adjunctive endovascular therapy, whereas radiosurgery with or without embolization is often used for smaller grade III lesions in eloquent locations.[92]

Staged Radiosurgery for Large Arteriovenous Malformations

Nearly all studies of AVMs treated with radiosurgery have found size to be a key determinant of outcome. This relates to adjusted prescription dose based on volume, as there is a direct relationship between volume and radiation-induced complications. One option for large AVMs is multistage radiosurgery to reduce the chances of complications and increase the opportunity for obliteration. In a series by Kano et al,[96] 47 AVMs undergoing volume staged radiosurgery had a mean target volume of 11.5 cm^3. The rates of total obliteration after two-stage stereotactic radiosurgery (SRS) were 7%, 20%, 28%, and 36% at 3, 4, 5, and 10 years, respectively, and overall rates of total obliteration after further repeat SRS were 18%, 45%, and 56% at 5, 7, and 10 years, respectively. Ten patients experienced hemorrhage after staged SRS, and 5 of these died. Cumulative annual hemorrhage rates ranged from 2.3 to 5.6% during follow-up. Series incorporating hypofractionated staged radiosurgery,[97] as well as other series regarding staged radiosurgery, have found similar rates of obliteration.[98–102]

Embolization and Radiosurgery for Large Arteriovenous Malformations

Cited reasons for preradiosurgery embolization include decreasing the size of AVMs to allow for better dose planning. Additional treatment goals may include staged reduction of blood flow in an AVM by stepwise occlusion of the AVM nidus over several weeks and elimination of deep-feeding arteries that could require dose planning to more critical locations. Despite

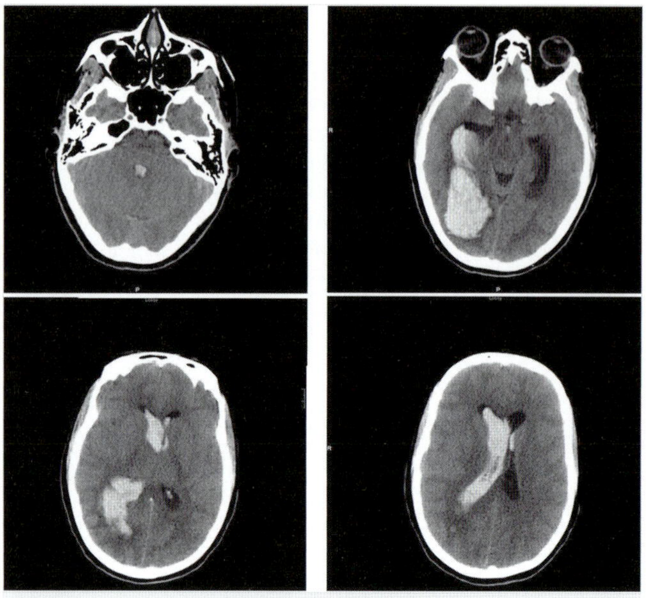

Fig. 13.1 Computed tomographic (CT) scans following early embolization. A 25-year-old woman experienced a cerebral hemorrhage early on while undergoing elective embolization. CT demonstrates a 56- × 43-mm hemorrhage in the right temporal occipital region extending into the right lateral ventricle with mild surrounding edema, asymmetric ventriculomegaly of the right lateral ventricle, mass effect on the midbrain, basilar cistern effacement, and 8 mm of midline shift.

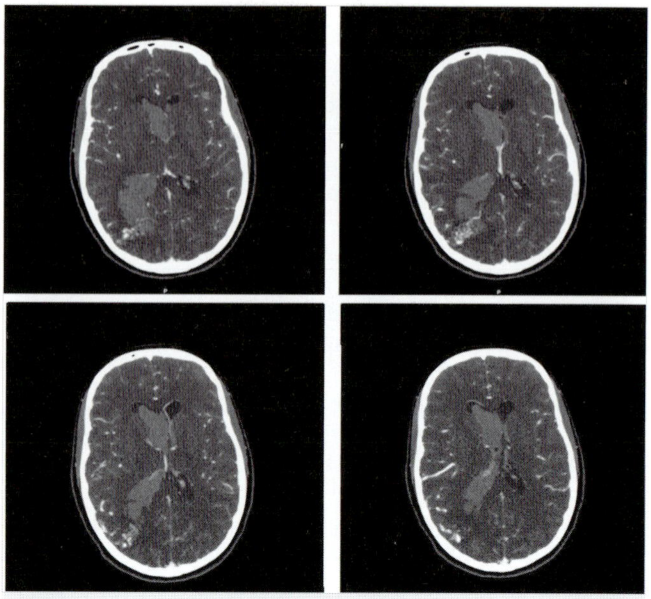

Fig. 13.2 CT angiography (CTA) on transfer. CTA demonstrates a Spetzler-Martin grade II arteriovenous malformation (AVM) nidus measuring 8 × 14 mm in the right parietal occipital region with arterial feeders from distal cortical branches of the right middle cerebral and right posterior cerebral arteries and both superficial and deep venous drainage.

these goals, embolization as an adjuvant to radiosurgery is controversial, as it may be associated with neoangiogenesis and worse outcomes. Also, studies have not found that embolization prior to radiosurgery allowed for radiation dose reduction.[103,104]

In the study by Blackburn et al,[105] 21 AVMs with a diameter > 3 cm were treated with embolization and radiosurgery, including 12 (57%) Spetzler-Martin grade IV or V lesions. Forty-three embolization procedures were performed, resulting in 8 embolization-related complications, of which 5 were transient and 3 minor. One patient experienced a permanent radiation-induced complication, and no patients experienced hemorrhage during the latency period. AVM obliteration was confirmed by catheter angiography in 13, magnetic resonance angiography in 2, and computed tomography angiography in 1. Other case series have reported similar outcomes, although few studies have found increased rates of hemorrhage following embolization during the latency period prior to radiation-induced obliteration.[70,71,90,106–109]

Thus far, two case control studies have been carried out in a retrospective fashion to compare patients treated with radiosurgery both with and without a history of embolization. In the study by Andrade-Souza et al,[110] 47 patients with a history of radiosurgery and embolization were matched according to volume, location, and marginal dose to 47 patients with radiosurgery and no history of embolization. Nidus obliteration was achieved in 47% of patients with a history of embolization and 70% of patients without a history of embolization. Permanent deficits related to hemorrhage or radiation occurred in 6% in both groups. Although two patients with no history of endovascular therapy died from hemorrhage, and two went on to receive surgical therapy, excellent outcome (obliteration and no associated deficit) was higher in those without a history of embolization (64% vs 47%). Similarly, a recent study using a case control -matched approach found that patients with a history of embolization in addition to radiosurgery were significantly less likely to achieve obliteration as compared to those treated with radiosurgery alone.[111]

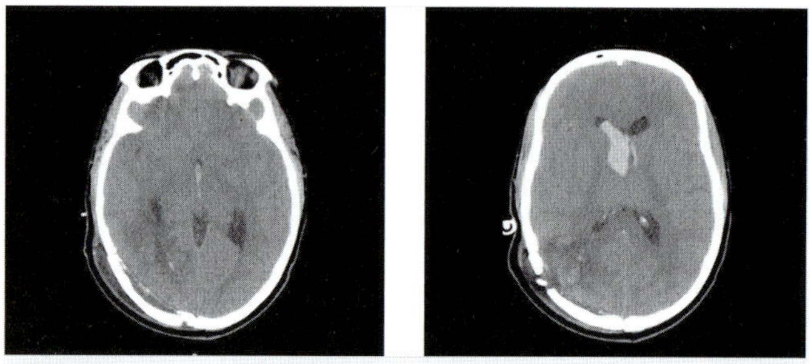

Fig. 13.3 Postoperative CT scan. The patient was taken to the operating room for evacuation of hemorrhage, and the AVM was safely removed during the same operation.

Along with prior studies,[102,109,112,113] we have found that embolization prior to radiosurgery is associated with lower obliteration rates and worse outcomes in multivariate analysis. At the University of Virginia, 1,012 patients undergoing planned single-session radiosurgery and a minimum of 2 years follow-up have received Gamma Knife radiosurgery. In Spetzler-Martin grade III or IV AVMs, 27% were treated with embolization prior to radiosurgery. We have found that Spetzler-Martin grade III or IV lesions have significantly lower rates of obliteration (64%)

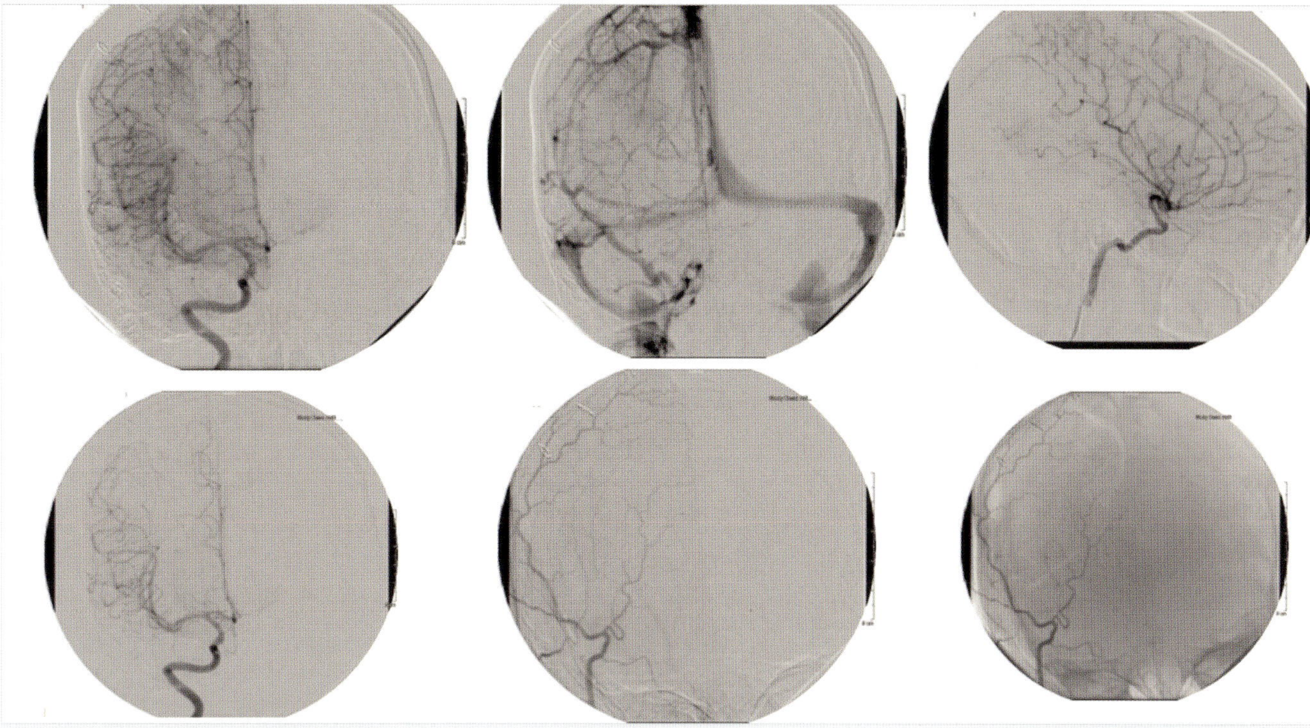

Fig. 13.4 Postoperative angiogram demonstrated no residual AVM. Postoperatively, the patient had a homonymous hemianopsia, generalized weakness, but symmetric strength and was discharged to a rehabilitation facility.

as compared to grade I and II lesions (74%). Transient symptomatic radiation-induced complications were significantly higher in larger lesions (11.6%) versus smaller lesions (8.5%), as were permanent complications (3.3% vs 1%).

Patients receiving embolization were also 3 times less likely to achieve obliteration (95% [CI] 2.20–4.20, $p < 0.001$) in multivariate analysis even after controlling for other predictive factors, including size. When assessing overall favorable outcome as a composite of obliteration and no radiation-induced complications, patients receiving embolization were 2 times less likely to achieve overall favorable outcomes (odds ratio 1.49–2.81, $p < 0.001$) in multivariate analysis.

In a review of 774 patients treated at Thomas Jefferson University, we found that those receiving endovascular therapy were also less likely to achieve obliteration and overall outcome.[unpublished] Additionally, in patients receiving embolization therapy, those receiving multiple endovascular treatments had lower rates of obliteration and favorable outcome. Although multivariate analysis was carried out, along with analysis for interaction and confounding, there are innate differences in patients treated with and without embolization that may not be taken into account.

Conclusion

Prior to treatment planning, all patient and AVM lesion characteristics need to be assessed to be sure the benefits of intervention outweigh the risks and to create the best treatment algorithm. Because there have been no randomized clinical trials to assess outcomes of AVM patients treated with and without embolization in the setting of radiosurgery, the best treatment modality remains unclear. Although each patient and lesion must be assessed individually, for the majority of small lesions requiring intervention, microsurgery may be the best option. For small lesions in patients with significant medical comorbidities or in patients unwilling to undergo surgical therapy, radiosurgery is an appropriate option. Although primary embolization is an option for select lesions that are accessible with a small number of feeders, embolization as either a primary or an adjunctive treatment is not the best option for small AVMs. For large lesions in superficial locations, surgery with or without embolization may be the best therapy. For large lesions in deep locations, staged radiosurgery or radiosurgery with embolization may be the best treatment modality, but further studies are necessary to dictate the best treatment option.

References

[1] Leblanc GG, Golanov E, Awad IA, Young WL Biology of Vascular Malformations of the Brain NINDS Workshop Collaborators. Biology of vascular malformations of the brain. Stroke 2009; 40: e694–e702

[2] Bulsara KR, Alexander MJ, Villavicencio AT, Graffagnino C. De novo cerebral arteriovenous malformation: case report. Neurosurgery 2002; 50: 1137–1140, discussion 1140–1141

[3] Sure U, Butz N, Siegel AM, Mennel HD, Bien S, Bertalanffy H. Treatment-induced neoangiogenesis in cerebral arteriovenous malformations. Clin Neurol Neurosurg 2001; 103: 29–32

[4] Sure U, Butz N, Schlegel J, et al. Endothelial proliferation, neoangiogenesis, and potential de novo generation of cerebrovascular malformations. J Neurosurg 2001; 94: 972–977

[5] Du R, Hashimoto T, Tihan T, Young WL, Perry V, Lawton MT. Growth and regression of arteriovenous malformations in a patient with hereditary hemorrhagic telangiectasia: case report. J Neurosurg 2007; 106: 470–477

[6] Shin M, Maruyama K, Kurita H, et al. Analysis of nidus obliteration rates after Gamma Knife surgery for arteriovenous malformations based on long-term follow-up data: the University of Tokyo experience. J Neurosurg 2004; 101: 18–24

[7] Pollock BE, Gorman DA, Coffey RJ. Patient outcomes after arteriovenous malformation radiosurgical management: results based on a 5- to 14-year follow-up study. Neurosurgery 2003; 52: 1291–1296, discussion 1296–1297

[8] Hashimoto T, Lawton MT, Wen G, et al. Gene microarray analysis of human brain arteriovenous malformations. Neurosurgery 2004;54(2):410–423, discussion 423–425

[9] Yuki I, Lee D, Murayama Y, et al. Thrombus organization and healing in an experimental aneurysm model, II: The effect of various types of bioactive bioabsorbable polymeric coils. J Neurosurg 2007; 107: 109–120

[10] Fabrikant JI, Lyman JT, Hosobuchi Y. Stereotactic heavy-ion Bragg peak radiosurgery for intra-cranial vascular disorders: method for treatment of deep arteriovenous malformations. Br J Radiol 1984; 57: 479–490

[11] Steiner L, Leksell L, Greitz T, Forster DM, Backlund EO. Stereotaxic radiosurgery for cerebral arteriovenous malformations: report of a case. Acta Chir Scand 1972; 138: 459–464

[12] Kiliç K, Konya D, Kurtkaya O, Sav A, Pamir MN, Kiliç T. Inhibition of angiogenesis induced by cerebral arteriovenous malformations using Gamma Knife irradiation. J Neurosurg 2007; 106: 463–469

[13] Akakin A, Ozkan A, Akgun E, et al. Endovascular treatment increases but gamma knife radiosurgery decreases angiogenic activity of arteriovenous malformations: an in vivo experimental study using a rat cornea model. Neurosurgery 2010; 66: 121–129, discussion 129–130

[14] Connors JJ, Wojak JC. Intervenional Neuroradiology: Strategies and Practical Techniques. Philadelphia, PA: WB Saunders; 1999

[15] Han PP, Ponce FA, Spetzler RF. Intention-to-treat analysis of Spetzler-Martin grades IV and V arteriovenous malformations: natural history and treatment paradigm. J Neurosurg 2003; 98: 3–7

[16] Miyamoto S, Hashimoto N, Nagata I, et al. Posttreatment sequelae of palliatively treated cerebral arteriovenous malformations. Neurosurgery 2000; 46: 589–594, discussion 594–595

[17] Wikholm G, Lundqvist C, Svendsen P. The Göteborg cohort of embolized cerebral arteriovenous malformations: a 6-year follow-up. Neurosurgery 2001; 49: 799–805, discussion 805–806

[18] Deruty R, Pelissou-Guyotat I, Mottolese C, Bascoulergue Y, Amat D. The combined management of cerebral arteriovenous malformations: experience with 100 cases and review of the literature. Acta Neurochir (Wien) 1993; 123: 101–112

[19] Arteriovenous malformations of the brain in adults. N Engl J Med 1999; 340: 1812–1818

[20] Hartmann A, Mast H, Mohr JP, et al. Determinants of staged endovascular and surgical treatment outcome of brain arteriovenous malformations. Stroke 2005; 36: 2431–2435

[21] Hartmann A, Pile-Spellman J, Stapf C, et al. Risk of endovascular treatment of brain arteriovenous malformations. Stroke 2002; 33: 1816–1820

[22] Hartmann A, Stapf C, Hofmeister C, et al. Determinants of neurological outcome after surgery for brain arteriovenous malformation. Stroke 2000; 31: 2361–2364

[23] Gobin YP, Laurent A, Merienne L, et al. Treatment of brain arteriovenous malformations by embolization and radiosurgery. J Neurosurg 1996; 85: 19–28

[24] Viñuela F, Dion JE, Duckwiler G, et al. Combined endovascular embolization and surgery in the management of cerebral arteriovenous malformations: experience with 101 cases. J Neurosurg 1991; 75: 856–864

[25] Morgan MK, Zurin AA, Harrington T, Little N. Changing role for preoperative embolisation in the management of arteriovenous malformations of the brain. J Clin Neurosci 2000; 7: 527–530

[26] Taylor CL, Dutton K, Rappard G, et al. Complications of preoperative embolization of cerebral arteriovenous malformations. J Neurosurg 2004; 100: 810–812

[27] Debrun GM, Aletich V, Ausman JI, Charbel F, Dujovny M. Embolization of the nidus of brain arteriovenous malformations with n-butyl cyanoacrylate. Neurosurgery 1997; 40: 112–120, discussion 120–121

[28] Deruty R, Pelissou-Guyotat I, Amat D, et al. Complications after multidisciplinary treatment of cerebral arteriovenous malformations. Acta Neurochir (Wien) 1996; 138: 119–131

[29] Fournier D, TerBrugge KG, Willinsky R, Lasjaunias P, Montanera W. Endovascular treatment of intracerebral arteriovenous malformations: experience in 49 cases. J Neurosurg 1991; 75: 228–233

[30] Frizzel RT, Fisher WS. Cure, morbidity, and mortality associated with embolization of brain arteriovenous malformations: a review of 1246 patients in 32 series over a 35-year period. Neurosurgery 1995; 37: 1031–1039, discussion 1039–1040

[31] Hurst RW, Berenstein A, Kupersmith MJ, Madrid M, Flamm ES. Deep central arteriovenous malformations of the brain: the role of endovascular treatment. J Neurosurg 1995; 82: 190–195

[32] Jafar JJ, Davis AJ, Berenstein A, Choi IS, Kupersmith MJ. The effect of embolization with N-butyl cyanoacrylate prior to surgical resection of cerebral arteriovenous malformations. J Neurosurg 1993; 78: 60–69

[33] Jahan R, Murayama Y, Gobin YP, Duckwiler GR, Vinters HV, Viñuela F. Embolization of arteriovenous malformations with Onyx: clinicopathological experience in 23 patients. Neurosurgery 2001; 48: 984–995, discussion 995–997

[34] Mathis JA, Barr JD, Horton JA, et al. The efficacy of particulate embolization combined with stereotactic radiosurgery for treatment of large arteriovenous malformations of the brain. AJNR Am J Neuroradiol 1995; 16: 299–306

[35] Meisel HJ, Mansmann U, Alvarez H, Rodesch G, Brock M, Lasjaunias P. Effect of partial targeted N-butyl-cyano-acrylate embolization in brain AVM. Acta Neurochir (Wien) 2002; 144: 879–887, discussion 888

[36] Merland JJ, Rüfenacht D, Laurent A, Guimaraens L. Endovascular treatment with isobutyl cyano acrylate in patients with arteriovenous malformation of the brain: indications, results and complications. Acta Radiol Suppl 1986; 369: 621–622

[37] Pasqualin A, Scienza R, Cioffi F, et al. Treatment of cerebral arteriovenous malformations with a combination of preoperative embolization and surgery. Neurosurgery 1991; 29: 358–368

[38] Paulsen RD, Steinberg GK, Norbash AM, Marcellus ML, Lopez JR, Marks MP. Embolization of rolandic cortex arteriovenous malformations. Neurosurgery 1999; 44: 479–484, discussion 484–486

[39] Paulsen RD, Steinberg GK, Norbash AM, Marcellus ML, Marks MP. Embolization of basal ganglia and thalamic arteriovenous malformations. Neurosurgery 1999; 44: 991–996, discussion 996–997

[40] Purdy PD, Samson D, Batjer HH, Risser RC. Preoperative embolization of cerebral arteriovenous malformations with polyvinyl alcohol particles: experience in 51 adults. AJNR Am J Neuroradiol 1990; 11: 501–510

[41] Schmutz F, McAuliffe W, Anderson DM, Elliott JP, Eskridge JM, Winn HR. Embolization of cerebral arteriovenous malformations with silk: histopathologic changes and hemorrhagic complications. AJNR Am J Neuroradiol 1997; 18: 1233–1237

[42] Viñuela F, Fox AJ, Debrun G, Drake CG, Peerless SJ, Girvin JP. Progressive thrombosis of brain arteriovenous malformations after embolization with isobutyl 2-cyanoacrylate. AJNR Am J Neuroradiol 1983; 4: 1233–1238

[43] Wikholm G, Lundqvist C, Svendsen P. Transarterial embolization of cerebral arteriovenous malformations: improvement of results with experience. AJNR Am J Neuroradiol 1995; 16: 1811–1817

[44] Lundqvist C, Wikholm G, Svendsen P. Embolization of cerebral arteriovenous malformations, II: Aspects of complications and late outcome. Neurosurgery 1996; 39: 460–467, discussion 467–469

[45] Wikholm G, Lundqvist C, Svendsen P. Embolization of cerebral arteriovenous malformations, I: Technique, morphology, and complications. Neurosurgery 1996; 39: 448–457, discussion 457–459

[46] Ledezma CJ, Hoh BL, Carter BS, Pryor JC, Putman CM, Ogilvy CS. Complications of cerebral arteriovenous malformation embolization: multivariate analysis of predictive factors. Neurosurgery 2006; 58: 602–611

[47] Spetzler RF, Martin NA, Carter LP, Flom RA, Raudzens PA, Wilkinson E. Surgical management of large AVM's by staged embolization and operative excision. J Neurosurg 1987; 67: 17–28

[48] Purdy PD, Batjer HH, Samson D. Management of hemorrhagic complications from preoperative embolization of arteriovenous malformations. J Neurosurg 1991; 74: 205–211

[49] Purdy PD, Batjer HH, Samson D, Risser RC, Bowman GW. Intraarterial sodium amytal administration to guide preoperative embolization of cerebral arteriovenous malformations. J Neurosurg Anesthesiol 1991; 3: 103–106

[50] Haw CS, terBrugge K, Willinsky R, Tomlinson G. Complications of embolization of arteriovenous malformations of the brain. J Neurosurg 2006; 104: 226–232

[51] Yu SC, Chan MS, Lam JM, Tam PH, Poon WS. Complete obliteration of intracranial arteriovenous malformation with endovascular cyanoacrylate embolization: initial success and rate of permanent cure. AJNR Am J Neuroradiol 2004; 25: 1139–1143

[52] Cronqvist M, Wirestam R, Ramgren B, et al. Endovascular treatment of intracerebral arteriovenous malformations: procedural safety, complications, and results evaluated by MR imaging, including diffusion and perfusion imaging. AJNR Am J Neuroradiol 2006; 27: 162–176

[53] Sorimachi T, Koike T, Takeuchi S, et al. Embolization of cerebral arteriovenous malformations achieved with polyvinyl alcohol particles: angiographic reappearance and complications. AJNR Am J Neuroradiol 1999; 20: 1323–1328

[54] Jayaraman MV, Marcellus ML, Hamilton S, et al. Neurologic complications of arteriovenous malformation embolization using liquid embolic agents. AJNR Am J Neuroradiol 2008; 29: 242–246

[55] n-BCA Trail Investigators. N-butyl cyanoacrylate embolization of cerebral arteriovenous malformations: results of a prospective, randomized, multi-center trial. AJNR Am J Neuroradiol 2002; 23: 748–755

[56] Oran I, Parildar M, Derbent A. Ventricular/paraventricular small arteriovenous malformations: role of embolisation with cyanoacrylate. Neuroradiology 2005; 47: 287–294

[57] Kim LJ, Albuquerque FC, Spetzler RF, McDougall CG. Postembolization neurological deficits in cerebral arteriovenous malformations: stratification by arteriovenous malformation grade. Neurosurgery 2006; 59: 53–59

[58] Davies JM, Yanamadala V, Lawton MT. Comparative effectiveness of treatments for cerebral arteriovenous malformations: trends in nationwide outcomes from 2000 to 2009. Neurosurg Focus 2012; 33: E11

[59] Starke RM, Komotar RJ, Otten ML, et al. Adjuvant embolization in the treatment of cerebral arteriovenous malformations: outcomes, complications, and predictors of neurologic deficits. Paper presented at: Congress of Neurological Surgeons; 2008; Orlando, FL

[60] Valavanis A, Yaşargil MG. The endovascular treatment of brain arteriovenous malformations. Adv Tech Stand Neurosurg 1998; 24: 131–214

[61] Valavanis A, Christoforidis G. Endovascular management of cerebral arteriovenous malformations. Neurointerventionist. 1999; 1: 34–40

[62] Wilms G, Goffin J, Plets C, et al. Embolization of arteriovenous malformations of the brain: preliminary experience. J Belge Radiol 1993; 76: 299–303

[63] Willinsky R, Goyal M, Terbrugge K, Montanera W, Wallace MC, Tymianski M. MC W, Tymianski M. Embolization of small (< 3 cm) brain arteriovnous malformations: correlation of angiographic results to a proposed angioarchitecture grading system. Interv Neuroradiol 2001; 7: 19–27

[64] Cockroft KM, Hwang SK, Rosenwasser RH. Endovascular treatment of cerebral arteriovenous malformations: indications, techniques, outcome, and complications. Neurosurg Clin N Am 2005; 16: 367–380, x.

[65] Katsaridis V, Papagiannaki C, Aimar E. Curative embolization of cerebral arteriovenous malformations (AVMs) with Onyx in 101 patients. Neuroradiology 2008; 50: 589–597

[66] Mounayer C, Hammami N, Piotin M, et al. Nidal embolization of brain arteriovenous malformations using Onyx in 94 patients. AJNR Am J Neuroradiol 2007; 28: 518–523

[67] van Rooij WJ, Sluzewski M, Beute GN. Brain AVM embolization with Onyx. AJNR Am J Neuroradiol 2007; 28: 172–177, discussion 178

[68] Weber W, Kis B, Siekmann R, Jans P, Laumer R, Kühne D. Preoperative embolization of intracranial arteriovenous malformations with Onyx. Neurosurgery 2007; 61: 244–252, discussion 252–254

[69] Florio F, Lauriola W, Nardella M, Strizzi V, Vallone S, Trossello MP. Endovascular treatment of intracranial arterio-venous malformations with Onyx embolization: preliminary experience. Radiol Med (Torino) 2003; 106: 512–520

[70] Xu F, Ni W, Liao Y, et al. Onyx embolization for the treatment of brain arteriovenous malformations. Acta Neurochir (Wien) 2011; 153: 869–878

[71] Lv X, Wu Z, Jiang C, et al. Complication risk of endovascular embolization for cerebral arteriovenous malformation. Eur J Radiol 2011; 80: 776–779

[72] Saatci I, Geyik S, Yavuz K, Cekirge HS. Endovascular treatment of brain arteriovenous malformations with prolonged intranidal Onyx injection technique: long-term results in 350 consecutive patients with completed endovascular treatment course. J Neurosurg 2011; 115: 78–88

[73] Heidenreich JO, Hartlieb S, Stendel R, et al. Bleeding complications after endovascular therapy of cerebral arteriovenous malformations. AJNR Am J Neuroradiol 2006; 27: 313–316

[74] Starke RM, Lavine SD, Meyers PM, Connolly ES. Endovascular Management of Arteriovenous Malformations for Cure. Winn R. Youmans Neurological Surgery: Expert Consult, 6th edition. New York, NY WB Saunders; 2012

[75] Heros RC, Korosue K, Diebold PM. Surgical excision of cerebral arteriovenous malformations: late results. Neurosurgery 1990; 26: 570–577, discussion 577–578

[76] Spetzler RF, Martin NA. A proposed grading system for arteriovenous malformations. J Neurosurg 1986; 65: 476–483

[77] Starke RM, Komotar RJ, Hwang BY, et al. Treatment guidelines for cerebral arteriovenous malformation microsurgery. Br J Neurosurg 2009; 23: 376–386

[78] DeMeritt JS, Pile-Spellman J, Mast H, et al. Outcome analysis of preoperative embolization with N-butyl cyanoacrylate in cerebral arteriovenous malformations. AJNR Am J Neuroradiol 1995; 16: 1801–1807

[79] Liscák R, Vladyka V, Simonová G, et al. Arteriovenous malformations after Leksell gamma knife radiosurgery: rate of obliteration and complications. Neurosurgery 2007; 60: 1005–1014, discussion 1015–1016

[80] McInerney J, Gould DA, Birkmeyer JD, Harbaugh RE. Decision analysis for small, asymptomatic intracranial arteriovenous malformations. Neurosurg Focus 2001; 11: e7

[81] Yen CP, Varady P, Sheehan J, Steiner M, Steiner L. Subtotal obliteration of cerebral arteriovenous malformations after Gamma Knife surgery. J Neurosurg 2007; 106: 361–369

[82] Pollock BE, Lunsford LD, Kondziolka D, Maitz A, Flickinger JC. Patient outcomes after stereotactic radiosurgery for "operable" arteriovenous malformations. Neurosurgery 1994; 35: 1–7, discussion 7–8

[83] Inoue HK, Ohye C. Hemorrhage risks and obliteration rates of arteriovenous malformations after gamma knife radiosurgery. J Neurosurg 2002; 97 (Suppl): 474–476

[84] Bollet MA, Anxionnat R, Buchheit I, et al. Efficacy and morbidity of arc-therapy radiosurgery for cerebral arteriovenous malformations: a comparison with the natural history. Int J Radiat Oncol Biol Phys 2004; 58: 1353–1363

[85] Chang JH, Chang JW, Park YG, Chung SS. Factors related to complete occlusion of arteriovenous malformations after Gamma Knife radiosurgery. J Neurosurg 2000; 93 (Suppl 3): 96–101

[86] Flickinger JC, Pollock BE, Kondziolka D, Lunsford LD. A dose-response analysis of arteriovenous malformation obliteration after radiosurgery. Int J Radiat Oncol Biol Phys 1996; 36: 873–879

[87] Lunsford LD, Kondziolka D, Flickinger JC, et al. Stereotactic radiosurgery for arteriovenous malformations of the brain. J Neurosurg 1991; 75: 512–524

[88] Ogilvy CS, Stieg PE, Awad I, et al. Special Writing Group of the Stroke Council, American Stroke Association. AHA Scientific Statement: Recommendations for the management of intracranial arteriovenous malformations. A statement for healthcare professionals from a special writing group of the Stroke Council, American Stroke Association. Stroke 2001; 32: 1458–1471

[89] Shin M, Kawamoto S, Kurita H, et al. Retrospective analysis of a 10-year experience of stereotactic radio surgery for arteriovenous malformations in children and adolescents. J Neurosurg 2002; 97: 779–784

[90] Starke RM, Komotar RJ, Hwang BY, et al. A comprehensive review of radiosurgery for cerebral arteriovenous malformations: outcomes, predictive factors, and grading scales. Stereotact Funct Neurosurg 2008; 86: 191–199

[91] Hamilton MG, Spetzler RF. The prospective application of a grading system for arteriovenous malformations. Neurosurgery 1994; 34: 2–6, discussion 6–7

[92] de Oliveira E, Tedeschi H, Raso J. Multidisciplinary approach to arteriovenous malformations. Neurol Med Chir (Tokyo) 1998; 38 (Suppl): 177–185

[93] Morgan MK, Drummond KJ, Grinnell V, Sorby W. Surgery for cerebral arteriovenous malformation: risks related to lenticulostriate arterial supply. J Neurosurg 1997; 86: 801–805

[94] de Oliveira E, Tedeschi H, Raso J. Comprehensive management of arteriovenous malformations. Neurol Res 1998; 20: 673–683

[95] Lawton MT UCSF Brain Arteriovenous Malformation Study Project. Spetzler-Martin Grade III arteriovenous malformations: surgical results and a modification of the grading scale. Neurosurgery 2003; 52: 740–748, discussion 748–749

[96] Kano H, Kondziolka D, Flickinger JC, et al. Stereotactic radiosurgery for arteriovenous malformations, VI: multistaged volumetric management of large arteriovenous malformations. J Neurosurg 2012; 116: 54–65

[97] Xiao F, Gorgulho AA, Lin CS, et al. Treatment of giant cerebral arteriovenous malformation: hypofractionated stereotactic radiation as the first stage. Neurosurgery 2010; 67: 1253–1259, discussion 1259

[98] Sirin S, Kondziolka D, Niranjan A, Flickinger JC, Maitz AH, Lunsford LD. Prospective staged volume radiosurgery for large arteriovenous malformations: indications and outcomes in otherwise untreatable patients. Neurosurgery 2008; 62 (Suppl 2): 744–754

[99] Huang PP, Rush SC, Donahue B, et al. Long-term outcomes after staged-volume stereotactic radiosurgery for large arteriovenous malformations. Neurosurgery 2012; 71: 632–643, discussion 643–644

[100] Hauswald H, Milker-Zabel S, Sterzing F, Schlegel W, Debus J, Zabel-du Bois A. Repeated linac-based radiosurgery in high-grade cerebral arteriovenous-malformations (AVM) Spetzler-Martin grade III to IV previously treated with radiosurgery. Radiother Oncol 2011; 98: 217–222

[101] Kim HY, Chang WS, Kim DJ, et al. Gamma Knife surgery for large cerebral arteriovenous malformations. J Neurosurg 2010; 113 (Suppl): 2–8

[102] Kano H, Kondziolka D, Flickinger JC, et al. Stereotactic radiosurgery for arteriovenous malformations, Part 3: outcome predictors and risks after repeat radiosurgery. J Neurosurg 2012; 116: 21–32
[103] Bing F, Doucet R, Lacroix F, et al. Liquid embolization material reduces the delivered radiation dose: clinical myth or reality? AJNR Am J Neuroradiol 2012; 33: 320–322
[104] Mamalui-Hunter M, Jiang T, Rich KM, Derdeyn CP, Drzymala RE. Effect of liquid embolic agents on Gamma Knife surgery dosimetry for arteriovenous malformations. Clinical article. J Neurosurg 2011; 115: 364–370
[105] Blackburn SL, Ashley WW, Rich KM, et al. Combined endovascular embolization and stereotactic radiosurgery in the treatment of large arteriovenous malformations. J Neurosurg 2011; 114: 1758–1767
[106] Darsaut TE, Guzman R, Marcellus ML, et al. Management of pediatric intracranial arteriovenous malformations: experience with multimodality therapy. Neurosurgery 2011; 69: 540–556, discussion 556
[107] Yuki I, Kim RH, Duckwiler G, et al. Treatment of brain arteriovenous malformations with high-flow arteriovenous fistulas: risk and complications associated with endovascular embolization in multimodality treatment. Clinical article. J Neurosurg 2010; 113: 715–722
[108] Lv X, Wu Z, Li Y, Yang X, Jiang C. Hemorrhage risk after partial endovascular NBCA and ONYX embolization for brain arteriovenous malformation. Neurol Res 2012; 34: 552–556
[109] Miyawaki L, Dowd C, Wara W, et al. Five year results of LINAC radiosurgery for arteriovenous malformations: outcome for large AVMS. Int J Radiat Oncol Biol Phys 1999; 44: 1089–1106
[110] Andrade-Souza YM, Ramani M, Scora D, Tsao MN, terBrugge K, Schwartz ML. Embolization before radiosurgery reduces the obliteration rate of arteriovenous malformations. Neurosurgery 2007; 60: 443–451, discussion 451–452
[111] Kano H, Kondziolka D, Flickinger JC, et al. Stereotactic radiosurgery for arteriovenous malformations after embolization: a case-control study. J Neurosurg 2012; 117: 265–275
[112] Pollock BE, Flickinger JC. A proposed radiosurgery-based grading system for arteriovenous malformations. J Neurosurg 2002; 96: 79–85
[113] Starke RM, Yen CP, Ding D, Sheehan JP. A practical grading scale for predicting outcome after radiosurgery for arteriovenous malformations: analysis of 1012 treated patients. J Neurosurg 2013 Jul 5. [Epub ahead of print]

Malignant Intrancranial Tumors

14 Resection of Solitary Brain Metastases

Ephraim W. Church, Elias B. Rizk, and Jonas M. Sheehan

Introduction

According to the American Cancer Society, 1.6 million Americans were expected to be diagnosed with cancer in 2012.[1] Up to 40% of these patients were expected to develop brain metastases, with approximately half of these being solitary.[2–4] Based on these estimates, up to 320,000 Americans will be diagnosed with solitary brain metastases during the year of this writing. It is generally acknowledged that epidemiological studies underestimate the true incidence of brain metastases. Moreover, it is likely that, as the population ages and diagnostic technologies continue to improve, metastatic tumors will become more common.[4]

Brain metastasis carries a poor prognosis. Without treatment, median survival is 4 to 6 weeks.[5] However, these data apply to all cases of newly discovered metastasis, whether solitary or multiple. In addition to surgical resection, there are alternative and complementary treatments, including whole-brain radiation therapy (WBRT) and stereotactic radiosurgery (SRS), both of which are commonly used in the treatment of brain metastasis. The benefit of SRS in contrast to WBRT is its ability to deliver a high, toxic radiation dose to the target tissue while delivering a much lower and safer dose to the surrounding healthy tissue. SRS has been used extensively with excellent results in patients with metastatic brain tumors. Indeed, the positive experience with SRS has raised important questions regarding the precise role of surgery in brain metastasis. The purpose of this chapter is to explore the role of surgical resection of solitary brain metastases, whether as an alternative or in addition to radiation. We evaluate and assess studies addressing this question for strength of evidence, assigning levels of evidence according to the U.S. Preventive Services Task Force guidelines (▶ Table 14.1).[6] Additionally, we review published consensus statements discuss our current practices and suggest areas for future investigation.

Table 14.1 U.S. Preventive Services Task Force level of evidence guidelines

Level of evidence	Definition
Level I	Evidence obtained from at least one properly designed randomized controlled trial
Level II-1	Evidence obtained from well-designed controlled trials without randomization
Level II-2	Evidence obtained from well-designed cohort or case control analytic studies
Level II-3	Evidence obtained from multiple time series with or without the intervention
Level III	Opinions of respected authorities based on clinical experience, descriptive studies, or reports of expert committees

Source: U.S. Preventive Task Force. Guide to clinical preventive services: report of the US Preventive Services Task Force. Darby, PA: DIANE Publishing; 1989.

It should be noted at the outset that some metastases, by nature of their location or because of patient characteristics (e.g., comorbidities, extent and pace of systemic disease), are not suitable for surgical consideration. For example, metastases located in the eloquent cortex or brainstem may be difficult to resect safely without loss of function and quality of life. Moreover, many patients with brain metastases are too infirm, whether from their primary disease or from medical comorbidities, to undergo surgery safely. Nevertheless, techniques such as functional imaging and intraoperative image guidance may allow surgeons to remove tumors that were considered inoperable previously.[2]

Level I and II Evidence

▶ Table 14.2 summarizes outcomes of ***level I*** and ***II*** studies of surgery, radiosurgery, and radiation therapy for brain metastases. For patients with single brain metastases amenable to surgical resection, surgery followed by WBRT was compared with WBRT alone in several randomized controlled trials (RCTs).[7–9] In 1990 Patchell et al conducted an RCT enrolling 48 patients with systemic cancer and a Karnofsky performance scale (KPS) of at least 70. They were randomized to undergo biopsy followed by WBRT (36 Gy in 12 daily fractions) or surgical resection followed by WBRT.[8] Survival was significantly increased in the resection group (40 vs 15 wk, $p < 0.01$). Recurrence, freedom from death due to neurologic causes, and duration of functional independence were also significantly improved in the surgical group.

A multicenter trial from the Netherlands with similar treatment arms and involving 63 patients also showed a mortality benefit for surgery plus WBRT (40 Gy in 2 Gy fractions) compared to WBRT alone.[9] In this study, the treatment effect was an additional 4 months' survival (10 vs 6 mo). The authors presented data to support their conclusion that surgery provided a survival benefit, particularly for patients younger than 60 years or with stable extracranial disease for at least 3 months. A similar multicenter trial from Canada involving 84 patients failed to show any survival benefit (5.6 mo in the surgery plus radiation group v 6.3 mo in the radiation-only group).[7] However, this study included more patients with progressive systemic disease and lower performance scores compared with its counterpart RCTs.

Several years later, Patchell et al conducted a well-designed RCT comparing resection alone versus resection plus WBRT.[10] Ninety-five adults with a KPS score of at least 70 who underwent complete resection of a single brain metastasis were randomized to receive postoperative WBRT (50.4 Gy in 28 fractions) or no radiation treatment. Prior to randomization, cases were stratified by the primary tumor type and the extent of extracranial disease. The treatment groups were comparable in terms of baseline characteristics. No patient was lost to follow-up, and the analysis was based on intention to treat. Eighteen percent of patients who received postoperative WBRT experienced a recurrence of brain metastasis compared to 70% of

Table 14.2 Outcomes of level I and II studies of surgery and radiation therapy for brain metastases

Study	Level of evidence	Survival	Decreased local recurrence	Decreased distant recurrence	Functional independence
Patchell et al[8]	I	S + WBRT > WBRT	S + WBRT > WBRT	S + WBRT ~ WBRT	S + WBRT > WBRT
Vecht et al[9]	I	S + WBRT > WBRT	NR	NR	S + WBRT > WBRT
Mintz et al[7]	I	S + WBRT ~ WBRT	NR	NR	S + WBRT ~WBRT
Lagerwaard et al[14]	II-2	S + WBRT > WBRT	NR	NR	NR
Patchell et al[10]	I	S + WBRT ~ S*	S + WBRT > S	S + WBRT > S	S + WBRT ~ S
Kocher et al[11]	I	S or SRS + WBRT ~ S or SRS	S or SRS + WBRT > S or SRS	S or SRS + WBRT > S or SRS	S or SRS + WBRT ~ S or SRS
Armstrong et al[15]	II-2	S + WBRT ~ S	S + WBRT ~ S	S + WBRT ~ S	NR
Hagen et al[16]	II-2	S + WBRT ~ S	NR	NR	NR
Skibber et al[17]	II-2	S + WBRT > S	NR	NR	NR
Muacevic et al[12]	I	S + WBRT ~ SRS*	S + WBRT ~ SRS*	S + WBRT > SRS*	NR
Muacevic et al[18]	II-2	S + WBRT ~ SRS	S + WBRT ~ SRS	S + WBRT > SRS	NR
Rades et al[19]	II-2	S + WBRT ~ SRS	S + WBRT ~ SRS	S + WBRT ~ SRS	NR
Roos et al[13]	I	S + WBRT ~ SRS + WBRT*	S + WBRT ~ SRS + WBRT*	S + WBRT ~ SRS + WBRT*	NR
Bindal et al[20]	II-2	S + WBRT > SRS + WBRT	NR	S + WBRT ~ SRS + WBRT	NR
Schöggl et al[21]	II-2	S + WBRT ~ SRS + WBRT	S + WBRT ~ SRS + WBRT	S + WBRT ~ SRS + WBRT	NR
O'Neill et al[22]	II-2	S + WBRT ~ SRS + WBRT	S + WBRT < SRS + WBRT	NR	NR
Garell et al[24]	II-2	S + WBRT ~ SRS + WBRT	NR	NR	NR
Wang et al[28]	II-2	S or WBRT or SRS < SRS + WBRT	S or WBRT or SRS ~ SRS + WBRT	NR	NR
Shinoura et al[27]	II-2	S + RT > SRS	S + RT ~SRS	NR	NR
Ikushima et al[26]	II-2	FSRT > S + RT or RT	FSRT ~ S + RT or RT	NR	NR

Abbreviations: FSRT, fractionated stereotactic radiosurgery; NR, not reported; RT, radiation therapy; S, surgery; SRS, stereotactic radiosurgery; WBRT, whole-brain radiation therapy; ~, no significant difference reported; *, low statistical power.

those who had surgery alone ($p < 0.001$, primary end point). There was decreased recurrence after WBRT at both local and distant sites, and the time to recurrence was significantly longer in the group that received WBRT. Although overall survival did not differ significantly between groups (48 wk in the surgery plus WBRT group vs 43 wk), the study was not powered to assess survival. Nevertheless, fewer patients in the WBRT group died from neurologic causes. The duration of functional independence (KPS ≥ 70) did not differ between groups. A second RCT involving 359 patients showed that WBRT (30 Gy) after either surgery or SRS (25 Gy marginal to each metastasis) did not affect overall survival or duration of functional independence (primary end point), but WBRT appeared to reduce intracranial relapse and neurologic death.[11] However, neurologic death was not included among the primary or secondary end points in the study design.

Muacevic et al performed an RCT that compared resection plus postoperative WBRT to SRS alone for patients with a newly diagnosed metastasis.[12] Unfortunately, this study was stopped early due to lack of accrual. Sixty-four patients (the planned accrual was 242) with a single metastasis no > 3 cm and a KPS of at least 70 were randomized to undergo surgery plus WBRT or SRS alone. Prognostic variables were comparable between groups. There was no crossover between groups, and no patients were lost to follow-up. There was no significant difference in overall survival between groups, which was the primary outcome measure. The groups did not differ in duration of freedom from local recurrence, but duration of freedom from recurrence at distant brain sites was longer in the surgery plus WBRT group compared to SRS alone. There was no difference in neurologic deaths. Another RCT comparing surgical resection plus WBRT versus SRS plus WBRT also suffered from low accrual, enrolling a total of 22 patients before study closure.[13] There was no statistical difference in survival time or quality of life, but these findings are difficult to interpret due to the low power.

Taken together, these trials provide ***level I evidence*** that, in patients with solitary brain metastases, surgery plus WBRT provides superior results compared to WBRT alone in terms of survival, recurrence, and functional independence.[7–9] This appears to be true for patients with good performance status and limited extracranial disease, but the best treatment for patients with a poor performance status, advanced systemic disease, or multiple brain metastases may involve combinations of WBRT and SRS, forgoing surgery.

The above ***level I evidence*** shows that the addition of WBRT following surgical treatment of a single, resectable metastasis appears to result in lower rates of recurrence in patients with a KPS score ≥ 70.[10] However, evidence that adjuvant WBRT prolongs survival is lacking at present. Also currently lacking is evidence that adjuvant WBRT delays loss of functional independence. Of course, this does not mean that adjuvant WBRT does not decrease mortality and functional dependence, but only that at present the data are lacking. In addition, the prematurely closed RCT by Muacevic et al failed to show a significant difference in mortality and local recurrence between surgical resection plus WBRT versus SRS, and it is difficult to draw firm conclusions regarding this comparison.[12] The authors acknowledge that this study was underpowered, but it did show improved distant brain recurrence in the group that received WBRT, which was attributed to the effect of radiation on micrometastases throughout the brain.

Level II Evidence

A landmark retrospective study of nearly 1,300 patients demonstrated an effect on survival for surgery plus radiotherapy compared to WBRT alone and to corticosteroids alone.[14] In this study, patients treated with surgical resection and WBRT survived 8.9 months compared to 3.6 months for patients treated with WBRT alone and 1.3 months for those treated with steroids only. These differences were statistically significant. The most commonly used fractionation schedules were 30 Gy in 10 fractions and 20 Gy in 5 fractions. The authors used multivariate analysis to identify prognostic factors affecting survival. Factors identified were performance status, response to steroid treatment, systemic tumor status and, to a lesser extent, site of primary tumor, age, and number of brain metastases.

There are at least three ***level II*** studies comparing surgery alone versus surgery plus WBRT. Unlike the ***level I evidence*** discussed above, few of these studies demonstrate a benefit of WBRT. Armstrong et al studied 185 lung cancer patients with resected brain metastases and found no difference attributable to WBRT in overall survival, brain failure (local or distant central nervous system [CNS] progression), and focal recurrence.[15] Hagen et al studied 35 melanoma patients with resected brain metastases and found no difference attributable to WBRT, although fewer patients who received radiation therapy died from neurologic causes.[16] Additionally, patients in the radiation therapy group experienced a significantly longer interval to relapse. Notably, these latter two findings were confirmed 8 years later in the RCT by Patchell et al.[10] Skibber et al studied 34 patients with melanoma and found increased survival in the 22 patients who received adjuvant radiation compared to the 12 who did not.[17] There was no difference between the groups for subsequent relapse rate.

Two retrospective cohort studies have been performed comparing surgery plus WBRT versus SRS alone. Muacevic et al studied 108 patients with a single tumor no > 3.5 cm who underwent either microsurgery and 50 Gy WBRT or single-dose Gamma Knife (Elekta AB, Stockholm, Sweden) radiosurgery with 22 Gy delivered to the target margin. They found no significant difference in median survival or local recurrence at 1 year, but, concordant with the RCT by Muacevic et al published 9 years later, patients who underwent surgery and WBRT were less likely to develop distant brain recurrence at 1 year.[12,18] Rades et al studied 206 patients who had one or two brain metastases and underwent either resection followed by WBRT or single-dose SRS with 18 to 25 Gy.[19] This study found no significant difference in overall survival, local recurrence, and brain recurrence (local and distant recurrence).

There are several retrospective cohort studies comparing surgery plus WBRT versus SRS plus WBRT. Bindal et al reviewed 93 patients who were treated with surgery plus WBRT or SRS (12–22 Gy) plus WBRT and found improved survival of 8.9 months in the surgery group.[20] Groups were matched according to histological characteristics of the primary tumor, extent of systemic disease, KPS score, time to brain metastasis, number of metastases, and patient age and gender. The median size of the lesion in the SRS group was 1.96 cm^3. The authors presented evidence that the difference in mortality was due to brain metastasis itself rather than progression of systemic disease. They also demonstrated that shorter survival in the SRS group was due to faster progression of treated lesions rather than development of new lesions. The variability of the marginal tumor dose in these patients may have contributed to the local failure rate in the SRS plus WBRT arm. Schöggl et al studied a total 133 patients who underwent surgical resection and WBRT (30 Gy/ 10 fractions) or SRS (17 Gy at the margin) plus WBRT and found no statistically significant difference in survival. Time to local recurrence was improved in the SRS group, whereas there was no difference for distant brain recurrence.[21] The median size of the lesions was 7,800 mm^3 in the SRS group compared to 12,500 mm^3 in the surgery group. O'Neill et al studied 97 patients who underwent WBRT and either surgery or SRS (dose not reported) and found no significant difference in survival.[22] However, the SRS group appeared to have improved local tumor control. Auchter et al compared 122 patients with single brain metastases treated with SRS to a historical control group treated with resection and WBRT.[23] Local recurrence and survival were similar in both groups. An additional study by Garell et al failed to show an outcome difference between resection plus WBRT and SRS plus WBRT.[24] An unpublished study that compared resection with SRS and included randomized and nonrandomized arms reported increased risk of local recurrence but not distant recurrence in the SRS group.[25]

Additional retrospective cohort studies compared surgery, SRS, WBRT, and alternative schedules of radiotherapy in various combinations for patients with metastases. In each of these studies, approximately two thirds of patients had solitary metastases. Ikushima et al investigated the use of fractionated stereotactic radiotherapy (FSRT) in patients with brain metastases from renal cell carcinoma.[26] Ten patients were treated with FSRT, 11 with surgery followed by radiotherapy (WBRT or local), and 14 with radiotherapy alone. Mortality was significantly improved in the FSRT group. Shinoura et al compared surgery plus radiotherapy (WBRT or local, 46.7 Gy) to SRS (28.9 Gy) among 63 patients and reported improved survival and time to recurrence at the original site in the surgery plus radiotherapy group.[27] Wang et al retrospectively reviewed 463 patients who were treated with surgery, WBRT, SRS, or WBRT plus SRS and reported survival to be greatest in the WBRT plus SRS group.[28]

Considered in toto, the studies above provide ***level II evidence*** that patients treated with WBRT in addition to surgery are less likely to die from neurologic causes than patients treated with surgery alone.[10,16] Similar to the ***level I*** data reviewed, there are no ***level II*** data that demonstrate an increase in overall survival with adjuvant WBRT. ***Level II*** data do not substantiate findings from the RCT by Patchell et al that adjuvant WBRT decreases the rate of local and distant recurrence, but one retrospective cohort study found that adjuvant WBRT increases time to CNS recurrence (local or distant).[15–17] Two ***level II*** studies examined surgery plus WBRT versus SRS and found no difference in survival or local recurrence between these treatments, but perhaps not surprisingly, one found a lower rate of distant brain recurrence at 1 year in the WBRT group.[18,19] Several retrospective cohort studies examined surgical resection plus WBRT versus SRS plus WBRT and yielded somewhat conflicting results. Nevertheless, it appears that surgery rather than SRS may be best for lesions at least 3 cm or producing significant mass effect in which dosing limitations may impair the effectiveness of SRS.[21] SRS is less invasive than surgery, can be performed on an outpatient basis, and does not carry the significant perioperative risks of general anesthesia and surgery. It may be cost-effective, and it appears to be particularly useful in the treatment of radiosensitive tumors (see below for further discussion).[21,29,30] Additionally, there is ***level II evidence*** that FSRT may have a role in the treatment of brain metastasis.[26] In summary, the addition of WBRT to surgical resection for a single metastasis does appear to decrease recurrence, particularly at distant brain sites, as well as death from neurologic cause. However, whether adjuvant WBRT increases overall survival remains unproven. Furthermore, the impact of delayed WBRT rather than WBRT delivered at the time of diagnosis remains unclear.

Consensus Statements

Several consensus statements regarding the treatment of brain metastasis have been published. Three statements that address the surgical management of single brain metastases will be reviewed briefly. In 2010 the Joint Guidelines Committee of the American Association of Neurological Surgeons (AANS) and the Congress of Neurological Surgeons (CNS) published a consensus statement in which they reviewed evidence regarding the management of patients with metastatic brain tumors, including data regarding surgical resection of single, newly diagnosed brain metastases in adults.[3] The committee reviewed RCTs, nonrandomized trials, cohort studies, and case-controlled studies that included one or more of the following comparisons: surgery versus WBRT, surgery versus surgery plus WBRT, surgery with or without WBRT versus SRS with or without WBRT, surgery versus surgery plus SRS, and surgery plus WBRT versus surgery plus SRS. Studies that met inclusion criteria were evaluated for quality using existing scales or modifications of existing scales. Quality and strength of recommendations were graded according to criteria established by the AANS and CNS.[31] Fifteen publications met the eligibility criteria.

The findings of the committee supported the following recommendations:

1. Surgical resection followed by WBRT compared with surgical resection alone is superior in local tumor control (***level I*** recommendation: reflecting a high degree of clinical certainty).
2. Surgical resection plus WBRT and SRS plus WBRT result in relatively equal survival rates (***level II*** recommendation: reflecting clinical certainty).
3. There is some evidence that SRS alone may be comparable to resection plus WBRT in terms of functional and survival outcomes if detection of distant site failure and salvage SRS are available (***level III*** recommendation: uncertain clinical utility due to inconclusive evidence).

The AANS/CNS brain metastases evidence-based clinical practice parameter guidelines included a second study by Gaspar et al that addressed the fundamental question of whether surgical resection in addition to WBRT improves outcomes when compared to WBRT alone.[32] The report concluded that surgical resection followed by WBRT is superior to WBRT alone with respect to survival and local tumor control for patients with a good performance status, defined as functionally independent and spending < 50% of time in bed, and limited extracranial disease (***level I*** recommendation).

The European Federation of Neurological Societies (EFNS) Task Force also provided evidence-based guidelines on the diagnosis and treatment of brain metastases.[33] This group searched numerous databases for relevant publications, assembled guidelines from national and European neuro-oncological societies from Italy, France, the Netherlands, Germany, and the UK, and surveyed attitudes of members of the task force from 10 countries regarding several critical issues. Papers were graded according to EFNS guidelines, and recommendations were graded A to C.[34] The levels of recommendation A to C roughly correspond to levels1 to 3 in the scheme used by Kalkanis et al.[3]

The EFNS report provided the following recommendations for the surgical treatment of single brain metastases:

1. Surgical resection should be considered when the tumor is accessible, large, when mass effect is considerable, or when obstructive hydrocephalus is present (agreed by all the members of the task force).
2. Surgical resection is recommended when KPS is at least 70 and systemic disease is absent or controlled (level A recommendation).
3. SRS should be considered when the tumor diameter is < 3.0 to 3.5 cm or the lesion is located in the eloquent cortex, basal ganglia, or brainstem (level B recommendation).

These guidelines also note that, in high-functioning patients with three or fewer lesions, either SRS, WBRT, or surgery may be considered.

Outcomes of Surgical Resection

Surgical resection of brain metastases in appropriate cases improves mortality and offers other benefits, such as a lower rate of relapse and an increased period of functional independence, as demonstrated by Patchell et al.[8] Of interest, the 1-month mortality in this study was no different in the surgery group than the comparison (4%). However, both groups did undergo a surgical procedure (surgical resection vs brain biopsy). For patients with single brain metastases who are functioning independently, surgical resection prior to WBRT appears to increase survival by as much as 25 weeks.[8,9] It remains unclear whether SRS offers a survival benefit over surgical resection for lesions < 3 cm or causing < 1 cm midline shift. Unlike radiotherapy, surgery allows rapid relief of symptoms of elevated intracranial pressure, focal neurologic deficits, and seizures, along with a rapid steroid taper.[33]

The common complications of surgical resection are in line with those of other intracranial procedures and include postoperative hematoma (3.2%), wound infection (1.6–3.0%), pneumonia (1.9%), and pulmonary embolus (1.5%). Depending on the size and location of a metastasis, the likelihood of a new postoperative neurologic deficit varies. Overall morbidity from surgical resection of metastases is reported to be approximately 8%, and 30-day mortality is 1.9 to 4.0%.[8,18,20,21] SRS has its own set of complications, including increased peritumor edema (7.5%), radiogenic necrosis (1.5–12.9%), intracranial hemorrhage (1.8–9.7%), treatment failure resulting in need for craniotomy (1.6–9.7%), deep venous thrombosis (12.9%), seizure (3.6%), and transient radiogenic complications such as nausea, dizziness, alopecia, and dermatitis (7.5%).[8,18,20,21,35] Overall morbidity from SRS treatment is reported to be 8.9%, although Patchell et al reported 30-day morbidity to be as high as 17%. Thirty-day mortality following SRS is reported to be 1.8 to 4.0%.[8,18] Thus, the morbidity and mortality rates of surgery and SRS are comparable.

Although there is evidence that surgical resection may as much as triple survival, the prognosis in brain metastasis remains very poor. Clearly, new therapies are needed. In response to this challenge, neurosurgeons are uniquely equipped to design, refine, and implement therapies that require access to the cranial cavity as well as the tumor bed. Surgery, in addition to the therapeutic benefit of resection itself, offers opportunities to sample tissues, implant devices, and directly administer medications, including biologics.

Our Clinical Experience

In our experience, patients presenting with brain metastases undergo a detailed neurologic examination, a thorough medical history review, and a contrast-enhanced magnetic resonance imaging (MRI) study and must have a recent staging of their systemic disease. These factors are considered before a treatment recommendation is made. When a patient presents with a possible brain metastasis with no history of primary disease, a tissue diagnosis is obtained before proceeding with treatment. Interestingly, in the study by Patchell et al, 11% of "tumors" detected by computed tomography (CT) were discovered to be primary brain tumors or an infectious etiology.[8] However, the patients in this study did not undergo routine MRI.

In our practice, surgical resection of brain metastases is offered to well-selected patients considering several factors. Initially, the location of the lesion and its size and mass effect are considered, along with the patient's symptoms. In keeping with the data presented in this chapter, metastases < 3 cm in diameter may be treated with SRS, especially within the eloquent cortex, basal ganglia, or brainstem. However, the addition of functional imaging and intraoperative guidance systems allow for resection in critical function areas in some cases.[36] In some instances, the clinical scenario may require surgery. For example, surgical resection may be necessary in the case of a comatose or seizing patient. Metastasis in the posterior fossa represents a special case in which surgical resection should be particularly considered, given the risk of fourth ventricle compression. There is a risk of sudden elevated intracranial pressure in patients with tumors > 3 cm associated with a significant amount of peritumoral edema narrowing the cerebrospinal fluid (CSF) drainage pathways, especially in the presence of untreated hydrocephalus.[32] Diffuse meningeal disease is a relative contraindication to surgery because it is a poor prognostic factor.[37] However, increasing experience with intrathecal chemotherapy suggests that leptomeningeal disease may be more treatable than previously thought.

The radiosensitivity of the metastasis is also considered. Although colon carcinoma, melanoma, and renal cell carcinoma typically respond poorly to FSRT, non-small-cell lung carcinoma and breast carcinomas generally respond well, and lymphomas and choriocarcinoma may be eradicated with radiotherapy.[5]

At every stage it is important to involve the patient and the family in the decision-making process so that their goals and preferences may be taken into account. Many cancer patients have strong opinions regarding their care and wish to direct it, considering previous experiences with surgery, radiation, and chemotherapy. The ultimate decision is in the hands of the patient. However, the patient should be presented with information and clear data as well as a recommendation from the treating physician(s). Merely counseling the patient without providing a recommendation is not enough; patients are unable to pool, comprehend, and evaluate the data accrued over the past 30 years in terms of managing metastatic tumors. That responsibility falls to the physicians. Cases are reviewed at our weekly tumor conference, which includes neurosurgeons, radiation oncologists, medical neuro-oncologists, neuroradiologists, and neuropsychologists.

Limitations and Future Studies

Although many of the questions reviewed above may be addressed effectively with RCTs, multiple approaches, including meta-analysis, well-designed cohort studies, and analyses of observational registries, will be useful. Examining every combination of surgery, WBRT, SRS, and fractionated SRS would require 72 separate treatment comparisons, and such a large number of comparisons by RCT are unlikely to be feasible. Although RCTs remain the gold standard in evidence-based medicine, they are subject to significant challenges, including cost, difficulty with blinding, pressure from therapeutic imperative, and study arm crossover.[38] There appears to be growing consensus that RCTs, though invaluable, are best viewed as complementary to observational approaches.[39]

As technology and experience with SRS for brain metastasis continue to advance, additional research will be needed. For example, there is some evidence that SRS plus WBRT may offer better local control rates than surgical resection plus WBRT in tumors such as small-cell lung cancer, leukemia, lymphoma, germ cell tumors, and multiple myeloma.[21] Moreover, surgical resection with adjuvant "resection bed" SRS has been investigated but will require additional study. It has been proposed that administration of SRS to the surgical resection cavity may improve outcomes.[3] Questions remain about the impact of subtotal versus total resection and about the management of recurrent metastases. A study by Agboola et al, which used the Radiation Therapy Oncology Group recursive partition analysis (RPA) subgroup classification scheme, demonstrated that complete surgical resection was an independent predictor of survival along with RPA criteria of age less than 65 years, KPS score of at least 70, and controlled primary disease.[40] Additionally, there is some evidence that reoperation for patients with relapse of a single brain metastasis who retain a high KPS score improves survival.[2] Further studies are needed to identify the most appropriate candidates for repeat resection.

In optimizing treatment approaches, quality of life including cognitive effects of treatments cannot be overlooked and in fact may be considered the primary end point goal. Although a treatment may affect outcomes such as mortality or recurrence, it may have more or less merit based on its effect on quality of life. For example, WBRT may cause early adverse effects, such as fatigue, alopecia, eustachian tube dysfunction, and, in the long term, cognitive neurotoxicity. Many patients develop clinical symptoms of memory loss progressing to dementia, frontal gait disorders, or urinary incontinence.[41] Likewise, treatments that do not appear to alter mortality should not be abandoned if they may improve quality of life. Studies that include quality of life measures are imperative in evaluating treatments for patients with brain metastases.

Finally, the treatment of brain metastases in children has not been fully studied. Although felt to be rare, pediatric metastasis is observed, with sarcoma and germ cell tumors accounting for most cases. Between 6 and 13% of pediatric brain tumors result from metastatic disease.[4] Additional investigation into these entities is warranted.

Conclusion

There is strong evidence that surgical resection of solitary brain metastases results in improved survival and that surgery may also improve rates of recurrence, freedom from death due to neurologic causes, and duration of functional independence. Postoperative adjuvant WBRT appears to improve recurrence and survival from neurologic causes, but at present there is no evidence that adjuvant WBRT improves overall survival. Based on the available data, surgical resection and SRS for metastases < 3 cm appear to offer equivalent survival benefit. However, there are currently no ***level I*** data that conclusively address this comparison. Multiple factors must be considered in the surgical resection of brain metastases, including location, size, mass effect, and histology. Patient symptomatology, the status of the primary disease, medical comorbidities, and the patient's goals should be considered.

It remains clear that each patient with a brain metastasis needs to be considered individually. Extent and trajectory of systemic disease, medical comorbidities, and patient desires affect the treatment decisions as much as size, location, and number of metastases. Valuable treatment options exist, but additional investigation to convincingly prove their merit is a necessary, valuable, and ongoing process.

References

[1] American Cancer Society. Cancer facts and figures 2012. http://www.cancer.org/Research/CancerFactsFigures/CancerFactsFigures/cancer-facts-figures-2012. Date accessed May 7, 2012

[2] Black PM, Johnson MD. Surgical resection for patients with solid brain metastases: current status. J Neurooncol 2004; 69: 119–124

[3] Kalkanis SN, Kondziolka D, Gaspar LE, et al. The role of surgical resection in the management of newly diagnosed brain metastases: a systematic review and evidence-based clinical practice guideline. J Neurooncol 2010; 96: 33–43

[4] Sul J, Posner JB. Brain metastases: epidemiology and pathophysiology. Cancer Treat Res 2007; 136: 1–21

[5] Cairncross JG, Posner JB. The management of brain metastases. In: Walker MD, ed. Oncology of the Nervous System. Boston, MA: Martinus Nijhoff; 1983: 342–377

[6] United States Preventive Task Force. Guide to clinical preventive services: report of the US Preventive Services Task Force. Darby, PA: DIANE Publishing; 1989

[7] Mintz AH, Kestle J, Rathbone MP, et al. A randomized trial to assess the efficacy of surgery in addition to radiotherapy in patients with a single cerebral metastasis. Cancer 1996; 78: 1470–1476

[8] Patchell RA, Tibbs PA, Walsh JW, et al. A randomized trial of surgery in the treatment of single metastases to the brain. N Engl J Med 1990; 322: 494–500

[9] Vecht CJ, Haaxma-Reiche H, Noordijk EM, et al. Treatment of single brain metastasis: radiotherapy alone or combined with neurosurgery? Ann Neurol 1993; 33: 583–590

[10] Patchell RA, Tibbs PA, Regine WF, et al. Postoperative radiotherapy in the treatment of single metastases to the brain: a randomized trial. JAMA 1998; 280: 1485–1489

[11] Kocher M, Soffietti R, Abacioglu U, et al. Adjuvant whole-brain radiotherapy versus observation after radiosurgery or surgical resection of one to three cerebral metastases: results of the EORTC 22952-26001 study. J Clin Oncol 2011; 29: 134–141

[12] Muacevic A, Wowra B, Siefert A, Tonn JC, Steiger HJ, Kreth FW. Microsurgery plus whole brain irradiation versus Gamma Knife surgery alone for treatment of single metastases to the brain: a randomized controlled multicentre phase III trial. J Neurooncol 2008; 87: 299–307

[13] Roos DE, Smith JG, Stephens SW. Radiosurgery versus surgery, both with adjuvant whole brain radiotherapy, for solitary brain metastases: a randomised controlled trial. Clin Oncol (R Coll Radiol) 2011; 23: 646–651

[14] Lagerwaard FJ, Levendag PC, Nowak PJ, Eijkenboom WM, Hanssens PE, Schmitz PI. Identification of prognostic factors in patients with brain metastases: a review of 1292 patients. Int J Radiat Oncol Biol Phys 1999; 43: 795–803

[15] Armstrong JG, Wronski M, Galicich J, Arbit E, Leibel SA, Burt M. Postoperative radiation for lung cancer metastatic to the brain. J Clin Oncol 1994; 12: 2340–2344

[16] Hagen NA, Cirrincione C, Thaler HT, DeAngelis LM. The role of radiation therapy following resection of single brain metastasis from melanoma. Neurology 1990; 40: 158–160

[17] Skibber JM, Soong SJ, Austin L, Balch CM, Sawaya RE. Cranial irradiation after surgical excision of brain metastases in melanoma patients. Ann Surg Oncol 1996; 3: 118–123

[18] Muacevic A, Kreth FW, Horstmann GA, et al. Surgery and radiotherapy compared with Gamma Nnife radiosurgery in the treatment of solitary cerebral metastases of small diameter. J Neurosurg 1999; 91: 35–43

[19] Rades D, Bohlen G, Pluemer A, et al. Stereotactic radiosurgery alone versus resection plus whole-brain radiotherapy for 1 or 2 brain metastases in recursive partitioning analysis class 1 and 2 patients. Cancer 2007; 109: 2515–2521

[20] Bindal AK, Bindal RK, Hess KR, et al. Surgery versus radiosurgery in the treatment of brain metastasis. J Neurosurg 1996; 84: 748–754

[21] Schöggl A, Kitz K, Reddy M, et al. Defining the role of stereotactic radiosurgery versus microsurgery in the treatment of single brain metastases. Acta Neurochir (Wien) 2000; 142: 621–626

[22] O'Neill BP, Iturria NJ, Link MJ, Pollock BE, Ballman KV, O'Fallon JR. A comparison of surgical resection and stereotactic radiosurgery in the treatment of solitary brain metastases. Int J Radiat Oncol Biol Phys 2003; 55: 1169–1176

[23] Auchter RM, Lamond JP, Alexander E, et al. A multiinstitutional outcome and prognostic factor analysis of radiosurgery for resectable single brain metastasis. Int J Radiat Oncol Biol Phys 1996; 35: 27–35

[24] Garell PC, Hitchon PW, Wen BC, Mellenberg DE, Torner J. Stereotactic radiosurgery versus microsurgical resection for the initial treatment of metastatic cancer to the brain. J Radiosurg. 1999; 2: 1–5

[25] Lang FF, Suki D, Maor M, et al. Conventional surgery versus stereotactic radiosurgery in the treatment of single brain metastases: a prospective study with both randomized and nonrandomized arms [abstract]. American Association of Neurological Surgeons; 2008

[26] Ikushima H, Tokuuye K, Sumi M, et al. Fractionated stereotactic radiotherapy of brain metastases from renal cell carcinoma. Int J Radiat Oncol Biol Phys 2000; 48: 1389–1393

[27] Shinoura N, Yamada R, Okamoto K, Nakamura O, Shitara N. Local recurrence of metastatic brain tumor after stereotactic radiosurgery or surgery plus radiation. J Neurooncol 2002; 60: 71–77

[28] Wang LG, Guo Y, Zhang X, et al. Brain metastasis: experience of the Xi-Jing hospital. Stereotact Funct Neurosurg 2002; 78: 70–83

[29] Lal LS, Byfield SD, Chang EL, et al. Cost-effectiveness analysis of a randomized study comparing radiosurgery with radiosurgery and whole brain radiation therapy in patients with 1 to 3 brain metastases. Am J Clin Oncol 2012; 35: 45–50

[30] Rutigliano MJ, Lunsford LD, Kondziolka D, Strauss MJ, Khanna V, Green M. The cost effectiveness of stereotactic radiosurgery versus surgical resection in the treatment of solitary metastatic brain tumors. Neurosurgery 1995; 37: 445–453, discussion 453–455

[31] Robinson PD, Kalkanis SN, Linskey ME, Santaguida PL. Methodology used to develop the AANS/CNS management of brain metastases evidence-based clinical practice parameter guidelines. J Neurooncol 2010; 96: 11–16

[32] Gaspar LE, Mehta MP, Patchell RA, et al. The role of whole brain radiation therapy in the management of newly diagnosed brain metastases: a systematic review and evidence-based clinical practice guideline. J Neurooncol 2010; 96: 17–32

[33] Soffietti R, Cornu P, Delattre JY, et al. EFNS guidelines on diagnosis and treatment of brain metastases: report of an EFNS Task Force. Eur J Neurol 2006; 13: 674–681

[34] Brainin M, Barnes M, Baron JC, et al. Guideline Standards Subcommittee of the EFNS Scientific Committee. Guidance for the preparation of neurological management guidelines by EFNS scientific task forces—revised recommendations 2004. Eur J Neurol 2004; 11: 577–581

[35] Jagannathan J, Bourne TD, Schlesinger D, et al. Clinical and pathological characteristics of brain metastasis resected after failed radiosurgery. Neurosurgery 2010; 66: 208–217

[36] Tan TC, Black PM. Image-guided craniotomy for cerebral metastases: techniques and outcomes. Neurosurgery 2007; 61 (Suppl): 349–356, discussion 356–357

[37] Wroński M, Arbit E, McCormick B. Surgical treatment of 70 patients with brain metastases from breast carcinoma. Cancer 1997; 80: 1746–1754

[38] Harbaugh RE. Class I evidence for the treatment of brain metastases: trial design issues [abstract]. Congress of Neurological Surgeons; 2011

[39] Mauri L. Why we still need randomized trials to compare effectiveness. N Engl J Med 2012; 366: 1538–1540

[40] Agboola O, Benoit B, Cross P, et al. Prognostic factors derived from recursive partition analysis (RPA) of Radiation Therapy Oncology Group (RTOG) brain metastases trials applied to surgically resected and irradiated brain metastatic cases. Int J Radiat Oncol Biol Phys 1998; 42: 155–159

[41] DeAngelis LM, Delattre JY, Posner JB. Radiation-induced dementia in patients cured of brain metastases. Neurology 1989; 39: 789–796

15 Radiosurgery for Solitary Metastases

Mark E. Linskey

Introduction

Metastatic spread of cancer to the brain is a significant problem in clinical oncology. Brain metastases are overwhelmingly the most common type of brain tumor, outnumbering primary brain tumors almost 5 to 1.[1,2] They are associated with poor prognosis from both a length and a quality of life standpoint. Brain metastases can occur as a single lesion or as multiple lesions. When brain metastases occur as a single lesion in the context of no other metastatic disease, they are called solitary metastases. When brain metastases occur as a single or one of a few detectable metastatic lesions, they are called oligometastatic tumors. When a single brain metastatic lesion occurs in the setting of significant known systemic disease, it is referred to as a single brain metastasis. These distinctions are important clinically, as more aggressive treatment options may be more appropriate, as well as potentially more successful, for patients with a solitary or oligometastatic brain tumor compared to those with a single brain metastasis. Metastatic brain tumors can also be described as either synchronous (diagnosed at the same time as the primary tumor or first sign of metastatic disease recurrence) or metachronous (identified a time interval after the diagnosis of the primary tumor or first sign of metastatic recurrence). Epidemiologic data indicate that single or solitary lesions are more likely to occur with breast, colorectal, and renal cell carcinoma, whereas lung cancer and melanoma are more likely to cause multiple metastases.[3]

Although metastatic spread of cancer to the brain includes the rarer forms of dural-based disease, leptomeningeal disease, and spinal cord metastases, for the purposes of this chapter, we will restrict ourselves to a discussion of solid parenchymal metastatic brain tumors, which represent 85 to 95% of the total.[1] Also, although stereotactic radiosurgery (SRS) includes single- as well as multisession procedures,[4] for the purposes of this chapter, we will restrict ourselves to a discussion of single-session SRS, as almost all published studies and clinical evidence using SRS for treating metastatic brain tumors is restricted to this form of delivery.[5]

Options for treating patients with metastatic brain tumors include whole-brain radiation therapy (WBRT), surgical resection, SRS, and systemic drug therapies (chemotherapy, biochemotherapy, targeted agents, experimental therapies, etc).[5–9] Deciding which treatment modality or combination of treatment modalities is optimal is far more controversial for patients with solitary, oligo-, or single metastatic brain tumors than their multiple metastatic brain tumor counterparts. Patients with solitary, oligo-, or single metastatic brain tumors are far more likely to have a potential for prolonged survival, or even potential cure, rather than solely targeting optimal local control, and/or functional status and quality of life optimization. More aggressive approaches for patients with solitary, oligo-, or single metastatic brain tumors and more extensive expenditure of health care resources in this patient subset are far more likely to be justifiable.

Evidence Base for Stereotactic Radiosurgery for Single Metastatic Brain Tumors

In the multidisciplinary clinical practice guidelines approved by the American Association of Neurological Surgery (AANS) and Congress of Neurological Surgeons (CNS) for treating patients with metastatic brain tumors, which were jointly developed with the McMasters Evidence-based Practice Center (EPC), the literature search extended through September 2008.[10] Thirty-two studies were included for analysis. This list has been subsequently updated by running the same search strategy[10] in Medline from August 2008 through May 15, 2012. The updated published evidence base in the English literature for SRS and metastatic brain tumors is summarized in ▶ Table 15.1.

The comparison of WBRT versus WBRT plus SRS included two ***level I*** prospective randomized controlled trials (RCTs),[11,12] one ***level II*** prospective cohort study,[13] one ***level II*** retrospective cohort study,[14] and one ***level III*** retrospective cohort study with historical controls,[15] for a total of five comparative studies. From September 2008 through May 2012, one additional ***level I*** RCT comparing WBRT to WBRT plus SRS for patients with one to three metastatic brain tumors with neurocognition rather than local control or patient survival, has been published.[16] Thus, there were six ***level I*** to ***III*** clinical studies comparing WBRT to WBRT plus SRS for patients with at least one metastatic brain tumor.

The comparison of SRS alone versus WBRT plus SRS included 1 ***level I*** prospective RCT with a companion article,[17,18] 1 ***level II*** prospective cohort study,[13] and 10 ***level II*** retrospective cohort studies.[14,19–27] From September 2008 through May 2012, one additional ***level I*** RCT comparing SRS alone to WBRT plus SRS for patients with one to three metastatic brain tumors was published.[28] Thus, there were 13 ***level I*** to ***III*** clinical studies comparing SRS alone to WBRT plus SRS for patients with at least one metastatic brain tumor.

Searching the comparison of SRS alone versus WBRT alone found only ***level II or III evidence***. No prospective RCTs have ever addressed this comparison. Searching this comparison yielded one prospective ***level II*** cohort study,[13] three retrospective ***level II*** cohort studies,[14,29,30] and two ***level III*** retrospective cohort studies with historical controls.[31,32] No additional clinical studies evaluating this comparison were published through May 2012. Thus, there were six ***level II*** or ***III*** clinical studies comparing SRS alone to WBRT alone for patients with at least one metastatic brain tumor.

Searching the comparison of SRS plus WBRT to surgical resection plus WBRT found only ***level II evidence.*** Through September 2008, no prospective RCTs assessed this comparison. Four ***level II*** retrospective cohort studies were identified addressing this comparison.[33–36] From September 2008 through May 2012, one ***level I*** RCT and one downgraded ***level II*** RCT (stopped early due to poor accrual) comparing SRS plus WBRT

Table 15.1 Published comparative evidence base (level I to III) in the English literature for stereotactic radiosurgery and metastatic brain tumors through May 13, 2012

Comparison (number of comparative clinical studies)	First author (year)	Study design (notes)	Evidence level
SRS + WBRT vs WBRT alone (*N* = 6)	Kondziolka et al[11]	RCT	I
	Andrews et al[12]	RCT	I
	Chang et al[16]	RCT	I
	Li et al[13]	Prospective cohort (2 of 3 study arms)	II
	Wang et al[14]	Retrospective cohort (2 of 4 study arms)	II
	Sanghavi et al[15]	Retrospective cohort (only historical controls)	III
SRS alone vs SRS + WBRT (*N* = 13)	Aoyama et al[17]	RCT	I
	Kocher et al[28]	RCT	I
	Li et al[13]	Prospective cohort (2 of 3 study arms)	II
	Wang et al[14]	Retrospective cohort (2 of 4 study arms)	II
	Chidel et al[19]	Retrospective cohort	II
	Coombs et al[20]	Retrospective cohort	II
	Hoffman et al[21]	Retrospective cohort	II
	Jawahar et al[22]	Retrospective cohort	II
	Noel et al[23]	Retrospective cohort	II
	Pirzkall et al[24]	Retrospective cohort	II
	Sneed et al[25]	Retrospective cohort	II
	Sneed et al[26]	Retrospective cohort	II
	Varlatto et al[27]	Retrospective cohort	II
SRS alone vs WBRT alone (*N* = 6)	Li et al[13]	Prospective cohort (2 of 3 study arms)	II
	Wang et al[14]	Retrospective Cohort (2 of 4 study arms)	II
	Lee et al[29]	Retrospective cohort	II
	Rades et al[30]	Retrospective cohort	II
	Datta et al[31]	Retrospective cohort (only historical controls)	III
	Kocher et al[32]	Retrospective cohort (only historical controls)	III
SRS + WBRT vs surgical resection + WBRT (*N* = 6)	Kocher et al[28]	RCT (2 of 4 study arms)	I
	Roos et al[37]	Downgraded RCT (stopped early/poor accrual)	II
	Bindal et al[33]	Retrospective cohort	II
	Garell et al[34]	Retrospective cohort	II
	O'Neill et al[35]	Retrospective cohort	II
	Schöggl et al[36]	Retrospective cohort	II
SRS alone vs surgical resection + WBRT (*N* = 5)	Kocher et al[28]	RCT (2 of 4 study arms)	I
	Muacevic et al[38]	RCT	I
	Muacevic et al[39]	Retrospective cohort	II
	Rades et al[40]	Retrospective cohort	II
	Shinoura et al[41]	Retrospective cohort (local radiotherapy not WBRT)	II
Surgical resection + SRS vs surgical resection + WBRT (*N* = 1)	Serizawa et al[42]	Retrospective cohort	II

Abbreviations: RCT, randomized controlled trial; SRS, stereotactic radiosurgery (single session only); WBRT, whole-brain radiation therapy.

to surgical resection plus WBRT for patients with one to three or solitary metastatic brain tumors were published.[28,37] Thus, there were six ***level I*** or ***II*** clinical studies comparing SRS plus WBRT to surgical resection plus WBRT for patients with at least one metastatic brain tumor.

Searching the comparison of SRS alone versus surgical resection plus WBRT found one ***level I*** RCT[38] and three ***level II*** retrospective cohort studies[39–41] assessing this comparison. From September 2008 through May 2012, one ***level I*** RCT included arms comparing SRS alone to surgical resection plus WBRT for patients with one to three metastatic brain tumors were published.[28] Thus, there were five ***level I*** or ***II*** clinical studies comparing SRS alone to surgical resection plus WBRT for patients with at least one metastatic brain tumor.

Searching the comparison of surgical resection plus SRS to surgical resection plus WBRT found only limited ***level II*** evidence. Through September 2008, no prospective RCTs assessed this comparison. There was one ***level II*** retrospective cohort study that did address this comparison.[42] From September 2008 through May 2012, no additional studies were published comparing surgical resection plus SRS to surgical resection plus WBRT. Thus, there is currently only one ***level II*** clinical study comparing surgical resection plus SRS to surgical resection plus WBRT for patients with at least one metastatic brain tumor.

Additional evidence will certainly become available as ongoing clinical trials reach conclusion, analysis, and publication. A listing of active comparative SRS metastatic brain tumor

Table 15.2 Active comparative stereotactic radiosurgery metastatic brain tumor clinical trials listed at http://clinicaltrials.gov as of May 13, 2012

ClinicalTrials.gov identifier	Sponsor	Status as of May 13, 2012	Clinical trial title
NCT00460395	MD Anderson Cancer Center	Completed, not yet published	Surgery versus stereotactic radiosurgery in the treatment of single brain metastases: A randomized trial
NCT00096265	RTOG	Completed, not yet published	Radiation therapy and stereotactic radiosurgery with or without temozolomide or erlotinib in treating patients with brain metastases secondary to non–small cell lung cancer
NCT01169129	Barretos Cancer Hospital, Brazil	Ongoing, not recruiting	Surgery and whole brain radiotherapy versus whole brain radiotherapy and radiosurgery for 1–3 resectable brain metastases
NCT01372774	NCCTG	Open, recruiting	Stereotactic radiosurgery or whole brain radiation therapy in treating patients with brain metastases that have been removed by surgery
NCT00377156	NCCTG	Open, recruiting	Stereotactic radiation therapy with or without whole brain radiation therapy in treating patients with brain metastases
NCT00280475	Japan Clinical Oncology Group	Open, recruiting	A trial of postoperative whole brain radiation therapy versus salvage radiosurgery therapy for metastases
NCT01535209	Maria Sklodowska-Curie Memorial Cancer Center, Poland	Open, recruiting	Stereotactic radiotherapy of resection cavity for single brain metastasis versus whole-brain radiotherapy after resection
NCT01295970	University Health Network, Toronto	Not yet open	Surgery versus radiosurgery for the treatment of single brain metastases

Abbreviations: NCCTG, North Central Cancer Treatment Group; RTOG, Radiation Therapy Oncology Group.

clinical trials listed at http://clinicaltrials.gov as of May 13, 2012, is given in ▶ Table 15.2.

Current Multidisciplinary, Evidence-linked Clinical Practice Guidelines for Stereotactic Radiosurgery

The AANS/CNS-approved multidisciplinary recommendations for treating patients with metastatic brain tumors, jointly developed with the McMasters EPC, published in January 2010 and based on literature published though September 2008, are currently our most complete, comprehensive, and up-to-date evidence-linked clinical practice guidelines available for treating patients with metastatic brain tumors.[2,5–10] They have not yet been updated and have not been superseded by any more recent, higher quality,[43–47] evidence-linked guidelines. SRS recommendations for patients with single metastatic brain tumors include[5]

a) SRS plus WBRT versus WBRT alone

- A ***level 1*** recommendation for SRS along with WBRT, rather than WBRT alone, for improving survival for patients with single metastatic brain tumors and Karnofsky performance scale (KPS) score ≥ 70
- A ***level II*** recommendation for SRS along with WBRT, rather than WBRT alone, for improving local tumor control for patients with single metastatic brain tumors and KPS ≥ 70
- A ***level III*** recommendation for SRS along with WBRT, rather than WBRT alone, for improving survival for patients with a single metastatic brain tumor and KPS < 70

b) SRS alone versus SRS plus WBRT

- A ***level II*** recommendation that SRS alone may provide equivalent survival advantage to SRS plus WBRT, calling into question the need for WBRT so long as active surveillance imaging follow-up allows for early detection of new disease distant to the SRS treatment volume

c) SRS with or without WBRT versus surgical resection plus WBRT

- A ***level II*** recommendation that SRS alone may provide equivalent survival advantage to SRS plus WBRT or surgical resection plus WBRT, calling into question the need for either surgical resection or WBRT so long as active surveillance imaging follow-up allows for early detection of new disease distant to the SRS treatment volume

d) SRS alone versus WBRT alone

- A ***level III*** recommendation that SRS alone appears to be superior to WBRT alone in terms of patient survival

Based on a to d above, for patients with solitary, oligo-, or even single metastatic brain tumors, there would seem to be very little support for continuing to treat these patients with WBRT alone. Indeed, cumulative ***level I*** to ***III evidence*** overwhelmingly supports a much more active and aggressive approach to local control in these patients. The controversy arises when considering SRS versus surgical resection for initial local control in these patients, as well as whether or not WBRT still has a role to play for patients with solitary, oligo-, or single metastatic brain tumors in the SRS era.

Should Patients with Solitary, Oligo-, or Single Metastatic Brain Tumors Still Receive Whole-Brain Radiation Therapy as Part of Their Treatment Strategy?

Certainly, the published evidence-based outlined above and in ▶ Table 15.1, as well as the 2010 multidisciplinary clinical practice guidelines for treating patients with metastatic brain tumors,[2,55,7–10] continue to support the use of WBRT to augment the superior local control achievable with SRS. However, this is largely because of the lack of studies comparing either SRS alone with SRS and WBRT or surgical resection with SRS to surgical resection followed by WBRT. Two recent RCTs published since the 2010 multidisciplinary clinical practice guidelines raise serious questions on the continued use of WBRT for patients with solitary, oligo-, or single metastatic brain tumors.[16,28] Pending results of the Japanese JLGK0901 study,[48] as well as likely results of clinical trials currently active and enrolling (▶ Table 15.2), will likely fill the evidence gap to further justify restricting the use of WBRT for patients with all but the most numerous multiple metastatic brain tumors.

Previously, Patchell et al clearly demonstrated that adding WBRT was necessary after surgical resection of a metastatic brain tumor in order to lower the chance of local resection cavity recurrence from ~ 40% to ~ 10%.[49] However, in the more recent Kocher et al European Organization for the Research and Treatment of Cancer (EORTC) trial, the local resection treatment volume recurrence rate was only 31% with SRS alone versus 59% with surgical resection alone, and all recurrences could be detected early for additional treatment with regular follow-up imaging.[28] Thus, second-stage WBRT may not be as necessary for local control for first-stage SRS as it is for first-stage surgical resection.

More importantly, the recent RCT by Chang et al at MD Anderson stunned the radiation oncology and general oncology world by confirming, and unequivocally objectively quantifying, the deleterious neurocognitive effects of WBRT, which had previously often been denied, downplayed, or even ascribed to the underlying malignancy rather than the therapy. Their RCT comparing SRS alone to WBRT plus SRS had to be stopped prematurely due to a 52% probability in cognitive decline 4 months after treatment in the WBRT plus SRS arm compared to a 24% probability of cognitive decline at 4 months in the SRS-alone arm.[16] Neurocognitive decline was objectively defined as a 5-point drop in the Hopkins Verbal Learning Test–Revised (HVLT-R). As a result of the MD Anderson study, there is increasing pressure to eliminate WBRT unless the results obtainable by using it are superior (rather than just not inferior).

The problem remains how best to augment surgical resection, which carries a 40 to 51% risk of resection cavity recurrence if used in isolation[28,49] for patients with metastatic brain tumors. SRS to the resection cavity is becoming increasingly more attractive to augment surgical resection based on not only results of SRS for metastatic brain tumors but also the potential to avoid the neurocognitive complications of WBRT while still potentially mitigating the high local recurrence rate of surgical resection used in isolation (▶ Fig. 15.1 and ▶ Fig. 15.2).

Are Solitary, Oligo-, and Single Metastatic Brain Tumors Best Treated with Stereotactic Radiosurgery or Surgical Resection?

This is perhaps the most controversial question of all. There are several very important issues to consider, and treatment must be individualized from patient to patient. First, there is excellent ***level I evidence*** supporting surgical resection followed by WBRT for improving survival rates as well as functional independence and performance status as compared to WBRT alone.[50,51] Indeed, the data for surgical resection are as strong as those for SRS plus WBRT, given multiple RCTs, as well as lesser quality comparative studies, confirming both survival and quality of life advantages.[7] Second, there are logistical and primary site cancer biology concerns regarding the need to begin or even suspend, systemic chemotherapy during the 2-week postoperative healing period for surgical resection that do not need to be considered for SRS. Thus, immediate SRS for a patient presenting with a synchronous solitary metastatic brain tumor has the potential advantage for ensuring that the brain metastasis remains solitary and that no new metastases do develop during a systemic therapy-free waiting period for surgical healing or recovery from a surgical complication (▶ Fig. 15.2). Furthermore, it allows a potential definitive primary resection to proceed with the least possible delay. This issue may not be as important for a patient presenting with a metachronous solitary brain metastasis who has already had the primary cancer source resected and who has already received an adequate course of systemic treatment, and might thus be more reasonably expected to have less to risk for going off therapy for a 2-week postsurgical healing period. Third, not all cancer patients are reasonable candidates for safe general anesthesia, based on cardiopulmonary or surgery risk factors. Fourth, patients will differ in their risk tolerance and life priority assessment when it comes to more invasive procedures such as open surgical resection, particularly when facing a diagnosis of cancer. Fifth, not all metastatic brain tumors arise in areas with low risk for surgical resection (▶ Fig. 15.3 and ▶ Fig. 15.4). Sixth, as will be discussed in the next section, solitary metastatic tumors represent a unique opportunity for

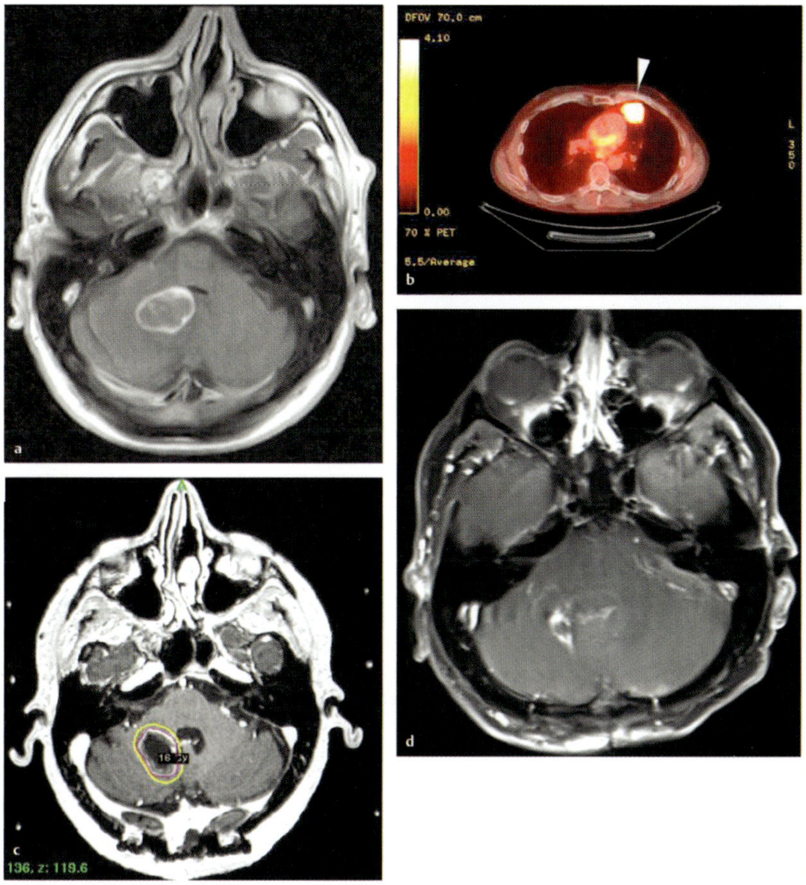

Fig. 15.1 A 62-year-old man with a 2.8 × 2.2 × 2.3-cm-deep right cerebellar cystic tumor. (a) T1-weighted contrast-enhanced axial magnetic resonance imaging (MRI) and (b) axial 18-fluorodeoxyglucose (FDG) positron emission tomography (PET) reveal a 3.4-cm primary non–small cell lung carcinoma (NSCLC). Without the synchronous solitary brain metastasis, the tumor would be considered stage 2 (T2a,N1,M0). The tumor was treated with surgical resection followed 10 days later with Gamma Knife (Elekta AB, Stockholm, Sweden) stereotactic radiosurgery (SRS). (c) T1-weighted contrast-enhanced MRI for targeting SRS that delivered 16 Gy to the resection cavity margin without whole-brain radiation therapy (WBRT). The patient went on to have the primary chest lesion resected followed by radiochemotherapy. (d) Three-year post-SRS T1-weighted contrast-enhanced MRI and 3-year PET/computed tomography (CT) (not shown) showed no evidence of disease.

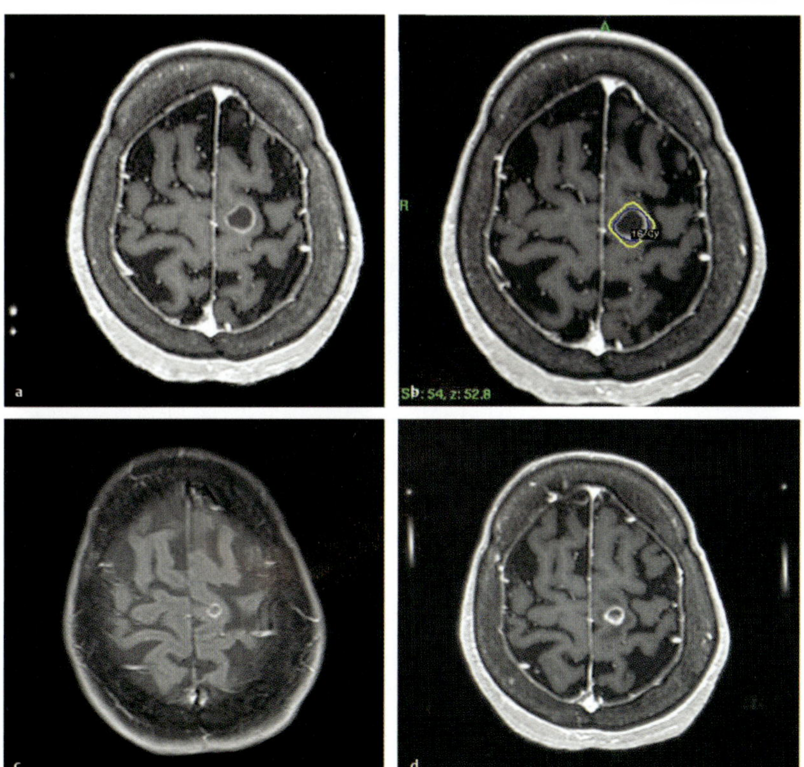

Fig. 15.2 A 72-year-old, left-handed man presenting with a seizure was found to have a 3-cm cystic dominant hemisphere primary sensory strip tumor. (a) T1-weighted contrast-enhanced MRI. A PET/CT scan revealed 5.5 × 6-cm primary NSCLC. (b) Coronal FDG PET. Without the synchronous solitary brain metastasis, the tumor would be considered stage II (T2b,N0,M0). The tumor was treated with surgical resection followed by Gamma Knife SRS to the resection bed with 18 Gy to the margin without WBRT. (c) T1-weighted contrast-enhanced SRS-targeting MRI. Unfortunately, the patient's postoperative course was complicated by a deep venous thrombosis and subsequent pulmonary embolus, which delayed the resection of the primary chest lesion by several months. Repeat prethoracotomy PET/CT showed a new vertebral body metastasis. Fortunately, the tumor had an epidermal growth factor receptor (EGFR) mutation, and he was able to be treated successfully with chest radiotherapy and erlotinib. (d) Nine-month postresection T1-weighted contrast-enhanced MRI showed no brain disease..

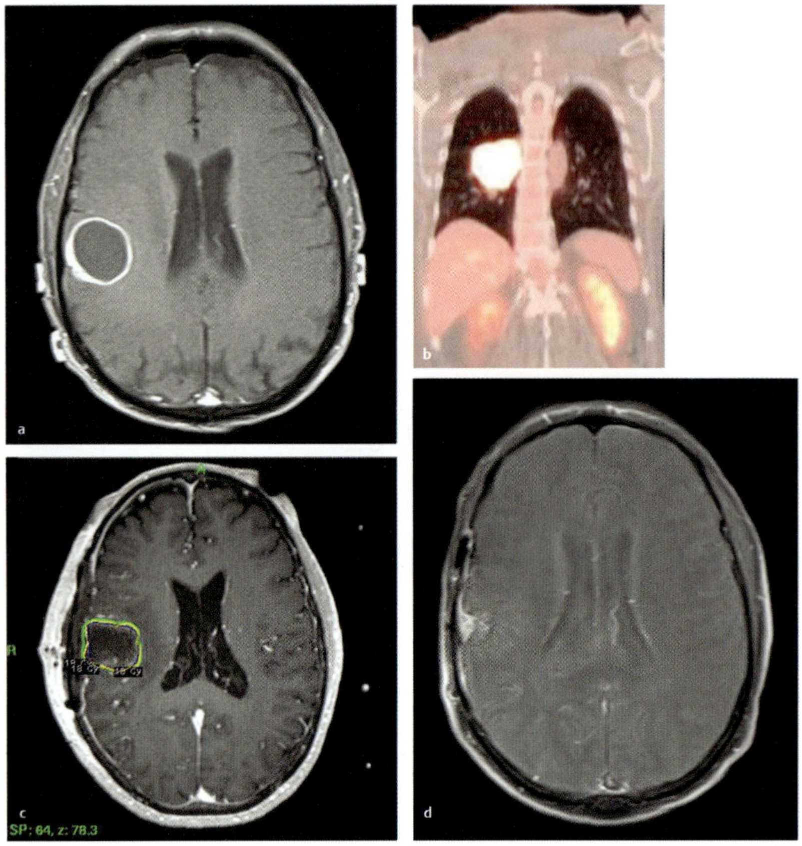

Fig. 15.3 A 67-year-old woman with stage 4 breast cancer and significant systemic disease presented with mild left foot clumsiness and weakness and a 1.4-cm cystic left perirolandic metastatic brain tumor. (a) She was treated with Gamma Knife SRS with 16 Gy to the tumor margin. (b) T1-weighted contrast-enhanced MRI for targeting SRS without WBRT. (c) T1-weighted contrast-enhanced MRI 12 months after SRS shows lesion shrinkage without any surrounding edema reaction. Four months later, the tumor started to regrow with new surrounding edema. It was retreated with a second round of Gamma Knife SRS 17 months after the first SRS. (d) T1-weighted contrast-enhanced MRI for targeting SRS with 16 Gy to the tumor margin. The patient has a stable brain lesion but continued systemic progression.

intervention for cure, rather than just long-term control at maximal functional status and quality of life (▶ Fig. 15.1).

The Special Case of Patients with an Unknown Primary Tumor

In up to 15% of cases where brain metastases are the first identified evidence of cancer, the primary tumor source is not found despite diligent systemic workup.[52–54] Many of these involve single metastases and should be considered special cases of isolated or oligometastases. Although limited published SRS results for patients with oligometastases and an unknown primary are encouraging,[55] in our opinion, this subset of patients is particularly attractive for a surgical resection approach, so long as the lesion is single.

For single brain lesions without proven primary cancer source, surgical confirmation of histology is critical to rule out primary brain tumor or even a nonneoplastic lesion. In one study of single brain masses in patients with a primary cancer source proven by histology within 2 years of brain lesion diagnosis, 11% of the brain lesions turned out not to be metastatic tumors.[50] For patients without a proven primary cancer histology or even workup-detected primary cancer source, this incidence is likely to be even higher. Although tissue diagnosis can certainly be obtained by stereotactic needle biopsy,[56] if the lesion is single, superficial, and/or surgically accessible with reasonably low risk of location-related neurologic morbidity, then surgical resection offers the advantage of obtaining the tissue diagnosis and treating the metastatic brain tumor at the same time. This avoids the need for, as well as the time commitment and potential additive morbidity of, two sequential procedures (stereotactic needle biopsy followed by SRS).

The Special Case of Patients with Solitary Brain Metastases

Patients with a solitary brain metastasis (either synchronous or metachronous) represent a unique subset of patients with single brain metastases. If one cannot make the case for an aggressive approach in treating this small patient subset, then an aggressive approach is never likely to be justified. Indeed, the unique opportunity to potentially achieve a cure, and not just long-term control or palliation, is extremely attractive (▶ Fig. 15.1).

Initial enthusiasm and the largest reported experience supporting this sort of aggressive approach for patients with solitary metastatic brain tumors come from experience with non-small-cell lung carcinoma (NSCLC). Multiple observational clinical studies as well as case series began to be published, demonstrating that patients with otherwise stage I or II disease (N0,1) (International Union Against Cancer [UICC] and American Joint Committee on Cancer [AJCC]), but a solitary

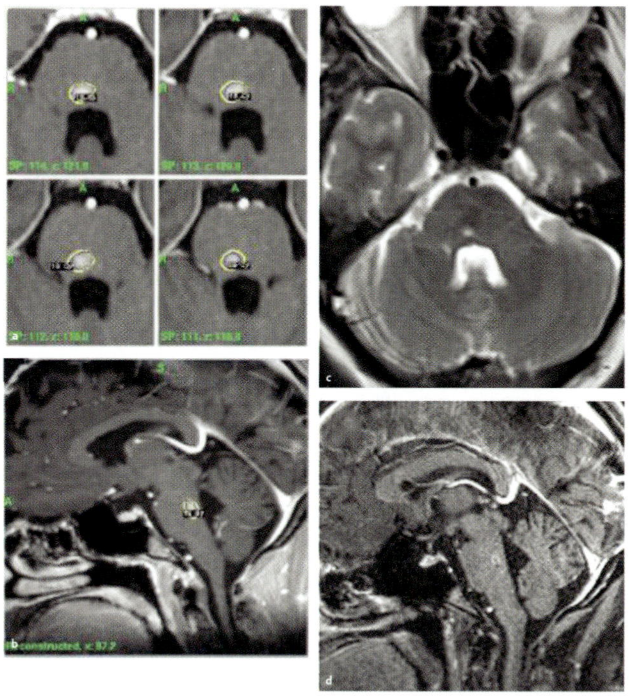

Fig. 15.4 A 44-year-old-woman with stage 4 infiltrating ductal breast cancer and systemic disease, including a hip metastasis, reducing her Karnofsky performance scale (KPS) score to 60. Complaints of diplopia led to a brain MRI revealing a 10 × 12 × 13-mm-deep dorsal pons/brainstem metastasis eccentric to the right. The patient was treated with Gamma Knife SRS with 18 Gy to the tumor margin. (a) Axial and (b) sagittal T1-weighted contrast-enhanced MRI for SRS with no WBRT. Follow-up imaging (c) Sagittal T1-weighted contrast-enhanced MRI and (d) T2-weighted noncontrast axial MRI 6 months after SRS show tumor shrinkage, and the patient is neurologically asymptomatic.

brain metastasis (technically stage 4–M1) fared as well as stage I or II counterparts so long as both the primary and the metastatic tumors were resected.[57–59] Soon additional observational clinical studies as well as case series began to be published, demonstrating that similar results were achievable substituting SRS for surgical resection.[59–62] The overall survival of these patients averaged 14% (range 8–21%), and the 5-year survival rate of these patients averaged 21% (range 16–30%).[59]

A Cochrane review published in 2006 and updated through March 2009 failed to find a single RCT comparing surgical resection with SRS for patients with NSCLC and solitary brain metastases.[63] However, enough strong observational clinical study data as well as weaker observational clinical study and clinical series data were available for the American College of Chest Physicians to arrive at evidence-linked clinical practice parameter guidelines, which were published in 2007.[64,65] For NSCLC patients with synchronous N0,1 disease, a strong recommendation (level 1C) based on observational studies or case series (low-quality evidence) was made for resection or SRS for the solitary brain metastasis coupled with resection of the primary brain tumor.[64] For NSCLC patients with metachronous N0,1 disease, a stronger recommendation (level 1B) based on strong observational studies (moderate-quality evidence), was made for resection or SRS for the solitary brain metastasis.[64] For instances where the brain metastasis is surgically resected, a weak recommendation (level 2B) was made for reinforcement with adjuvant WBRT based on strong observational studies that the pros and cons of adding WBRT were about equally balanced.

The strongest results were obtained in this aggressive approach for metachronous solitary metastasis rather than synchronous metastasis.[59,64] The biggest predictor of worse outcome was if the solitary brain metastasis was aggressively treated, but somehow the primary cancer failed to be resected, or had delayed resection, despite best original intentions.[59] Thus, at our institution, we prefer SRS for synchronous solitary metastatic NSCLC to allow the primary resection to proceed as quickly as possible. We can always consider delayed brain metastasis resection for cure assuming all goes well, and the treated brain lesion remains the only evidence of disease over time. For metachronous isolated NSCLC brain metastases identified after successful primary tumor resection, we prefer brain tumor resection followed by SRS to the brain resection bed if the lesion is in a suitable location, the patient is a good candidate for general anesthesia, and the patient is willing. This approach maximizes the chance of potential cure. We need to keep in mind that tumor control with SRS is not necessarily a "cure." Living tumor cells are usually present in SRS-controlled tumors, despite their failure to grow. Delayed SRS failures do occur (▶ Fig. 15.3) and are usually associated with biologically active tumors, as indicated by the postresection MIB-1 labeling proliferation index.[66]

A search of the National Library of Medicine database shows that, in addition to NSCLC, solitary brain metastases have been reported for breast cancer, thyroid cancer, ovarian cancer, renal cell carcinoma, bladder cancer, esophageal cancer, colon cancer, intestinal cancer, cervical cancer, osteosarcoma, and Ewing sarcoma. There is no reason to believe that outcomes will be different for an aggressive approach to these histologies corresponding to that justified with NSCLC. Indeed, preliminary data on breast cancer–related solitary brain metastasis are consistent with those reported for NSCLC.[67]

Conclusion

In the setting of single, oligo-, and solitary metastatic brain tumors, SRS has an important and increasing role for patient management, whereas the role of WBRT is steadily declining. In certain patient settings, it is the initial treatment of choice for many brain tumor and oncology programs. In settings where surgical resection maintains priority, it is now the preferred secondary treatment, in lieu of WBRT for sterilizing the resection cavity. Ongoing clinical trials hold promise for providing the evidence base necessary to place current management paradigms on even more solid footing.

References

[1] Alexandru D, Bota D, Linskey ME. Epidemiology of central nervous system metastases. Prog Neurol Surg 2012; 25: 13–29

[2] Kalkanis SN, Linskey ME. Evidence-based clinical practice parameter guidelines for the treatment of patients with metastatic brain tumors: introduction. J Neurooncol 2010; 96: 7–10

[3] Delattre JY, Krol G, Thaler HT, Posner JB. Distribution of brain metastases. Arch Neurol 1988; 45: 741–744

[4] Barnett GH, Linskey ME, Adler JR, Cozzens JW, Friedman WA, Heilbrun MP, Lunsford LD, Schulder M, Sloan AE American Association of Neurological Surgeons, Congress of Neurological Surgeons Washington Committee Stereotactic Radiosurgery Task Force. Stereotactic radiosurgery—an organized neurosurgery-sanctioned definition. J Neurosurg 2007; 106: 1–5

[5] Linskey ME, Andrews DW, Asher AL, et al. The role of stereotactic radiosurgery in the management of patients with newly diagnosed brain metastases: a systematic review and evidence-based clinical practice guideline. J Neurooncol 2010; 96: 45–68

[6] Gaspar LE, Mehta MP, Patchell RA, et al. The role of whole brain radiation therapy in the management of newly diagnosed brain metastases: a systematic review and evidence-based clinical practice guideline. J Neurooncol 2010; 96: 17–32

[7] Kalkanis SN, Kondziolka D, Gaspar LE, et al. The role of surgical resection in the management of newly diagnosed brain metastases: a systematic review and evidence-based clinical practice guideline. J Neurooncol 2010; 96: 33–43

[8] Mehta MP, Paleologos NA, Mikkelsen T, et al. The role of chemotherapy in the management of newly diagnosed brain metastases: a systematic review and evidence-based clinical practice guideline. J Neurooncol 2010; 96: 71–83

[9] Olson JJ, Paleologos NA, Gaspar LE, et al. The role of emerging and investigational therapies for metastatic brain tumors: a systematic review and evidence-based clinical practice guideline of selected topics. J Neurooncol 2010; 96: 115–142

[10] Robinson PD, Kalkanis SN, Linskey ME, Santaguida PL. Methodology used to develop the AANS/CNS management of brain metastases evidence-based clinical practice parameter guidelines. J Neurooncol 2010; 96: 11–16

[11] Kondziolka D, Patel A, Lunsford LD, Kassam A, Flickinger JC. Stereotactic radiosurgery plus whole brain radiotherapy versus radiotherapy alone for patients with multiple brain metastases. Int J Radiat Oncol Biol Phys 1999; 45: 427–434

[12] Andrews DW, Scott CB, Sperduto PW, et al. Whole brain radiation therapy with or without stereotactic radiosurgery boost for patients with one to three brain metastases: phase III results of the RTOG 9508 randomised trial. Lancet 2004; 363: 1665–1672

[13] Li B, Yu J, Suntharalingam M, et al. Comparison of three treatment options for single brain metastasis from lung cancer. Int J Cancer 2000; 90: 37–45

[14] Wang LG, Guo Y, Zhang X, et al. Brain metastasis: experience of the Xi-Jing hospital. Stereotact Funct Neurosurg 2002; 78: 70–83

[15] Sanghavi SN, Miranpuri SS, Chappell R, et al. Radiosurgery for patients with brain metastases: a multi-institutional analysis, stratified by the RTOG recursive partitioning analysis method. Int J Radiat Oncol Biol Phys 2001; 51: 426–434

[16] Chang EL, Wefel JS, Hess KR, et al. Neurocognition in patients with brain metastases treated with radiosurgery or radiosurgery plus whole-brain irradiation: a randomised controlled trial. Lancet Oncol 2009; 10: 1037–1044

[17] Aoyama H, Shirato H, Tago M, et al. Stereotactic radiosurgery plus whole-brain radiation therapy vs stereotactic radiosurgery alone for treatment of brain metastases: a randomized controlled trial. JAMA 2006; 295: 2483–2491

[18] Aoyama H, Tago M, Kato N, et al. Neurocognitive function of patients with brain metastasis who received either whole brain radiotherapy plus stereotactic radiosurgery or radiosurgery alone. Int J Radiat Oncol Biol Phys 2007; 68: 1388–1395

[19] Chidel MA, Suh JH, Reddy CA, Chao ST, Lundbeck MF, Barnett GH. Application of recursive partitioning analysis and evaluation of the use of whole brain radiation among patients treated with stereotactic radiosurgery for newly diagnosed brain metastases. Int J Radiat Oncol Biol Phys 2000; 47: 993–999

[20] Combs SE, Schulz-Ertner D, Thilmann C, Edler L, Debus J. Treatment of cerebral metastases from breast cancer with stereotactic radiosurgery. Strahlenther Onkol 2004; 180: 590–596

[21] Hoffman R, Sneed PK, McDermott MW, et al. Radiosurgery for brain metastases from primary lung carcinoma. Cancer J 2001; 7: 121–131

[22] Jawahar A, Willis BK, Smith DR, Ampil F, Datta R, Nanda A. Gamma Knife radiosurgery for brain metastases: do patients benefit from adjuvant external-beam radiotherapy? An 18-month comparative analysis. Stereotact Funct Neurosurg 2002; 79: 262–271

[23] Noel G, Medioni J, Valery CA, et al. Three irradiation treatment options including radiosurgery for brain metastases from primary lung cancer. Lung Cancer 2003; 41: 333–343

[24] Pirzkall A, Debus J, Lohr F, et al. Radiosurgery alone or in combination with whole-brain radiotherapy for brain metastases. J Clin Oncol 1998; 16: 3563–3569

[25] Sneed PK, Lamborn KR, Forstner JM, et al. Radiosurgery for brain metastases: is whole brain radiotherapy necessary? Int J Radiat Oncol Biol Phys 1999; 43: 549–558

[26] Sneed PK, Suh JH, Goetsch SJ, et al. A multi-institutional review of radiosurgery alone vs. radiosurgery with whole brain radiotherapy as the initial management of brain metastases. Int J Radiat Oncol Biol Phys 2002; 53: 519–526

[27] Varlotto JM, Flickinger JC, Niranjan A, Bhatnagar A, Kondziolka D, Lunsford LD. The impact of whole-brain radiation therapy on the long-term control and morbidity of patients surviving more than one year after Gamma Knife radiosurgery for brain metastases. Int J Radiat Oncol Biol Phys 2005; 62: 1125–1132

[28] Kocher M, Soffietti R, Abacioglu U, et al. Adjuvant whole-brain radiotherapy versus observation after radiosurgery or surgical resection of one to three cerebral metastases: results of the EORTC 22952–26001 study. J Clin Oncol 2011; 29: 134–141

[29] Lee YK, Park NH, Kim JW, Song YS, Kang SB, Lee HP. Gamma Knife radiosurgery as an optimal treatment modality for brain metastases from epithelial ovarian cancer. Gynecol Oncol 2008; 108: 505–509

[30] Rades D, Pluemer A, Veninga T, Hanssens P, Dunst J, Schild SE. Whole-brain radiotherapy versus stereotactic radiosurgery for patients in recursive partitioning analysis classes 1 and 2 with 1 to 3 brain metastases. Cancer 2007; 110: 2285–2292

[31] Datta R, Jawahar A, Ampil FL, Shi R, Nanda A, D'Agostino H. Survival in relation to radiotherapeutic modality for brain metastasis: whole brain irradiation vs. gamma knife radiosurgery. Am J Clin Oncol 2004; 27: 420–424

[32] Kocher M, Maarouf M, Bendel M, Voges J, Müller RP, Sturm V. Linac radiosurgery versus whole brain radiotherapy for brain metastases. A survival comparison based on the RTOG recursive partitioning analysis. Strahlenther Onkol 2004; 180: 263–267

[33] Bindal AK, Bindal RK, Hess KR, et al. Surgery versus radiosurgery in the treatment of brain metastasis. J Neurosurg 1996; 84: 748–754

[34] Garell PC, Hitchon PW, Wen BC, Mellenberg DE, Torner J. Stereotactic radiosurgery versus microsurgical resection for the initial treatment of metastatic cancer to the brain. J Radiosurg 1999; 2: 1–5

[35] O'Neill BP, Iturria NJ, Link MJ, Pollock BE, Ballman KV, O'Fallon JR. A comparison of surgical resection and stereotactic radiosurgery in the treatment of solitary brain metastases. Int J Radiat Oncol Biol Phys 2003; 55: 1169–1176

[36] Schöggl A, Kitz K, Reddy M, et al. Defining the role of stereotactic radiosurgery versus microsurgery in the treatment of single brain metastases. Acta Neurochir (Wien) 2000; 142: 621–626

[37] Roos DE, Smith JG, Stephens SW. Radiosurgery versus surgery, both with adjuvant whole brain radiotherapy, for solitary brain metastases: a randomised controlled trial. Clin Oncol (R Coll Radiol) 2011; 23: 646–651

[38] Muacevic A, Wowra B, Siefert A, Tonn JC, Steiger HJ, Kreth FW. Microsurgery plus whole brain irradiation versus Gamma Knife surgery alone for treatment of single metastases to the brain: a randomized controlled multicentre phase III trial. J Neurooncol 2008; 87: 299–307

[39] Muacevic A, Kreth FW, Horstmann GA, et al. Surgery and radiotherapy compared with Gamma Knife radiosurgery in the treatment of solitary cerebral metastases of small diameter. J Neurosurg 1999; 91: 35–43

[40] Rades D, Bohlen G, Pluemer A, et al. Stereotactic radiosurgery alone versus resection plus whole-brain radiotherapy for 1 or 2 brain metastases in recursive partitioning analysis class 1 and 2 patients. Cancer 2007; 109: 2515–2521

[41] Shinoura N, Yamada R, Okamoto K, Nakamura O, Shitara N. Local recurrence of metastatic brain tumor after stereotactic radiosurgery or surgery plus radiation. J Neurooncol 2002; 60: 71–77

[42] Serizawa T, Iuchi T, Ono J, et al. Gamma Knife treatment for multiple metastatic brain tumors compared with whole-brain radiation therapy. J Neurosurg 2000; 93 (Suppl 3): 32–36

[43] Linskey ME. Evidence-based medicine for neurosurgeons: introduction and methodology. Prog Neurol Surg 2006; 19: 1–53

[44] Linskey ME. Neurosurgery quality: pay-for-performance, guidelines, and outcome measures. Clin Neurosurg 2007; 54: 157–179

[45] Linskey ME. The emergence of clinical practice parameter guidelines in neuro-oncology: promise of utility tempered with caution. J Neurooncol 2008; 89: 359–362

[46] Linskey ME, Kalkanis SN. Evidence-linked, clinical practice guidelines-getting serious; getting professional. J Neurooncol 2010; 96: 1–5

[47] Linskey ME. Defining excellence in evidence-based medicine clinical practice guidelines. Clin Neurosurg 2010; 57: 28–37

[48] Serizawa T, Hirai T, Nagano O, et al. Gamma Knife surgery for 1–10 brain metastases without prophylactic whole-brain radiation therapy: analysis of cases meeting the Japanese prospective multi-institute study (JLGK0901) inclusion criteria. J Neurooncol 2010; 98: 163–167

[49] Patchell RA, Tibbs PA, Regine WF, et al. Postoperative radiotherapy in the treatment of single metastases to the brain: a randomized trial. JAMA 1998; 280: 1485–1489

[50] Patchell RA, Tibbs PA, Walsh JW, et al. A randomized trial of surgery in the treatment of single metastases to the brain. N Engl J Med 1990; 322: 494–500

[51] Vecht CJ, Haaxma-Reiche H, Noordijk EM, et al. Treatment of single brain metastasis: radiotherapy alone or combined with neurosurgery? Ann Neurol 1993; 33: 583–590

[52] Nussbaum ES, Djalilian HR, Cho KH, Hall WA. Brain metastases: histology, multiplicity, surgery, and survival. Cancer 1996; 78: 1781–1788

[53] Bartelt S, Lutterbach J. Brain metastases in patients with cancer of unknown primary. J Neurooncol 2003; 64: 249–253

[54] Polyzoidis KS, Miliaras G, Pavlidis N. Brain metastasis of unknown primary: a diagnostic and therapeutic dilemma. Cancer Treat Rev 2005; 31: 247–255

[55] Niranjan A, Kano H, Khan A, et al. Radiosurgery for brain metastases from unknown primary cancers. Int J Radiat Oncol Biol Phys 2010; 77: 1457–1462

[56] Owen CM, Linskey ME. Frame-based stereotaxy in a frameless era: current capabilities, relative role, and the positive- and negative predictive values of blood through the needle. J Neurooncol 2009; 93: 139–149

[57] Wroński M, Arbit E, Burt M, Galicich JH. Survival after surgical treatment of brain metastases from lung cancer: a follow-up study of 231 patients treated between 1976 and 1991. J Neurosurg 1995; 83: 605–616

[58] Hall WA, Djalilian HR, Nussbaum ES, Cho KH. Long-term survival with metastatic cancer to the brain. Med Oncol 2000; 17: 279–286

[59] Detterbeck FC, Bleiweis MS, Ewend MG. Surgical treatment of stage IV non-small cell lung cancer. In: Detterbeck FC, Rivera MP, Socinski MA, et al, eds. Diagnosis and Treatment of Lung Cancer: An Evidence-based Guide for the Practicing Clinician. Philadelphia, PA: WB Saunders; 2001; 326–338

[60] O'Neill BP, Iturria NJ, Link MJ, Pollock BE, Ballman KV, O'Fallon JR. A comparison of surgical resection and stereotactic radiosurgery in the treatment of solitary brain metastases. Int J Radiat Oncol Biol Phys 2003; 55: 1169–1176

[61] Hu C, Chang EL, Hassenbusch SJ, et al. Nonsmall cell lung cancer presenting with synchronous solitary brain metastasis. Cancer 2006; 106: 1998–2004

[62] Flannery TW, Suntharalingam M, Regine WF, et al. Long-term survival in patients with synchronous, solitary brain metastasis from non-small-cell lung cancer treated with radiosurgery. Int J Radiat Oncol Biol Phys 2008; 72: 19–23

[63] Fuentes R, Bonfill X, Exposito J. Surgery versus radiosurgery for patients with a solitary brain metastasis from non-small cell lung cancer. Cochrane Database Syst Rev 2006; 25: CD004840

[64] Shen KR, Meyers BF, Larner JM, Jones DR. American College of Chest Physicians. Special treatment issues in lung cancer: ACCP evidence-based clinical practice guidelines. Chest 2007; 132: 290S–305S

[65] McCrory DC, Lewis SZ, Heitzer J, Colice G, Alberts WM American College of Chest Physicians. Methodology for lung cancer evidence review and guideline development: ACCP evidence-based clinical practice guidelines (2nd Edition). Chest 2007; 132 (Suppl): 23S–28S

[66] Jagannathan J, Bourne TD, Schlesinger D, et al. Clinical and pathological characteristics of brain metastasis resected after failed radiosurgery. Neurosurgery 2010; 66: 208–217

[67] Niwińska A, Pogoda K, Murawska M, Niwiński P. Factors influencing survival in patients with breast cancer and single or solitary brain metastasis. Eur J Surg Oncol 2011; 37: 635–642

16 Radiosurgery for More than Four Brain Metastases

Igor J. Barani and David A. Larson

Introduction

In 1989 Lindquist[1] reported the first case of stereotactic radiosurgery (SRS) for brain metastasis in a patient treated for a cerebral hypernephroma. By the mid-1990s, numerous reports of SRS alone or following whole-brain radiation therapy (WBRT) had been published, and strong opinions developed regarding selection criteria for patients treated with WBRT, SRS, or both. Some practitioners adopted formulaic recommendations based on tumor size, the Karnofsky performance scale (KPS), age, status of extracranial disease, and number of brain metastases while giving no formulaic weight to potential brain toxicity.[2] Others used the KPS together with a strict cutoff limit on the number of brain metastases that could be treated with SRS. Yet others adopted a less rigid approach that allows SRS for almost any number of targets, depending in a flexible manner on tumor location, degree of edema, and likelihood of clinical complications, among other things. Ideally, one might have hoped that published guidelines based mainly on interpretations of phase III studies would lead to unanimity among experts regarding treatment recommendations for one to four brain metastases and, by extrapolation, recommendations for more than four brain metastases. They have not, for reasons outlined below. For more than four brain metastases, WBRT despite the lack of randomized trials comparing WBRT to SRS, despite the relative lack of detailed outcome data for WBRT (other than overall survival and clinical response), and despite the small but favorable literature on SRS for multiple metastases.

Stereotactic Radiosurgery versus Whole-Brain Radiation Therapy for More than Four Brain Metastases

Some physicians recommend WBRT for more than four brain metastases, whereas others recommend SRS alone. Physicians who favor combined therapy (SRS plus WBRT) for four or fewer metastases cite the widely accepted phase III finding that brain control with combined therapy is significantly better than that with SRS or WBRT alone.[3–7] Those who favor SRS alone cite the phase III finding that risk of neurocognitive deficit is doubled with the addition of WBRT to SRS.[7] Whether SRS is used alone or combined with WBRT, these studies lend strong support for SRS, at least as a component of management; they lend little support for WBRT alone for patients meeting phase III selection criteria. This suggests that SRS is underused.[8]

Most physicians recognize that WBRT for brain metastases provides improved survival and symptom relief compared to observation or corticosteroids even if the degree of benefit relative to the number of brain metastases is not known. Nevertheless, given the lack of phase III outcome data, it seems counterintuitive to blindly favor WBRT alone as the best currently available alternative for more than four brain metastases. Those who favor WBRT over SRS argue that (1) WBRT prevents some of the distant brain metastases that would otherwise develop after SRS alone,[5] (2) that brain recurrences after initial SRS alone are associated with a high rate of clinical neurologic deficits,[9] (3) that there are methodological flaws[10] associated with the phase III finding that SRS-alone patients fare better than SRS plus WBRT patients on the Hopkins Verbal Learning Tests,[5] and (4) that salvage therapy, widely known to be more frequently required in SRS-alone patients, could be less effective than initial therapy.

Physicians who favor SRS alone have several counterarguments. (1) They cite the phase III findings of Chang et al[7] that, although the addition of WBRT decreases distant brain failure compared to SRS alone, the addition of WBRT doubles the risk for significant verbal learning and memory deficits at 4 months. (2) They argue that the finding of Ayoma et al[11] that the addition of WBRT to SRS leads to a significantly longer time to Mini-Mental State Examination (MMSE) decline is based on the flawed assumption[12] that MMSE is an adequate measure of neurocognitive function changes related to radiation, and they further note that posttherapy leukoencephalopathy was seen on magnetic resonance imaging (MRI) in some patients in the combined arm and in no patients in the SRS-alone arm.[11] (3) They question the conclusion of Regine et al[9] that brain recurrences after SRS alone are associated with a high rate of neurologic deficits, as their reported rate of serious neurologic complications affecting language, memory, cranial nerve, gait, and motor function is far higher than that reported by other authors, which may reflect unfortunate target selection. (4) They believe the acknowledged brain control advantages of SRS plus WBRT are not outweighed by the acknowledged side effects of WBRT[13–15]—side effects that have motivated proponents of WBRT to develop intensity-modulated radiation therapy (IMRT)-based hippocampal-sparing WBRT techniques for multiple metastases[16,17]. (5) They argue that salvage SRS, although needed more frequently in patients treated initially with SRS alone rather than with combined therapy, is safe, efficient, and effective, even for more than four brain metastases.[18] It is further argued that the four-metastasis limit for SRS techniques is a historical relic reflecting technological and practical limitations of early SRS technology, limitations that have since been overcome.

Given the state of this controversy, the majority of our patients prefer SRS alone for more than four metastases to avoid hair loss and to minimize fears of WBRT-related neurocognitive deficits, and because they prefer a 1-day rather than a multi-week procedure. Additionally, SRS patients (and their physicians) often express the desire to minimize interruptions in systemic therapy, leading them to prefer SRS treatment. For many physicians who favor SRS alone for one to four brain metastases, the recommendation for SRS for more than four brain metastases seems reasonable, especially when they are committed to obtaining frequent follow-up exams and providing salvage therapy as needed, as they do for patients with fewer than four metastases. That recommendation has been supported by the development of commercial radiosurgery apparatus that is capable of treating a large number of brain metastases, so that physicians using currently available apparatus are faced with few technical limitations in the number of lesions that can be treated with SRS. Our own clinical experience suggests that treating a large number of lesions is safe. Nevertheless, physicians should be mindful that the normal tissue dose increases with the number of tumors treated with SRS, and that normal tissue dose is apparatus-dependent.[19]

Literature Review

There are as yet no published phase III data directly addressing the current controversy. Despite that, several professional medical organizations have published consensus documents that include reference to management of more than four brain metastases. In addition, there are several published retrospective studies on SRS for multiple brain metastases that relate overall survival and/or local or distant brain control and/or clinical or radiographic complications to the number of brain metastases. There are few similar WBRT publications.

Consensus Documents

Most consensus statements do not address more than four brain metastases, except tangentially or by implication. Below we review relevant statements from recent consensus documents.

In 2006 the European Federation of Neurological Societies published an evidence-based guidelines document.[20] The authors state, without reference:

"In patients with more than three brain metastases WBRT with hypofractionated regimens is the treatment of choice."

In 2011 the American College of Neurological Surgeons and the Congress of Neurosurgeons published a consensus summary of evidence-based guidelines for management of brain metastases.[21] The report states:

"A risk to consider when giving WBRT is the development of neurocognitive deficits. These deficits can be subtle and easily missed on many routine medical examinations or basic mental evaluations, such as the Mini-Mental Status Examination. Nevertheless they can be disturbing to both patients and families."

The authors of the report further note that

"SRS alone may be an advantage to patients in that one therapy session is required. The entire brain is not exposed to radiation in SRS; furthermore, there is a risk of potential neurocognitive deficits with the use of WBRT, although this has not been well studied because the effects may be subtle and variable."

They reviewed 11 observational studies that support the recommendation that SRS alone may provide an equivalent survival advantage compared to combined WBRT and SRS. However, the consensus statement does not specifically address multiple brain metastases in any detail.

In 2011 the American College of Radiology reviewed and updated a 2009 critical literature review that used the formal Delphi consensus process to develop appropriateness criteria for the treatment of multiple brain metastases.[22] The document states that "effectiveness of SRS for patients with multiple metastases may be primarily a function of proper patient selection but it probably cannot replace the benefits of WBRT." The authors list an appropriateness scale from 1 to 9 (least to most appropriate) to score therapies as applied to different clinical variants. The document includes five clinical variants encompassing from two to six brain metastases, KPS score of 50 to 100, and various extents of extracranial disease. Only one variant is for more than four metastases: a patient, age 50, with non–small-cell lung carcinoma (NSCLC), KPS score of 90, with primary tumor resected, no systemic metastases, and six newly diagnosed, asymptomatic brain metastases. This variant received a Delphi score of 1 (least appropriate) for SRS alone, 2 for SRS plus WBRT, and 8 for WBRT alone, accompanied by the statement that "Number of lesions and absence of evidence do not support SRS in this patient." Clinical evidence for or against those scores was not presented. A similar patient with only two brain metastases rather than six received a Delphi score of 6 for SRS alone, 7 for WBRT, and 8 for SRS with WBRT. For both variants, the Delphi scores in 2011 were similar to those obtained in 2000.[23]

In 2012 the American Society for Therapeutic Radiology and Oncology published an evidence-based guideline on the role of radiation for newly diagnosed brain metastases.[24] The only mention of SRS for multiple metastases is stated as follows: "It is unknown if there is a cutoff for the maximum number of targets appropriate for radiosurgery. Total target volume as well as number of targets may be important for safety and efficacy."

In summary, the above consensus statements offer mixed enthusiasm for SRS alone for more than four brain metastases while offering little information to support those same consensus statements' management recommendations. However, there may be a higher degree of enthusiasm for SRS for multiple targets than is reflected in the consensus documents. Knisely et al[25] surveyed radiosurgery practitioners at two international radiosurgery congresses to determine willingness to use SRS for multiple brain metastases. In 2007 in San Francisco, 55% of those surveyed considered it reasonable to use SRS for 5 or more metastases and 22% for 10 or more. In 2009 in Japan, the percentages were 83% and 57%, respectively.

Stereotactic Radiosurgery for More than Four Brain Metastases

In 2007 Bhatnagar et al[26] reported results for 205 patients treated with SRS for 4 to 18 (64% with > 4) brain metastases, 17% of whom had SRS alone, 46% SRS with WBRT, and 38% SRS after WBRT failure. The median treatment volume was 6.8 cm^3 (range 0.6–51.0 cm^3). Median overall survival was 8 months, time to progression or time to new brain metastases was 9 months, and local control was 71% at 1 year and 49% at 2 years. Multivariate analysis showed that significant factors for overall survival included total treatment volume, age, recursive partitioning analysis (RPA) class, and marginal dose. The number of intracranial metastases was not significant ($p = 0.333$). For local control, total treatment volume was significant, and the number of intracranial metastases was not significant. The authors proposed that total treatment volume instead of (or together with) number of metastases should be a selection factor.

In 2010 Chang et al[27] reported results for 323 patients treated with SRS, an unspecified number of whom received WBRT. Total treatment volumes were not specified. Patients were retrospectively placed in groups based on the number of brain metastases, with 1 to 5, 6 to 10, 11 to 15, and more than 15 lesions in groups 1 to 4, respectively. Median survivals were not significantly different at 10, 10, 13, and 8 months, respectively ($p = 0.554$). Local tumor control rates were not significantly different among the groups. Median progression-free survivals were 9, 11, 8, and 6 months and were significantly shorter for group 4 ($p = 0.03$), as was distant brain progression ($p = 0.014$). Follow-up radiologic changes did not differ significantly among the groups (7.9%, 10.3%, 11.8%, and 3.0%, respectively). The authors concluded that SRS is a reasonable treatment for patients with multiple brain metastases, even for more than 15 lesions.

Hunter et al[28] focused on overall survival in 64 patients treated with SRS for more than 4 brain metastases, of whom 63% had received WBRT more than 1 month prior to SRS, 14% had received concurrent WBRT within 1 month of SRS, and 23% had received no WBRT. The median number of lesions treated was 6 (range 5–10). The median total lesion volume was 4.1 cm^3 (range 0.003–25.5 cm^3). The median overall survival was 7.5 months, and survival was significantly improved ($p = 0.008$). "Prior WBRT" patients had significantly improved survival compared to "concurrent WBRT" patients ($p = 0.034$). However, omitting WBRT showed no disadvantage, in that no significant survival differences were seen when comparing "no WBRT" with either "prior WBRT" or "concurrent WBRT." Median survival for lesions (6.6 months) was not significantly different from that for lesions (9.9 mo). Local control, distant brain control, and radiographic changes were not addressed.

Chang et al[29] reported a series of 26 patients treated with SRS for more than 10 brain metastases (range 10–37), of whom 13 had failed prior WBRT, 5 had received SRS and concurrent WBRT, 2 had received WBRT for SRS failure, and 6 had received SRS alone. Overall survival was significantly longer for synchronous brain metastases compared to metachronous metastases, for KPS score 80 compared to 70, for primary disease controlled compared to uncontrolled, and for two or more cycles of systemic chemotherapy compared to fewer than two cycles. Local control in a subset of 17 patients with 263 lesions was 79.5%. Radiation necrosis was observed in only one lesion (in a patient who had 19 target lesions and did not receive WBRT). The lesion had largely resolved at 38 months.

Nath et al[30] reported clinical results for 26 patients who received SRS for a median of 5 brain metastases (range 2–13), 23% of whom had received prior WBRT. Actuarial 1-year survival was 38%. Actuarial 1-year local control was 83%, with significantly improved local control at 6 months for lesion size ≤ 1.5 cm. Local control was not significantly affected by use of WBRT. Distant brain failures developed in 7 patients and were salvaged in 5 patients with WBRT and in 2 with SRS.

Serizawa et al[31] analyzed results of SRS as sole treatment for 1,508 patients who met the inclusion criteria of the otherwise unrelated Japanese multi-institutional trial JLGK0901 (a trial designed to assess noninferiority of SRS as sole treatment of 5 to 10 brain metastases compared to 2 to 4 brain metastases): patients with 1 to 10 newly diagnosed brain metastases, largest tumor volume $< 10\,cm^3$, total brain metastases volume $< 15\,cm^3$, no cerebrospinal fluid dissemination, and excluding patients with KPS score ≤ 70 due to extracranial disease. Patients were divided into three groups based on number of tumors: groups A (1 tumor), B (2–4 tumors), and C (5–10 tumors). Univariate analysis revealed mean survivals of 0.99 year for group A, 0.68 year for group B, and 0.62 year for group C, and they were significantly different (A vs B, $p < 0.0001$; B vs C, $p = 0.0312$). However, multivariate analysis showed significantly worse survival for group B compared to group A but no survival difference for group B compared to group C. This analysis did not address local and distant brain control or complications.

In a somewhat different analysis than that discussed above, Serizawa et al[32] described a study involving 778 similarly selected patients who were placed in five analysis groups according to number of tumors: groups A (1 tumor), B (2), C (3 or 4), D (5 or 6), and E (7–10). The median maximum tumor volume was 1.8 cm^3 (range 0.1–9.9 cm^3), and the median total tumor volume was 2.8 cm^3 (range 0.1–15.0 cm^3). Extracranial disease was controlled in 84 patients and uncontrolled in 694. Lesions were synchronous in 201 patents and metachronous in 577. Mean survival times were in the range of 0.83 to 0.59 but were not significantly different between any two groups. As expected, mean survival was significantly ($p < 0.0001$) related to RPA class: class 1 (2.2 y) versus class 2 (0.7 y) versus class 3 (0.3 y). One-year neurologic death-free survival rates in groups A to E were 96.8%, 95.5%, 84.7%, 91.2%, and 89.2%, respectively, with no significant differences between any two groups. One-year local control was significantly ($p = 0.0001$) related to tumor size: 98% (tiny) versus 92.3% (small) versus 77.9% (medium-sized). One-year distant brain control rates were 71.6%, 53.7%, 43.6%, 50.7%, and 66.3% for groups A to E, respectively. Significant differences were seen when comparing A and B, and also when comparing C and D. The authors concluded that the number of brain lesions treated with SRS alone did not influence overall survival, local control, neurologic death-free survival, or functional survival.

In 2012 Yamamoto et al[33] analyzed 1,676 patients treated with SRS and made pairwise comparisons of actuarial survival based on 14 pairs of treated metastases (1 vs 2, 2 vs 3, 3 vs 4 … 14 vs 15). They found a significant difference in median survival only for the 1 versus 2 pair ($p = 0.0002$).

Caballero et al[18] analyzed prognostic factors for survival in 310 patients treated with salvage SRS for new, progressive, or recurrent brain metastases after WBRT. The median number of brain metastases treated was 4 (range 1–31), and 53% of patients had 4 to 31 brain metastases treated. Patients treated with SRS for a single tumor had longer median survival than those treated for more than one tumor (12.0 vs 7.9 mo, $p = 0.001$), but among patients with multiple lesions treated, there was no significant trend toward shorter survival with increasing number of brain metastases. The authors concluded that, for multiple metastases, the median survival of 7.9 months made SRS a worthwhile therapy for patients who had failed or progressed after WBRT, and they found no evidence to support the use of a cutoff for number of brain metastases appropriate for salvage therapy.

Whole-Brain Radiation Therapy for More than Four Brain Metastases

Until recently, most physicians accepted that WBRT represents the standard of care for patients with more than four brain metastases, and most would agree that WBRT is preferable to observation or corticosteroids. For over 50 years innumerable patients have received WBRT, and numerous phase III trials have examined various WBRT outcomes with various dose-fractionation schemes but without regard to the number of brain metastases. Surprisingly, there are few publications relating the relative number of lesions to outcomes for patients with more than four tumors. Some information is available from Nieder et al,[34] who studied 113 patients with a median of 6 (range 4–50) brain metastases treated with WBRT. They found that the number of brain metastases had no appreciable influence on survival. Direct comparisons with SRS-alone series cannot be made, as there is no way to know if Nieder et al's patients might have met reasonable SRS selection criteria.

Do Outcomes Depend on the Number of Metastases?

▶ Table 16.1 summarizes the above reports on SRS for a large number of brain metastases. It should be kept in mind that variable numbers of patients in each series may have received WBRT or surgery either before or after SRS, and that selection factors for SRS varied from series to series. Nevertheless, the tabulated data lend support to the notion that survival, local control, progression-free survival, neurologic death-free survival, and functional survival are not significantly diminished as increasing numbers of tumors are treated, except with the caveat that survival after SRS for a very small number of tumors is probably superior to that for a larger number of tumors. Likewise, survival after WBRT alone is not significantly affected by the number of tumors in the range 4 to 50.[34] Radiologic changes after SRS for multiple metastases occur at a low rate,[27] not unlike that reported in patients treated with SRS for one to four brain metastases. However, detailed information on neurocognitive changes as a function of number of brain metastases is lacking.

Conclusion

Numerous pre-computed tomography studies have demonstrated that survival time in patients with symptomatic brain metastases is improved with corticosteroids and further improved with WBRT. Patients with more than four brain metastases and massive edema or impending herniation or large intracranial tumor burden are well served by WBRT. For less dramatic cases with more than four brain metastases, arguments for SRS alone or for WBRT alone have merit. However, absent randomized SRS versus WBRT comparisons of survival, local control, distant brain control, neurocognitive function, and quality of life figures, physicians must rely on currently available retrospective data or on extrapolation of phase III data. Those phase III data favor either SRS alone or SRS plus WBRT, depending on interpretation; they do not support WBRT alone. That fact and the retrospective data summarized in ▶ Table 16.1 lead us to favor SRS over WBRT for more than four brain metastases. We await future phase III results for more definitive guidance.

Table 16.1 Relationship of the number of brain metastases to various outcomes

Study*	No. of patients	Outcome	No. metastases (p = ns)	No. metastases ($p < 0.05$)
Bhatnagar et al[26]	205	Survival Local control	4–18 4–18	
Chang et al[27]	323	Survival Local control Progression-free survival MRI changes	1–> 15 1–> 15 1–15 1–> 15	> 15 worse than ≤ 15
Hunter et al[28]	64	Survival	5–10	
Serizawa et al[31]	1,508	Survival	2–10	2–4 worse than 1
Serizawa et al[32]	778	Survival Local control Neurologic death-free survival Functional survival	1–10 1–10 1–10 1–10	
Yamamoto et al[33]	1,676	Survival	2–15	2 worse than 1
Caballero et al[18]	310	Survival	2–31	> 1 worse than 1
Nieder et al[34]	113	Survival	4–50	

* In most cases, the number of metastases was not a significant factor (p = ns). Variable numbers of patients in each series may have received WBRT or surgery before or after SRS. Selection criteria for SRS varied.
Data from Caballero et al[18] are for salvage SRS after WBRT failure.
Data from Nieder et al[34] are for WBRT without SRS.
Abbreviations: MRI, magnetic resonance imaging; ns: non-significant; SRS: stereotactic radiosurgery; WBRT, whole-brain radiation therapy.

References

[1] Lindquist C. Gamma Knife surgery for recurrent solitary metastasis of a cerebral hypernephroma: case report. Neurosurgery 1989; 25: 802–804
[2] Eichler AF, Loeffler JS. Multidisciplinary management of brain metastases. Oncologist 2007; 12: 884–898
[3] Kondziolka D, Patel A, Lunsford LD, Kassam A, Flickinger JC. Stereotactic radiosurgery plus whole brain radiotherapy versus radiotherapy alone for patients with multiple brain metastases. Int J Radiat Oncol Biol Phys 1999; 45: 427–434
[4] Andrews DW, Scott CB, Sperduto PW, et al. Whole brain radiation therapy with or without stereotactic radiosurgery boost for patients with one to three brain metastases: phase III results of the RTOG 9508 randomised trial. Lancet 2004; 363: 1665–1672
[5] Aoyama H, Shirato H, Tago M, et al. Stereotactic radiosurgery plus whole-brain radiation therapy vs stereotactic radiosurgery alone for treatment of brain metastases: a randomized controlled trial. JAMA 2006; 295: 2483–2491
[6] Kocher M, Soffietti R, Abacioglu U, et al. Adjuvant whole-brain radiotherapy versus observation after radiosurgery or surgical resection of one to three cerebral metastases: results of the EORTC 22952-26001 study. J Clin Oncol 2011; 29: 134–141
[7] Chang EL, Wefel JS, Hess KR, et al. Neurocognition in patients with brain metastases treated with radiosurgery or radiosurgery plus whole-brain irradiation: a randomised controlled trial. Lancet Oncol 2009; 10: 1037–1044
[8] Halasz LM, Weeks JC, Neville BA, Taback N, Punglia RS. Use of stereotactic radiosurgery for brain metastases: a SEER-Medicare analysis. Int J Radiat Oncol Biol Phys 2011; 81: S550–S551
[9] Regine WF, Huhn JL, Patchell RA, et al. Risk of symptomatic brain tumor recurrence and neurologic deficit after radiosurgery alone in patients with newly diagnosed brain metastases: results and implications. Int J Radiat Oncol Biol Phys 2002; 52: 333–338
[10] Mahmood U, Kwok Y, Regine WF, Patchell RA. Whole-brain irradiation for patients with brain metastases: still the standard of care. Lancet Oncol 2010; 11: 221–222, author reply 223
[11] Aoyama H, Tago M, Kato N, et al. Neurocognitive function of patients with brain metastasis who received either whole brain radiotherapy plus stereotactic radiosurgery or radiosurgery alone. Int J Radiat Oncol Biol Phys 2007; 68: 1388–1395
[12] Meyers CA, Wefel JS. The use of the Mini-Mental State Examination to assess cognitive functioning in cancer trials: no ifs, ands, buts, or sensitivity. J Clin Oncol 2003; 21: 3557–3558
[13] Shrieve DC, Loeffler JS. Human Brain Injury. Philadelphia, PA: Lippincott Williams & Wilkins; 2011
[14] Sun A, Bae K, Gore EM, et al. Phase III trial of prophylactic cranial irradiation compared with observation in patients with locally advanced non-small-cell lung cancer: neurocognitive and quality-of-life analysis. J Clin Oncol 2011; 29: 279–286
[15] Marsh JC, Gielda BT, Herskovic AM, Abrams RA. Cognitive sparing during the administration of whole brain radiotherapy and prophylactic cranial irradiation: current concepts and approaches. J Oncol 2010; 2010: 198208. doi: 10.1155/2010/198208
[16] Prokic V, Wiedenmann N, Fels F, Schmucker M, Nieder C, Grosu AL. Whole brain irradiation with hippocampal sparing and dose escalation on multiple brain metastases: a planning study on treatment concepts. Int J Radiat Oncol Biol Phys 2013; 85: 264–270
[17] Gondi V, Tomé WA, Mehta MP. Why avoid the hippocampus? A comprehensive review. Radiother Oncol 2010; 97: 370–376
[18] Caballero JA, Sneed PK, Lamborn KR, et al. Prognostic factors for survival in patients treated with stereotactic radiosurgery for recurrent brain metastases after prior whole brain radiotherapy. Int J Radiat Oncol Biol Phys 2012; 83: 303–309
[19] Ma L, Petti P, Wang B, et al. Apparatus dependence of normal brain tissue dose in stereotactic radiosurgery for multiple brain metastases. J Neurosurg 2011; 114: 1580–1584
[20] Soffietti R, Cornu P, Delattre JY, et al. EFNS guidelines on diagnosis and treatment of brain metastases: report of an EFNS Task Force. Eur J Neurol 2006; 13: 674–681
[21] Bhangoo SS, Linskey ME, Kalkanis SN American Association of Neurologic Surgeons (AANS). Congress of Neurologic Surgeons (CNS). Evidence-based guidelines for the management of brain metastases. Neurosurg Clin N Am 2011; 22: 97–104, viii
[22] Videtic GM, Gaspar LE, Aref AM, et al. Expert Panel on Radiation Oncology-Brain Metastases. American College of Radiology appropriateness criteria on multiple brain metastases. Int J Radiat Oncol Biol Phys 2009; 75: 961–965
[23] Shaw EG, Gaspar LE, Gibbs FA, et al. Multiple brain metastases: American College of Radiology appropriateness criteria. Radiology 2000; 215 (Suppl): 1121–1128
[24] Tsao MN, Rades D, Wirth A, et al. Radiotherapeutic and surgical management for newly diagnosed brain metastasis(es): an american society for radiation oncology evidence-based guideline. Practical Radiation Oncology. 2012; 2: 210–225
[25] Knisely JP, Yamamoto M, Gross CP, Castrucci WA, Jokura H, Chiang VL. Radiosurgery alone for 5 or more brain metastases: expert opinion survey. J Neurosurg 2010; 113 (Suppl): 84–89
[26] Bhatnagar AK, Kondziolka D, Lunsford LD, Flickinger JC. Recursive partitioning analysis of prognostic factors for patients with four or more intracranial metastases treated with radiosurgery. Technol Cancer Res Treat 2007; 6: 153–160
[27] Chang WS, Kim HY, Chang JW, Park YG, Chang JH. Analysis of radiosurgical results in patients with brain metastases according to the number of brain lesions: is stereotactic radiosurgery effective for multiple brain metastases? J Neurosurg 2010; 113 (Suppl): 73–78
[28] Hunter GK, Suh JH, Reuther AM, et al. Treatment of five or more brain metastases with stereotactic radiosurgery. Int J Radiat Oncol Biol Phys 2012; 83: 1394–1398
[29] Chang WS, Kim HY, Chang JW, Park YG, Chang JH. Analysis of radiosurgical results in patients with brain metastases according to the number of brain lesions: is stereotactic radiosurgery effective for multiple brain metastases? J Neurosurg 2010; 113 (Suppl): 73–78
[30] Nath SK, Lawson JD, Simpson DR, et al. Single-isocenter frameless intensity-modulated stereotactic radiosurgery for simultaneous treatment of multiple brain metastases: clinical experience. Int J Radiat Oncol Biol Phys 2010; 78: 91–97
[31] Serizawa T, Yamamoto M, Sato Y, et al. Gamma Knife surgery as sole treatment for multiple brain metastases: 2-center retrospective review of 1508 cases meeting the inclusion criteria of the JLGK0901 multi-institutional prospective study. J Neurosurg 2010; 113 (Suppl): 48–52
[32] Serizawa T, Hirai T, Nagano O, et al. Gamma Knife surgery for 1–10 brain metastases without prophylactic whole-brain radiation therapy: analysis of cases meeting the Japanese prospective multi-institute study (JLGK0901) inclusion criteria. J Neurooncol 2010; 98: 163–167
[33] Yamamoto M, Kawabe T, Barfod BE. How many metastases can be treated with radiosurgery? Prog Neurol Surg 2012; 25: 261–272
[34] Nieder C, Andratschke N, Grosu AL, Molls M. Recursive partitioning analysis (RPA) class does not predict survival in patients with four or more brain metastases. Strahlenther Onkol 2003; 179: 16–20

17 Whole-Brain Radiation Therapy for More than Five Metastases

Usama Mahmood, Zain Husain, Young Kwok, and William F. Regine

Introduction

Brain metastases represent a significant cause of morbidity and mortality among cancer patients. In the US, there are over 200,000 cases of brain metastases annually, afflicting 10 to 30% of all cancer patients and outnumbering primary brain tumors by a ratio of 10:1.[1,2] Whether the result of improved detection via novel imaging techniques or improved control of extracranial disease due to more potent systemic therapies (which less effectively traverse the blood–brain barrier), the incidence of brain metastases is increasing.[3]

Historically, brain metastases were rapidly fatal, with most patients surviving ~ 1 month. The use of steroids to decrease mass effect and peritumoral edema nearly doubled survival to about 2 months. Over the last several decades, advancements in surgery and radiation therapy, combined with other strides in the general management of patients with cancer, have significantly improved these results. In fact, there have even been some reports of cure among select patients with solitary metastases who undergo aggressive treatment to both their intracranial and their extracranial disease sites.[4]

The initial approach to the patient with brain metastases must take into account not only the status of disease within the brain but also the status of the patient as a whole. The number and location of metastases within the brain, associated symptoms, the site and histology of the primary, the presence of other extracranial metastases, and the patient's overall performance status and comorbidities all need to be taken into account when making treatment decisions. Several prognostic systems for patients with brain metastases have been created that incorporate such factors and can help tailor treatment to an appropriate level of aggressiveness.[1,5,6]

Ultimately, the primary goals of the management of the patient with brain metastases are to provide effective palliation, improve quality of life, and, if at all possible, extend survival. To this end, whole-brain radiation therapy (WBRT) is an effective treatment modality that often plays a significant role in the management of patients with brain metastases. In this chapter, we discuss the role of WBRT in the management of patients with multiple brain metastases. Also, we elaborate on the association of WBRT with neurotoxicity in the setting of brain metastasis, an area of controversy and confusion.

Upfront Whole-Brain Radiation Therapy in Patients with Multiple Brain Metastases

The role of WBRT in patients with limited (one to four) brain metastases continues to be elucidated. ***Level I evidence*** in the form of randomized trials for patients with limited brain metastases have shown not only that the addition of surgery and/or stereotactic radiosurgery (SRS) to WBRT improves outcomes[7–9] but also that the addition of WBRT to surgery and/or SRS results in improved local and elsewhere intracranial control and—in some trials—lower rates of neurologic death.[10–13] Nonetheless, the favorable local control with surgery and/or SRS combined with concerns about neurotoxicity related to WBRT (further discussed below) have led some investigators to treat patients with limited brain metastases with surgery and/or SRS alone, delaying WBRT until time of progression.

Whereas there is some controversy regarding the optimal management of patients with limited brain metastases, WBRT is the cornerstone of management of patients with five or more brain metastases. This is not to say that surgery plays no role for these patients. It can provide histologic confirmation of metastatic disease, relieve mass effect, if present, and improve local tumor control and therefore should be considered in the appropriate circumstances. SRS is even more selectively employed in this setting, given the concern for irradiating large volumes of intracranial disease to high doses. The University of Pittsburgh published their experience, reporting on the results of 205 patients with more than four brain metastases treated with SRS during one session.[14] Within this subset, patients with treatment volume < 7 cm^3 and fewer than seven brain metastases fared better, whereas all others had a median survival of 6 months.

In the setting of multiple brain metastases, WBRT can provide palliative as well as survival benefits. Responses to radiation can be seen early in the treatment course, with 50% of patients experiencing an improvement in neurologic symptoms by the second week of treatment.[15] Moreover, as demonstrated by serial imaging studies, the maximum response to WBRT occurs within 3 months for the vast majority of patients.[16] Overall, the clinical and radiographic response to brain radiation ranges from 50 to 75%.[2] The addition of WBRT to steroids is also generally felt to improve the survival for patients with multiple brain metastases from 2 to 4 months.[17] To our knowledge, only one randomized trial (performed in the pre–computed tomography era) has evaluated the addition of WBRT to supportive care.[18] In this trial, 48 patients with presumed brain metastases were randomized to steroids with or without 40 Gy WBRT. Although probability values were not given, the addition of WBRT led to improved duration of remission (11 vs 5 wk) as well as median survival (14 vs 10 wk).

Unfortunately, despite multiple randomized trials, we have been unable to improve upon standard fractionated WBRT for such patients. Multiple randomized trials evaluating altered fractionation of WBRT have been attempted without any difference in survival;[2] similarly, multiple randomized trials have failed to identify a benefit to the addition of radiosensitizers or chemotherapy to WBRT.[2] A complete list of such trials would be exhaustive—if not discouraging—and beyond the scope of this chapter. Interested readers are therefore directed to more comprehensive reviews of the subject.[2]

Repeat Whole-Brain Radiation Therapy for Recurrent/Progressive Brain Metastases

Treatment of patients with recurrent/progressive brain metastases should be individualized, taking into consideration the patient's functional status, extent of intracranial and systemic disease, previous treatment, and histology. Options in this setting include supportive care, reirradiation (WBRT and/or SRS), surgery, or chemotherapy. Several retrospective series largely in the form of ***level III evidence*** have demonstrated that repeat WBRT can provide palliative benefit, although, as expected, prognosis is dismal. In one of the earliest and largest series, investigators from the Mayo Clinic noted 70% improvement among 86 patients with recurrent/progression brain metastases.[19] Median survival, however, was 4 months. Similarly, Son et al from the Massachusetts General Hospital noted improvement of symptoms in 8 out of 10 patients treated with repeat WBRT.[20] Again, the overall prognosis of these patients was poor, with a median survival of 5.2 months. Importantly, whereas the most common dose for upfront WBRT is 30 Gy, repeat WBRT is typically less intense (~ 20 Gy in 1.8–2.0 Gy/fraction).

Whole-Brain Radiation Therapy and Neurocognitive Toxicity

The debate about the risks and benefits of WBRT in patients with brain metastases must keep in mind the original goals of therapy. The primary intent of WBRT is to effectively palliate symptoms associated with brain metastases, to improve quality of life, and, perhaps to a lesser degree, to improve overall survival. We feel that the toxicities of WBRT—specifically, the risk of neurocognitive dysfunction—are overstated, and, for the majority of patients with brain metastases, WBRT provides an overall benefit in terms of palliation and improved quality of life.

When discussing neurotoxicity, it is important to note that nearly all patients with brain metastases present with neurocognitive deficits prior to beginning WBRT.[21] Meyers et al reported the most extensive study evaluating neurocognitive function for patients with brain metastases. This detailed work examined neurocognitive function in patients with brain metastases randomized to WBRT with or without the radiation sensitizer motexafin gadolinium. In the study, 401 patients were enrolled, and each patient underwent a battery of eight neurocognitive function tests at baseline and following treatment. At baseline, 91% of patients had a deficit, and 42% had deficits seen in four or more tests. Lesion volume was predictive of initial neurocognitive deficit. These data are critical, as most studies do not describe baseline neurocognitive deficits.

When considering withholding WBRT, one must be mindful that patients not receiving WBRT are more likely to have tumor progression at local and distant brain sites. Withholding WBRT results in a significantly increased risk of local and elsewhere failure in the brain. Such progression is often accompanied by irreversible neurologic symptoms requiring invasive salvage treatments. As an example, researchers at the University of Kentucky detailed their experience with 36 consecutive patients with limited brain metastases treated with SRS alone.[22] In this study, patients were followed with serial magnetic resonance imaging (MRI) ~ 3 months apart, despite which nearly half (17 patients, 47%) had in-brain tumor recurrence; of these, 12 (71%) presented with symptoms, and 10 (59%) presented with neurologic deficits. This study demonstrated a 1-year neurologicdeficit-free survival with this approach of only ~50%.

Not only does recurrence of intracranial disease result in significant symptoms, it is also one of the most important predictors of neurocognitive dysfunction. In the study cited above, Li et al noted a correlation between tumor progression and worsening neurocognitive function.[23] Following treatment, patients with tumor shrinkage at 2 months greater than the population median had improved survival as well as a longer time to neurocognitive dysfunction. Patients with a partial response also had an improvement in execution function and visual motor scanning from baseline. In comparison, patients with progressive disease had a significant worsening of neurocognitive symptoms. Similar results were seen in the Radiation Therapy Oncology Group (RTOG) 9104 study.[24] This trial randomized patients to two different radiation schedules and examined changes related to Mini-Mental Status Examination (MMSE) scores. The study demonstrated that, at 3 months, the average change in MMSE for patients with brain metastases that were controlled was −0.5, while it was −6.3 for patients with uncontrolled metastases, again suggesting that control of metastases plays a large role in the maintenance of neurocognitive function. These data suggest that the most significant threat to neurocognitive function is the recurrence/progression of brain metastases, and, much less likely, radiation-related toxicity. In addition, patients who respond to therapy can in fact have neurocognitive improvement.

Perhaps the most cited work regarding the risks of neurotoxicity in patients receiving WBRT is the retrospective series from Memorial Sloan-Kettering published by DeAngelis et al.[25] This study evaluated 47 long-term survivors (≥ 1 y following the diagnosis of brain metastases) and noted that 5 patients (11%) developed severe dementia associated with ataxia, as well as urinary incontinence. It should be remembered, however, that these patients represented a select subgroup of patients who are long-term survivors; therefore, the 11% severe dementia rate does not apply to those newly diagnosed with brain metastasis. Moreover, on closer examination, each of these five patients was treated using a nonstandard treatment regimen, placing them at higher risk of neurotoxicity. Four of the five patients received high-dose per fraction radiation therapy (5 −6 Gy/fraction), which is concerning, given that fraction size is one of the most important predictors of late toxicity. The fifth patient received a standard dose per fraction of 3 Gy but was treated with concurrent chemotherapy. Importantly, and not often discussed, is that no patient treated with 3 Gy or less per fraction without concurrent chemotherapy developed dementia. Perhaps, then, the most valuable finding from this study is to be wary of both the use of large fraction sizes and concurrent chemotherapy when delivering WBRT.

Concerns regarding the neurotoxicity associated with WBRT have once again been raised, given the publication of a randomized trial including patients with one to three brain metastases, reported by Chang et al from MD Anderson.[13] Patients in this study were randomized to 15 to 24 Gy SRS with or without 30-Gy WBRT in 12 fractions. The primary end point was a decline in the Hopkins Verbal Learning Test–Revised (HVLT-R) at 4 months. The trial closed early after accrual of only 58 patients based on concern for significantly worse neurocognitive outcomes secondary to the addition of WBRT. WBRT patients were found to have a 52% decline in HVLT-R at 4 months, whereas patients in the SRS-alone arm had only a 24% decline. Once again, the addition of WBRT resulted in decreased 1-year intracranial recurrence (27% vs 73%, $p = 0.0003$), including both improved local (100% vs 67%, $p = 0.012$) and elsewhere (73% vs 45%, $p = 0.02$) brain tumor control. Paradoxically, and unprecedented in similar randomized trials, patients in the WBRT arm had a significantly compromised median survival (5.7 vs 15.2 mo, $p = 0.003$).

The trial, though commendable for its effort to prospectively study neurocognitive function following central nervous system (CNS)–directed WBRT, has several shortcomings that make its findings difficult to generalize.[26] First, the study used patient stratification variables not prognostic of the study's primary neurocognitive end point. In this study, patients were stratified by recursive partitioning analysis (RPA) class, number of brain metastases, and histology, which are factors linked to survival rather than neurocognitive function. The authors did not stratify by baseline neurocognitive function, examination of which suggests at least a trend toward increased neurocognitive dysfunction in the WBRT group. Also important is the fact that the authors failed to account/stratify for many medications commonly prescribed to cancer patients—including opioids, sedatives, anticonvulsants, and steroids—that are known to cause neurocognitive dysfunction. Second, the authors chose an end point with questionable clinical relevance. The primary end point of their study was an assessment of neurocognitive function using only the HVLT-R at a single point of 4 months; however, given the complexity of cognitive function, a battery of tests over time is required to accurately depict the neurocognitive effects of radiation therapy.[27] In addition, this primary end point inadvertently biased the trial against WBRT, as previous work had already shown that radiation therapy has a transient effect on memory, as measured by verbal learning tests. In serial neuropsychological studies, Armstrong et al assessed patients with low-grade glioma who received radiation therapy and found a transient decline in verbal memory, with the nadir after radiation therapy corresponding exactly to the 4-month time interval used by Chang and colleagues.[28] Finally, as mentioned above, patients receiving WBRT inexplicably had a significantly shorter median survival than those who received SRS alone, on the order of a 3-fold difference (5.7 vs 15.2 mo). This is particularly perplexing, given the improved CNS disease control with WBRT (27% vs 73% at 1 y). Moreover, three previous randomized studies reported equivalent survival with the addition of WBRT to local therapy.[10–12] What specifically led to such a survival difference is unclear, although close inspection of the baseline patient characteristics suggests at least a trend toward more favorable factors (RPA class I, female gender, and lower median tumor volume) in the SRS-alone group. The authors suggested that the survival difference may be due in part to more frequent surgical salvage in patients who received SRS alone; however, the greater use of surgical salvage is more likely to be the result of increased CNS disease recurrence rather than a disproportionate rationing of salvage treatments. Also, although patients receiving WBRT had a higher proportion of systemic deaths, this is due to a delay in neurologic mortality rather than an increased systemic disease burden, a finding originally reported by Patchell et al.[10] Perhaps the survival difference was simply the result of statistical anomaly due to small patient numbers. Regardless, this survival difference could in itself explain the neurocognitive dysfunction found in patients receiving WBRT. The primary end point of this study was an assessment of neurocognitive function at 4 months (~1 mo prior to the median date of death of patients in the WBRT group). Many studies suggest that patients with terminal cancer experience profound neurocognitive dysfunction.[29,30] For example, Pereira et al followed 348 cancer patients using the serial MMSE and found that patients who died had a trend toward decreased scores, with 68% of patients having abnormal MMSE scores before death.[29] The decline in MMSE score was most profound 1 month before death. As such, the higher neurocognitive dysfunction noted in the WBRT group cannot be confidently ascribed to radiation, given the large survival difference noted between treatment groups, along with the timing of death in the WBRT group, in relation to the single 4-month study end point (~ 1 mo prior to median survival in the WBRT group).

It is not to say that WBRT is not associated with some risk of neurotoxicity. The RTOG published the results of a randomized trial in which patients with stage 3 non–small-cell lung cancer were randomized to prophylactic cranial radiation therapy (30 Gy) versus observation.[31] Although the trial failed to meet accrual goals, the authors noted that WBRT resulted in a decreased incidence of 1-year brain metastases (8% vs 18%); however, overall survival was not different. Relevant to our discussion regarding neurocognitive dysfunction, patients receiving prophylactic cranial radiation therapy did have a slightly worse immediate and delayed recall, albeit without an effect on global quality of life; this required sensitive neurocognitive testing to detect (and again did not stratify for all factors known to affect neurocognitive dysfunction). As such, the question is not whether WBRT alone results in any neurotoxicity but rather whether its overstated risks are outweighed by the benefits of reduced intracranial failure with associated neurocognitive dysfunction. In our view, it generally is. When discussing the pros and cons of WBRT with patients, it is important that the physician maintains an appropriate perspective regarding the toxicities associated with WBRT. For instance, recently, there have been accumulating data suggesting that many systemic chemotherapies are associated with long-term neurotoxicities.[32,33] That is not to say that all chemotherapy need be abandoned, but rather that, whenever prescribing treatment, one must make sure that the benefits outweigh the risks.

Researchers are exploring many avenues to potentially decrease the neurotoxicity associated with WBRT for the treatment of brain metastases. The RTOG completed accrual on a phase III trial randomizing patients to WBRT with or without memantine, an *N*-methyl-*D*-aspartate (NMDA) receptor antagonist that has proven to be effective in the treatment of vascular and Alzheimer dementia.[34] The drug has minimal side effects and, if proven successful, would represent an important step forward in reducing radiation-induced neurotoxicity. Other groups are taking a different approach, by limiting dose to regions of the brain thought to be central to radiation therapy-induced neurocognitive toxicity. A retrospective analysis from

Tata Memorial Hospital of patients with low-grade gliomas demonstrated that, following radiation therapy, one third of patients had > 10% decrease in intelligence quotient (IQ).[35] Dosimetric analysis demonstrated that dose to the left temporal lobe was correlated with the decline in IQ. A separate analysis from MD Anderson of patients with low-grade or anaplastic brain tumors demonstrated a dose response, with hippocampal dose correlated with decline in learning and delayed recall.[36] These studies, along with preclinical data, have brought the hippocampus forward as the prime target of current investigations. This has led the RTOG to develop a trial, 0933, which will test a hippocampus-sparing WBRT technique for patients with brain metastases. The primary outcome will be delayed recall using the HVLT-R at 4 months posttreatment, which is an unfortunate limitation, as previously critiqued in our discussion above regarding the trial by Chang et al.[13] Although specifically avoiding dose to regions of the brain does raise concern for potentially resulting in high failure rates at these sites, retrospective analyses have shown that ~ 8% of metastases occur near the hippocampus.[37] Were the trial to be successful in reducing neurocognitive dysfunction compared to a planned cohort of historical controls, the trade-off of a slightly higher failure rate in return for decreased neurotoxicity would likely be acceptable to most practitioners. Unfortunately, there are several reasons to be skeptical of such an approach; namely, hippocampus-sparing WBRT requires time-intensive contouring, planning, quality assurance, and increased cost; sparing of the hippocampus by currently available techniques may not lead to a clinically significant benefit; and hippocampus-sparing WBRT downplays the importance of other parts of the brain (i.e., the remainder of the limbic circuit and cerebral cortex) in memory function.

Conclusion

Brain metastases remain a common problem in cancer patients, and, as systemic therapies improve, leading patients to live longer, the brain's role as a "sanctuary" site will make this an even more frequent occurrence. Randomized, prospective trials and retrospective trials (***levels of evidence I*** to ***III***) demonstrate enhanced survival and intracranial disease control with WBRT for patients with multiple brain metastases. Although there is some variation in the management of patients with limited brain metastases, WBRT remains the cornerstone of management of patients with multiple (more than five) brain metastases. Future developments, including radiosensitizers, radioprotectors, alternative fractionation schemes, and techniques to reduce dose to sensitive brain tissues, may lead to improved results.

References

[1] Sperduto PW, Chao ST, Sneed PK, et al. Diagnosis-specific prognostic factors, indexes, and treatment outcomes for patients with newly diagnosed brain metastases: a multi-institutional analysis of 4,259 patients. Int J Radiat Oncol Biol Phys 2010; 77: 655–661

[2] Kwok Y, Patchell RA, Regine WF. Management of overt central nervous system metastases: brain and spinal cord. In: Pass HI, Carbone DP, Johnson DH et al eds. Principles and Practice of Lung Cancer. 4th ed. Pass, HI: Lippincott Williams & Wilkins; 2010: 911–926

[3] Wen PY, Loeffler JS. Overview of the clinical manifestations, diagnosis, and management of patients with brain metastases. UpToDate. http://www.uptodate.com. Accessed May 29, 2012

[4] Flannery TW, Suntharalingam M, Regine WF, et al. Long-term survival in patients with synchronous, solitary brain metastasis from non-small-cell lung cancer treated with radiosurgery. Int J Radiat Oncol Biol Phys 2008; 72: 19–23

[5] Gaspar L, Scott C, Rotman M, et al. Recursive partitioning analysis (RPA) of prognostic factors in three Radiation Therapy Oncology Group (RTOG) brain metastases trials. Int J Radiat Oncol Biol Phys 1997; 37: 745–751

[6] Sperduto PW, Berkey B, Gaspar LE, Mehta M, Curran W. A new prognostic index and comparison to three other indices for patients with brain metastases: an analysis of 1,960 patients in the RTOG database. Int J Radiat Oncol Biol Phys 2008; 70: 510–514

[7] Patchell RA, Tibbs PA, Walsh JW, et al. A randomized trial of surgery in the treatment of single metastases to the brain. N Engl J Med 1990; 322: 494–500

[8] Kondziolka D, Patel A, Lunsford LD, Kassam A, Flickinger JC. Stereotactic radiosurgery plus whole brain radiotherapy versus radiotherapy alone for patients with multiple brain metastases. Int J Radiat Oncol Biol Phys 1999; 45: 427–434

[9] Andrews DW, Scott CB, Sperduto PW, et al. Whole brain radiation therapy with or without stereotactic radiosurgery boost for patients with one to three brain metastases: phase III results of the RTOG 9508 randomised trial. Lancet 2004; 363: 1665–1672

[10] Patchell RA, Tibbs PA, Regine WF, et al. Postoperative radiotherapy in the treatment of single metastases to the brain: a randomized trial. JAMA 1998; 280: 1485–1489

[11] Aoyama H, Shirato H, Tago M, et al. Stereotactic radiosurgery plus whole-brain radiation therapy vs stereotactic radiosurgery alone for treatment of brain metastases: a randomized controlled trial. JAMA 2006; 295: 2483–2491

[12] Kocher M, Soffietti R, Abacioglu U, et al. Adjuvant whole-brain radiotherapy versus observation after radiosurgery or surgical resection of one to three cerebral metastases: results of the EORTC 22952-26001 study. J Clin Oncol 2011; 29: 134–141

[13] Chang EL, Wefel JS, Hess KR, et al. Neurocognition in patients with brain metastases treated with radiosurgery or radiosurgery plus whole-brain irradiation: a randomised controlled trial. Lancet Oncol 2009; 10: 1037–1044

[14] Bhatnagar AK, Kondziolka D, Lunsford LD, Flickinger JC. Recursive partitioning analysis of prognostic factors for patients with four or more intracranial metastases treated with radiosurgery. Technol Cancer Res Treat 2007; 6: 153–160

[15] Borgelt B, Gelber R, Kramer S, et al. The palliation of brain metastases: final results of the first two studies by the Radiation Therapy Oncology Group. Int J Radiat Oncol Biol Phys 1980; 6: 1–9

[16] Nieder C, Berberich W, Schnabel K. Tumor-related prognostic factors for remission of brain metastases after radiotherapy. Int J Radiat Oncol Biol Phys 1997; 39: 25–30

[17] Sneed PK, Larson DA, Wara WM. Radiotherapy for cerebral metastases. Neurosurg Clin N Am 1996; 7: 505–515

[18] Horton J, Baxter DH, Olson KB. The management of metastases to the brain by irradiation and corticosteroids. Am J Roentgenol Radium Ther Nucl Med 1971; 111: 334–336

[19] Wong WW, Schild SE, Sawyer TE, Shaw EG. Analysis of outcome in patients reirradiated for brain metastases. Int J Radiat Oncol Biol Phys 1996; 34: 585–590

[20] Son CH, Jimenez R, Niemierko A, Loeffler JS, Oh KS, Shih HA. Outcomes after whole brain reirradiation in patients with brain metastases. Int J Radiat Oncol Biol Phys 2012; 82: e167–e172

[21] Meyers CA, Smith JA, Bezjak A, et al. Neurocognitive function and progression in patients with brain metastases treated with whole-brain radiation and motexafin gadolinium: results of a randomized phase III trial. J Clin Oncol 2004; 22: 157–165

[22] Regine WF, Huhn JL, Patchell RA, et al. Risk of symptomatic brain tumor recurrence and neurologic deficit after radiosurgery alone in patients with newly diagnosed brain metastases: results and implications. Int J Radiat Oncol Biol Phys 2002; 52: 333–338

[23] Li J, Bentzen SM, Renschler M, Mehta MP. Regression after whole-brain radiation therapy for brain metastases correlates with survival and improved neurocognitive function. J Clin Oncol 2007; 25: 1260–1266

[24] Regine WF, Scott C, Murray K, Curran W. Neurocognitive outcome in brain metastases patients treated with accelerated-fractionation vs. accelerated-hyperfractionated radiotherapy: an analysis from Radiation Therapy Oncology Group Study 91-04. Int J Radiat Oncol Biol Phys 2001; 51: 711–717

[25] DeAngelis LM, Mandell LR, Thaler HT, et al. The role of postoperative radiotherapy after resection of single brain metastases. Neurosurgery 1989; 24: 798–805

[26] Mahmood U, Kwok Y, Regine WF, Patchell RA. Whole-brain irradiation for patients with brain metastases: still the standard of care. Lancet Oncol 2010; 11: 221–222, author reply 223

[27] Regine WF, Schmitt FA, Scott CB, et al. Feasibility of neurocognitive outcome evaluations in patients with brain metastases in a multi-institutional cooperative group setting: results of Radiation Therapy Oncology Group trial BR-0018. Int J Radiat Oncol Biol Phys 2004; 58: 1346–1352

[28] Armstrong CL, Corn BW, Ruffer JE, Pruitt AA, Mollman JE, Phillips PC. Radiotherapeutic effects on brain function: double dissociation of memory systems. Neuropsychiatry Neuropsychol Behav Neurol 2000; 13: 101–111

[29] Pereira J, Hanson J, Bruera E. The frequency and clinical course of cognitive impairment in patients with terminal cancer. Cancer 1997; 79: 835–842

[30] Lawlor PG, Gagnon B, Mancini IL, et al. Occurrence, causes, and outcome of delirium in patients with advanced cancer: a prospective study. Arch Intern Med 2000; 160: 786–794

[31] Sun A, Bae K, Gore EM, et al. Phase III trial of prophylactic cranial irradiation compared with observation in patients with locally advanced non-small-cell lung cancer: neurocognitive and quality-of-life analysis. J Clin Oncol 2011; 29: 279–286

[32] Koppelmans V, Breteler MM, Boogerd W, Seynaeve C, Gundy C, Schagen SB. Neuropsychological performance in survivors of breast cancer more than 20 years after adjuvant chemotherapy. J Clin Oncol 2012; 30: 1080–1086

[33] Deprez S, Amant F, Smeets A, et al. Longitudinal assessment of chemotherapy-induced structural changes in cerebral white matter and its correlation with impaired cognitive functioning. J Clin Oncol 2012; 30: 274–281

[34] Orgogozo JM, Rigaud AS, Stöffler A, Möbius HJ, Forette F. Efficacy and safety of memantine in patients with mild to moderate vascular dementia: a randomized, placebo-controlled trial (MMM 300). Stroke 2002; 33: 1834–1839

[35] Jalali R, Mallick I, Dutta D, et al. Factors influencing neurocognitive outcomes in young patients with benign and low-grade brain tumors treated with stereotactic conformal radiotherapy. Int J Radiat Oncol Biol Phys 2010; 77: 974–979

[36] Mahajan A, Dong L, Prabhu S, et al. Application of deformable image registration to hippocampal doses and neurocognitive outcomes. Soc Neuro Oncol 2007; 9: 538

[37] Gondi V, Tome WA, Marsh J, et al. Estimated risk of perihippocampal disease progression after hippocampal avoidance during whole-brain radiotherapy: safety profile for RTOG 0933. Radiother Oncol 2010; 95: 327–331

18 Radiosurgery for Glioblastoma

Hideyuki Kano, Douglas Kondziolka, Ajay Niranjan, John C. Flickinger, and L. Dade Lunsford

Introduction

Glioblastoma multiforme (GBM) is the most common primary brain tumor in adults, with nearly 10,000 cases diagnosed annually in the United States. Despite aggressive surgery when feasible, radiation therapy, and chemotherapy, the prognosis for this disease is poor. The extent of resection of the initial lesion, which is related to the location and invasiveness of the tumor, correlates with survival.[1,2] In addition, the volume of locally recurrent disease correlates inversely with survival.[3] In an analysis of data from the Brain Tumor Study Group protocols, an improvement in median survival time was demonstrated with increasing radiation therapy dose (delivered conventionally): from 18 weeks without radiation, to 28 weeks with 50 Gy, 36 weeks with 55 Gy, and 42 weeks with 60 Gy.[4] Unfortunately, efforts to increase radiation dose beyond 60 Gy have not improved outcomes but did increase toxicity.[5]

A meta-analysis for randomized controlled trials to assess the clinical impact of adjuvant chemotherapy in patients with GBM was performed.[6] In this study, nitrosoureas, local therapy using carmustine-loaded wafers, and temozolomide (TMZ) were all more effective than no chemotherapy. Stupp et al performed a randomized, multicenter, phase III clinical trial (***level I evidence***) in 573 patient with newly diagnosed GBM.[7] The median survival benefit was 2.5 months; the median survival was 14.6 months (95% confidence interval [CI], range 13.2–16.8 mo) with radiotherapy plus TMZ and 12.1 months (95% CI, range 11.2 –13.0 mo) with radiotherapy alone. Thus, radiotherapy plus concomitant and adjuvant TMZ was superior to radiotherapy alone, establishing this regimen as the current standard of care.

Even with optimal treatment, nearly all malignant gliomas recur. The 6-month progression-free survival varies from 6 to 16%.[8–10] Recurrence and disease progression are generally adjacent to the surgical treatment volume. Local recurrences are located within 2 cm of the enhancing edge of the original tumor (▶ Fig. 18.1).[11,12] The treatment of recurrent GBM is challenging. Reirradiation using conventional fractionated stereotactic radiotherapy (FSRT), either alone or combined with chemotherapy, is potentially associated with a higher risk of adverse radiation effects (AREs).[13]

The Rationale for Radiosurgery in Patients with Glioblastoma Multiforme

Stereotactic radiosurgery (SRS) is a minimally invasive surgical procedure that is usually performed on an outpatient basis. Numerous review articles discuss this delivery method.[14–16] SRS can selectively boost the radiation effect within a designated volume where most recurrences develop. Some reports described the potential efficacy and toxicity of SRS for recurrent GBM.[17–19] There is sufficient ***level III*** evidence to support the use of SRS for the treatment of GBM. There is no ***level I*** or ***II*** evidence that compares SRS to other treatment modalities (e.g., repeat radiation therapy, chemotherapy alone) for primary or recurrent GBMs.

In the early 1990s, retrospective studies demonstrated encouraging outcomes with improved survival of patients with GBM when SRS was added as an adjuvant treatment (▶ Table 18.1). Loeffler et al reported (***level III evidence***) that 23 GBM patients with residual tumor after surgical resection and conventional radiation therapy underwent boost SRS and had a median survival of 26 months.[20] Kondziolka et al (***level III evidence***) reported 45 GBM patients who underwent Gamma Knife (Elekta AB, Stockholm, Sweden) radiosurgery as part of initial management and 19 who underwent Gamma Knife radiosurgery at the time of tumor progression.[21] The SRS target was the contrast-enhanced portion of the tumor. The median survival after SRS was 16 months. In comparison to historical controls of outcome after radiation therapy, the 2-year survival in Radiation Therapy Oncology Group (RTOG) class V patients was extended from 6 to > 20%.

Shrieve et al (***level III evidence***) reported 78 patients who underwent SRS as a boost for a residual GBM after surgical resection or biopsy and conventional radiation therapy.[22] Their target was the magnetic resonance imaging (MRI) contrast-enhanced residual tumor with < 4 cm diameter. Seven of 78 patients had no enhancing tumor on postoperative imaging. In these cases, the surgical cavity was treated with a 5-mm margin. The median survival time from diagnosis was 19.9 months. Patients in this series fell into RTOG classes III (27 patients), IV (29 patients), or V (22 patients). Class III patients had a median survival time of 29.5 months following diagnosis; this was significantly longer than median survival times for classes IV and V, which were 19.2 and 18.2 months, respectively ($p = 0.001$). Only patient age (< 40 y) was a significant prognostic factor according to multivariate analysis.

Masciopinto et al (***level III evidence***) reported a median survival of 9.5 months after surgery or biopsy, conventional radiation therapy, and SRS as part of their primary treatment.[23] They interpreted these results to suggest that SRS provided no survival benefit. Villavicencio et al (***level III evidence***) reported 46 patients who underwent SRS at multiple institutions.[24] Twenty patients (43.5%) had CyberKnife (Accuray Inc., Sunnyvale, CA) radiosurgery at the time of initial diagnosis (during the first 3 mo of their initial clinical treatment), and 26 (56.5%) were treated at the time of tumor recurrence or progression. The median overall survival as an initial clinical therapy was 11.5 months, compared to 24 months for patients treated at the time of tumor recurrence or progression ($p < 0.0004$).

Pannullo et al (***level III evidence***) performed a meta-analysis of SRS for GBMs covering 456 patients in 11 studies.[25] The median overall survival from diagnosis was 13.5 to 26.0 months, and the overall complication rate was 11.4% (95% CI, 5.1–23.6%). The authors compared the median overall survival from studies in which SRS was used as a boost to the median overall survival from studies in which SRS was used as salvage for recurrent tumor. They found that the reported ranges of median overall survival were similar (9.5–25.0 vs 10.2–26.0 mo, respectively).

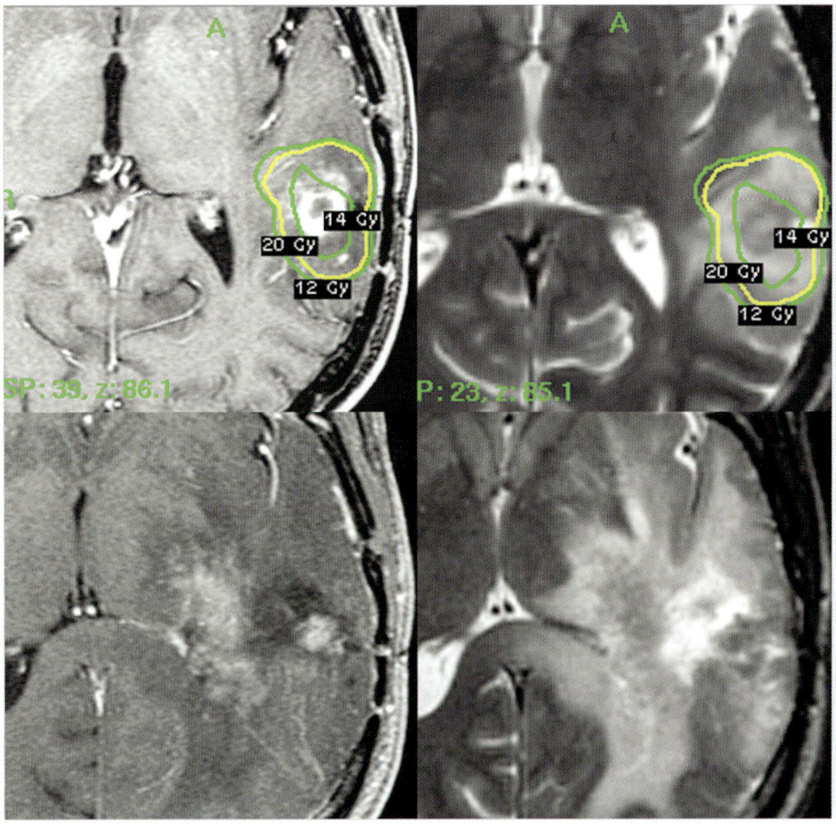

Fig. 18.1 40 year-old man with a recurrent left temporal glioblastoma multiforme underwent SRS after resection, external radiotherapy, and temozolomide chemotherapy. Axial T1-weighted contrast enhanced (Upper Left) and T2-weighted (Upper Right) MR images show at stereotactic radiosurgery. The margin dose was 12 Gy (outer green line). The yellow line shows 14 Gy volume and the inner green line shows 20 Gy volume. Sixteen months later axial T1-weighted contrast enhanced (Lower Left) and T2-weighted (Lower Right) MR images show marginal tumor progression.

The safety of SRS has been investigated by the RTOG in a phase I dose escalation study (RTOG 90–05) for the treatment of recurrent primary brain tumors and central nervous system metastases in patients who have previously received fractionated brain radiation therapy. The maximal tolerable dose based on overall toxicity was determined to be 24 Gy for ≤ 20-mm tumors, 18 Gy for 21- to 30-mm tumors, and 15 Gy for 31- to 40-mm tumors.[26]

Appropriate targeting is essential to improve the success and safety of boost SRS for GBM. Emerging evidence suggests that defining the contrast-enhancing tumor as the target is unsatisfactory. Image-guided stereotactic biopsies have shown infiltrating tumor cells in the adjacent high T2 signal region that surrounds the contrast-enhancing tumor.[27] In addition, work with glioma cell lines has shown that diffuse astrocytoma, especially GBM, invades the brain preferentially along white matter fiber tracts.[28–30] Because this property is shared with human fetal brain cells that have been transplanted into the adult brain, it has been hypothesized that glioma cells share migratory features similar to cells found during embryonic development. The Cadherin superfamily is associated with glioma invasion, embryonic development, and maintenance of tissue architecture in adults.[31] Invasion of white matter pathways begins regionally but then spreads contralaterally via the corpus callosum.[30] Based on such invasive and migratory properties of glioma cells, it is not surprising that dose escalation focused on the contrast-enhancing portion of glioblastoma tumor has not been successful.

Retrospective studies provide initial ***level II*** or ***III*** data, but they may be affected by patient selection bias. To reduce bias, the RTOG 93–05 protocol was established as a randomized control study using an unusual clinical paradigm of upfront SRS. In this study, Souhami et al (***level Ia evidence***) reported that SRS followed by external beam radiation therapy and carmustine, or bis-chloroethylnitrosourea (BCNU), does not improve the outcome in patients with GBM, nor does it change the quality of life or cognitive functioning.[32] In this study, GBM patients with residual tumor after surgical resection were included. The authors did not use SRS for recurrent GBMs. Tsao et al stated that SRS followed by external beam radiotherapy (EBRT) and BCNU does not confer benefit in terms of overall survival, local tumor control, or quality of life.[33] They noted that there is insufficient evidence regarding either benefit or toxicity in the use of FSRT for patients with newly diagnosed or progressive/recurrent high-grade glioma. Such reports are limited by the wide variation in technologies, target volume, patient selection, and doses that are used to administer boost radiation to patients who have failed initial GBM management. Such studies also fail to differentiate both methodological and radiobiological differences between fractionated radiation therapy boosts and SRS.

Multiple clinical trials of TMZ in combination with FSRT have sufficient evidence that its addition to radiotherapy after surgical resection provides a statistically significant longer median survival (of several months) compared to postoperative radiation therapy alone.[7,34,36] Concurrent and adjuvant TMZ chemotherapy has been widely adopted as the initial management for malignant glioma.

The RTOG recursive partitioning analysis (RPA) classification of malignant gliomas is a method to reduce the effects of patient

Table 18.1 Summary of stereotactic radiosurgery for glioblastoma multiforme studies (level III evidence)

Study	No. patients	SRS timing	Type of SRS	Median tumor volume (cm³) (range)	Median margin dose (Gy) (range)	Median survival after SRS (months)
Loeffler et al[20]	23	Residual	LINAC	4.8 (1.2–72)	12 (10–20)	26.0
Masciopinto et al[23]	31	Residual	LINAC	16.4 (2.3–59.7)	11.7* (10.0–20.0)	9.5
Hall et al[58]	26	Recurrent	LINAC	28.0 (2.4–98.0)	20 (7.5–40.0)	18.0
Sarkaria et al[39]	96	Residual + Recurrent	LINAC	10	12 (6–20)	22.0
Larson et al[59]	97	Residual + Recurrent	GK	6.4 (0.3–96)	16.0 (5.0–37.5)	13.3
Kondziolka et al[21]	64	Residual + Recurrent	GK	6.5[a] (0.9–31.2)	15.5[a] (12.0–25.0)	16.0
Shrieve et al[22]	78	Residual	LINAC	9.4 (0.86–72)	12 (6–24)	19.9
Nwokedi et al[60]	31	Residual	GK	18.5 (1.6–62.2)	17.1 (10.0–28.0)	25.0
Souhami et al[32]	89	Residual	LINAC + GK	0.7–6.0 cm[b]	15–24	13.5
Combs et al[18]	32	Recurrent	Linac	10.0 (1.2–59.2)	15 (10–20)	10.0
Hsieh et al[61]	51	Residual + Recurrent	GK	13.6 (0.6–64.4)	12	9.3
Patel et al[62]	26	Recurrent	LINAC	10.4 (0.3–60.1)	18 (12–20)	8.5
Villavicencio et al[24]	20	Residual	Cyber	5.8 (0.7–47.3)	20 (12–25)	9.5
	26	Recurrent	Cyber	7.0 (0.4–48.5)	20 (8–-25)	7.0
Pouratian et al[38]	22	Residual	GK	13.4 (4.4–56)	5.6 (4–10)	10.0
	26	Recurrent	GK	21.3 (0.3–110.0)	6.0 (3.0–15.0)	9.4
Conti et al[63]	11	Recurrent	Cyber	15.1	20	12 (SRS + TMZ)
	12	Recurrent	Cyber	13.1	20	7 (SRS alone)
Park et al[57]	11	Recurrent	GK	13.6 (1.2–45.1)	16 (13–18)	17.9 (SRS + bevacizumab)
	44 [c]	Recurrent	GK	9.5 (1.5–48.9)	15 (10–20)	12.2 (SRS alone)

[a]mean, [b]tumor diameter, [c]case match control
SRS, stereotactic radiosurgery; GK, gamma knife; TMZ, temozolomide

selection bias. The RTOG RPA classification includes age, Karnofsky performance scale (KPS) score, prior surgical resection, prior fractionated radiation therapy, and employment status. The RPA classification is a significant predictor of patient survival. Mirimanoff et al (***level III evidence***) reported that the overall survival was 17 months for RPA class III, 15 months for RPA class IV, and 10 months for RPA class V ($p < 0.0001$).[37] Survival with combined TMZ/radiation therapy was higher in RPA class III, with 21-month median survival time and a 43% 2-year survival rate versus 15-month median survival time and 20% 2-year survival for radiation therapy alone ($p = 0.006$). In RPA class IV, the survival advantage remained significant, with median survival times of 16 months and 2-year survival rates of 28%. In RPA class V, however, the survival advantage of radiation therapy/TMZ was of borderline significance ($p = 0.054$). RPA classification is also a significant predictor of survival in patients with GBMs who underwent SRS after surgical resection, radiation therapy, and TMZ chemotherapy. Pouratin et al (***level III evidence***) reported RPA class III patients with recurrent GBM who underwent SRS had a median overall survival of 34.5 months.[38] The benefit of SRS was as great in RPA class IV and V patients. Sarkaria et al (***level III evidence***)[39] reported that RPA class III patients who underwent additional SRS had a longer overall survival. RPA class III GBM patients may be the best candidates for SRS.

■ The Role of Stereotactic Radiosurgery for Glioblastoma Multiforme

At most centers, SRS is used for progressive or recurrent GBM, in part because a randomized controlled study showed no clear benefit to SRS prior to conventional fractionated radiation therapy.[22] Patterns of recurrence following SRS are similar to patterns reported for FSRT, that is, regional recurrence in 83.5% of patients.[40] Patients tend to fail within 1 to 2 cm from the contrast-enhancing border of the tumor being treated, in keeping with the biology of this tumor, which is highly infiltrative and invasive. One potential reason for the high rate of subsequent local recurrence after SRS is inadequate targeting of tumor when SRS is performed. It is standard practice to use the region of gadolinium enhancement on T1-weighted MRI as the basis for the treatment plan for SRS. However, it is known that gadolinium enhancement does not correspond fully to active tumor; there are often regions of nonenhancing tumor that extend beyond the areas of contrast enhancement. These areas may be better defined using magnetic resonance spectroscopy (MRS); elevation of choline levels and an increased ratio between choline and *N*-acetyl-acetate (NAA) correlate with tumor presence.[41] In addition, several series reported that the outcome of patients with recurrent GBM treated with SRS is correlated with the degree of overlap between treatment target (based on gadolinium-enhanced MRI) and presence of tumor as assessed by MRS.[42–44] Areas of tumor detected by MRS that are not included in the SRS target volume are likely to recur, and there is a trend toward poorer survival in these patients. The role of MRS for SRS targeting in patients with recurrent GBM will require further studies, possibly including randomized prospective studies.

Koga et al (***level III evidence***) reported extended field SRS for recurrent GBMs.[45] The target volume was extended by adding a 0.5- to 1.0-cm margin to the periphery of the gadolinium-enhanced lesion. The target tumor volume was extended up to a maximum of 1 cm in all directions. Nine patients (GBM: 8, anaplastic astrocytoma:1) underwent conventional SRS after surgical resection, EBRT, and chemotherapy (3-[(4-amino-2-methyl-5-pyrimidinyl)methyl]-l-(chloroethyl)-l-nitrosourea [ACNU]: 6, TMZ: 2, carboplatin and etoposide: 1). Nine patients (GBM: 7, anaplastic astrocytoma: 1, diffuse astrocytoma: 1) underwent extended field SRS after surgical resection, EBRT, and chemotherapy (TMZ: 9). The median overall survival after conventional SRS and extended field SRS was 10.5 months and 9.0 months, respectively (no statistical significance). However, the local control rate in patients treated by extended field SRS was significantly better than that with conventional SRS (93 vs 47%, $p = 0.0035$). AREs were observed in two patients (6.5%) with conventional SRS and four patients (29%) with extended field SRS (no statistical significance: $p = 0.052$). All AREs were asymptomatic and resolved their imaging abnormalities using corticosteroid administration. The authors concluded that extended field SRS was well tolerated and superior to conventional SRS in the local control of small recurrent lesions of GBM, although a further device to suppress remote recurrences may be necessary to improve survival.

Stereotactic Radiosurgery and Bevacizumab

GBMs are innately hypoxic tumors with strong endogenous expression of vascular endothelial growth factor (VEGF) and consequently demonstrate vigorous angiogenesis. Bevacizumab, a humanized monoclonal antibody to VEGF, has been used with safety and clinical success with concomitant chemotherapy in solid tumors,[46–48] including GBM.[49–51] Several reasons exist to combine bevacizumab and radiation therapy. These include the ability of antiangiogenic agents to sensitize the tumor endothelium by depletion of VEGF and the reduction of its prosurvival signaling.[52,53] Recently, a phase II trial of single-agent bevacizumab at tumor progression in patients with recurrent GBM who underwent conventional radiation therapy and TMZ chemotherapy reported that 6 (12.5%) of 48 patients had drug-associated toxicity (five thromboembolic events, one bowel perforation). The median progression-free survival (PFS) and overall survival were 16 and 31 weeks, respectively. The 6-month PFS and overall survival were 29% and 57%, respectively (***level III evidence***).[54]

The combination of SRS and bevacizumab was reported by Gutin et al (***level III evidence***) in the management of 25 patients with recurrent malignant glioma.[55] For 20 patients with GBM, the overall tumor response rate was 50%, and median PFS and overall survival were 7.3 and 12.5 months, respectively. The rationale for combining bevacizumab and SRS is based on the potential radiosensitizing benefit of bevacizumab. The potential for such synergistic effects has been proposed both for the ability of antiangiogenic agents to normalize blood vessels and for its ability to counteract the effects of radiation-induced VEGF secretion from tumor cells.

Cuneo et al (***level III evidence***) reported 49 patients with recurrent GBM.[56] Thirty-three patients received bevacizumab before or after linear accelerator (LINAC)–based radiosurgery, and 16 underwent SRS without bevacizumab. The authors demonstrated that patients who underwent SRS followed by bevacizumab administration had significantly longer PFS and overall survival compared to patients who had SRS without bevacizumab (median PFS 5.2 vs 2.1 mo; median overall survival 11.2 vs 3.9 mo). Recently, our center reported a case control study of salvage Gamma Knife radiosurgery followed by bevacizumab for recurrent GBMs comparing it to recurrent GBM without bevacizumab chemotherapy (***level III evidence***).[57] Compared to patients who did not receive bevacizumab, those who received bevacizumab had significantly prolonged PFS (6-mo PFS: 73% vs 58%, median PFS: 15 vs 7 mo, $p = 0.035$) and overall survival (6-mo overall survival: 100% vs 89%, median overall survival: 18 vs 12 mo, $p = 0.005$) and were less likely to develop an ARE (9% vs 46%, $p = 0.037$). We believe that a combination of salvage Gamma Knife SRS followed by bevacizumab provided additional benefit but little toxicity in this series of patients with progressive GBM.

Conclusion

Management of recurrent GBM remains an ongoing clinical challenge. Despite initial standard management of GBM that includes surgical resection, EBRT, and chemotherapy using TMZ, virtually all patients recur. Our approach has been to maximize the benefit of the one treatment modality that is required to have any meaningful improvement of outcomes: radiation. Most GBMs progress in the vicinity of the resection cavity. Some patients may be candidates for additional surgical resection and others for SRS. The combination of bevacizumab and SRS may add value. Progression after initial management first develops 1 to 2 cm from the contrast-enhancing edge, in keeping with the biology of this tumor, which is highly infiltrative and invasive. The future will likely include a combination of aggressive surgery and radiation therapy coupled with adjuvant TMZ. For residual or recurrent disease, adjuvant radiosurgery remains an option, likely in concert with agents that improve the radiobiological response or reduce the risk of treatment toxicity.

References

[1] Nitta T, Sato K. Prognostic implications of the extent of surgical resection in patients with intracranial malignant gliomas. Cancer 1995; 75: 2727–2731

[2] Daneyemez M, Gezen F, Canakçi Z, Kahraman S. Radical surgery and reoperation in supratentorial malignant glial tumors. Minim Invasive Neurosurg 1998; 41: 209–213

[3] Keles GE, Lamborn KR, Chang SM, Prados MD, Berger MS. Volume of residual disease as a predictor of outcome in adult patients with recurrent supratentorial glioblastomas multiforme who are undergoing chemotherapy. J Neurosurg 2004; 100: 41–46

[4] Walker MD, Strike TA, Sheline GE. An analysis of dose-effect relationship in the radiotherapy of malignant gliomas. Int J Radiat Oncol Biol Phys 1979; 5: 1725–1731

[5] Butowski NA, Sneed PK, Chang SM. Diagnosis and treatment of recurrent high-grade astrocytoma. J Clin Oncol 2006; 24: 1273–1280

[6] Spiegel BM, Esrailian E, Laine L, Chamberlain MC. Clinical impact of adjuvant chemotherapy in glioblastoma multiforme: a meta-analysis. CNS Drugs 2007; 21: 775–787

[7] Stupp R, Mason WP, van den Bent MJ, et al. European Organisation for Research and Treatment of Cancer Brain Tumor and Radiotherapy Groups. National Cancer Institute of Canada Clinical Trials Group. Radiotherapy plus concomitant and adjuvant temozolomide for glioblastoma. N Engl J Med 2005; 352: 987–996

[8] Ballman KV, Buckner JC, Brown PD, et al. The relationship between six-month progression-free survival and 12-month overall survival end points for phase II trials in patients with glioblastoma multiforme. Neuro-oncol 2007; 9: 29–38

[9] Lamborn KR, Yung WK, Chang SM, et al. North American Brain Tumor Consortium. Progression-free survival: an important end point in evaluating therapy for recurrent high-grade gliomas. Neuro-oncol 2008; 10: 162–170

[10] Wong ET, Hess KR, Gleason MJ, et al. Outcomes and prognostic factors in recurrent glioma patients enrolled onto phase II clinical trials. J Clin Oncol 1999; 17: 2572–2578

[11] Hochberg FH, Pruitt A. Assumptions in the radiotherapy of glioblastoma. Neurology 1980; 30: 907–911

[12] Wallner KE, Galicich JH, Krol G, Arbit E, Malkin MG. Patterns of failure following treatment for glioblastoma multiforme and anaplastic astrocytoma. Int J Radiat Oncol Biol Phys 1989; 16: 1405–1409

[13] Bauman GS, Sneed PK, Wara WM, et al. Reirradiation of primary CNS tumors. Int J Radiat Oncol Biol Phys 1996; 36: 433–441

[14] McKenzie MR, Souhami L, Podgorsak EB, Olivier A, Caron JL, Villemure JG. Photon radiosurgery: a clinical review. Can J Neurol Sci 1992; 19: 212–221

[15] Podgorsak EB. Physics for radiosurgery with linear accelerators. Neurosurg Clin N Am 1992; 3: 9–34

[16] Wu A. Physics and dosimetry of the gamma knife. Neurosurg Clin N Am 1992; 3: 35–50

[17] Biswas T, Okunieff P, Schell MC, et al. Stereotactic radiosurgery for glioblastoma: retrospective analysis. Radiat Oncol 2009; 4: 11

[18] Combs SE, Widmer V, Thilmann C, Hof H, Debus J, Schulz-Ertner D. Stereotactic radiosurgery (SRS): treatment option for recurrent glioblastoma multiforme (GBM). Cancer 2005; 104: 2168–2173

[19] Kong DS, Lee JI, Park K, Kim JH, Lim DH, Nam DH. Efficacy of stereotactic radiosurgery as a salvage treatment for recurrent malignant gliomas. Cancer 2008; 112: 2046–2051

[20] Loeffler JS, Alexander E, Shea WM, et al. Radiosurgery as part of the initial management of patients with malignant gliomas. J Clin Oncol 1992; 10: 1379–1385

[21] Kondziolka D, Flickinger JC, Bissonette DJ, Bozik M, Lunsford LD. Survival benefit of stereotactic radiosurgery for patients with malignant glial neoplasms. Neurosurgery 1997; 41: 776–783, discussion 783–785

[22] Shrieve DC, Alexander E, Black PM, et al. Treatment of patients with primary glioblastoma multiforme with standard postoperative radiotherapy and radiosurgical boost: prognostic factors and long-term outcome. J Neurosurg 1999; 90: 72–77

[23] Masciopinto JE, Levin AB, Mehta MP, Rhode BS. Stereotactic radiosurgery for glioblastoma: a final report of 31 patients. J Neurosurg 1995; 82: 530–535

[24] Villavicencio AT, Burneikiene S, Romanelli P, et al. Survival following stereotactic radiosurgery for newly diagnosed and recurrent glioblastoma multiforme: a multicenter experience. Neurosurg Rev 2009; 32: 417–424

[25] Pannullo SC, Fraser JF, Moliterno J, Cobb W, Stieg PE. Stereotactic radiosurgery: a meta-analysis of current therapeutic applications in neuro-oncologic disease. J Neurooncol 2011; 103: 1–17

[26] Shaw E, Scott C, Souhami L, et al. Single dose radiosurgical treatment of recurrent previously irradiated primary brain tumors and brain metastases: final report of RTOG protocol 90–05. Int J Radiat Oncol Biol Phys 2000; 47: 291–298

[27] Kelly PJ, Daumas-Duport C, Kispert DB, Kall BA, Scheithauer BW, Illig JJ. Imaging-based stereotaxic serial biopsies in untreated intracranial glial neoplasms. J Neurosurg 1987; 66: 865–874

[28] Beliën AT, Paganetti PA, Schwab ME. Membrane-type 1 matrix metalloprotease (MT1-MMP) enables invasive migration of glioma cells in central nervous system white matter. J Cell Biol 1999; 144: 373–384

[29] Giese A, Kluwe L, Laube B, Meissner H, Berens ME, Westphal M. Migration of human glioma cells on myelin. Neurosurgery 1996; 38: 755–764

[30] Pedersen PH, Edvardsen K, Garcia-Cabrera I, et al. Migratory patterns of lac-z transfected human glioma cells in the rat brain. Int J Cancer 1995; 62: 767–771

[31] Demuth T, Berens ME. Molecular mechanisms of glioma cell migration and invasion. J Neurooncol 2004; 70: 217–228

[32] Souhami L, Seiferheld W, Brachman D, et al. Randomized comparison of stereotactic radiosurgery followed by conventional radiotherapy with carmustine to conventional radiotherapy with carmustine for patients with glioblastoma multiforme: report of Radiation Therapy Oncology Group 93–05 protocol. Int J Radiat Oncol Biol Phys 2004; 60: 853–860

[33] Tsao MN, Mehta MP, Whelan TJ, et al. The American Society for Therapeutic Radiology and Oncology (ASTRO) evidence-based review of the role of radiosurgery for malignant glioma. Int J Radiat Oncol Biol Phys 2005; 63: 47–55

[34] Athanassiou H, Synodinou M, Maragoudakis E, et al. Randomized phase II study of temozolomide and radiotherapy compared with radiotherapy alone in newly diagnosed glioblastoma multiforme. J Clin Oncol 2005; 23: 2372–2377

[35] Stupp R, Dietrich PY, Ostermann Kraljevic S, et al. Promising survival for patients with newly diagnosed glioblastoma multiforme treated with concomitant radiation plus temozolomide followed by adjuvant temozolomide. J Clin Oncol 2002; 20: 1375–1382

[36] Stupp R, Hegi ME, Mason WP, et al. European Organisation for Research and Treatment of Cancer Brain Tumour and Radiation Oncology Groups. National Cancer Institute of Canada Clinical Trials Group. Effects of radiotherapy with concomitant and adjuvant temozolomide versus radiotherapy alone on survival in glioblastoma in a randomised phase III study: 5-year analysis of the EORTC-NCIC trial. Lancet Oncol 2009; 10: 459–466

[37] Mirimanoff RO, Gorlia T, Mason W, et al. Radiotherapy and temozolomide for newly diagnosed glioblastoma: recursive partitioning analysis of the EORTC 26981/22981-NCIC CE3 phase III randomized trial. J Clin Oncol 2006; 24: 2563–2569

[38] Pouratian N, Crowley RW, Sherman JH, Jagannathan J, Sheehan JP. Gamma Knife radiosurgery after radiation therapy as an adjunctive treatment for glioblastoma. J Neurooncol 2009; 94: 409–418

[39] Sarkaria JN, Mehta MP, Loeffler JS, et al. Radiation Therapy Oncology Group. Radiosurgery in the initial management of malignant gliomas: survival comparison with the RTOG recursive partitioning analysis. Int J Radiat Oncol Biol Phys 1995; 32: 931–941

[40] McDermott MW, Sneed PK, Chang SM, Gutin PH, Wara WM, Verhey LJ, Smith V, Petti PL, Ho M, Park E, Edwards MSB, Prados MD, Larson DA. Results of radiosurgery for recurrent gliomas. In Kondziolka D (ed.): Radiosurgery 1995, Karger, Basel. Radiosurgery, vol. 1, pp. 102–112, 1996

[41] McKnight TR, von dem Bussche MH, Vigneron DB, et al. Histopathological validation of a three-dimensional magnetic resonance spectroscopy index as a predictor of tumor presence. J Neurosurg 2002; 97: 794–802

[42] Chan AA, Lau A, Pirzkall A, et al. Proton magnetic resonance spectroscopy imaging in the evaluation of patients undergoing Gamma Knife surgery for Grade IV glioma. J Neurosurg 2004; 101: 467–475

[43] Chuang CF, Chan AA, Larson D, et al. Potential value of MR spectroscopic imaging for the radiosurgical management of patients with recurrent high-grade gliomas. Technol Cancer Res Treat 2007; 6: 375–382

[44] Graves EE, Nelson SJ, Vigneron DB, et al. A preliminary study of the prognostic value of proton magnetic resonance spectroscopic imaging in Gamma Knife radiosurgery of recurrent malignant gliomas. Neurosurgery 2000; 46: 319–326, discussion 326–328

[45] Koga T, Maruyama K, Tanaka M, et al. Extended field stereotactic radiosurgery for recurrent glioblastoma. Cancer 2012; 118: 4193–4200
[46] Levin VA, Crafts DC, Norman DM, Hoffer PB, Spire JP, Wilson CB. Criteria for evaluating patients undergoing chemotherapy for malignant brain tumors. J Neurosurg 1977; 47: 329–335
[47] Macdonald DR, Cascino TL, Schold SC, Cairncross JG. Response criteria for phase II studies of supratentorial malignant glioma. J Clin Oncol 1990; 8: 1277–1280
[48] Prados MD, Lamborn K, Yung WK, et al. North American Brain Tumor Consortium. A phase 2 trial of irinotecan (CPT-11) in patients with recurrent malignant glioma: a North American Brain Tumor Consortium study. Neuro-oncol 2006; 8: 189–193
[49] Buckner JC. Factors influencing survival in high-grade gliomas. Semin Oncol 2003; 30 (Suppl 19): 10–14
[50] Lamborn KR, Chang SM, Prados MD. Prognostic factors for survival of patients with glioblastoma: recursive partitioning analysis. Neuro-oncol 2004; 6: 227–235
[51] Therasse P, Le Cesne A, Van Glabbeke M, Verweij J, Judson I EORTC Soft Tissue and Bone Sarcoma Group. RECIST vs. WHO: prospective comparison of response criteria in an EORTC phase II clinical trial investigating ET-743 in advanced soft tissue sarcoma. Eur J Cancer 2005; 41: 1426–1430
[52] Ahn GO, Brown JM. Matrix metalloproteinase-9 is required for tumor vasculogenesis but not for angiogenesis: role of bone marrow-derived myelomonocytic cells. Cancer Cell 2008; 13: 193–205
[53] Gorski DH, Beckett MA, Jaskowiak NT, et al. Blockage of the vascular endothelial growth factor stress response increases the antitumor effects of ionizing radiation. Cancer Res 1999; 59: 3374–3378
[54] Kreisl TN, Kim L, Moore K, et al. Phase II trial of single-agent bevacizumab followed by bevacizumab plus irinotecan at tumor progression in recurrent glioblastoma. J Clin Oncol 2009; 27: 740–745
[55] Gutin PH, Iwamoto FM, Beal K, et al. Safety and efficacy of bevacizumab with hypofractionated stereotactic irradiation for recurrent malignant gliomas. Int J Radiat Oncol Biol Phys 2009; 75: 156–163
[56] Cuneo KC, Vredenburgh JJ, Sampson JH, et al. Safety and efficacy of stereotactic radiosurgery and adjuvant bevacizumab in patients with recurrent malignant gliomas. Int J Radiat Oncol Biol Phys 2012; 82: 2018–2024
[57] Park KJ, Kano H, Iyer A, et al. Salvage Gamma Knife stereotactic radiosurgery followed by bevacizumab for recurrent glioblastoma multiforme: a case-control study. J Neurooncol 2012; 107: 323–333
[58] Hall WA, Djalilian HR, Sperduto PW, et al. Stereotactic radiosurgery for recurrent malignant gliomas. J Clin Oncol 1995; 13: 1642–1648
[59] Larson DA, Gutin PH, McDermott M, et al. Gamma Knife for glioma: selection factors and survival. Int J Radiat Oncol Biol Phys 1996; 36: 1045–1053
[60] Nwokedi EC, DiBiase SJ, Jabbour S, Herman J, Amin P, Chin LS. Gamma Knife stereotactic radiosurgery for patients with glioblastoma multiforme. Neurosurgery 2002; 50: 41–46, discussion 46–47
[61] Hsieh PC, Chandler JP, Bhangoo S, et al. Adjuvant gamma knife stereotactic radiosurgery at the time of tumor progression potentially improves survival for patients with glioblastoma multiforme. Neurosurgery 2005; 57: 684–692, discussion 684–692
[62] Patel M, Siddiqui F, Jin JY, et al. Salvage reirradiation for recurrent glioblastoma with radiosurgery: radiographic response and improved survival. J Neurooncol 2009; 92: 185–191
[63] Conti A, Pontoriero A, Arpa D, et al. Efficacy and toxicity of CyberKnife re-irradiation and "dose dense" temozolomide for recurrent gliomas. Acta Neurochir (Wien) 2012; 154: 203–209

19 The Argument against Radiosurgery for Glioblastoma

Alireza M. Mohammadi, Pablo F. Recinos, and Michael A. Vogelbaum

Introduction

Long-term survival for patients with high-grade glioma remains an elusive goal despite the use of aggressive, multimodality treatment for this disease. Standard of care for high-grade glioma includes maximum safe resection, postoperative external beam radiotherapy (EBRT), and chemotherapy.[1–4] Although stereotactic radiosurgery (SRS) has never been studied as a definitive treatment for high-grade gliomas, its role as an adjunct therapy, in combination with other therapies, or as a salvage therapy has been studied. A critical, evidence-based evaluation of the current literature does not reveal a clear role for SRS in the treatment of high-grade gliomas. In this chapter, we examine the role of SRS for high-grade gliomas as upfront or salvage treatment and review the evidence supporting each role.

Stereotactic Radiosurgery as an Upfront Treatment for Newly Diagnosed High-Grade Glioma

Randomized Controlled Studies

The Radiation Therapy Oncology Group (RTOG) 93–05 trial, which was published in 2004, is the only randomized controlled study that has evaluated SRS as an upfront treatment for newly diagnosed high-grade glioma.[5] In this study, 203 adult patients with pathologically confirmed glioblastomas (GBMs) without prior radiation or chemotherapy were randomized into two arms: standard therapy (EBRT + chemotherapy with bis-chloroethylnitrosourea [BCNU]) and standard therapy with adjuvant upfront SRS. Relevant inclusion criteria included a maximum tumor dimension ≤ 4 cm, a Karnofsky performance scale (KPS) score ≥ 60, and no brainstem lesions. The primary end point was survival, and secondary end points were treatment toxicity and quality of life. Patients were treated with an SRS dose range of 15 to 24 Gy, stratified by tumor size, and had a median follow-up time of 61 months. Median survival was not statistically different between the two groups (13.6 mo in the standard therapy group vs 13.5 mo in the standard therapy + SRS group). One year actuarial survivals were 19% (standard group) and 21% (standard + SRS group). In addition, a decline was seen in the Spitzer Quality of Life Index and Mini-Mental State Examination in both groups, with no significant difference between them. Late grade 3 radiation-related toxicity occurred in four patients of the SRS group. Three patients in the standard group and seven patients in the SRS group had pathologically confirmed radiation necrosis. Radiographic tumor progression occurred in ~ 80% of patients in each group, with > 90% of failures occurring locally in both groups. Salvage surgery was performed in one third of patients in each arm. Notably, in this study 18% of patients in the SRS group were found to have unacceptable deviations from the protocol. It is unclear how much these deviations may have affected outcomes of treatment in the SRS group.

Prospective, Nonrandomized Studies

Five prospective, nonrandomized studies have been published reporting the results of an SRS boost for newly diagnosed high-grade glioma.

The first study was by Loeffler et al.[6] In this study, 23 patients with GBM and 14 with anaplastic gliomas (AGs) were treated with SRS after completing EBRT. Inclusion criteria were a well-defined tumor without radiographic evidence of subependymal spread, a KPS score ≥ 70, and no brainstem lesions. There was no age limitation. SRS was performed 2 to 4 weeks after completion of EBRT, with a median dose of 12 Gy (10–20 Gy) and a 2- to 4-mm margin to the enhancing lesion. Median survival for GBM patients was 26 months. Median survival was not reached for the AG patients at the time of last follow-up (median follow-up 19 months, range 7–41 mo). One-year actuarial survival was 79% for GBM and 82% for AG. No acute toxicity related to SRS was reported, and the reoperation rate was 20%. There were two cases of radiation necrosis. Quality of life and local progression were not assessed in this study. Given the high median survival, the authors concluded that SRS could be considered as a useful adjunct for upfront treatment. However, the study had a selection bias, as it included only small (median volume 4.8 cm^3), well-defined lesions in patients with high KPS scores (which is predictive of better prognosis). In addition, inclusion of pediatric patients could have contributed to longer survival, as pediatric patients with GBM have a longer life expectancy than adults.[7]

Mehta et al reported on a series of 31 adult GBM patients who underwent SRS in conjunction with EBRT.[7] Patients with a supratentorial lesion ≤ 4 cm in maximum dimension were included. Notably, performance status was not used as a selection criterion. Patients were treated with a median SRS dose of 12 Gy (range 10–20 Gy). Median overall survival was 10.5 months, and 1-year actuarial survival was 38%. No central failures occurred, but 79% of failures occurred within a 2-cm margin of the lesion and had a median time to progression of 5.5 months. There was no acute toxicity, but delayed radiation necrosis did occur in 13% of patients. One third of patients had salvage surgery. In this study, the inclusion of poor performance status patients, treatment of relatively larger lesions (median volume 17.4 cm^3), and exclusion of pediatric patients contributed to shorter survival. Of note, the timing of SRS treatment was not consistent, as some patients had SRS before EBRT, whereas others had it after EBRT. This contrasts with the Loeffler et al study, in which all patients had SRS after EBRT.[6]

Stea et al reported the results of a prospective study comparing SRS to stereotactic radiation implants.[8] Nineteen patients with a high-grade glioma (12 GBM and 7 AG) were treated with SRS 2 to 4 weeks after EBRT, and 33 patients underwent brachytherapy. Adult patients with a KPS score ≥ 50 and supratentorial lesions were included. The median dose of SRS was 10 Gy (range 6.5–15 Gy). After 4- to 24-months' follow-up, median survival was not reached, and 1-year actuarial survival was 51% in the SRS group. No acute toxicity was reported, and 16% needed salvage surgery after SRS. The authors concluded that

SRS was as effective as brachytherapy with a lower rate of morbidity and mortality. However, the study was small, subject to selection bias, and lacked a suitable control group for its mix of GBM and AG patients.

Gannett et al reported a study of 30 patients with a pathologically confirmed high-grade glioma (17 GBM, 10 AG, 1 mixed glioma, and 2 gliosarcoma) treated with SRS within 8 weeks after completion of EBRT.[9] Patients were included if their tumor volume was ≤ 115 cm^3 (median 24 cm^3) and if they had a KPS score ≥ 70. There was no age restriction. Median survival was 28 months for AG and 13 months for GBM, with a 1-year actuarial survival of 64% and 53%, respectively. Median time to radiographic progression was 7 months. No acute toxicity or radiation necrosis was reported. Reoperation rate was 33%. Although it appeared that survival was comparable to other large series with high-grade gliomas treated with surgery and radiation therapy, selection bias introduced several potential confounders (e.g., inclusion of the pediatric patients, higher performance status, and high rate of reoperation for SRS failures) that prevented any definitive conclusion regarding the effect of SRS.

Shenouda et al reported another prospective study of 14 GBM patients treated with SRS almost 2 weeks after EBRT.[10] With a median SRS dose of 20 Gy, median survival was 10 months with a 1-year actuarial survival of 43%. Median time to radiographic progression was 6 months, and radiation necrosis occurred in 14% of patients.

Retrospective Studies

Twelve retrospective studies have been published that examined SRS as upfront therapy for newly diagnosed high-grade glioma.[11–22] The sample size of those treated with SRS ranged from 10 to 78 patients. The median survival after SRS ranged from 10 to 25 months for GBM and 12 to 24 months for AG. The effect of SRS on quality of life was mixed, as two studies reported stable/improved KPS,[19,20] and one study reported a gradual decline.[16] Eight studies evaluated radiographic progression, with local failure rates ranging from 38 to 92% and progression-free survival (PFS) ranging from 4 to 8 months.[11,15–17,19–22] Acute toxicity was reported in nine studies and ranged from 0 to 64%.[11,13,15–18,20–22]

In summary, among these 12 retrospective series, favorable survival (without adequate control groups) was seen in 4 series, while no benefit from SRS was seen in 8 series. Local failure was the most prominent pattern of failure. As in prospective studies, selection bias was an important concern in these series. Most patients in the retrospective studies had a high KPS score, a unifocal location, and a small tumor. To evaluate how SRS eligibility criteria related to survival, Curran et al explored whether patients who could be candidates to receive SRS had a higher expected survival than those who could not receive SRS.[1] They applied the SRS eligibility criteria used by Loeffler et al (well-circumscribed, ≤ 4 cm in maximum diameter, KPS score ≥ 70, away from chiasm or brainstem, and no subependymal spread) to 778 patients with high-grade gliomas included in the RTOG 83–02 trial. They noticed a survival advantage in the SRS-eligible group compared to the SRS-ineligible patients (14.4 vs 11.7 mo, respectively; $p = 0.04$).[1,6] Irish et al reported similar results after dividing a group of 101 GBM patients treated with conventional treatment into SRS-eligible and SRS-ineligible subgroups (16 vs 6 mo survival, respectively; $p = 0.0001$).[23] In one of the reported series, patients were divided into two groups of brachytherapy-eligible (arm 1) or -ineligible (arm 2) with patients who were younger (< 70 years), higher KPS score (> 60), and with unifocal supratentorial lesions < 5 cm enrolled in arm 1.[12]As shown in ▶ Table 19.1, the results were much better in arm 1 than in arm 2.

In conclusion, the only ***level I evidence*** available regarding the use of upfront SRS for high-grade gliomas showed no difference in overall survival, local control rate, and quality of life measures. The relatively small prospective series (14–37 patients per series) reported a median survival of 10 to 26 months for GBM and 19 to 28 months for AG. Three studies showed no benefit by adding SRS to EBRT, one study showed improved survival, and one had no conclusion because of possible confounding factors. The most important factor that yielded different results among these studies was selection bias. The variability of patient selection criteria, treatment protocols used, and conclusions makes it difficult to make definitive recommendations based on these ***level II*** data. This selection bias problem also exists in the retrospective studies, again making it difficult to make recommendations based on them. Of note, in the nonrandomized prospective studies and in the retrospective studies, SRS was used after EBRT rather than before, as it had been done in the randomized trial (RTOG 93-05). Hence, the post-EBRT KPS became a selection criterion in the nonrandomized studies. Consequently, the selection of patients with a better post-EBRT KPS may have identified a group of patients with a better overall response to radiation. It is possible but still unclear whether this subgroup of patients may have preferentially benefited from SRS.[11,12,14,15]

Stereotactic Radiosurgery as a Salvage Treatment for Recurrent Malignant Glioma

Prospective Studies

There were no randomized controlled studies that addressed this issue. Three prospective series, however, did evaluate the role of SRS as a salvage treatment for recurrent malignant glioma.

Chamberlain et al reported a series of 20 cases of recurrent malignant glioma (5 GBM, 10 AG, and 5 World Health Organization [WHO] grade II) treated by SRS.[24] All patients had a lesion ≤ 4 cm in maximum dimension, a KPS score ≥ 50, and had been treated with EBRT as part of their initial treatment. The median interval between initial treatment and SRS was 16 months. After SRS treatment with a median dose of 13 Gy (range 12–15 Gy), the median survival was 7 months, with a 1-year actuarial survival of 33%. The median time to progression was 4 months, and acute toxicity was observed in 7 patients. No radiation necrosis was reported. Notably, the investigators did not separate survival results by tumor grade, and the median overall survival was only 7 months despite the inclusion of WHO grade II and III gliomas.

Table 19.1 Use of stereotactic radiosurgery as an upfront treatment for newly diagnosed high-grade gliomas

Study	No. patients	Median KPS	Target volume (cm^3) (range)	SRS dose (Gy) (range)	Median post-SRS survival (mo)	Local failure (PFS)	Toxicity (RN)	Median f/u (mo) (range)
Randomized controlled study								
Souhami et al[5]	GBM: 89	90	NA	(15–24)	13.5	91%	5% (8%)	61
Prospective studies								
Loeffler et al[6]	GBM: 23 AG: 14	85	4.8 (1.2–72)	12 (10–20)	GBM: 26 AG: > 36	NA	0 (5%)	19 (7–41)
Mehta et al[7]	GBM: 31	70	17.4 (2.3–59)	12 (10–20)	10.5	79% (5.5 mo)	0 (13%)	> 3 (4–42)
Stea et al[8]	GBM: 12 AG: 7	NA	50.5 (11–157)	10 (6.5–15)	NA	NA	0	(4–24)
Gannett et al[9]	GBM: 17 AG: 10	90	24 (< 115)	10 (5–18)	GBM: 13 AG: 28	(7 mo)	0 (0)	30 (12–45)
Shenouda et al[10]	GBM: 14	80	NA	20	10	(6 mo)	7% (14%)	9
Retrospective studies								
Buatti et al[11]	GBM: 6 AG: 5	90	14 (5.5–22.0)	12.5 (10–15)	10.2	81% (4 mo)	27%	10.2 (6–25)
Larson et al[12]	GBM: 31 AG: 16	90	5.9 (1.3–52.0)	16 Gy (8–30)	A1: GBM: 21 AG: 24 A2: GBM: 10 AG: 20	NA	NA	17 (0–85)
Nwokedi et al[13]	GBM: 31	80	18.5 (1.6–62.0)	17 (10–28)	25	NA	0 (6%)	17.5
Prisco et al[14]	GBM: 14 AG: 1	70	15 (2.9–70.0)	10 (8–12.5)	21.4	NA	(27%)	> 10 (10–68)
Selch et al[15]	GBM: 12 AG: 7	90	14 (3–65)	30 (15–37)	GBM: 14 AG: 12	89%	16%	14 (6–47)
Shrieve et al[16]	GBM: 78	90	9.4 (0.8–72.0)	12 (6–24)	19.9	38%	0 (26%)	40 (25–79)
Cho et al[17]	GBM: 14	70	27 (9–57)	10.5 (10–18)	16	29%	64% (14%)	12 (4–54)
Hsieh et al[18]	GBM: 25	70	23.6 (0.6–64.0)	12	10	NA	0	21
Kong et al[19]	GBM: 10	80	11.1 (4–26)	12 (9–16)	12	NA	NA	7.2
Smith et al[20]	GBM: 27	NA	34.6 (13–73)	12	11.5	44%	0 (33%)	11.5 (4–56)
Pouratian et al[21]	GBM: 22	80	13.4 (4–56)	5.6 (4–10)	10	(8 mo)	0	10.4 (4–45)
Biswas et al[22]	GBM: 15	NA	13.2 (1.5–85.0)	13 (6–20)	10.3	92% (6 mo)	0 (6%)	NA

Abbreviations: *A1, arm 1; A2, arm 2; AG, anaplastic glioma; f/u, follow up; GBM, glioblastoma multiforme; KPS, Karnofsky performance scale; PFS, progression-free survival; RN, radiation necrosis; SRS, stereotactic radiosurgery.*

Hall et al published the results of a prospective study of 35 recurrent high-grade gliomas (26 GBM, 9 AG) treated with SRS.[25] After treatment with a median dose of 20 Gy (range 7.5–40.0 Gy), median survival was 8 months in GBM patients and 12 months in AG patients. In total, 85% of patients had local failure, and reoperation was performed in 20%. No acute toxicity was reported.

Larson et al reported the results of a phase II study of high-dose SRS and the matrix metalloproteinase inhibitor Marimastat in a series of 26 patients (14 GBM, 12 AG).[26] Patients were included if they had a tumor that was well defined, supratentorial in location, and ≤ 3 cm in maximum diameter. In addition, previous surgery, EBRT as the primary treatment, and a KPS score ≥ 50 were required. The median peripheral dose of SRS was 12 to 18 Gy. The median overall survival was 9.5 months for GBM and 17 months for AG patients, and median time to progression was 4 and 7 months, respectively. A minor survival advantage was observed in the AG group using this treatment strategy, but no advantage was seen in the GBM group.

Retrospective Studies

There have been 14 publications of retrospective series that evaluated the results of SRS as a salvage treatment for recurrent high-grade glioma.[12,15,18,21,22,27–35] Median overall survival ranged from 5 to 18 months for GBM (all 14 series) and 8 to 12 months for AG (3 series).[12,15,27] Local failure occurred in 7 to 92%, with a median PFS of 2 to 15 months.[15,21,22,27–33] (▶ Table 19.2).

Survival after recurrence of high-grade glioma has been reported to range between 5 and 11 months after conventional treatment using a variety of systemic agents, including chemotherapy and anti–vascular endothelial growth factor (VEGF)) therapy.[29,36,37] As was seen in studies that evaluated SRS as an upfront treatment for high-grade glioma, the patient inclusion criteria were variable in retrospective studies evaluating SRS as a salvage therapy. Most of the patients selected for these trials had smaller tumor volumes and better performance status, making comparison of outcomes to all patients with recurrent malignant gliomas difficult.

It has been proposed that SRS may act synergistically with other agents as a salvage therapy. Park et al used SRS in conjunction with bevacizumab for treatment of recurrent GBM and reported a median of 18 months' survival after treatment.[33] Amplifying the field of treatment has also been studied. Koga et al studied extended field (0.5- to 1-cm margin) SRS compared to normal field SRS.[32] Marginal improvement of survival was reported in the extended field group (10.5 vs 9 mo, statistically not significant). In the rest of the reported series, the survival was reported as being ~ 10 months. Acute toxicity was 0 to 45%.[15,18,21,22,27,28,30–35]

In summary, the three prospective series reported a median overall survival of 7.0 to 9.5 months for GBM and 7 to 17 months for AG; compared to other therapies, these studies showed no or modest benefit from use of SRS. In the retrospective series, there is insufficient evidence to support SRS as a salvage treatment for recurrent malignant glioma. Newer systemic treatments used in conjunction with SRS may have some potential for benefit and need to be evaluated by prospective studies.

Our Experience

In our institution, 92 patients with high-grade glioma (81 GBM, 11 AG) have been treated with SRS since 1990 (57 with Gamma Knife, Elekta AB, Stockholm Sweden, and 35 with linear accelerator [LINAC]) out of almost 1,400 patients treated with high-grade glioma over the same period of time (~ 6.6%). SRS was used as an upfront treatment in 40 patients and as a salvage treatment for recurrence in 52 patients. A majority of patients (83%) were treated before the results of the RTOG 93-05 clinical trial were published. Since then, SRS has been used rarely, and when used, exclusively as a salvage therapy for highly select glioma patients. Most recently, we have been enrolling these patients in a prospective trial of dose escalation of SRS in combination with bevacizumab.

Overall, 80 patients (87%) with high-grade glioma treated with SRS at our institution have died. With a median follow-up period of 11.2 months (range 0–244 mo), median survival was 10.6 months (11.1 for upfront, 10.4 for salvage) for GBM patients and 18.4 months (11.2 for upfront, 27 for salvage) for AG patients. Because of the change in standard chemotherapy over the past 2 decades, it is difficult to make a direct comparison with the results of conventional therapy. However, we do not suspect that there was a survival advantage associated with the use of SRS in these patients, but this was likely due to a selection bias. We did observe some lengthy survivals in patients with AG, but this was a small number of patients,[11] and 4 of these had anaplastic oligodendrogliomas. Hence, the prolonged survivals in these patients are more likely to be explained by favorable tumor biology than by therapeutic benefit from SRS. Indeed, we have previously reported that the overall survival for anaplastic astrocytoma (215 patients) treated at our hospital was 17 months, while for anaplastic oligodendroglioma (65 patients), it was 74 months.[38]

Future Directions

Most high-grade gliomas recur locally after surgery, within a 2-cm margin of a surgical resection cavity.[39] This finding has generated interest in the use of intensive local therapies (both in lieu of and adjuvant to open surgery). Experimental studies have shown that when gliomas are treated with SRS, the tumors become hypocellular and more edematous, especially in the center of the treatment field.[40,41] Temporary early cell cycle arrest, induction of apoptosis, and dose-dependent growth inhibition after SRS have also been observed.[41–43] On the other hand, cell migration has not been shown to meaningfully change after SRS.[44] These effects suggest that SRS may be useful as a local treatment, although they also raise the concern that it may not be effective in preventing further tumor infiltration into the surrounding brain. Hence, although future work is likely to focus on improving the ability to use SRS to achieve local control, its overall clinical benefit will likely depend on its combination with other therapies designed to prevent or treat tumor infiltration.

The sharp radiation-dose margin of SRS can be considered to be a limitation for its use in treating high-grade gliomas. Treatment of wider tumor margins with single-fraction radiosurgery would be associated with an unacceptable risk of significant

Table 19.2 Use of stereotactic radiosurgery as a salvage treatment for recurrent high-grade gliomas

Study	No. patients	Median KPS	Time to SRS (months)	Target volume (cm^3) (range)	SRS dose (Gy) (range)	Median post-SRS survival (mo)	Local failure (PFS)	Acute toxicity	Median f/u (mo) (range)
Prospective studies									
Chamberlain et al[24]	GBM: 5 AG: 10	80	16	17 (3–53)	13.4 (12.0–15.7)	7	(4 mo)	35%	8 (2–29)
Hall et al[25]	GBM: 26 AG: 9	70	10	28 (2.8–98)	20 (7.5–40.0)	GBM: 8 AG: 12	85%	0	(>1 mo)
Larson et al[26]	GBM: 14 AG: 12	90	GBM: 43 AG: 12	GBM: 4.8 AG: 2.7	15 (12–18)	GBM: 9.5 AG: 17	(GBM: 4 mo, AG: 7 mo)	NA	NA
Retrospective studies									
Larson et al[12]	GBM: 66 AG: 27	90	3.5	6.7 (0.3–96.0)	16 (5–37)	A1: GBM: 13 AG: not reached A2: GBM: 10 AG: 12	NA	NA	16 (0–224)
Sanghavi et al[27]	GBM: 22 AG: 8	80	16	7.2 (0.4–35.0)	12 (10–20)	AG: 11 GBM: 7	(4 mo)	10% (3%)	70 (6–116)
Selch et al[15]	GBM: 12 AG: 6	NA	NA	20 (6–113)	27 Gy (15–37)	AG: 8 GBM: 7	89%	16%	7.5 (4–20)
Shrieve et al[28]	GBM: 86	80	NA	10.1 (2.2–83.0)	13 (6–20)	10.2	31%	12% (2%)	17.5 (6–45)
Mahajan et al[29]	GBM: 41	90	11	4.7 (0.1–16.0)	NA	11	56% (2 mo)	(2%)	21 (3–61)
Combs et al[30]	GBM: 32	80	10	10 (1.2–59.0)	15 (10–20)	10	(5 mo)	0 (0)	10 (1–25)
Hsieh et al[18]	GBM: 26	70	6	21.6 (0.6–64.0)	12	10	NA	0	22
Pouratian et al[21]	GBM: 26	80	NA	21 (0.3–110.0)	6 (3–15)	9.4	(7.1 mo)	0	8.3 (2–51)
Patel et al[31]	GBM: 26	80	12.5	10.4 (0.3–60.0)	18 (12–20)	8.4	69%	0 (4%)	NA
Biswas et al[22]	GBM: 18	NA	12	8.4 (0.2–32.0)	15 (9–20)	5.3	92% (3.4 mo)	5%	(2–50)
Koga et al[32]	GBM: 18	A1: 90 A2: 70	14	A1: 15 A2: 13 (3–47)	20	A1: 10.5 A2: 9.0	A1: 53% A2: 7%	0 (33%)	8 (3–29)
Park et al[33]	GBM: 11	90	17	13.6 (1.2–45.0)	16 (13–18)	18	27% (14.9 mo)	45% (9%)	13.7 (4–28)
Maranzano et al[34]	GBM: 13	90	9	5.3 (6–14)	17 (14–22)	11	NA	15% (23%)	8.5 (5–41)
Sirin et al[35]	GBM: 19	90	9	13 (7–19)	16 (10–19)	9.3	21% (7 mo)	0	13 (2–59)

Abbreviations: A1, arm 1; A2, arm 2; AG, anaplastic glioma; f/u, follow-up; GBM, glioblastoma multiforme; KPS, Karnofsky performance scale; PFS, progression-free survival; RN, radiation necrosis; SRS, stereotactic radiosurgery.

injury to normal brain. Theoretically, SRS could be useful as a local radiation boost to the "worst" part of the tumor, which can be defined in multiple ways, including but not limited to the enhancing volume, the region of highest cerebral blood volume on magnetic resonance perfusion imaging, or the areas with highest creatine:choline ratio on magnetic resonance spectroscopy. Another strategy that may help to boost local tumor control is to increase the prescription dose while providing therapy that may reduce the risk of radiation injury. This strategy is currently undergoing prospective evaluation at our hospital.

It is important to recognize that patients with tumor recurrence who previously had a robust response to EBRT may be predisposed to having a better response to salvage SRS compared to those who never responded well to the radiation. Hence, SRS may have a role as a salvage therapy in a select group of patients. This idea needs to be validated in prospective, randomized studies. Until such studies are performed, interpretation of single-arm prospective or retrospective studies must include consideration of the impact that prior response to radiation has had on the patient selection process.

Conclusion

Level I evidence does not support the addition of SRS as an upfront treatment for high-grade gliomas in addition to conventional EBRT and chemotherapy. For patients with recurrent gliomas, ***level II evidence*** suggests a modest survival benefit after SRS, which is likely to be seen only in a small subgroup of patients with high KPS scores and small, well-defined recurrences. Future prospective studies, such as those that combine SRS with systemically or locally administered antitumor drugs, may better define a role for SRS in a combined local-regional treatment strategy for these malignant tumors.

References

[1] Curran WJ, Scott CB, Weinstein AS, et al. Survival comparison of radiosurgery-eligible and -ineligible malignant glioma patients treated with hyperfractionated radiation therapy and carmustine: a report of Radiation Therapy Oncology Group 83–02. J Clin Oncol 1993; 11: 857–862

[2] Walker MD, Alexander E, Hunt WE, et al. Evaluation of BCNU and/or radiotherapy in the treatment of anaplastic gliomas: a cooperative clinical trial. J Neurosurg 1978; 49: 333–343

[3] Andersen AP. Postoperative irradiation of glioblastomas: results in a randomized series. Acta Radiol Oncol Radiat Phys Biol 1978; 17: 475–484

[4] Fine HA, Dear KB, Loeffler JS, Black PM, Canellos GP. Meta-analysis of radiation therapy with and without adjuvant chemotherapy for malignant gliomas in adults. Cancer 1993; 71: 2585–2597

[5] Souhami L, Seiferheld W, Brachman D, et al. Randomized comparison of stereotactic radiosurgery followed by conventional radiotherapy with carmustine to conventional radiotherapy with carmustine for patients with glioblastoma multiforme: report of Radiation Therapy Oncology Group 93–05 protocol. Int J Radiat Oncol Biol Phys 2004; 60: 853–860

[6] Loeffler JS, Alexander E, Shea WM, et al. Radiosurgery as part of the initial management of patients with malignant gliomas. J Clin Oncol 1992; 10: 1379–1385

[7] Mehta MP, Masciopinto J, Rozental J, et al. Stereotactic radiosurgery for glioblastoma multiforme: report of a prospective study evaluating prognostic factors and analyzing long-term survival advantage. Int J Radiat Oncol Biol Phys 1994; 30: 541–549

[8] Stea B, Rossman K, Kittelson J, et al. A comparison of survival between radiosurgery and stereotactic implants for malignant astrocytomas. Acta Neurochir Suppl (Wien) 1994; 62: 47–54

[9] Gannett D, Stea B, Lulu B, Adair T, Verdi C, Hamilton A. Stereotactic radiosurgery as an adjunct to surgery and external beam radiotherapy in the treatment of patients with malignant gliomas. Int J Radiat Oncol Biol Phys 1995; 33: 461–468

[10] Shenouda G, Souhami L, Podgorsak EB, et al. Radiosurgery and accelerated radiotherapy for patients with glioblastoma. Can J Neurol Sci 1997; 24: 110–115

[11] Buatti JM, Friedman WA, Bova FJ, Mendenhall WM. Linac radiosurgery for high-grade gliomas: the University of Florida experience. Int J Radiat Oncol Biol Phys 1995; 32: 205–210

[12] Larson DA, Gutin PH, McDermott M, et al. Gamma Knife for glioma: selection factors and survival. Int J Radiat Oncol Biol Phys 1996; 36: 1045–1053

[13] Nwokedi EC, DiBiase SJ, Jabbour S, Herman J, Amin P, Chin LS. Gamma Knife stereotactic radiosurgery for patients with glioblastoma multiforme. Neurosurgery 2002; 50: 41–46, discussion 46–47

[14] Prisco FE, Weltman E, de Hanriot RM, Brandt RA. Radiosurgical boost for primary high-grade gliomas. J Neurooncol 2002; 57: 151–160

[15] Selch MT, Desalles AAF, Goetsch SJ, et al. Single-fraction radiosurgery for primary and recurrent malignant gliomas. J Radiosurg 1998; 1: 155–168

[16] Shrieve DC, Alexander E, Black PM, et al. Treatment of patients with primary glioblastoma multiforme with standard postoperative radiotherapy and radiosurgical boost: prognostic factors and long-term outcome. J Neurosurg 1999; 90: 72–77

[17] Cho KH, Hall WA, Lo SS, Dusenbery KE. Stereotactic radiosurgery versus fractionated stereotactic radiotherapy boost for patients with glioblastoma multiforme. Technol Cancer Res Treat 2004; 3: 41–49

[18] Hsieh PC, Chandler JP, Bhangoo S, et al. Adjuvant Gamma Knife stereotactic radiosurgery at the time of tumor progression potentially improves survival for patients with glioblastoma multiforme. Neurosurgery 2005; 57: 684–692, discussion 684–692

[19] Kong D-S, Nam D-H, Lee J-I, Park K, Kim JH. Preservation of quality of life by preradiotherapy stereotactic radiosurgery for unresectable glioblastoma multiforme. J Neurosurg 2006; 105 (Suppl): 139–143

[20] Smith KA, Ashby LS, Gonzalez LF, et al. Prospective trial of gross-total resection with Gliadel wafers followed by early postoperative Gamma Knife radiosurgery and conformal fractionated radiotherapy as the initial treatment for patients with radiographically suspected, newly diagnosed glioblastoma multiforme. J Neurosurg 2008; 109 (Suppl): 106–117

[21] Pouratian N, Crowley RW, Sherman JH, Jagannathan J, Sheehan JP. Gamma Knife radiosurgery after radiation therapy as an adjunctive treatment for glioblastoma. J Neurooncol 2009; 94: 409–418

[22] Biswas T, Okunieff P, Schell MC, et al. Stereotactic radiosurgery for glioblastoma: retrospective analysis. Radiat Oncol 2009; 4: 11

[23] Irish WD, Macdonald DR, Cairncross JG. Measuring bias in uncontrolled brain tumor trials—to randomize or not to randomize? Can J Neurol Sci 1997; 24: 307–312

[24] Chamberlain MC, Barba D, Kormanik P, Shea WM. Stereotactic radiosurgery for recurrent gliomas. Cancer 1994; 74: 1342–1347

[25] Hall WA, Djalilian HR, Sperduto PW, et al. Stereotactic radiosurgery for recurrent malignant gliomas. J Clin Oncol 1995; 13: 1642–1648

[26] Larson DA, Prados M, Lamborn KR, et al. Phase II study of high central dose Gamma Knife radiosurgery and marimastat in patients with recurrent malignant glioma. Int J Radiat Oncol Biol Phys 2002; 54: 1397–1404

[27] Sanghavi S, Skrupky R, Badie B, et al. Recurrent malignant gliomas treated with radiosurgery. Surgery 1999; 2: 1–6

[28] Shrieve DC, Alexander E, Wen PY, et al. Comparison of stereotactic radiosurgery and brachytherapy in the treatment of recurrent glioblastoma multiforme. Neurosurgery 1995; 36: 275–282, discussion 282–284

[29] Mahajan A, McCutcheon IE, Suki D, et al. Case-control study of stereotactic radiosurgery for recurrent glioblastoma multiforme. J Neurosurg 2005; 103: 210–217

[30] Combs SE, Widmer V, Thilmann C, Hof H, Debus J, Schulz-Ertner D. Stereotactic radiosurgery (SRS): treatment option for recurrent glioblastoma multiforme (GBM). Cancer 2005; 104: 2168–2173

[31] Patel M, Siddiqui F, Jin J-Y, et al. Salvage reirradiation for recurrent glioblastoma with radiosurgery: radiographic response and improved survival. J Neurooncol 2009; 92: 185–191

[32] Koga T, Maruyama K, Tanaka M, et al. Extended field stereotactic radiosurgery for recurrent glioblastoma. Cancer 2012; 118(17): 4193–4200

[33] Park K-J, Kano H, Iyer A, et al. Salvage Gamma Knife stereotactic radiosurgery followed by bevacizumab for recurrent glioblastoma multiforme: a case-control study. J Neurooncol 2012; 107: 323–333

[34] Maranzano E, Anselmo P, Casale M, et al. Treatment of recurrent glioblastoma with stereotactic radiotherapy: long-term results of a mono-institutional trial. Tumori 2011; 97: 56–61

[35] Sirin S, Oysul K, Surenkok S, et al. Linear accelerator-based stereotactic radiosurgery in recurrent glioblastoma: a single center experience. Vojnosanit Pregl 2011; 68: 961–966

[36] Wong ET, Hess KR, Gleason MJ, et al. Outcomes and prognostic factors in recurrent glioma patients enrolled onto phase II clinical trials. J Clin Oncol 1999; 17: 2572–2578

[37] Vauleon E, Mesbah H, Gedouin D, et al. Retrospective analysis of 24 recurrent glioblastoma after chemoradiation and treated with nitrosoureas or irinotecan and bevacizumab [in French]. Bull Cancer 2012; 99: 121–126

[38] Hashemi-Sadraei NBH, Satra A, Rahmathulla G, et al. Prognostic factors in patients with WHO grade III gliomas: the Cleveland Clinic experience. American Society of Clinical Oncology (ASCO) Annual Meeting; June 3–7, 2011. J Clin Oncol 2011; 29 (15-suppl): 2053

[39] Hochberg FH, Pruitt A. Assumptions in the radiotherapy of glioblastoma. Neurology 1980; 30: 907–911

[40] Kondziolka D, Lunsford LD, Claassen D, Pandalai S, Maitz AH, Flickinger JC. Radiobiology of radiosurgery, II: The rat C6 glioma model. Neurosurgery 1992; 31: 280–287, discussion 287–288

[41] Shinoda J, Yano H, Ando H, et al. Radiological response and histological changes in malignant astrocytic tumors after stereotactic radiosurgery. Brain Tumor Pathol 2002; 19: 83–92

[42] Fehlauer F, Stalpers LJ, Panayiotides J, et al. Effect of single dose irradiation on human glioblastoma spheroids in vitro. Oncol Rep 2004; 11: 477–485

[43] Thorsen F, Enger PØ, Wang J, Bjerkvig R, Pedersen P-H. Human glioblastoma biopsy spheroids xenografted into the nude rat brain show growth inhibition after stereotactic radiosurgery. J Neurooncol 2007; 82: 1–10

[44] Kleynen CE, Stoter TR, Tadema TM, et al. The effects of irradiation on cell migration from glioblastoma multiforme biopsy spheroids. Anticancer Res 2003; 23 6C: 4907–4912

Functional Radiosurgery

20 Radiosurgical Root Entry Zone Targeting for Trigeminal Neuralgia

Ajay Niranjan, Douglas Kondziolka, John C. Flickinger, and L. Dade Lunsford

Introduction

Gamma Knife (Elekta AB, Stockholm, Sweden) surgery is a minimally invasive surgical approach for managing trigeminal neuralgia (TN). The goal of TN radiosurgery is to eliminate or reduce face pain in order to improve the quality of life and preserve sensory function. Several reports have documented the efficacy of Gamma Knife radiosurgery for TN.[1–22] Because radiosurgery is the least invasive procedure for TN, it is a good treatment option for patients with comorbidities, advanced age, high-risk medical illness, or pain refractory to prior surgical procedures. Radiosurgery is an attractive alternative, especially for those who do not want to accept the greater risks associated with other, more invasive surgical procedures.

Several factors have been associated with the positive results achieved by radiosurgery in treating TN: the absence of multiple sclerosis, greater radiation dose, no previous surgery, typical pain features, and proximity of the isocenters to the brainstem edge.[23,24] In a population of 54 patients, Rogers et al[25] found a higher Barrow Neurological Institute (BNI) grade I outcome (no pain, off medications) in patients with idiopathic typical TN in comparison to those with atypical features: 49% (21 out of 43) as opposed to 9% (1 out of 11). In their series of 179 patients, Brisman et al[24] reported 41% of their patients with a grade I outcome and 17% with a grade II outcome. Better results were achieved in patients with no previous surgery (60% [35 out of 58]). Similar results were reported by Young et al[26] and Maesawa et al,[27] who described the presence of atypical pain as the most important factor yielding a poor response to radiosurgery (84.4 vs 43.8%). Several authors have reported similar results using linear accelerator (LINAC)-based radiosurgery.[28–33]

Recent reports suggest that the dominant factor that predicted improved treatment efficacy was the development of numbness following Gamma Knife radiosurgery.[34] Previous radiosurgery series had also highlighted this factor both in the primary setting[35,36] and after a second application of Gamma Knife radiosurgery for recurrent TN.[37,38] Pollock et al reported their results at the Mayo Clinic in which patients were treated with either 70 or 90 Gy.[36] Patients treated with the higher dose experienced a higher rate of TN dysfunction following Gamma Knife radiosurgery. These patients also had an improved rate of pain relief. Similarly, Aubuchon et al found that the most significant factor predicting pain relief after a second application of Gamma Knife radiosurgery was the development of postprocedural numbness.[37]

The Controversy

To date, the largest reported series are still characterized by a wide spectrum of success rates after radiosurgery. Grade I outcomes are reported in 21 to 76.8% of the patients and grade II outcomes in 65 to 88%.[1,11,13,23,26,27,39–41] Three methods have been used to improve facial pain outcomes after TN radiosurgery. The first is to keep the radiation dose constant, but to increase the length of the trigeminal nerve that is irradiated (short vs long). The second method is to increase the maximum radiation dose (lower vs higher dose). The third method used to improve the results is the target position (proximal vs distal). It is also possible that a proximal versus distal isocenter location is less important than accurately targeting the trigeminal nerve at some point along its path to provide pain relief. Current evidence to support proximal or distal targeting of the trigeminal nerve is ***level III*** in nature.

Is the Proximal (More Posterior) Target Better?

Despite the widespread use of Gamma Knife radiosurgery for TN, there remains debate on target selection. The reason for the comparisons of the anterior and posterior targets is to achieve higher rates of pain control and lower rates of associated complications. Initial results were based on a posterior target directed at the trigeminal nerve in the Obersteiner-Redlich zone, where peripheral myelin formed by Schwann cells transforms to central myelin formed by oligodendroglia. This target, well defined at the time of microvascular decompression, tends to be closer to the nerve entry into the pons. Kondziolka et al recommended the proximal trigeminal nerve and root entry zone as an appropriate anatomical target for Gamma Knife radiosurgery based on the extensive series of microvascular cross-compression operations for TN performed at the University of Pittsburgh between 1971 and 2012.[42] They reported that 56% of patients had excellent results (100% pain free), and 32% reported good relief (50–90% improvement), when targeting the dorsal root entry zone (DREZ).[1] In a study by Sheehan et al, 34% patients were pain free, and 70% had pain relief with the DREZ target.[13]

Brisman and Mooij performed dose-volume histogram analysis on the nerve and brainstem and suggested that the target structure of radiation effect was in close proximity to the brainstem.[43] In this series, patients with greater brainstem volumes who received a dose of at least 15 Gy experienced improved pain relief.

More recently, the pars triangularis has been considered an attractive isocenter location. Multiple series have supported the observation that placement of the radiosurgical isocenter at the pars triangularis yields a lower rate of trigeminal nerve dysfunction and equivalent pain relief compared to more proximal isocenter locations.[16,44]

Marshall et al tried to determine a potential target of radiation effect within the trigeminal nerve, specifically, the optimal location of the treatment isocenter.[34] Their analysis supports the concept that better pain relief occurs when the isocenter is placed closer to the brainstem. On univariate analysis, these authors noted a statistically significant difference between the doses delivered to the DREZ in patients who benefited from Gamma Knife radiosurgery compared to those who did not benefit. The authors showed that, with more denervation, there was a higher chance of better and longer pain relief. The isocenter position closer to the brainstem is likely to cause more denervation. The shorter cisternal segment of the nerve, whereby more of the DREZ of the brainstem was radiated, was associated with better pain relief. Placing the isocenter farther away from the brainstem (distally) may allow a higher dose, which can give comparable denervation and pain relief, but it is not clear what the exact distal dose is that may correspond to a smaller proximal dose (nearer the brainstem). The DREZ has been described in the literature as a potential target of radiation effect after Gamma Knife radiosurgery because of the change in radiosensitivity at this location based on the transition from Schwann cells distally to oligodendrocytes centrally.[1]

Matsuda et al studied 100 patients with typical and medically refractory TN.[49] Fifty-one patients received 80 Gy at the proximal trigeminal nerve, including the DREZ (posterior group), and 49 were treated using the anterior target (7 patients received 80 Gy, 1 received 85 Gy, and 41 received 90 Gy). The dose rate at Gamma Knife radiosurgery was higher and the follow-up duration shorter in the anterior group. In the anterior group, the prescription dose was higher, the irradiated volume of brainstem > 12 Gy was smaller, and the integrated energy of the trigeminal nerve root was greater. Their analysis of initial pain control showed that patients in the posterior target group were more likely to have an excellent result ($p = 0.003$). The total complication rate, as well as the bothersome complication rate, was significantly higher in the anterior target group ($p = 0.009$ and $p = 0.014$, respectively).

A Case for Distal (Anterior) Target

Regis et al started to target the retrogasserian zone (RGZ), which is just posterior to the gasserian ganglion, and documented the efficacy and safety of the RGZ target.[10,44] They reported that 87% of patients were initially free of pain in their series of 57 patients treated with a maximum dose of 75 to 90 Gy.[11,45] In most patients, they used the higher maximum dose of 90 Gy, and their target was placed at a more anterior site (closer to the retrogasserian portion).

Massager et al performed Gamma Knife SRS using a far-anterior cisternal target and a high dose.[16] In their study, excellent pain control (excellent or good pain relief) was achieved in 68% of patients, and pain relief was satisfactory in 83%.[16] These authors opined that Gamma Knife radiosurgery using the RGZ target had a lower rate of complications compared to the DREZ target with the same irradiation dose. They suggested that the nerve should be targeted at a distance of 5 to 8 mm from the brainstem for an optimal balance between better pain control achieved by a higher dose and concomitant complications, such as trigeminal dysfunction. Although these investigators used the more anterior target, they noted that a shorter distance between the target and brainstem, a higher radiation dose delivered to the brainstem, and the development of mild facial numbness are statistically significant factors of effective pain control.

Park et al compared the RGZ with the DREZ target to determine which is more effective for Gamma Knife radiosurgery.[46] These authors retrospectively reviewed 39 patients who had stereotactic radiosurgery (SRS) for TN. The DREZ target was used as the primary target point in 23 patients, and the RGZ was targeted in 16 patients. Fifteen (93.8%) RGZ and 20 (87.0%) DREZ cases achieved treatment success (BNI pain score I–IIIb); however, this difference was not statistically significant ($p = 0.631$). The time to a response after the Gamma Knife radiosurgery was significantly shorter in the RGZ group (mean 4.1 wk) than in the DREZ group (mean 6.4 wk, $p = 0.044$). The complication rate (~ 25%) was similar for both groups. The frequency of bothersome facial numbness and dry eye syndrome was lower in the RGZ group compared to the DREZ group (13.1% vs. 8.7%); however, it was not significant ($p = 0.255$ and $p = 0.503$, respectively). The trend toward better outcome in the RGZ group could be due to the higher prescription dose (85.6 vs 82.6) compared to the DREZ group.

The University of Pittsburgh Experience

We evaluated our TN radiosurgery experience by retrospectively reviewing outcomes in 503 medically refractory patients with TN.[47] A single 4-mm isocenter was used in 498 patients (99%), and two 4-mm isocenters were used in 5 patients (1%). With a single isocenter, the target was 3 to 8 mm anterior from the junction of the trigeminal nerve and pons. The isocenter was usually located so that the brainstem surface was irradiated at the 20% isodose line or less. Initial nonpublished studies on TN radiosurgery targeted the root entry zone and included the brainstem surface. At our institution, we select the trigeminal nerve target just anterior to the brainstem. This target is not too anterior (with a high risk of cell body injury in the gasserian ganglion) but not so proximal that it delivers a high dose to the brainstem (▶ Fig. 20.1). We do this for the following reasons:

1. Selecting the trigeminal nerve target in this way reduces the risk of trigeminal sensory loss.
2. The nerve can be identified well using magnetic resonance imaging (MRI) in the cistern as it enters the brainstem.
3. All three divisions (V_1, V_2, and V_3) are located within this section of the postganglionic nerve.
4. This target includes the critical nerve region where central myelin produced by oligodendroglia transitions to peripheral myelin formed by Schwann cells. This region may be especially radiosensitive.
5. It is close to the location of the causative vascular compression.

Maximum doses of 60 (in 2% of patients), 70 (in 4%), 75 (in 3%), 80 (in 88%), 85 (in 2%), and 90 Gy (in 2% of patients) was administered. Four hundred forty-nine patients (89%) responded to Gamma Knife radiosurgery after the procedure at a median latency of 1 month. Significant pain relief (BNI scores I–IIIa) was achieved in 73% at 1 year, 65% at 2 years, and 41% at 5 years. Eighty-nine percent of patients achieved initial pain relief with or without medications (BNI scores I–IIIb). Including score IIIb (pain adequately controlled with medication), a BNI score of I to

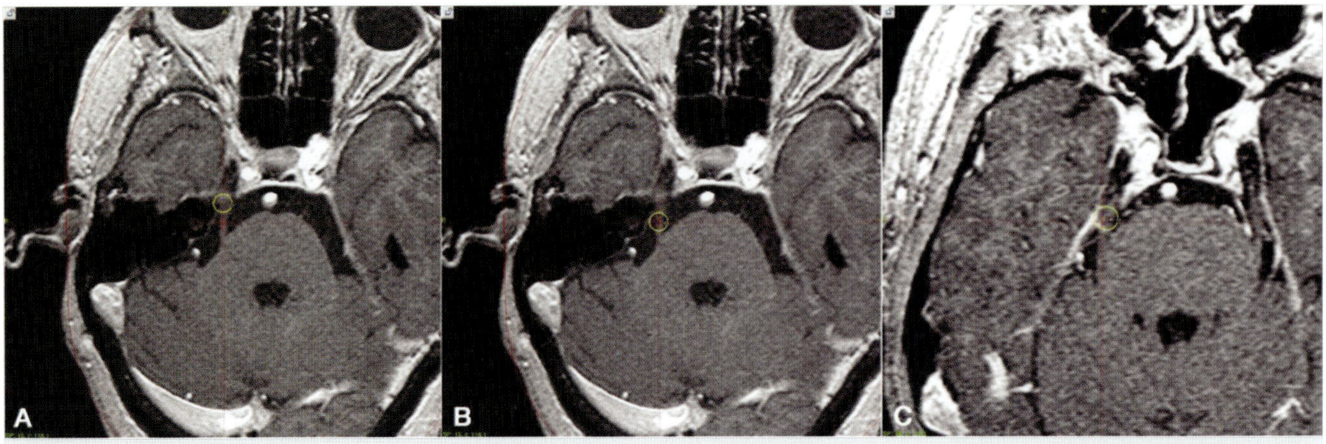

Fig. 20.1 Axial magnetic resonance imaging (MRI) showing the 50% isodose line using (a) anterior target and (b) posterior target selection for trigeminal neuralgia radiosurgery. Target selection is possible only when there is a long nerve segment on MRI. (c) In some patients, a short cisternal nerve component anterior versus posterior target selection may be irrelevant.

IIIb was found in 80% at 1 year, 71% at 3 years, 46% at 5 years, and 30% at 10 years. A faster initial pain response including adequate and some pain relief was seen in patients with TN without additional symptoms, patients without prior surgery, and patients with a pain duration 3 years or less. One hundred ninety-three (43%) of 450 patients who achieved initial pain relief reported some recurrence at a median of 50 months after initial relief. Factors associated with earlier pain recurrence that failed to maintain adequate or some pain relief were TN with additional symptoms and three or more prior failed surgical procedures. Fifty-three patients (10.5%) developed new facial numbness, and 1 developed deafferentation pain; these symptoms resolved in 17 patients. Patients who developed sensory loss had better long-term pain control (78% at 5 y).

One hundred ninety-three (43%) underwent repeat radiosurgery.[48] One-year complete (BNI grade I), significant (BNI grade I–IIIa), and adequate (BNI grade I–IIIb) pain relief rates were 26%, 78%, and 81%, respectively. The median interval until significant pain relief (BNI grade I–IIIa) was 45 days, and adequate pain relief (BNI grade I–IIIb) was 30 days. Patients with fewer than three previous operations had a greater chance of complete or adequate pain relief. The probability of maintaining adequate pain relief (BNI grade I–IIIb) was 80% at 1 year, 74% at 2 years, 66% at 3 years, and 55% at 5 years. Eighteen patients (9.3%) developed increased trigeminal sensory loss or paresthesia during the first 2 years after radiosurgery. The 1-, 3-, and 5-year rates for maintenance of adequate pain relief (BNI grade I–IIIb) in patients who observed new sensory dysfunction were 94%, 86%, and 86%, respectively, whereas the 1-, 3-, and 5-year rates for maintenance of adequate pain relief in patients without new sensory loss were 78%, 64%, and 51%, respectively.

Conclusion

The role of radiosurgery in the management of medically refractory TN has evolved. The posterior target closer to the brainstem is well established. Targeting the nerve is best achieved by high-definition MRI done with the stereotactic frame. Prospective, randomized, multicenter studies comparing the two targeting techniques may be necessary to determine the optimal radiosurgical target zone. The controversy may also be irrelevant in patients with a short cisternal nerve component (as seen in scaphocephalic cranial vaults) compared to those with dolicocephalic vaults, which are more commonly seen in European populations. Targeting then becomes largely dependent on the length of the nerve, the distance between the pons and the gasserian ganglion, and the fall-off of the isocenter into either the lateral pons or the medial temporal lobe.

References

[1] Kondziolka D, Lunsford LD, Flickinger JC, et al. Stereotactic radiosurgery for trigeminal neuralgia: a multiinstitutional study using the gamma unit. J Neurosurg 1996; 84: 940–945

[2] Zheng LG, Xu DS, Kang CS, et al. Stereotactic radiosurgery for primary trigeminal neuralgia using the Leksell Gamma unit. Stereotact Funct Neurosurg 2001; 76: 29–35

[3] Pollock BE, Phuong LK, Gorman DA, Foote RL, Stafford SL. Stereotactic radiosurgery for idiopathic trigeminal neuralgia. J Neurosurg 2002; 97: 347–353

[4] Tawk RG, Duffy-Fronckowiak M, Scott BE, et al. Stereotactic Gamma Knife surgery for trigeminal neuralgia: detailed analysis of treatment response. J Neurosurg 2005; 102: 442–449

[5] Li K, Ma L. Selective source blocking for Gamma Knife radiosurgery of trigeminal neuralgia based on analytical dose modelling. Phys Med Biol 2004; 49: 3455–3463

[6] Guo S, Chao ST, Reuther AM, Barnett GH, Suh JH. Review of the treatment of trigeminal neuralgia with Gamma Knife radiosurgery. Stereotact Funct Neurosurg 2008; 86: 135–146

[7] Gellner V, Kurschel S, Kreil W, Holl EM, Ofner-Kopeinig P, Unger F. Recurrent trigeminal neuralgia: long term outcome of repeat Gamma Knife radiosurgery. J Neurol Neurosurg Psychiatry 2008; 79: 1405–1407

[8] Massager N, Lorenzoni J, Devriendt D, Levivier M. Radiosurgery for trigeminal neuralgia. Prog Neurol Surg 2007; 20: 235–243

[9] Pollock BE, Ecker RD. A prospective cost-effectiveness study of trigeminal neuralgia surgery. Clin J Pain 2005; 21: 317–322

[10] Régis J, Metellus P, Hayashi M, Roussel P, Donnet A, Bille-Turc F. Prospective controlled trial of Gamma Knife surgery for essential trigeminal neuralgia. J Neurosurg 2006; 104: 913–924

[11] Régis J, Metellus P, Dufour H, et al. Long-term outcome after Gamma Knife surgery for secondary trigeminal neuralgia. J Neurosurg 2001; 95: 199–205

[12] Régis J. High-dose trigeminal neuralgia radiosurgery associated with increased risk of trigeminal nerve dysfunction. Neurosurgery 2002; 50: 1401–1402, author reply 1402–1403

[13] Sheehan J, Pan HC, Stroila M, Steiner L. Gamma Knife surgery for trigeminal neuralgia: outcomes and prognostic factors. J Neurosurg 2005; 102: 434–441

[14] Alpert TE, Chung CT, Mitchell LT, et al. Gamma Knife surgery for trigeminal neuralgia: improved initial response with two isocenters and increasing dose. J Neurosurg 2005; 102 (Suppl): 185–188

[15] Keep MF, DeMare PA, Ashby LS. Gamma Knife surgery for refractory postherpetic trigeminal neuralgia: targeting in one session both the retrogasserian trigeminal nerve and the centromedian nucleus of the thalamus. J Neurosurg 2005; 102 (Suppl): 276–282

[16] Massager N, Lorenzoni J, Devriendt D, Desmedt F, Brotchi J, Levivier M. Gamma Knife surgery for idiopathic trigeminal neuralgia performed using a far-anterior cisternal target and a high dose of radiation. J Neurosurg 2004; 100: 597–605

[17] Nicol B, Regine WF, Courtney C, Meigooni A, Sanders M, Young B. Gamma Knife radiosurgery using 90 Gy for trigeminal neuralgia. J Neurosurg 2000; 93 (Suppl 3): 152–154

[18] Longhi M, Rizzo P, Nicolato A, Foroni R, Reggio M, Gerosa M. Gamma Knife radiosurgery for trigeminal neuralgia: results and potentially predictive parameters, I: Idiopathic trigeminal neuralgia. Neurosurgery 2007; 61: 1254–1260, discussion 1260–1261

[19] McNatt SA, Yu C, Giannotta SL, Zee CS, Apuzzo ML, Petrovich Z. Gamma Knife radiosurgery for trigeminal neuralgia. Neurosurgery 2005; 56: 1295–1301, discussion 1301–1303

[20] Kang JH, Yoon YS, Kang DW, Chung SS, Chang JW. Gamma Knife radiosurgery for medically refractory idiopathic trigeminal neuralgia. Acta Neurochir Suppl (Wien) 2008; 101: 35–38

[21] Dhople A, Kwok Y, Chin L, et al. Efficacy and quality of life outcomes in patients with atypical trigeminal neuralgia treated with gamma-knife radiosurgery. Int J Radiat Oncol Biol Phys 2007; 69: 397–403

[22] Balamucki CJ, Stieber VW, Ellis TL, et al. Does dose rate affect efficacy? The outcomes of 256 Gamma Knife surgery procedures for trigeminal neuralgia and other types of facial pain as they relate to the half-life of cobalt. J Neurosurg 2006; 105: 730–735

[23] Brisman R. Gamma Knife radiosurgery for primary management for trigeminal neuralgia. J Neurosurg 2000; 93 (Suppl 3): 159–161

[24] Brisman R, Khandji AG, Mooij RB. Trigeminal nerve-blood vessel relationship as revealed by high-resolution magnetic resonance imaging and its effect on pain relief after Gamma Knife radiosurgery for trigeminal neuralgia. Neurosurgery 2002; 50: 1261–1266, discussion 1266–1267

[25] Rogers CL, Shetter AG, Fiedler JA, Smith KA, Han PP, Speiser BL. Gamma Knife radiosurgery for trigeminal neuralgia: the initial experience of the Barrow Neurological Institute. Int J Radiat Oncol Biol Phys 2000; 47: 1013–1019

[26] Young RF, Vermulen S, Posewitz A. Gamma Knife radiosurgery for the treatment of trigeminal neuralgia. Stereotact Funct Neurosurg 1998; 70 (Suppl 1): 192–199

[27] Maesawa S, Salame C, Flickinger JC, Pirris S, Kondziolka D, Lunsford LD. Clinical outcomes after stereotactic radiosurgery for idiopathic trigeminal neuralgia. J Neurosurg 2001; 94: 14–20

[28] Frighetto L, De Salles AA, Smith ZA, Goss B, Selch M, Solberg T. Noninvasive linear accelerator radiosurgery as the primary treatment for trigeminal neuralgia. Neurology 2004; 62: 660–662

[29] Richards GM, Bradley KA, Tomé WA, Bentzen SM, Resnick DK, Mehta MP. Linear accelerator radiosurgery for trigeminal neuralgia. Neurosurgery 2005; 57: 1193–1200, discussion 1193–1200

[30] Gerbi BJ, Higgins PD, Cho KH, Hall WA. Linac-based stereotactic radiosurgery for treatment of trigeminal neuralgia. J Appl Clin Med Phys 2004; 5: 80–92

[31] Patil CG, Veeravagu A, Bower RS, et al. CyberKnife radiosurgical rhizotomy for the treatment of atypical trigeminal nerve pain. Neurosurg Focus 2007; 23: E9

[32] Villavicencio AT, Lim M, Burneikiene S, et al. Cyberknife radiosurgery for trigeminal neuralgia treatment: a preliminary multicenter experience. Neurosurgery 2008; 62: 647–655, discussion 647–655

[33] Lim M, Villavicencio AT, Burneikiene S, et al. CyberKnife radiosurgery for idiopathic trigeminal neuralgia. Neurosurg Focus 2005; 18: E9

[34] Marshall K, Chan MD, McCoy TP, et al. Predictive variables for the successful treatment of trigeminal neuralgia with Gamma Knife radiosurgery. Neurosurgery 2012; 70: 566–572, discussion 572–573

[35] Massager N, Murata N, Tamura M, Devriendt D, Levivier M, Régis J. Influence of nerve radiation dose in the incidence of trigeminal dysfunction after trigeminal neuralgia radiosurgery. Neurosurgery 2007; 60: 681–687, discussion 687–688

[36] Pollock BE, Phuong LK, Foote RL, Stafford SL, Gorman DA. High-dose trigeminal neuralgia radiosurgery associated with increased risk of trigeminal nerve dysfunction. Neurosurgery 2001; 49: 58–62, discussion 62–64

[37] Aubuchon AC, Chan MD, Lovato JF, et al. Repeat Gamma Knife radiosurgery for trigeminal neuralgia. Int J Radiat Oncol Biol Phys 2011; 81: 1059–1065

[38] Dvorak T, Finn A, Price LL, et al. Retreatment of trigeminal neuralgia with Gamma Knife radiosurgery: is there an appropriate cumulative dose? Clinical article. J Neurosurg 2009; 111: 359–364

[39] Brisman R. Gamma Knife surgery with a dose of 75 to 76.8 Gy for trigeminal neuralgia. J Neurosurg 2004; 100: 848–854

[40] Hasegawa T, Kondziolka D, Spiro R, Flickinger JC, Lunsford LD. Repeat radiosurgery for refractory trigeminal neuralgia. Neurosurgery 2002; 50: 494–500, discussion 500–502

[41] Pollock BE, Foote RL, Stafford SL, Link MJ, Gorman DA, Schomberg PJ. Results of repeated Gamma Knife radiosurgery for medically unresponsive trigeminal neuralgia. J Neurosurg 2000; 93 (Suppl 3): 162–164

[42] Kondziolka D, Flickinger JC, Lunsford LD, Habeck M. Trigeminal neuralgia radiosurgery: the University of Pittsburgh experience. Stereotact Funct Neurosurg 1996; 66 (Suppl 1): 343–348

[43] Brisman R, Mooij R. Gamma Knife radiosurgery for trigeminal neuralgia: dose-volume histograms of the brainstem and trigeminal nerve. J Neurosurg 2000; 93 (Suppl 3): 155–158

[44] Régis J, Bartolomei F, Metellus P, et al. Radiosurgery for trigeminal neuralgia and epilepsy. Neurosurg Clin N Am 1999; 10: 359–377

[45] Régis J, Métellus P, Lazorthes Y, Porcheron D, Peragut JC. Effect of Gamma Knife on secondary trigeminal neuralgia. Stereotact Funct Neurosurg 1998; 70 (Suppl 1): 210–217

[46] Park SH, Hwang SK, Kang DH, Park J, Hwang JH, Sung JK. The retrogasserian zone versus dorsal root entry zone: comparison of two targeting techniques of Gamma Knife radiosurgery for trigeminal neuralgia. Acta Neurochir (Wien) 2010; 152: 1165–1170

[47] Kondziolka D, Zorro O, Lobato-Polo J, et al. Gamma Knife stereotactic radiosurgery for idiopathic trigeminal neuralgia. J Neurosurg 2010; 112: 758–765

[48] Kano H, Kondziolka D, Yang HC, et al. Outcome predictors after Gamma Knife radiosurgery for recurrent trigeminal neuralgia. Neurosurgery 2010; 67: 1637–1644, discussion 1644–1645

[49] Matsuda S, Nagano O, Serizawa T, Higuchi Y, Ono J. Trigeminal nerve dysfunction after Gamma Knife surgery for trigeminal neuralgia: a detailed analysis. J Neurosurg 2010 Dec; 113 (Suppl): 184–90

21 Distal Radiosurgical Targeting for Trigeminal Neuralgia

Jean Régis, Romain Carron, Constantin Tuleasca, and Anne Donnet

Introduction

Results of radiosurgery for trigeminal neuralgia (TN), or tic douloureux, as reported in the literature seem related to variability in the dose-planning strategy. That strategy involves selecting the target, whether the dorsal root entry zone (DREZ), plexus triangularis, or retrogasserian. Also variable is the level of dosing. The use of a higher maximum dose appears to be related to a higher chance of pain freedom and toxicity. Conversely, a larger volume of nerve treated is related to a higher risk of cranial nerve V (CN V) disturbance.

In our experience, high-dose (80- to 90-Gy), retrogasserian (7–8 mm from the brainstem) Gamma Knife (Elekta AB, Stockholm, Sweden) radiosurgery provides patients with a higher chance of long-term pain relief and a lower risk of trigeminal nerve functional disturbance. In the very long term, the probability of pain freedom with our strategy seems to be higher and the rate of CN V disturbance lower. Patient-related parameters (e.g., age and atrophy) and operative technical nuances (e.g., maximum dose, volume of nerve treated, and target location) have a major influence on the probability of pain freedom and the risk of toxicity

In this chapter, we review the results in the literature and our own experience to highlight the potential pros and cons of this dose-planning strategy.

A Brief History of Targeting Location in Trigeminal Neuralgia Surgery

The surgical treatment of TN started far before the development of adjuvant medical therapies for this disease. The Meckel cave was the first surgical target, with the gasserectomy proposed by Wears in 1885 and performed by Roos in 1890.[1] However, because of the association of keratitis and anesthesia dolorosa with the approach, this target was soon abandoned. Next, the cisternal portion of the trigeminal nerve was targeted. In 1901 Frazier and Spiller described a retrogasserian neurotomy at the level of the plexus triangularis using an extradural suprapetrous approach.[2] In 1920 Dandy developed a neurotomy at the level of the entrance in the pons via a suboccipital approach.[3] In the brainstem, in the 1930s, Sjöqvist proposed a trigeminal tractotomy at the level of the obex, and Dogliotti and Walker a trigeminal tractotomy at the level of the mesencephalon. Then neurosurgeons came back to the gasserian ganglion. The decompression of the gasserian ganglion by the opening of the roof of the Meckel cave, as proposed by Taarnhoj in 1952, was also rapidly abandoned due to its poor efficacy. Subsequently, first through a direct approach, then through a percutaneous approach, physical treatments of the gasserian ganglion were investigated.[4] Thermocoagulation,[5,6] compression,[7] and alcoholization were developed and extensively practiced.[8–10] Microvascular decompression of the cisternal trigeminal nerve, which attempted to treat the main cause of TN,[11] as performed by Gardner in 1959 and popularized by Janetta in 1966, became the reference technique.[12–14]

In the 1960s, the first cases of radiosurgery for TN were reported by Lars Leksell targeting the gasserian ganglion on X-ray films.[15] After treating a series of 40 patients, Leksell's team abandoned this approach due to the discovery of the efficacy of glycerol injection,[8] which was used for the visualization of the Meckel cave and turned out to be sufficient to stop the pain in a significant percentage of patients.[8] The clear limitation of the other medical and surgical therapeutic options, on the one hand, and the possibility, based on magnetic resonance imaging (MRI), of an accurate direct targeting of the nerve, on the other, accounted for the reappraisal of the idea of radiosurgery for TN in the early 1990s.

At this time, Rand et al proposed moving the target from the Meckel cave to the trigeminal cistern.[16] In 1993 Alexander and Lindquist promoted the elegant idea of targeting the DREZ with the following definition of this target: "a 4-mm shot centered on the trigeminal REZ treated with a dose of 70 Gy to the center, including the nerve root and adjacent brainstem within the 50% isodose surface (35 Gy)."[17]

Worried about the potential hazard of brainstem injury, we proposed a far more anterior retrogasserian target at the level of the plexus triangularis (▶ Fig. 21.1), which is a common target for microsurgical rhizotomy[2] and thermocoagulation. A retrospective analysis showed an optimum outcome in patients with

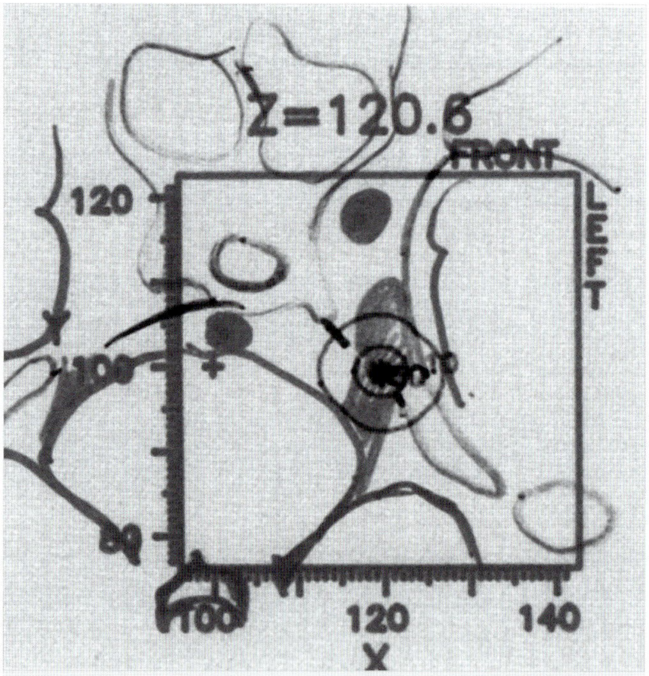

Fig. 21.1 Plexus triangularis target The 4-mm shot is positioned on the nerve at the level of the trigeminal incisura of the petrous bone apex. The targeting is based both on constructive interference in steady state magnetic resonance imaging (MRI) and computed tomography (CT) bony window.

the target positioned slightly more posteriorly.[18] Then we moved to the anterior cisternal segment of the nerve, that is, 7 to 8 mm anteriorly to the emergence of CN V.[19,20] Nowadays, the optimum targeting remains a matter of controversy in the literature.

Review of the Literature

What Level of Evidence Exists for Anterior Targeting?

No ***level I*** or ***II evidence*** exists in favor of either an anterior or a posterior target. The evidence for safety and efficacy is based on retrospective case studies and one prospective trial.[20–23] The only prospective, randomized, comparative study in the literature addresses a technical issue (1 vs 2 shots) and does not really contribute to the demonstration of safety efficacy of radiosurgery as compared to other treatment modalities.[24] It does demonstrate that the enlargement of the volume of nerve treated does not improve the efficacy but dramatically increases the toxicity (Flickinger effect). The evidence supporting the use of other modalities of surgical treatment for TN is based on retrospective case studies.[22] Additionally, the numerous studies published to date have not used uniform outcome measures, making comparison between techniques difficult.[25] Globally, studies frequently report results with very heterogeneous methodology. Due to the delayed effect of radiosurgery, efficacy can be appreciated very differently, for instance, if instead of long-term pain freedom without medication, only the initial pain cessation or pain freedom with or without medication (▶ Table 21.1) is reported. Sometime pain-free patients are mixed in with patients presenting a > 90% reduction in the number of attacks. We consider it mandatory to separate patients who are pain free with or without medication from patients who are improved but not completely pain free. Additionally, the rates of recurrence after surgery (whatever the approach) are significant and must prompt researchers to report actuarial rates of pain freedom at 1, 2, and 3 years instead of pain freedom at the last follow-up. The only prospective trial was published in the *Journal of Neurosurgery* by our group in 2006.[20] This study fulfilled all the major criteria for "quality reporting in surgery for trigeminal neuralgia," as published by Zakrzewska and Lopez in 2003.[25] It must be acknowledged that none of the currently available surgical techniques are perfect, thus explaining the continuing effort of neurosurgeons to develop new treatment methods. All these treatments must be rigorously evaluated in order to know how to best help these patients. However, the heterogeneity of the clinical results after radiosurgery suggests the strong impact of pre- and perioperative parameters.

Critical Review of Anatomical Terminology in the Literature

A cautious analysis of the literature reveals that anatomical terms do not always refer to the same targets.

Retrogasserian Target

One of the very first papers about radiosurgery for trigeminal neuralgia was published in 1993 by Rand reporting a preliminary series of 12 patients treated with a variety of dose-volumes and targets.[16] In patient number 8, the target is presented as retrogasserian (8-mm shot; maximum dose 64.3 Gy). In 1994, our group reported our preliminary experience in a small group of 20 patients.[26] The target for essential trigeminal neuralgia was described as the cisternal retrogasserian part of the root of CN V (4 mm shot; maximum dose 90 Gy). ▶ Fig. 21.2 shows that the same retrogasserian anatomical term was used to refer to a quite different targeting.

DREZ Target

The DREZ target is an appealing concept in pain-relief surgery. The dorsal root entry zone, also known as the Obersteiner-Redlich (OR) zone, is histologically defined as the area where the peripheral myelination (Schwann cells) transitions to the central type of myelination (oligodendrocytic) in cranial nerves. De Ridder et al demonstrated the fact that the location of this zone is highly variable and can spread more distally in some patients.[27] Conversely, McLaughlin et al emphasized the fact that the OR zone can be variable in length, particularly in the case of the trigeminal nerve, and may extend to a more distal portion of the nerve than previously described.[28] The variability of the limit between the Schwann cells and the glial environment of the nerve as it exits the brainstem, typically located 3 mm from the emergence, must be kept in mind.[27] Of course, there is no in vivo possibility to evaluate individually the extent of this zone on the nerve, which makes the term *DREZ target* somewhat inappropriate. The term *emergence target* should definitely be preferred. In 1994 Alexander and Lindquist (▶ Fig. 21.3) defined the DREZ anatomical target from a dose-planning point of view, as follows: "a 4 mm collimator centered on the trigeminal root entry zone treated with a dose of 70 Gy to the center, including the nerve root and the adjacent brainstem within the 50% isodose surface (35 Gy)."[17] According to this definition, a significant part of the brainstem is included in the 50% isodose line. However, the majority of teams using the term *DREZ target* have shifted their shot outside the brainstem and are now reporting the 20% isodose line as being the highest isodose touching the brainstem.[17] The Pittsburgh group described their targeting method as follows: "[T]he 4 mm isocenter was placed 2 to 4 mm anterior to the junction of the trigeminal nerve and pons," which looks to be much more posterior than our 7- to 8-mm zone. However, their fine-tuning is described as follows: "[T]he isocenter was positioned so that the brainstem surface was usually irradiated at no more than the 30% isodose." In our understanding, this second rule frequently leads to displacement of the shot anteriorly. The same team in 1996 provided postoperative magnetic resonance imaging (MRI) scans, giving the location of the contrast enhancement that was more likely to be at 7 mm than at 2 to 4 mm. It was thus clear that this team, with one of the largest experiences of the so-called DREZ target, did not actually use the same target as described initially by Alexander and Lindquist (▶ Fig. 21.4). Interestingly, in their more recent studies, the target is described as a "single 4 mm isocenter targeted to the midposterior portion of the trigeminal nerve, anterior to the pons."[29] Gorgulho et al reported a series of patients apparently treated according to the Alexander and Lindquist definition of the DREZ target as demonstrated by some of their postoperative MR images (▶ Fig. 21.5).[30]

Table 21.1 Main series of the literature, comparing published studies according to the device used, either Gamma Knife, CyberKnife, Novalis or adapted linear accelerator (Linac)

Study	No. patients	Age (years)	Device	% Maximum dose (Gy)			DE (mm)	Median f/u (months)	% Patients			
				<70	70– 80	>80			Without pain (%)	Pain alleviated > 90%(%)	Side effects (%, G–NG)	Recurrence (%)
Tuleasca et al (in progress)	497 (f/u>1 yr)	68.3	GK			Med 85 (70–90)	7.6	43.8	91.75		21.1	34.4
Lee et al[103]	22	61.5	GK				0	92.2	27.3	68.3	4.54	
Loescher et al[104]	72	65.6	GK	0	100	0	0		39	71	31	
Dos Santos et al[105]	52		LINAC	46.2	53.8	0	Cisternal (11.5%), near gasser (36.5%), between previous (51.9%)	26.6	17.3	53.8	36	28.8
Park et al[106]	17	62.7	GK	0	100	0	2–4				23.5	35.3
Verheul et al[107]	365	65 +/- 13	GK	0	100	0	0	28	75	60	35.05	25 at 5 y
Matsuda et al[33]	104	74	GK	0	100	0	0 (50.9, 6%), proximal target (49.0, 3%)	37	98		49	16.34
Kondziolka et al[39]	503	72	GK	1.6	94.9	3.4	0		89	89	10.5	42.9
Riesenburger et al[108]	53	65.8	GK	0			0 (72%), proximal target (28%)	48		83	35.8	27
Dhople et al[38]	112	64	GK			0	Adjacent REZ	67.2	70	81	6	56
Arkha et al[91]	262	68	GK	0	33.2	66.8	8.5	37.5 (12 –147)	88.9	60	12.9 (12.5/0.4)	21–34
Longhi et al[59]	160	63.4	GK	0	Med 85 (75–95)		2–5	37.4	61 (without med)	90	9.5	18
Fountas et al[46]	106	72.3	GK	0	94.4	5.6	0	36 (12–72)	82.5/69.4	91.3/77.6	16	
Pusztaszeri et al[68]	17	71	LINAC	17	0	0	0	12 (2–60)	35	70	5.8	29.4
Réegis et al[20]	110	68.2	GK	0		Med 85 (70–90)	7.84	>12	83	97	10 (55)	17
Yomo et al[78]	86	76	GK	0	97	3	27 post					
Urgosik et al[76]	107	75	GK	0	100	0	58 ant	40	-4	87	15	8
Sheehan et al[73]	136	68	GK	1.4	98	0.7	0	60 (6–94)	80.4	96.3	20	25
Lim et al[96]	41	68	CyK	0	70.7	29.3	2–4	19	44	70	19	24
McNatt et al[62]	49	68	GK	0	100	0	2–3	11 (6–15)	87.8	92.7	51.2 (28.6 –32.6)	15.8
Richards et al[70]	28	74	LINAC	0	100	0	0	49 (12–70)	46	61	52 (52–0)	23

Table 21.1 continued

Study	No. patients	Age (years)	Device	% Maximum dose (Gy) <70	70– 80	>80	DE (mm)	Median f/u (months)	% Patients Without pain (%)	Pain alleviated> 90%(%)	Side effects (%, G-NG)	Recurrence (%)
Massager et al[34]	47	69	GK	0	0	100	0	12 (1–40)	57	75	14.2	46 (11 –24)
Brisman[41]	293	70	GK	0	100	0	10	16 (6–42)	59	71	4–38	4
Shaya et al[72]	40	64.3	GK	0	90	10	2	23 (5–55)	21.8	68.3	10.5–11.1	23.9
Chen et al[44]	32	67	LINAC	37	0	67	2–4	14.1 (3–31)	40	70	17.5	17
Cheuk et al[45]	112	62.02	GK	60–80 Med 75	0			8	78	87	0–9.3	
Frighetto et al[47]	22	22	LINAC	5 pts 70–85	17		2–4		80.2	89.6	5.2–10.4	
Goss et al[48]	25	65	LINAC	0	0	25	0	18 (8–52)	76	100	32	0–44
Petit et al[65]	112	64	GK	0	100	0	2–4	30 (8–66)	77	86	3.1–4.2	29
Kondziolka et al	220	70	GK	2.7	94.6	2.7	2–4	24 (6–78)	40	69.1	0.4–10	13,6
Pollock et al[67]	117	67.8	GK	0	56	44	5,9	26 (1–48)	58	85	37 (12–25)	16
Maesawa et al[61]	220	70	GK	2.7	94.6	2.7	2–4	22 (6–78)	40	69.1	0.4–10.0	13.6
Rogers et al[83]	54	67	GK	0	100	0	0	12 (3–28)	41	71	0–14	21
Kannan et al[50]	6	56	GK	0	100	0	2–4	10 (5–16)	66	100	0	0
Young et al[81]	110	64.7	GK	7	93	0		19.8 (4–49)	76.4	88	0–2.7	34
Kondziolka et al	106	67	GK	0	94	6	2–4	18 (6–48)	60	77	10	0–10

Abbreviations: *ant, anterior; CyK, CyberKnife; DE, the distance between the center of the shot and the emergence of the nerve; f/u, follow-up; GK, Gamma Knife; LINAC, linear accelerator; med, median; post, posterior; pts, patients; REZ, root entry zone.*

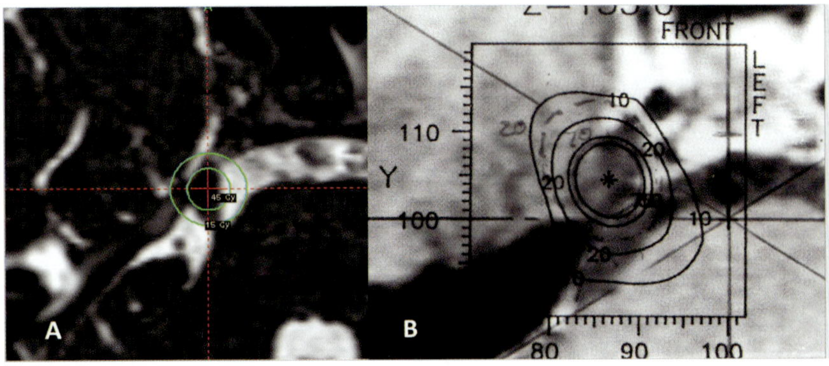

Fig. 21.2 Retrogasserian target as reported by our group (a) and by Rand et al (b). In Rand's approach, an 8-mm shot is placed at the posterior aspect of the Meckel cave. In our group's approach, a 4-mm shot is positioned at the most anterior aspect of the cisternal segment of the trigeminal nerve.

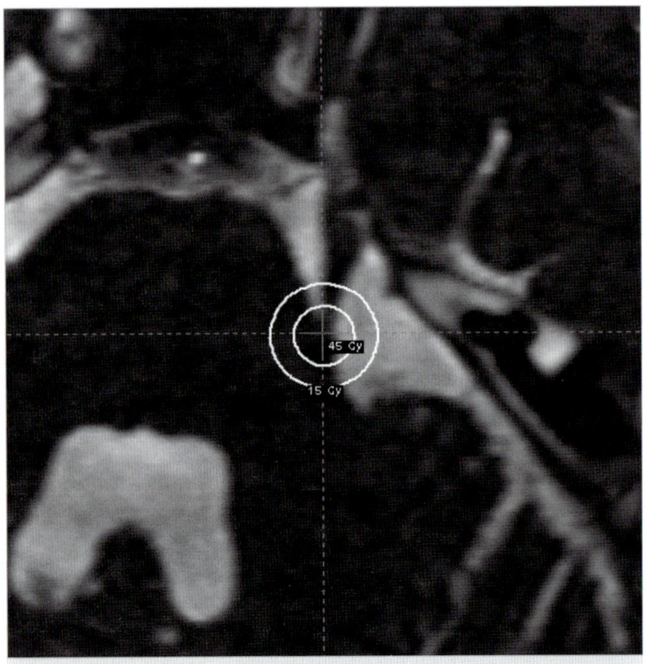

Fig. 21.3 Dorsal root entry zone (DREZ) target according to Alexander and Lindquist's definition. The 50% isodose (35-Gy) line must generously overlap the brainstem.

Park et al[31] published a retrospective comparative study of the DREZ target and the plexus triangularis target (retrogasserian zone, RGZ). They found that patients treated with the RGZ target were more likely to be pain free (per Barrow Neurological Institute [BNI] pain intensity score I–IIIb) than those treated at the DREZ (93.8% for RGZ, 87.0% for DREZ; $p = 0.631$). Seven (43.8%) RGZ and four (17.4%) DREZ patients reported complete pain relief without medications (BNI I). The time to a response after Gamma Knife radiosurgery was significantly shorter in the RGZ group (mean 4.1 wk) than in the DREZ group (mean 6.4 wk, $p = 0.044$). The frequency of bothersome facial numbness and dry eye syndrome was lower in the RGZ group (0%, 0%) as compared to the DREZ group (13.1%, 8.7%). Park et al's conclusion was that the RGZ targeting technique had a better treatment success, with fewer bothersome complications, compared to the DREZ target. These findings are perfectly in line with our institutional experience.[32]

Matsuda et al published a comparison of a posterior and an anterior targeting.[33] They found improved safety and efficacy with the posterior target. A cautious analysis of their study demonstrates that their anterior target corresponds to the plexus triangularis target that we used initially in the early 1990s,[33] and their posterior target proves to be very close to our anterior cisternal target, which is the target that we have been using for the majority of our patients.[20] This cisternal targeting is quite far anterior from the so-called DREZ target according to the definition by Alexander and Lindquist (► Fig. 21.6). Thus, this study tends to confirm the relevance of our policy to move from the plexus triangularis to the cisternal, anterior target, as confirmed by other groups.[34]

The terms *DREZ target, plexus triangularis target,* and *RGZ target* are obviously used with very different definitions; this must be taken into account when analyzing the literature. Also, the variability in size of the posterior fossa and in the anatomy of the trigeminal cistern is usually not mentioned in studies. The cerebellopontine angle (CPA) cistern in patients with TN is

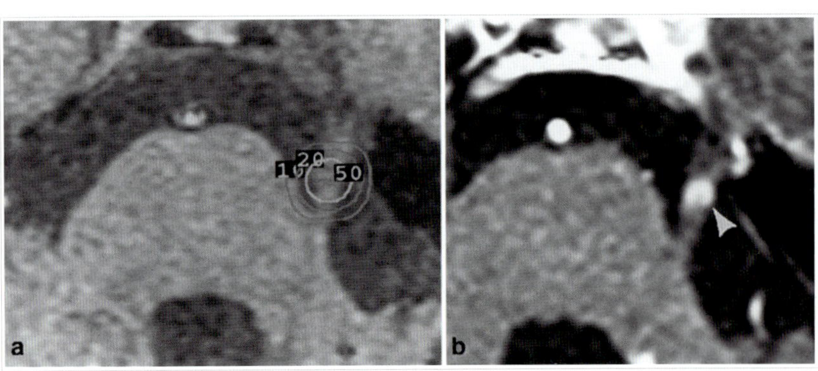

Fig. 21.4 DREZ target according to Kondziolka et al's multicentric study.[55] Obviously, the targeting used is more anterior than the DREZ target as defined by Alexander and Lindquist. (**a**) Targeting. (**b**) Contrast enhancement seen on the trigeminal nerve on follow-up magnetic resonance imaging (MRI).

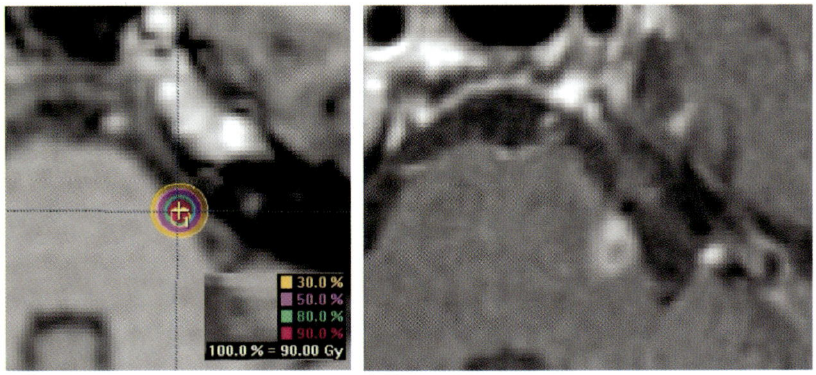

Fig. 21.5 DREZ target according to Gorgulho et al.[30] The targeting is very close to Alexander and Lindquist's definition.

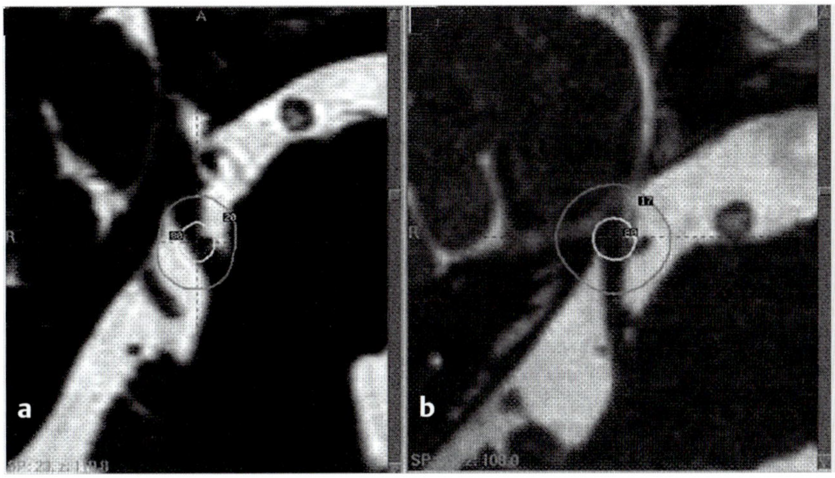

Fig. 21.6 Illustration of anterior (a) and posterior (b) targets according to Matsuda et al in a comparative study of two different targeting modes.[33] In fact, the anterior target is close to the retrogasserian target, and the "posterior" target is close to our anterior target and much more anterior than the DREZ target as defined by Alexander and Lindquist.

usually smaller, leaving little room for truly different anatomical targeting.[35]

Comparison of Long-term Results

The only complication reported after radiosurgery for TN is a more or less disabling disturbance of the trigeminal nerve function, including dry eye in Matsuda et al.[36] An evidence-based review of the literature published in *Neurology* by the Federation of Neurological Societies clearly establishes the fact that the rate of hypesthesia in the literature is not significantly different between microvascular decompression (MVD) and radiosurgery but is much rarer compared to percutaneous treatments.[37] Other complications (cerebellar lesion, cerebrospinal fluid leak, aseptic or bacterial meningitis, diplopia, deafness, and facial palsy) described with MVD and/or percutaneous treatments are not reported after radiosurgery.[37]

Dhople et al[38] and Kondziolka et al[39] reported their long-term results (more than 100 patients with a follow-up longer than 5 y for Kondziolka et al's series). Both teams, using the DREZ target with low doses, reported a steady rate of late failures: 22% still pain free at 7 years for Dhople et al, and Kondziolka et al recorded a rate of 30% for BNI score I to IIIb at 10 years.

Our Long-term Results

We recently analyzed our long-term results using high doses and an anterior cisternal target.[40] Between 1993 and 2010, we treated 737 patients with Gamma Knife radiosurgery for TN (median maximum dose 85.0 Gy); among these, 497 had no history of multiple sclerosis, did not have a megadolicho basilar artery, and had not undergone previous radiosurgery. All were assessable for more than 1-year follow-up. The median follow-up was 43.8 months (range 12–174.4 mo), with 225 males and 272 females; age range was 28 to 93 years (median age 68.3 y). The median of the distance between the center of the isocenter and the emergence was 7.6 mm (4–14 mm). Initial pain relief occurred in 91.75% of patients in a median time of 10 days (range 1–459 d). Their probability of remaining pain free at 10 years was 45.3%. The rate of sufficiently severe pain recurrence requiring new surgery was 67.8% at 10 years. The hypesthesia actuarial rate at 5 years was 20.4% with a median delay of onset of 12 months (range 1–65 mo). A bothersome facial hypesthesia was reported in 11 patients (2.21%). These results compare favorably with results of low-dose DREZ target series. In the absence of a prospective comparative study, conclusions about the superiority of one target over another remain speculative.

Influence of Preoperative and Operative Parameters

There are large discrepancies among centers in terms of reported results (▶ Table 21.1). The range of reported results proved as high as 35 to 100% for initial pain cessation, 0 to 42% for pain recurrence, and 0 to 57% for trigeminal nerve injury.[24,34,41–81] These differences may reflect the lack of homogeneity in the methodology of evaluation and the scoring techniques used. Frequently, the rates of complete pain freedom and of drug cessation are not explicitly indicated. The reported follow-up is often very heterogeneous, with some studies including very short-term follow-up in the final analysis. However, several retrospective studies have identified some pre- and perioperative parameters that appear to influence the outcome significantly. A diagnosis of multiple sclerosis[82,83] and a past history of surgery for the treatment of TN on the same side[20,38,61,67] have both been linked to a lower rate of pain control, as have younger age, shorter nerve, and less atrophic nerve.[20] The presence of a conflict is described as a predictor of success by Brisman et al,[84] a predictor of failure by Shaya et al,[72] and having no influence by Sheehan et al.[85] Atypical features of the pain correlate with less successful outcomes.[42]

On several occasions, we have found inconsistencies between our series and series from the literature, but each time we have finally found clear explanations in technical nuances that cover these apparent contradictions; however, these discrepancies were superficial, and the influence of some dose-planning parameters is rising.

The Dose Rate

Arai et al[29] and Balamucki et al,[86] found that the dose rate has no significant influence on the outcome, but Matsuda et al[33] reported a higher risk of toxicity when the dose rate is higher.

The Maximum Dose

The maximum dose is clearly related to the probability of pain cessation in our series and the literature.[59,72] Pollock et al published a study comparing 70 Gy in 27 patients and 90 Gy in 41 patients.[66] In this study, high-dose radiosurgery was associated with a higher chance of pain freedom (61% vs 41%) but also a higher chance of trigeminal nerve injury (54% vs 15%).[66] While demonstrating the influence of the maximum dose on the probability of pain freedom, this study did not confirm the very low rate of hypesthesia we observed in our population. Between our two series, there is one major difference that is not discussed by the authors: the anatomical location of the target.[19] We hypothesized on the occasion of a comment published in the *Journal of Neurosurgery* [19] that this lower toxicity in our series could be due to the longer distance between the center of the isocenter and the anatomical emergence of CN V.

The Location of the Shot

The location of the shot on the nerve turns out to be a crucial predictor, especially for toxicity. What makes the difference between the two anatomical targets? The dose to the DREZ and the dose to the brainstem (or more precisely, to the trigeminal nerve pathways within the brainstem) are dramatically increased with the DREZ target. In essential TN using very high dosage, the rate of hypesthesia in our experience is much lower than in the typical experience with CPA tumors.[87,88] Here again, the dose to the pathways of the trigeminal nerve in the brainstem is much higher in the second group of patients.[87,88] This is another argument for the role of the central trigeminal pathways in radiosurgically induced hypesthesia. Similarly, in a series of vestibular schwannomas treated by linear accelerator (LINAC) radiosurgery, Foote and colleagues[89] demonstrated the direct relationship between the risk of trigeminal nerve dysfunction and the dose to the brainstem (but the absence of a relationship with the dose delivered to the nerve itself). Marshall et al found a significantly higher dose to the DREZ (57.6 vs 47.3 Gy) in patients with numbness.[90] Goss et al, using LINAC, reported facial numbness in 32% of their patients, with a significantly higher risk of numbness in patients with a higher brainstem volume inside the 50% isodose line.[48] Finally, the complication of dry eye syndrome reported by Matsuda et al[36] never occurred in our series.[91] These authors used a posterior target and correlated this complication with the delivery of high doses to the brainstem.[36,48]

The Integrated Dose to the Nerve

The integrated dose to the nerve (the volume of the nerve irradiated and/or the average dose) has been found to correlate with the risk of trigeminal nerve dysfunction (Flickinger effect). In a trial comparing two 4-mm isocenters with one, Flickinger et al found a dramatic increase in the level of toxicity.[24] Kanner et al, using 4- and 8-mm superimposed isocenters, observed similar toxicity.[92] Interestingly, these two groups found no benefit in terms of the pain-freedom rate. Massager et al[34] published results comparable to ours in terms of pain cessation but with a much higher incidence of hypesthesia: 43% versus 20% in our overall series.[91] After a careful analysis, we discovered that in the case of a narrow cistern with a high dosage delivered to the brainstem, the attitude of the two teams differed. In these cases, our attitude was to lower the maximum dose, and Massager et al's approach was to keep the 90-Gy maximum dose and rely on shielding for reduction of the brainstem dose. At the time, we hypothesized that this plugging strategy accounted for the differences in toxicity. To confirm this hypothesis, we allowed Massager's team to view our materials in order to allow them to test for the influence of this parameter in our two series. Massager et al found that in patients with a large cistern, our methods were similar and resulted in comparable results, with ~ 20% of patients showing trigeminal nerve disturbance.[93] In "narrow cistern" patients, the shielding strategy led to a dramatic increase ($p < 0.05$) of the mean dose (42.86 Gy instead of 38.01) and integrated dose (3.28 instead of 2.76), with the rate of hypesthesia rising from 15% with no bothersome hypesthesia to 50%, including 10% with bothersome hypethesia ($p < 0.05$).[93] In this study, as in Flickinger et al's and Kanner et al's studies, no significant benefit was associated with the increased volume of nerve treated.[24,92,93] Thus, the dose-volume rate to the nerve can account for huge differences in the hypesthesia rate. The study by Massager et al confirmed our results in terms of efficacy and safety and the influence of the Flickinger effect (integrated dose), showing how much technical nuances can dramatically influence the results.[93] Thus, the mean dose to the nerve is linked to two other parameters. Of course, the volume of the nerve influences the average dose to the nerve, and it has to be kept in mind that both the toxicity and the safety turn out to be influenced by the degree of atrophy of the nerve. This also indicates how much the variability of cisternal anatomy can affect the clinical outcome, especially for those who are not aware of these technical nuances.

Predictions Based on Results in the Literature

Based on the influence of the presented preoperative and operative parameters, one could predict- with a high reliability- the results in terms of safety-efficacy in the main series of the literature. Gorgulho et al at UCLA reported a series of 126 patients with follow-up of 196 treated between 1996 and 2006.[94] A 4-mm shot was placed on the emergence of the trigeminal nerve, with 90 Gy at the center.[44] As predicted, the short-term successful pain outcome was high (90–95%), with 10 to 35% recurrence and 70% long-term pain relief. Because of the location of the shot, not surprisingly, the rate of numbness was very high (58.3%), including 19.4% of patients with severely bothersome numbness, 30.5% with subjective dry eyes, and 30.5% with decreased corneal reflex. The toxicity to the brainstem was well illustrated by the four of six patient investigated with postoperative MRI demonstrating high signal and contrast enhancement in the brainstem. Lim et al reported a series of 83 patients treated between 2002 and 2006.[95] The maximum dose was between 71.4 and 86.4 Gy, with a special strategy of covering all the cisternal segment of the nerve.[96] As predicted by the volume of nerve treated, the rate of hypesthesia was high (74% of patients with numbness, with 39% having severe numbness). The authors demonstrated that the longer nerve length resulted in higher rates of numbness. The patients treated with a maximum dose > 75 Gy had a much higher chance to be pain free. Spencer et al reported their results in 350 patients with follow-up available in 320.[97] They tested the role of the anatomical position of the shot (separating groups by location of the shot: into the brainstem, touching and not touching). The location had no influence on the quality of the results, but the closer the shot was to the brainstem, the more likely the patient was to experience numbness (from 16.7% to 40.0%), confirming our hypothesis on the role of the central trigeminal nerve pathway on the incidence of radiosurgically induced hypesthesia.

Our Group's Perspective

Concerned about the delivery of a high dosage to the brainstem, we decided to use a cisternal target more anterior than the DREZ as described by Alexander and Lindquist.[17] The plexus triangularis made sense because of the thermocoagulation study by Sindou et al demonstrating that when the tip of the probe was located at the level of the plexus, the rate of pain cessation was high, and the risk of toxicity was low.[1] Groups using balloon microcompression found comparable results (when the balloon extends into the posterior fossa with a strong compression of the plexus triangularis displaying a pear shape).[9,98] Finally, retrogasserian section was historically performed at the location of the plexus triangularis.[2] Reviewing our experience, the optimal distance from the emergence has in fact turned out in our material to be 7 mm (range 5 –8 mm).[18] The inaccurate use of anatomical terminology for targeting and the existence of numerous other confounding factors (age, atrophy, morphology of the cistern, volume of nerve treated, etc) tend to preclude a clear confirmation of the relevance of our target.

Globally, two clinical strategies are possible. Our conviction is that a conservative approach tends to yield the best results in terms of pain control with, rarely, hypesthesia. Such an approach requires that a high dose be delivered anteriorly. A more radical approach is to use a similar dosage posteriorly at the level of the emergence,[30,99] based on the argument that hypesthesia increases the chance of pain freedom.[100] Our position is that with radiosurgery as opposed to percutaneous treatment, very good pain control is obtained in the majority of patients without any hypesthesia. Clearly, a small subgroup of patients with hypesthesia have a higher probability of long-lasting pain relief,[100,101] but the most important point is that the vast majority of patients experiencing long-term pain control do not have any kind of trigeminal nerve dysfunction.[20,38,39]

Our recommendation is to place a single 4-mm shot on the cisternal portion of the nerve 7 mm (range 5–8 mm) from the emergence of the brainstem with a maximum dose of 90 Gy (▶ Fig. 21.7b). In cases where the dose to the brainstem proves too high, we start by decreasing the maximum dose; if insufficient, a plugging strategy is employed. In the DREZ target, a 4-mm shot is centered on the emergence of the nerve or at 2 mm anteriorly (▶ Fig. 21.7a). The plexus triangularis target was used at the very beginning of our experience (▶ Fig. 21.7c); due to the morphology of the cistern, the shot is placed 14 mm anterior to the emergence.

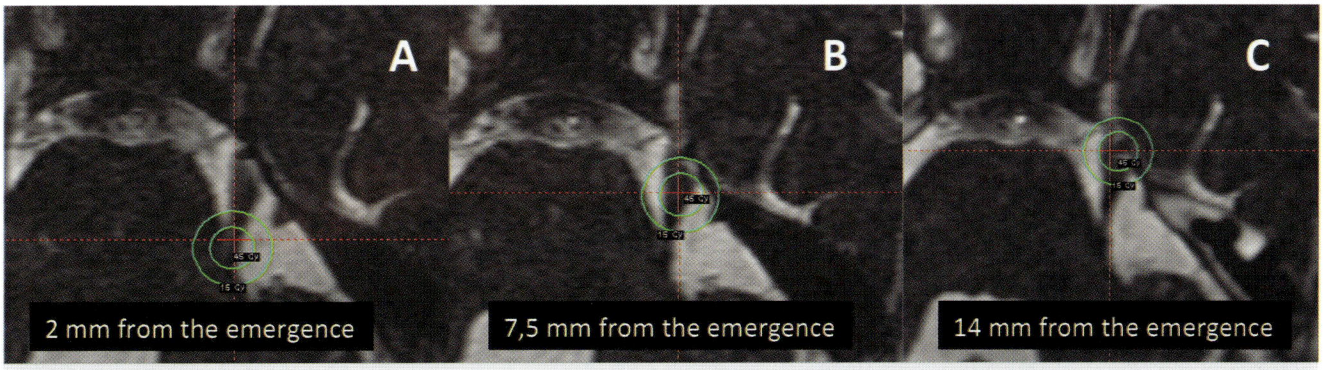

Fig. 21.7 The three main anatomical targeting modes. (a) In the DREZ target, a 4-mm shot is centered on the emergence of the brainstem or 2 mm anteriorly. (b) With the anterior cisternal target, we usually focus 7.5 mm anterior to the emergence of cranial nerve V. (c) The plexus triangularis target (due to the morphology of the cistern, the focus is 14 mm anterior to the emergence).

Conclusion

Radiosurgery is considered the least invasive surgical technique for the treatment of trigeminal neuralgia. Our prospective trial has established Gamma Knife radiosurgery as a safe and effective treatment for TN. However, there is still some controversy in the literature regarding pain relief and toxicity. It is our hypothesis that technical nuances can nicely explain differences in study results. In our experience, high-dose (80–90 Gy), retrogasserian (7–8 mm from the brainstem) Gamma Knife radiosurgery provides the patient with a better chance of long-term pain relief and a lower risk of trigeminal nerve dysfunction. Radiosurgery directed to a more anterior portion of the cisternal nerve may allow the safe use of a higher dose while still affording a low risk of sensory loss. However, this recommendation is supported by a low level of evidence.

To further refine the role of stereotactic radiosurgery compared with other techniques, a randomized controlled, comparative study fulfilling stringent quality criteria is required.[21]

Acknowledgments

Supported by Timone University Hospital (Assistance Publique des Hôpitaux de Marseille).

References

[1] Sindou M, Keravel Y, Abdennebi B, Szapiro J. Neurosurgical treatment of trigeminal neuralgia. Neurochirurgie 1987; 33: 89–111

[2] Frazier CH. Operation for the radical cure of trigeminal neuralgia: analysis of five hundred cases. Ann Surg 1928; 88: 534–547

[3] Dandy WE. The treatment of trigeminal neuralgia by the cerebellar route. Ann Surg 1932; 96: 787–795

[4] Shelden CH, Pudenz RH, Freshwater DB, Crue BL. Compression rather than decompression for trigeminal neuralgia. J Neurosurg 1955; 12: 123–126

[5] Kirschner M. The technique of punctioning and the electrocoagulation of the Gassers's ganglion: about operations with target. Arch Klin Chir. 1933; 176: 581–620

[6] Sweet WH, Wepsic JG. Controlled thermocoagulation of trigeminal ganglion and rootlets for differential destruction of pain fibers:1.Trigeminal neuralgia J Neurosurg 1974; 40: 143–156

[7] Mullan S, Lichtor T. Percutaneous microcompression of the trigeminal ganglion for trigeminal neuralgia. J Neurosurg 1983; 59: 1007–1012

[8] Håkanson S. Trigeminal neuralgia treated by the injection of glycerol into the trigeminal cistern. Neurosurgery 1981; 9: 638–646

[9] Mullan S, Lichtor T. Percutaneous microcompression of the trigeminal ganglion for trigeminal neuralgia. J Neurosurg 1983; 59: 1007–1012

[10] Sweet WH. The treatment of trigeminal neuralgia (tic douloureux). N Engl J Med 1986; 315: 174–177

[11] Love S, Coakham HB. Trigeminal neuralgia: pathology and pathogenesis. Brain 2001; 124: 2347–2360

[12] Barker FG, Jannetta PJ, Bissonette DJ, Jho HD. Trigeminal numbness and tic relief after microvascular decompression for typical trigeminal neuralgia. Neurosurgery 1997; 40: 39–45

[13] Barker FG, Jannetta PJ, Bissonette DJ, Larkins MV, Jho HD. The long-term outcome of microvascular decompression for trigeminal neuralgia. N Engl J Med 1996; 334: 1077–1083

[14] Broggi G, Ferroli P, Franzini A, Servello D, Dones I. Microvascular decompression for trigeminal neuralgia: comments on a series of 250 cases, including 10 patients with multiple sclerosis. J Neurol Neurosurg Psychiatry 2000; 68: 59–64

[15] Leksell L. Sterotaxic radiosurgery in trigeminal neuralgia. Acta Chir Scand 1971; 137: 311–314

[16] Rand RW, Jacques DB, Melbye RW, Copcutt BG, Levenick MN, Fisher MR. Leksell Gamma Knife treatment of tic douloureux. Stereotact Funct Neurosurg 1993; 61 (Suppl 1): 93–102

[17] Alexander E, Lindquist C. Special indications: radiosurgery for functional neurosurgery and epilepsy. In: Alexander E III, Loeffler J, Lunsford L, eds. Stereotactic Radiosurgery. New York, NY: McGraw-Hill; 1993: 221–225

[18] Régis J, Bartolomei F, Metellus P, et al. Radiosurgery for trigeminal neuralgia and epilepsy. Neurosurg Clin N Am 1999; 10: 359–377

[19] Régis J. High-dose trigeminal neuralgia radiosurgery associated with increased risk of trigeminal nerve dysfunction. Neurosurgery 2002; 50: 1401–1402, author reply 1402–1403

[20] Régis J, Metellus P, Hayashi M, Roussel P, Donnet A, Bille-Turc F. Prospective controlled trial of Gamma Knife surgery for essential trigeminal neuralgia. J Neurosurg 2006; 104: 913–924

[21] Lopez BC, Hamlyn PJ, Zakrzewska JM. Stereotactic radiosurgery for primary trigeminal neuralgia: state of the evidence and recommendations for future reports. J Neurol Neurosurg Psychiatry 2004; 75: 1019–1024

[22] Merrison AF, Fuller G. Treatment options for trigeminal neuralgia. BMJ 2003; 327: 1360–1361

[23] Zakrzewska JM, Akram H. Neurosurgical interventions for the treatment of classical trigeminal neuralgia. Cochrane Database Syst Rev 2011; 9: CD007312

[24] Flickinger JC, Pollock BE, Kondziolka D, et al. Does increased nerve length within the treatment volume improve trigeminal neuralgia radiosurgery? A prospective double-blind, randomized study. Int J Radiat Oncol Biol Phys 2001; 51: 449–454

[25] Zakrzewska JM, Lopez BC. Quality of reporting in evaluations of surgical treatment of trigeminal neuralgia: recommendations for future reports. Neurosurgery 2003; 53: 110–120, discussion 120–122

[26] Régis J, Manera L, Dufour H, Porcheron D, Sedan R, Peragut JC. Effect of the Gamma Knife on trigeminal neuralgia. Stereotact Funct Neurosurg 1995; 64 (Suppl 1): 182–192

[27] De Ridder D, Moller A, Verlooy J, Cornelissen M, De Ridder L. Is the root entry/exit zone important in microvascular compression syndromes? Neurosurgery 2002;51:427–433, discussion 433–424

[28] McLaughlin MR, Jannetta PJ, Clyde BL, Subach BR, Comey CH, Resnick DK. Microvascular decompression of cranial nerves: lessons learned after 4400 operations. J Neurosurg 1999; 90: 1–8

[29] Arai Y, Kano H, Lunsford LD, et al. Does the Gamma Knife dose rate affect outcomes in radiosurgery for trigeminal neuralgia? J Neurosurg 2010; 113 (Suppl): 168–171

[30] Gorgulho A, De Salles AA, McArthur D, et al. Brainstem and trigeminal nerve changes after radiosurgery for trigeminal pain. Surg Neurol 2006; 66: 127–135, discussion 135

[31] Park SH, Hwang SK, Kang DH, Park J, Hwang JH, Sung JK. The retrogasserian zone versus dorsal root entry zone: comparison of two targeting techniques of Gamma Knife radiosurgery for trigeminal neuralgia. Acta Neurochir (Wien) 2010; 152: 1165–1170

[32] Régis J, Arkha Y, Yomo S, et al. Radiosurgery in trigeminal neuralgia: long-term results and influence of operative nuances [in French] Neurochirurgie 2009; 55: 213–222

[33] Matsuda S, Nagano O, Serizawa T, Higuchi Y, Ono J. Trigeminal nerve dysfunction after Gamma Knife surgery for trigeminal neuralgia: a detailed analysis. J Neurosurg 2010; 113 (Suppl): 184–190

[34] Massager N, Lorenzoni J, Devriendt D, Desmedt F, Brotchi J, Levivier M. Gamma Knife surgery for idiopathic trigeminal neuralgia performed using a far-anterior cisternal target and a high dose of radiation. J Neurosurg 2004; 100: 597–605

[35] Park SH, Hwang SK, Lee SH, Park J, Hwang JH, Hamm IS. Nerve atrophy and a small cerebellopontine angle cistern in patients with trigeminal neuralgia. J Neurosurg 2009; 110: 633–637

[36] Matsuda S, Serizawa T, Sato M, Ono J. Gamma Knife radiosurgery for trigeminal neuralgia: the dry-eye complication. J Neurosurg 2002; 97 (Suppl): 525–528

[37] Gronseth G, Cruccu G, Alksne J, et al. Practice parameter: the diagnostic evaluation and treatment of trigeminal neuralgia (an evidence-based review): report of the Quality Standards Subcommittee of the American Academy of Neurology and the European Federation of Neurological Societies. Neurology 2008; 71: 1183–1190

[38] Dhople AA, Adams JR, Maggio WW, Naqvi SA, Regine WF, Kwok Y. Long-term outcomes of Gamma Knife radiosurgery for classic trigeminal neuralgia: implications of treatment and critical review of the literature. Clinical article. J Neurosurg 2009; 111: 351–358

[39] Kondziolka D, Zorro O, Lobato-Polo J, et al. Gamma Knife stereotactic radiosurgery for idiopathic trigeminal neuralgia. J Neurosurg 2010; 112: 758–765

[40] Régis J, Tuleasca C, Resseguier N, Carron R, Donnet A, Roussel P. Long-term outcome of radiosurgery for essential trigeminal neuralgia: a prospective series of 130 consecutive patients with more than 7 years of follow-up. Stereotact Funct Neurosurg 2012; 90 s1: 82

[41] Brisman R. Gamma Knife radiosurgery for primary management for trigeminal neuralgia. J Neurosurg 2000; 93 (Suppl 3): 159–161

[42] Brisman R. Gamma Knife surgery with a dose of 75 to 76.8 Gy for trigeminal neuralgia. J Neurosurg 2004; 100: 848–854

[43] Chang JW, Chang JH, Park YG, Chung SS. Gamma Knife radiosurgery for idiopathic and secondary trigeminal neuralgia. J Neurosurg 2000; 93 (Suppl 3): 147–151

[44] Chen JC, Girvigian M, Greathouse H, Miller M, Rahimian J. Treatment of trigeminal neuralgia with linear accelerator radiosurgery: initial results. J Neurosurg 2004; 101 (Suppl 3): 346–350

[45] Cheuk AV, Chin LS, Petit JH, Herman JM, Fang HB, Regine WF. Gamma Knife surgery for trigeminal neuralgia: outcome, imaging, and brainstem correlates. Int J Radiat Oncol Biol Phys 2004; 60: 537–541

[46] Fountas KN, Smith JR, Lee GP, Jenkins PD, Cantrell RR, Sheils WC. Gamma Knife stereotactic radiosurgical treatment of idiopathic trigeminal neuralgia: long-term outcome and complications. Neurosurg Focus 2007; 23: E8

[47] Frighetto L, De Salles AA, Smith ZA, Goss B, Selch M, Solberg T. Noninvasive linear accelerator radiosurgery as the primary treatment for trigeminal neuralgia. Neurology 2004; 62: 660–662

[48] Goss BW, Frighetto L, DeSalles AA, Smith Z, Solberg T, Selch M. Linear accelerator radiosurgery using 90 Gy for essential trigeminal neuralgia: results and dose volume histogram analysis. Neurosurgery 2003; 53: 823–828, discussion 828–830

[49] Han PP, Shetter AG, Smith KA, et al. Gamma Knife radiosurgery for trigeminal neuralgia: experience at the Barrow Neurological Institute. Stereotact Funct Neurosurg 1999; 73: 131–133

[50] Kannan V, Deopujari CE, Misra BK, Shetty PG, Shroff MM, Pendse AM. Gamma Knife radiosurgery for trigeminal neuralgia. Australas Radiol 1999; 43: 339–341

[51] Kondziolka D, Flickinger JC, Lunsford LD, Habeck M. Trigeminal neuralgia radiosurgery: the University of Pittsburgh experience. Stereotact Funct Neurosurg 1996; 66 (Suppl 1): 343–348

[52] Kondziolka D, Lunsford LD, Flickinger JC. Gamma Knife radiosurgery as the first surgery for trigeminal neuralgia. Stereotact Funct Neurosurg 1998; 70 (Suppl 1): 187–191

[53] Kondziolka D, Lunsford LD, Habeck M, Flickinger JC. Gamma Knife radiosurgery for trigeminal neuralgia. Neurosurg Clin N Am 1997; 8: 79–85

[54] Kondziolka D, Lunsford LD, Flickinger JC. Stereotactic radiosurgery for the treatment of trigeminal neuralgia. Clin J Pain 2002; 18: 42–47

[55] Kondziolka D, Lunsford LD, Flickinger JC, et al. Stereotactic radiosurgery for trigeminal neuralgia: a multiinstitutional study using the Gamma unit. J Neurosurg 1996; 84: 940–945

[56] Kondziolka D, Lunsford LD, Habeck M, Flickinger JC. Gamma Knife radiosurgery for trigeminal neuralgia. Neurosurg Clin N Am 1997; 8: 79–85

[57] Kondziolka D, Perez B, Flickinger JC, Habeck M, Lunsford LD. Gamma Knife radiosurgery for trigeminal neuralgia: results and expectations. Arch Neurol 1998; 55: 1524–1529

[58] Kondziolka D, Perez B, Flickinger JC, Lunsford LD. Gamma Knife radiosurgery for trigeminal neuralgia. Prog Neurol Surg 1998; 14: 212–221

[59] Longhi M, Rizzo P, Nicolato A, Foroni R, Reggio M, Gerosa M. Gamma Knife radiosurgery for trigeminal neuralgia: results and potentially predictive parameters—part I: Idiopathic trigeminal neuralgia. Neurosurgery 2007; 61: 1254–1260, discussion 1260–1261

[60] Lunsford LD, Young RF. Radiosurgery for trigeminal neuralgia. Surg Neurol 2000; 54: 285–287

[61] Maesawa S, Salame C, Flickinger JC, Pirris S, Kondziolka D, Lunsford LD. Clinical outcomes after stereotactic radiosurgery for idiopathic trigeminal neuralgia. J Neurosurg 2001; 94: 14–20

[62] McNatt SA, Yu C, Giannotta SL, Zee CS, Apuzzo ML, Petrovich Z. Gamma Knife radiosurgery for trigeminal neuralgia. Neurosurgery 2005; 56: 1295–1301, discussion 1301–1303

[63] Mehta V, Meier R, Gilrein J, Vermeulen S, Young R. Gamma Knife radiosurgery for treatment of trigeminal neuralgia. Int J Radiat Oncol Biol Phys 2003; 57: S136

[64] Nicol B, Regine WF, Courtney C, Meigooni A, Sanders M, Young B. Gamma Knife radiosurgery using 90 Gy for trigeminal neuralgia. J Neurosurg 2000; 93 (Suppl 3): 152–154

[65] Petit JH, Herman JM, Nagda S, DiBiase SJ, Chin LS. Radiosurgical treatment of trigeminal neuralgia: evaluating quality of life and treatment outcomes. Int J Radiat Oncol Biol Phys 2003; 56: 1147–1153

[66] Pollock BE, Phuong LK, Foote RL, Stafford SL, Gorman DA. High-dose trigeminal neuralgia radiosurgery associated with increased risk of trigeminal nerve dysfunction. Neurosurgery 2001; 49: 58–62, discussion 62–64

[67] Pollock BE, Phuong LK, Gorman DA, Foote RL, Stafford SL. Stereotactic radiosurgery for idiopathic trigeminal neuralgia. J Neurosurg 2002; 97: 347–353

[68] Pusztaszeri M, Villemure JG, Regli L, Do HP, Pica A. Radiosurgery for trigeminal neuralgia using a linear accelerator with BrainLab system: report on initial experience in Lausanne, Switzerland. Swiss Med Wkly 2007; 137: 682–686

[69] Rand RW. Leksell Gamma Knife treatment of tic douloureux. Neurosurg Clin N Am 1997; 8: 75–78

[70] Richards GM, Bradley KA, Tomé WA, Bentzen SM, Resnick DK, Mehta MP. Linear accelerator radiosurgery for trigeminal neuralgia. Neurosurgery 2005; 57: 1193–1200, discussion 1193–1200

[71] Romanelli P, Heit G, Chang SD, Martin D, Pham C, Adler J. CyberKnife radiosurgery for trigeminal neuralgia. Stereotact Funct Neurosurg 2003; 81: 105–109

[72] Shaya M, Jawahar A, Caldito G, Sin A, Willis BK, Nanda A. Gamma Knife radiosurgery for trigeminal neuralgia: a study of predictors of success, efficacy, safety, and outcome at LSUHSC. Surg Neurol 2004; 61: 529–534, discussion 534–535

[73] Sheehan J, Pan HC, Stroila M, Steiner L. Gamma Knife surgery for trigeminal neuralgia: outcomes and prognostic factors. J Neurosurg 2005; 102: 434–441

[74] Shetter AG, Rogers CL, Ponce F, Fiedler JA, Smith K, Speiser BL. Gamma Knife radiosurgery for recurrent trigeminal neuralgia. J Neurosurg 2002; 97 (Suppl): 536–538

[75] Smith ZA, De Salles AA, Frighetto L, et al. Dedicated linear accelerator radiosurgery for the treatment of trigeminal neuralgia. J Neurosurg 2003; 99: 511–516

[76] Urgosik D, Liscak R, Novotny J, Vymazal J, Vladyka V. Treatment of essential trigeminal neuralgia with Gamma Knife surgery. J Neurosurg 2005; 102 (Suppl): 29–33

[77] Urgosik D, Vymazal J, Vladyka V, Liscák R. Gamma Knife treatment of trigeminal neuralgia: clinical and electrophysiological study. Stereotact Funct Neurosurg 1998; 70 (Suppl 1): 200–209

[78] Yomo S, Takihana T, Hatano M, Hirai T. Gamma Knife surgery for trigeminal neuralgia. Noshinkeigekasokuho 2006; 16: 501–509

[79] Young RF. Functional neurosurgery with the Leksell Gamma Knife. Stereotact Funct Neurosurg 1996; 66: 19–23

[80] Young RF, Vermeulen SS, Grimm P, Blasko J, Posewitz A. Gamma Knife radiosurgery for treatment of trigeminal neuralgia: idiopathic and tumor related. Neurology 1997; 48: 608–614

[81] Young RF, Vermulen S, Posewitz A. Gamma Knife radiosurgery for the treatment of trigeminal neuralgia. Stereotact Funct Neurosurg 1998; 70 (Suppl 1): 192–199

[82] Huang E, Teh BS, Zeck O, et al. Gamma Knife radiosurgery for treatment of trigeminal neuralgia in multiple sclerosis patients. Stereotact Funct Neurosurg 2002; 79: 44–50

[83] Rogers CL, Shetter AG, Ponce FA, Fiedler JA, Smith KA, Speiser BL. Gamma Knife radiosurgery for trigeminal neuralgia associated with multiple sclerosis. J Neurosurg 2002; 97 (Suppl): 529–532

[84] Brisman R, Khandji AG, Mooij RBM. Trigeminal nblood vessel relationship as revealed by high-resolution magnetic resonance imaging and its effect on pain relief after Gamma Knife radiosurgery for trigeminal neuralgia. Neurosurgery 2002; 50: 1261–1266, discussion 1266–1267

[85] Sheehan JP, Ray DK, Monteith S, et al. Gamma Knife radiosurgery for trigeminal neuralgia: the impact of magnetic resonance imaging-detected vascular impingement of the affected nerve. J Neurosurg 2010; 113: 53–58

[86] Balamucki CJ, Stieber VW, Ellis TL, et al. Does dose rate affect efficacy? The outcomes of 256 Gamma Knife surgery procedures for trigeminal neuralgia and other types of facial pain as they relate to the half-life of cobalt. J Neurosurg 2006; 105: 730–735

[87] Régis J, Metellus P, Dufour H, et al. Long-term outcome after Gamma Knife surgery for secondary trigeminal neuralgia. J Neurosurg 2001; 95: 199–205

[88] Régis J, Métellus P, Lazorthes Y, Porcheron D, Peragut JC. Effect of Gamma Knife on secondary trigeminal neuralgia. Stereotact Funct Neurosurg 1998; 70 (Suppl 1): 210–217

[89] Foote KD, Friedman WA, Buatti JM, Meeks SL, Bova FJ, Kubilis PS. Analysis of risk factors associated with radiosurgery for vestibular schwannoma. J Neurosurg 2001; 95: 440–449

[90] Marshall K, Chan MD, McCoy TP, et al. Predictive variables for the successful treatment of trigeminal neuralgia with Gamma Knife radiosurgery. Neurosurgery 2012; 70: 566–572, discussion 572–573

[91] Arkha Y, Murata N, Yomo S, Roussel P, Donnet A, Régis J. Gamma Knife surgery for essential trigeminal neuralgia: long-term results in a series of 262 patients. J Neurosurg 2008
[92] Kanner AA, Neyman G, Suh JH, Weinhous MS, Lee SY, Barnett GH. Gamma Knife radiosurgery for trigeminal neuralgia: comparing the use of a 4-mm versus concentric 4- and 8-mm collimators. Stereotact Funct Neurosurg 2004; 82: 49–57
[93] Massager N, Murata N, Tamura M, Devriendt D, Levivier M, Régis J. Influence of nerve radiation dose in the incidence of trigeminal dysfunction after trigeminal neuralgia radiosurgery. Neurosurgery 2007; 60: 681–687, discussion 687–688
[94] Gorgulho A, Mitchell E, De Salles A, et al. Stereotactic radiosurgery (SRS) for trigeminal neuralgia: clinical, radiological and dosimetric characteristics of patients presenting immediate pain relief. Presented at: 8th International Stereotactic Radiosurgery Society Congress; San Francisco, California; June 23–27, 2007
[95] Lim M, Bower R, Soltys S, et al. Treating trigeminal neuralgia with the CyberKnife: single center experience. Presented at: 8th International Stereotactic Radiosurgery Society Congress; San Francisco, California; June 23–27, 2007
[96] Lim M, Villavicencio AT, Burneikiene S, et al. CyberKnife radiosurgery for idiopathic trigeminal neuralgia. Neurosurg Focus 2005; 18: E9
[97] Spencer S, Swaid S, Young P, Guthrie B, et al. The impact of dose rate on outcomes of Gamma Knife radiosurgery in patients with face pain. Presented at: 8th International Stereotactic Radiosurgery Society Congress; San Francisco, California; June 23–27, 2007
[98] Lichtor T, Mullan JF. A 10-year follow-up review of percutaneous microcompression of the trigeminal ganglion. J Neurosurg 1990; 72: 49–54
[99] Gorgulho AA, De Salles AA. Impact of radiosurgery on the surgical treatment of trigeminal neuralgia. Surg Neurol 2006; 66: 350–356
[100] Rogers CL, Shetter AG, Fiedler JA, Smith KA, Han PP, Speiser BL. Gamma Knife radiosurgery for trigeminal neuralgia: the initial experience of the Barrow Neurological Institute. Int J Radiat Oncol Biol Phys 2000; 47: 1013–1019
[101] Pollock BE. Radiosurgery for trigeminal neuralgia: is sensory disturbance required for pain relief? J Neurosurg 2006; 105 (Suppl): 103–106
[102] Régis J, Manera L, Dufour H, Porcheron D, Sedan R, Peragut JC. Effect of the Gamma Knife on trigeminal neuralgia. Stereotact Funct Neurosurg 1995; 64 (Suppl 1): 182–192
[103] Lee JK, Choi HJ, Ko HC, Choi SK, Lim YJ, J Korean Neurosurg Soc. Long term outcomes of gamma knife radiosurgery for typical trigeminal neuralgia-minimum 5-year follow-up. Neurosurg Soc 2012 May; 51: 276–80
[104] Loescher AR, Radatz M, Kemeny A, Rowe J. Stereotactic radiosurgery for trigeminal neuralgia: outcomes and complications. Br J Neurosurg 2012 Feb; 26: 45–52
[105] Dos Santos MA, Perez de Salcedo JB, Guiterrez Diaz JA, Nagore G, Calvo FA, Samblas J, Marsiglia H, Sallabanda K. Outcome for patients with essential trigeminal neuralgia treated with linear accelerator stereotactic radiosurgery. Stereotac Funct Neurosurg 2011; 89: 220–5
[106] Park SH, Hwang SK. Outcomes of gamma knife radiosurgery for trigeminal neuralgia after a minimum 3-year follow-up. J Clin Neurosci 2011 May; 18: 645–8
[107] Verheul JB, Hanssens PE, Lie ST, Leenstra S, Persma H, Beute GN. Gamma Knife surgery for trigeminal neuralgia: a review of 450 consecutive cases. J Neurosurg 2010 Dec; 113 (Suppl): 160–7
[108] Riesenburger RI, Hwang SW, Schirmer CM, Zerris V, Wu JK, Mahn K, et al. Outcomes following single-treatment Gamma Knife surgery for trigeminal neuralgia with a minimum 3-year follow-up. J Neurosurg 2010; 112: 766–771

22 Mesial Temporal Lobe Epilepsy: Surgical Resection

Robert A. McGovern and Guy M. McKhann II

Introduction

Epilepsy is one of the most common neurologic disorders, accounting for ~ 1% of worldwide disease burden.[1] Of patients with epilepsy, 20 to 30% will be unable to control their seizures with medication.[2,3] These medically intractable, or pharmacoresistant, patients account for the majority of the costs associated with epilepsy.[4] Mesial temporal lobe epilepsy (MTLE) is the most common cause of pharmacoresistant epilepsy and has been shown to respond well to surgical resection with rates of seizure freedom ranging from 60 to 70% at 2 to 5 years.[5,6] Surgical resection entails either removal of the anterior two thirds of the temporal lobe (standard anterior temporal lobe resection) or a more selective resection of mesial temporal structures via selective amygdalohippocampectomy. Both procedures are well defined and lead to high rates of seizure freedom when compared to medical therapy alone. However, surgical resection is associated with short-term memory loss in dominant temporal lobe surgery, as well as low rates of death, infection, hemiparesis, visual field deficits, and cranial nerve palsies.

Because surgical resection for MTLE is essentially an ablative procedure, the question arises whether a noninvasive method such as stereotactic radiosurgery (SRS) may provide the same benefit as surgical resection while minimizing the complications associated with traditional open surgical approaches such as those described above. Here we discuss the rationale for open surgical resection, including the process for selecting MTLE patients; the evidence supporting surgical resection; our personal experience with this approach; the circumstances under which it should be used, and the choice of surgical procedure.

Rationale for Temporal Lobe Epilepsy Surgery

The complex partial seizures typically seen in MTLE were suspected to arise from mesial temporal lobe structures as early as 1941, when Herbert Jasper began using electroencephalography (EEG) to investigate seizures.[7] Indeed, Wilder Penfield had already begun his initial series of temporal lobe resections in 1939, although these mainly consisted of anterior and lateral temporal cortex resections.[8] A series of experiments in the 1950s showed that the amygdala and hippocampus were intimately involved in the genesis of typical temporal lobe seizures.[7] As a result, Penfield and Baldwin published a classic study of temporal lobectomies, including resection of the amygdala and hippocampus.[9] They described hippocampal atrophy in two thirds of the cases and named it "incisural sclerosis."[9] Since that time, advances in surgical techniques have made MTLE surgery a safe and effective choice for pharmacoresistant MTLE patients. Two randomized controlled trials have shown convincing evidence that MTLE surgery is superior to continuing medical therapy in these patients.[6,10] To maximize the efficacy of MTLE surgery, however, selecting the correct patients is paramount.

Proceeding to Surgical Resection

Patient Selection

For surgical resection to be successful in patients with MTLE, they must be selected carefully. First, patients must have established pharmacoresistance. Although studies have defined this in many different ways over time, a generally accepted definition of pharmacoresistance is the presence of at least monthly or bimonthly seizures, on average, over a 1- to 2-year period, despite having tried at least two antiepileptic drugs (AEDs), one of which must have a monotherapy indication.[5,6,10,11] The AEDs must be used at appropriate therapeutic dosages. Seizure semiology helps localize the epileptogenic zone in the majority of epilepsy patients, including MTLE.[12] MTLE seizures are most commonly complex partial in nature, often involving an aura experienced as a rising abdominal sensation, as well as head and hand automatisms, such as contralateral forced head version prior to secondary generalization, lip smacking, and dystonia.[12,13] The presence of postictal language difficulties can also indicate a dominant lobe lesion.[12,13]

Video EEG is frequently used to lateralize and localize interictal activity and ictal onset, as well as to correlate the seizure semiology with ictal EEG activity. MTLE patients typically show lateralized interictal spikes;[14] those with recorded bilateral interictal discharges or lateralized discharges with contralateral spread have been associated with worse surgical outcomes.[15] Multiple concordant unilateral seizures are typically recorded from an individual patient to complete the electrographic lateralization and localization of MTLE.[16]

Imaging in MTLE consists mainly of brain magnetic resonance imaging (MRI) sequences aimed at revealing the effects of hippocampal sclerosis (HS), the main pathology seen in MTLE. Thin-cut T1-weighted sequences as well as coronal T2- and fluid attenuation inversion recovery (FLAIR)–weighted sequences perpendicular to the long axis of the hippocampus reveal hippocampal and temporal lobe atrophy,[17] increased hippocampal T2/FLAIR signal,[18,19] and loss of normal hippocampal architecture.[20] Because MTLE patients often have coexisting focal cortical dysplasia (FCD),[17,21] the entirety of the temporal lobes should be closely examined on these sequences, looking for subtle gray-white junction blurring or other features of FCD. Magnetic resonance spectroscopy (MRS), magnetoencephalography (MEG), diffusion tractography–based MRI, and other advanced imaging techniques are used as adjuvant studies in TLE, but they are not usually required to make the diagnosis.

Finally, neuropsychological testing should be included as part of every patient evaluation. Testing serves to diagnose any preexisting cognitive impairment, evaluate an individual's cognitive outcome postsurgery, and potentially serve as a tool to predict which patients will be best served by surgery. In general, patients with left-sided MTLE tend to show verbal memory deficits, whereas patients undergoing right-sided resection show little in the way of specific cognitive impairments.[22,23] In addition, patients with HS on MRI have worse verbal memory scores preoperatively but decline less postoperatively than those without HS.[22] Patients with higher neuropsychological function preoperatively, particularly in the verbal memory domain, have greater function at risk as a result of dominant MTLE surgery. Seizure freedom is likely one of the most important factors in determining long-term cognitive outcome, as patients undergoing surgical resection for MTLE but still suffering seizures show similar outcomes as medically treated intractable MTLE patients.[24]

Sodium Amobarbital (Wada) Testing

In the Wada test, cerebral angiography is combined with sequential unilateral intracarotid injection of sodium amobarbital in an awake, functioning patient who is undergoing language and memory testing. It is used for two main purposes: (1) to determine cerebral language dominance and (2) to ascertain whether each side of the brain has sufficient ability to support short-term memory function when the other side has been "anesthesized" with the short-acting barbiturate. Although many centers still routinely carry out Wada testing in all potential MTLE patients, functional MRI to determine language dominance together with neuropsychological testing has largely supplanted Wada testing in many centers for nondominant MTLE patients and in some centers for all MTLE patients.

Surgical Approach

Once an MTLE patient has met the above criteria for planned surgical resection, the neurosurgeon must decide on the appropriate approach. The two major approaches currently used are the "standard" anterior temporal lobectomy (ATL) and the selective amygdalohippocampectomy (SAH). Both procedures are aimed at removing nonfunctional, sclerotic, epileptogenic tissue in the offending mesial temporal lobe, including primarily the parahippocampal gyrus, hippocampus, and amygdala. ATL of the language-dominant side involves removing 3 to 4 cm of the lateral temporal lobe, including the middle and inferior temporal gyri, as measured from the most anterior aspect of the middle fossa. Most centers avoid resection of the dominant superior temporal gyrus to minimize the risk of a postoperative language deficit. On the nondominant side, resection can extend up to 4.5 to 6.0 cm posteriorly, with the position of the vein of Labbé being the posteriorly limiting factor.[13] However, even on the nondominant side, most surgeons limit their lateral temporal resection to the anterior 3 to 4 cm of the middle and inferior temporal gyri in ATL surgery. Although the efficacy of ATL has been well established,[6,10,25] the presence of neuropsychological complications, in particular, persistent verbal memory decline in dominant temporal lobe surgery, as mentioned above, suggests that ATL involves the resection of functional tissue that may be spared. The multiple techniques of SAH evolved as a way to limit the resection of potentially functional but nonepileptogenic tissue.

In SAH, the medial temporal structures are removed with minimal resection of the lateral neocortical structures. A transsylvian SAH approach, as initially applied by Yasargil,[70] has the advantage of completely avoiding lateral temporal neocortex but adds the surgical complexity and risk of a wide sylvian fissure dissection. Though appealing due to its lack of cortical resection, the dissection complexity of the transsylvian approach, combined with the need to transect the temporal stem to get to the temporal horn of the lateral ventricle, has turned most surgeons to other SAH approaches. A lateral transcortical or transsulcal SAH approach may be taken, which is simpler, more direct, and avoids excessive retraction. The use of frameless stereotactic navigation systems has made a lateral SAH approach minimally invasive, allowing for preoperative planning and intraoperative confirmation of the most favorable transgyral or transsulcal route to the temporal horn of the lateral ventricle. The mesial temporal structures are then resected from within the temporal horn in an inside-out fashion. A direct comparison of the two approaches has shown little difference in cognitive outcome, with the transcortical approach actually showing improved verbal fluency, a measure of executive function and thought to be a result of the lower amount of retraction used in this approach.[26]

During the transcortical approach, a cortical incision in the middle temporal gyrus is used to enter the temporal horn and resect the parahippocampal gyrus, amygdala, and hippocampus. Frameless stereotactic guidance is used to both select the correct entry point and ensure a complete resection of the medial temporal structures.[13] Although the evidence for SAH as a preferred strategy is equivocal,[27,28] most studies have shown at least equivalent outcomes to ATL in terms of seizure freedom[29,30] and neuropsychological outcomes,[24,30] with SAH offering a potential benefit in short-term verbal recall tasks but similar declines in long-term verbal memory deficits.[24,30]

■ Literature Supporting the Use of Surgical Resection in Temporal Lobe Epilepsy

Surgical Resection versus Continued Medical Therapy in Temporal Lobe Epilepsy

In 2003, a practice parameter from the American Academy of Neurology (AAN) in association with the American Epilepsy Society (AES) and the American Association of Neurological Surgeons (AANS) regarding surgical treatment of MTLE was published[5] and included a comprehensive review of the literature that revealed 1 class I study comparing surgical resection with continued medical treatment for pharmacoresistant MTLE,[6] as well as 24 class IV studies between 1990 and 2001. The parameter stated that patients with persistent, disabling complex partial seizures due to MTLE should be offered ATL, as the benefits for resection were greater than medical therapy and the risks comparable. The practice parameter also called for a randomized controlled trial examining early surgical resection for MTLE, as the majority of studies have shown a large gap between age at onset of seizures and time to resection (~ 20 y). In response to that statement, another class I study comparing "early" surgical resection to continued medical treatment for pharmacoresistant MTLE has been published.[10] In addition, a number of observational studies comparing seizure and neuropsychological and imaging outcomes, typically between different surgical approaches, have also been published.[23,24,28,29,31–37]

Both class I studies have shown a significant benefit in terms of seizure freedom from surgical resection for pharmacoresistant TLE. Wiebe et al[6] randomized patients who were having, on average, monthly seizures for at least 1 year while taking at least two AEDs, one of which had to be phenytoin, valproic acid, or carbamazepine, to either continued medical treatment or surgical resection with ATL. Medical therapy resulted in freedom from seizures impairing awareness (Engel class I) in only 8% of patients, and 58% of patients undergoing ATL were seizure-free at 1 year postop.

Engel et al, in the Early Randomized Surgical Epilepsy Trial (ERSET), attempted to test the hypothesis that early surgery could potentially be more beneficial to patients, as there is some evidence that persistent seizures lead to long-term cognitive deficits;[10] also, Wiebe et al had shown significant seizure freedom in this population.[6] ERSET randomized TLE patients who had persistently disabling seizures for no more than 2 consecutive years following two brand-name AED trials to either continued medical therapy or ATL. Although the target goal for this trial was 200 patients, enrollment was slow, with 76 eligible patients identified and only 38 patients enrolled, with 23 patients randomized to the medical group and 15 to the surgical group. Nonetheless, the researchers found that 11 of 15 patients randomized to early ATL were seizure free, whereas 0 of 23 patients in the medical group were seizure free 2 years postoperatively.[10] Surgery patients also had significantly higher quality of life (QOL) scores at 9, 12, and 18 months postoperatively. The main limitation of this study was its low enrollment and early termination. Studies that are terminated early because of beneficial treatment effects can suffer from positive bias, but this study was ended solely due to the lack of enrollment. Indeed, the results from this study are so striking that they not only support Wiebe et al's claim that ATL is significantly more beneficial than continued medical therapy in pharmacoresistant TLE but also that clinicians should consider surgery as an initial option once a patient has failed two AEDs.

Anterior Temporal Lobectomy versus Selective Amygdalohippocampectomy

Because ATL entails the resection of approximately two thirds of the anterior lateral temporal lobe in addition to the mesial temporal structures, the possibility for postoperative language and verbal deficits has always been a concern, particularly in patients with dominant ATL. Indeed, the result of years of cognitive outcomes research has shown that patients undergoing dominant temporal ATL tend to have persistent verbal memory and word-finding deficits.[22,38] In addition, those with HS generally have worse cognitive baselines and decline less than those without HS on MRI and pathology, whereas those without HS tend to have higher baseline cognitive scores and decline more severely postoperatively.[39] This indicates that patients without HS likely have more functional tissue that is being resected during an ATL. Partly in response to these data, the SAH has been used as a way to minimize lateral temporal neocortical resection and maximize resection of presumably nonfunctional mesial temporal structures.

There have been no prospective, controlled trials randomizing patients to either ATL or SAH, but there have been a number of studies comparing both seizure and/or neuropsychological outcomes. Most of these studies are retrospective in nature and suffer from the fact that many neurosurgeons in the field began performing mostly SAH surgeries over the past decade. Thus, these retrospective studies mainly compare data from ATL surgeries performed at the beginning of the study period and SAH surgeries toward the end of the study period.[29,35] Nevertheless, there have been consistent themes that have emerged from the bevy of studies performed.

First, almost every direct comparison study has shown equivalent seizure freedom rates (60–90% at 3–6 y of follow-up) between SAH and ATL,[29,30,33,34,37,40] although there have been exceptions.[28] In addition, studies describing only SAH[26,32,41–43] have shown similar seizure freedom rates to historic ATL data.[44] Interestingly, Helmstaedter et al found that seizure control significantly affected cognitive outcome regardless of surgical approach, implying that verbal memory and language impairments may be more related to seizure freedom rates than the amount or type of tissue resected.[24] Other studies have not corroborated these findings.[34]

Most cognitive outcome studies comparing SAH and ATL have shown slightly better results for SAH, although a meta-analysis was unable to detect a difference between surgical approaches.[45] The most consistent finding across multiple retrospective studies is a smaller decline in verbal memory in dominant lobe surgical resection than that seen in ATL,[29,30,46] with some studies showing a higher percentage of patients actually improving in verbal memory postoperatively.[33] For example, Clusmann et al found 43% of dominant lobe ATL patients had worse verbal memory scores postoperatively, whereas only 31% of SAH patients worsened.[29] Other studies found improved nonverbal memory in nondominant SAH compared to ATL[35,47] and improved immediate recall.[30] To try to determine why SAH patients still showed significant verbal and language difficulties despite sparing of the lateral temporal neocortex, one group characterized tissue undergoing "collateral damage" (T2/FLAIR signal change) along the surgical approach corridor. They concluded that this "collateral damage" was responsible for SAH-related verbal memory decline, as an increase in damage predicted worse memory outcome.[48] Finally, it should be noted that none of these studies have examined these issues in a rigorous, randomized, controlled fashion. There are several examples of studies showing no difference in cognitive or seizure-free outcomes between SAH and ATL techniques.[49–51]

Surgical Resection versus Stereotactic Radiosurgery in Mesial Temporal Lobe Epilepsy

Given that surgical resection has been proven to be a successful treatment option for pharmacoresistant MTLE over a number of studies in the last 30 years, including two class I randomized controlled trials, SRS must clear a high therapeutic bar to be considered a competing treatment option. First, SRS studies should show equivalent rates of seizure freedom, arguably the most important outcome in MTLE patients. Because there are no published randomized controlled trials directly comparing the two treatments, one can only attempt to draw conclusions from the noncontrolled observational studies currently representing the published literature.

Bartolomei et al and Barbaro et al published the two largest, best characterized prospective studies with long-term follow-up[52,53] in groups of 15 and 30 MTLE patients, respectively. Both studies used similar treatment protocols with a marginal dose of 24 Gy and the total volume of the 50% isodense target area between 5.5 and 9 mL. The Barbaro et al multicenter study randomized its 30 patients to either a standard dose of 24 Gy or a low dose of 20 Gy. Overall, both studies showed similar outcomes, with 60 and 67% seizure freedom (Engel class IA/B) rates at 8 and 2 years' follow-up, respectively. Notably, the low-dose group in the Barbaro et al study showed lower seizure freedom rates (59%) than the standard dose group (77%). For comparison, the two class I surgical resection trials showed seizure freedom rates of 58% and 73% at 1 and 2 years' follow-up, respectively. Similarly, a recent decision analysis used a figure of 71.9% for 1-year seizure freedom rates based on 13 studies published after 1999.[71]

There are two important aspects of these studies to note. First, the effect of SRS on seizure frequency is delayed, with a maximum reduction in seizures typically seen 12 to 24 months posttreatment.[54] During this time, seizures continue to occur, and the risk of associated morbidity and mortality (sudden unexplained death in epilepsy) likely remains.[55,56] In fact, auras actually tend to increase during the intervening time, peaking during 9 to 12 months posttreatment. Second, there are many studies that have shown minimal or no efficacy for SRS in TLE,[55,57–61] although these all suffer from flaws, including small sample size, low treatment dose (a recognized factor in efficacy[54]), and retrospective design.

Thus, based on the best available evidence, seizure freedom rates in MTLE following SRS may be comparable to postsurgical outcomes if SRS is performed with a 24-Gy dose. The Radiosurgery or Open Surgery for Epilepsy (ROSE) trial is a prospective, randomized, controlled trial that is ongoing (in its follow-up phase) and may help answer some of these important questions, as it is planned to report seizure freedom, cognitive outcomes, and cost with 3 years of follow-up. Unfortunately, like the ERSET trial of early surgery, the ROSE trial was recently closed for new enrollment by the National Institutes of Health due to the lack of patient accrual. The ROSE trial will provide important useful information but will likely not definitively answer the important comparison questions between SRS and open surgery.

If we assume comparable seizure freedom rates, then the next major factor in deciding between these two treatments is cognitive outcome. There have been few neuropsychological outcome studies performed in SRS for TLE. Initial studies indicated that SRS could potentially lead to poorer cognitive outcomes, particularly in verbal memory.[55,59] The larger, prospective studies since then have mainly shown no difference in cognitive outcomes post-SRS.

The most detailed data come from the Quigg et al multicenter prospective trial that revealed potential benefits in verbal memory performance following dominant temporal SRS in comparison to historical postsurgical results.[62] In the 24-Gy treated patients, there were mild decreases in confrontation naming and noncontextual verbal memory. In addition, 36% of dominant lobe SRS patients showed a significant impairment in at least one test. By comparison, a meta-analysis of 22 studies reporting neuropsychological outcomes in TLE surgery described a risk of verbal memory loss in 44% and naming impairment in 34% of dominant lobe surgery patients.[45] Verbal fluency was more likely to be improved in these patients, with essentially no overall change in intelligence quotient (IQ) or executive functioning.

In the European SRS study, Régis et al reported stable or improved cognitive outcomes in all of their patients.[56] However, detailed neuropsychological data were not made available. The patients were divided into six groups (0–5) ranging from "far below average" (0) to "far above average" (5) based on the testing. The majority (55%) of these patients had a baseline score of 0; thus, it would be impossible for them to decline by this measure.

The issue of long-term cognitive outcome remains in question following SRS for the treatment of MTLE. There is insufficient evidence to conclude whether or not SRS represents an improvement over TLE surgery in cognitive outcome. Although there have been enough surgical studies to reasonably evaluate the cognitive effects of TLE surgery, the same cannot be said of SRS. The most recent studies suggest that SRS may represent an improvement over surgery in terms of long-term cognition, but the ROSE trial and future SRS studies detailing neuropsychological outcomes will be needed to help further delineate differences between the two treatments.

In terms of other complications following open surgical or SRS treatment in MTLE, the comparison for patients is really one of personal choice. Open surgical procedures carry a very small but real risk of general anesthesia, stroke, and retraction injury that are not seen following SRS. In contrast, SRS carries the risk of postoperative headaches and steroid dependence not seen in the surgical group. In addition, SRS may have an extremely low risk of delayed malignancy in the irradiated field.

Personal Experience

My (GMM) personal decision on what treatment to recommend for a given MTLE patient depends on a variety of factors. There are actually two levels of decision: whether to recommend a less invasive but experimental treatment option versus open surgical resection and what type of open surgical procedure, ATL versus SAH. The "standard" remains open surgical resection, based on decades of epilepsy surgery experience and class I medical evidence. Although these randomized trials were carried out using ATL as the surgical procedure, the majority of accumulated clinical experience to date suggests that ATL and SAH are at least equally effective in providing seizure freedom in MTLE patients.

So, when should SAH be the procedure of choice? This question depends on whether the seizures arise from the dominant temporal lobe, the neuropsychological and occupational status of the patient, the concordance of the preoperative epilepsy evaluation data, and the personal preference and experience of the operating surgeon. SAH, depending on the technique used, likely provides some potential neuropsychological benefit for dominant TLE surgery. If a patient has dominant MTLE with some degree of preserved neuropsychological function, SAH is a logical procedure to choose. If, however, the preoperative data are less than completely concordant for mesial temporal sclerosis, suggesting the possibility of neocortical TLE as well as MTLE, then ATL is the more logical surgical procedure to choose.

It is important to realize that SAH is not a single surgical procedure. It was initially developed as a sylvian fissure–splitting procedure that transgresses the temporal stem to get to the temporal horn of the lateral ventricle. Since then, many variations have been described incorporating frameless stereotactic navigation to access the temporal horn from lateral temporal or basal temporal approaches. These approaches have a variable degree of interruption of white matter pathways within the temporal lobe, impacting the potential for neuropsychological decline and visual field deficit. Lateral approaches through the middle temporal sulcus or inferior temporal gyrus or basal approaches through the inferior temporal or collateral sulci may carry lower neuropsychological risk but are technically more demanding of the surgeon than ATL surgery.

In addition to radiosurgical treatment for MTLE, there are a growing number of other options to focally treat the mesial temporal structures in MTLE. Even more selective surgical approaches using various types of hippocampal transections, at times combined with anteromesial temporal subpial transections, have been promoted as potentially superior in patients with preserved neuropsychological function. Recently, an MRI-compatible laser has been stereotactically placed down the long axis of the hippocampus and then been used to ablate the mesial temporal structures under MR thermographic guidance. In comparison to Gamma Knife (Elekta AB, Stockholm, Sweden) radiosurgery, this technique has several potential advantages, including (1) MRI-based confirmation of target damage; (2) immediate damage to the target structures, with no long delay to therapeutic benefit; and (3) no delayed radiobiological risks. Future studies will be necessary to better understand which individual patients will most benefit from the various treatment options for MTLE, balancing seizure freedom with procedural risk.

Conclusion

The decision to commit to surgical resection for TLE is best taken when the patient fulfills the clinical, radiological, and neuropsychological criteria described above. Although some studies have shown equivalent outcomes in groups of patients who do not conform to the above criteria,[63] in general, patients who do not fulfill those criteria (e.g., bitemporal seizure onset, normal MRI, nondominant verbal memory function) have worse outcomes postoperatively.[15,64] It should be kept in mind, however, that these outcomes may still be better than continued medical therapy, as multiple studies have shown that only 0 to 5% of patients who have failed two AEDs will become seizure free,[6,65–67] and that persistent seizures have long-term detrimental cognitive and psychiatric effects.[68,69] This evidence, combined with the results of the ERSET trial, make a strong argument for reducing the time between the development of pharmacoresistance and surgical resection. As such, each decision should be made on an individual basis, with the patient well informed as to the risks and benefits of both surgical resection and continued medical therapy.

Because there have been no direct trials comparing surgical resection to SRS, the ROSE trial will answer many of the questions regarding the equivalence and relative benefits of these two therapies. Current practice based on the available evidence, however, dictates that surgical resection remain the first option in pharmacoresistant TLE patients. If a patient is not a surgical candidate, then he or she may be considered for SRS under a clinical research protocol. Although some may advocate for SRS in high-functioning patients who have dominant lobe TLE and are at higher risk for verbal memory decline,[60] we consider the evidence too scant to currently recommend this. Other new options, including hippocampal transections and laser-based ablation of mesial temporal structures, hold potential promise in the treatment of MTLE and should be further studied in direct comparison to MTLE surgery using ATL and/or SAH.

References

[1] Murray CJL, Lopez AD, Jamison DT. The global burden of disease in 1990: summary results, sensitivity analyses and future directions. Bulletin of the World Health Organization 1994; 72: 495–508

[2] Hauser WA, Hesdorffer DC. Epilepsy: Frequency, Causes and Consequences. New York, NY: Demos Press; 1990

[3] Berg AT. Understanding the delay before epilepsy surgery: who develops intractable focal epilepsy and when? CNS Spectr 2004; 9: 136–144

[4] Begley CE, Famulari M, Annegers JF, et al. The cost of epilepsy in the United States: an estimate from population-based clinical and survey data. Epilepsia 2000; 41: 342–351

[5] Engel J, Wiebe S, French J, et al. Practice parameter: temporal lobe and localized neocortical resections for epilepsy. Epilepsia 2003; 44: 741–751

[6] Wiebe S, Blume WT, Girvin JP, Eliasziw M Effectiveness and Efficiency of Surgery for Temporal Lobe Epilepsy Study Group. A randomized, controlled trial of surgery for temporal-lobe epilepsy. N Engl J Med 2001; 345: 311–318

[7] de Almeida AN, Teixeira MJ, Feindel WH. From lateral to mesial: the quest for a surgical cure for temporal lobe epilepsy. Epilepsia 2008; 49: 98–107

[8] Penfield W, Flanigin H. Surgical therapy of temporal lobe seizures. AMA Arch Neurol Psychiatry 1950; 64: 491–500

[9] Penfield W, Baldwin M. Temporal lobe seizures and the technic of subtotal temporal lobectomy. Ann Surg 1952; 136: 625–634

[10] Engel J, McDermott MP, Wiebe S, et al. Early Randomized Surgical Epilepsy Trial (ERSET) Study Group. Early surgical therapy for drug-resistant temporal lobe epilepsy: a randomized trial. JAMA 2012; 307: 922–930

[11] Engel J, McDermott MP, Wiebe S, et al. Early Randomized Surgical Epilepsy Trial (ERSET) Study Group. Design considerations for a multicenter randomized controlled trial of early surgery for mesial temporal lobe epilepsy. Epilepsia 2010; 51: 1978–1986

[12] Rosenow F, Lüders H. Presurgical evaluation of epilepsy. Brain 2001; 124: 1683–1700

[13] Winn HR. Youmans Neurological Surgery. 6th ed. Vol. 1. Philadelphia, PA: Elsevier Health Science; 2011

[14] Chee MW, Morris HH, Antar MA, et al. Presurgical evaluation of temporal lobe epilepsy using interictal temporal spikes and positron emission tomography. Arch Neurol 1993; 50: 45–48

[15] Schulz R, Lüders HO, Hoppe M, Tuxhorn I, May T, Ebner A. Interictal EEG and ictal scalp EEG propagation are highly predictive of surgical outcome in mesial temporal lobe epilepsy. Epilepsia 2000; 41: 564–570

[16] Blum D. Prevalence of bilateral partial seizure foci and implications for electroencephalographic telemetry monitoring and epilepsy surgery. Electroencephalogr Clin Neurophysiol 1994; 91: 329–336

[17] Diehl B, Najm I, LaPresto E, et al. Temporal lobe volumes in patients with hippocampal sclerosis with or without cortical dysplasia. Neurology 2004; 62: 1729–1735

[18] Berkovic SF, Andermann F, Olivier A, et al. Hippocampal sclerosis in temporal lobe epilepsy demonstrated by magnetic resonance imaging. Ann Neurol 1991; 29: 175–182

[19] Van Paesschen W, Sisodiya S, Connelly A, et al. Quantitative hippocampal MRI and intractable temporal lobe epilepsy. Neurology 1995; 45: 2233–2240

[20] Lencz T, McCarthy G, Bronen RA, et al. Quantitative magnetic resonance imaging in temporal lobe epilepsy: relationship to neuropathology and neuropsychological function. Ann Neurol 1992; 31: 629–637

[21] Prayson RA, Reith JD, Najm IM. Mesial temporal sclerosis: a clinicopathologic study of 27 patients, including 5 with coexistent cortical dysplasia. Arch Pathol Lab Med 1996; 120: 532–536

[22] Hamberger MJ, Drake EB. Cognitive functioning following epilepsy surgery. Curr Neurol Neurosci Rep 2006; 6: 319–326

[23] Helmstaedter C. Neuropsychological aspects of epilepsy surgery. Epilepsy Behav 2004; 5 (Suppl 1): S45–S55
[24] Helmstaedter C, Kurthen M, Lux S, Reuber M, Elger CE. Chronic epilepsy and cognition: a longitudinal study in temporal lobe epilepsy. Ann Neurol 2003; 54: 425–432
[25] Wyler AR, Hermann BP, Somes G. Extent of medial temporal resection on outcome from anterior temporal lobectomy: a randomized prospective study. Neurosurgery 1995; 37: 982–990, discussion 990–991
[26] Lutz MT, Clusmann H, Elger CE, Schramm J, Helmstaedter C. Neuropsychological outcome after selective amygdalohippocampectomy with transsylvian versus transcortical approach: a randomized prospective clinical trial of surgery for temporal lobe epilepsy. Epilepsia 2004; 45: 809–816
[27] Olivier A. Transcortical selective amygdalohippocampectomy in temporal lobe epilepsy. Can J Neurol Sci 2000; 27 (Suppl 1): S68–S76, discussion S92–S96
[28] Bate H, Eldridge P, Varma T, Wieshmann UC. The seizure outcome after amygdalohippocampectomy and temporal lobectomy. Eur J Neurol 2007; 14: 90–94
[29] Clusmann H, Schramm J, Kral T, et al. Prognostic factors and outcome after different types of resection for temporal lobe epilepsy. J Neurosurg 2002; 97: 1131–1141
[30] Helmstaedter C, Elger CE, Hufnagel A, Zentner J, Schramm J. Different effects of left anterior temporal lobectomy, selective amygdalohippocampectomy, and temporal cortical lesionectomy on verbal learning, memory, and recognition. J Epilepsy 1996; 9: 39–45
[31] de Tisi J, Bell GS, Peacock JL, et al. The long-term outcome of adult epilepsy surgery, patterns of seizure remission, and relapse: a cohort study. Lancet 2011; 378: 1388–1395
[32] Georgakoulias NV, Mitsos AP, Konstantinou EA, Nicholson C, Jenkins A. Transsylvian selective amygdalohippocampectomy for medically intractable temporal lobe epilepsy: a single-centre experience. Br J Neurosurg 2008; 22: 535–541
[33] Paglioli E, Palmini A, Portuguez M, et al. Seizure and memory outcome following temporal lobe surgery: selective compared with nonselective approaches for hippocampal sclerosis. J Neurosurg 2006; 104: 70–78
[34] Sagher O, Thawani JP, Etame AB, Gomez-Hassan DM. Seizure outcomes and mesial resection volumes following selective amygdalohippocampectomy and temporal lobectomy. Neurosurg Focus 2012; 32: E8
[35] Tanriverdi T, Dudley RW, Hasan A, et al. Memory outcome after temporal lobe epilepsy surgery: corticoamygdalohippocampectomy versus selective amygdalohippocampectomy. J Neurosurg 2010; 113: 1164–1175
[36] Tanriverdi T, Olivier A. Cognitive changes after unilateral cortico-amygdalohippocampectomy unilateral selective-amygdalohippocampectomy mesial temporal lobe epilepsy. Turk Neurosurg 2007; 17: 91–99
[37] Tanriverdi T, Olivier A, Poulin N, Andermann F, Dubeau F. Long-term seizure outcome after mesial temporal lobe epilepsy surgery: corticalamygdalohippocampectomy versus selective amygdalohippocampectomy. J Neurosurg 2008; 108: 517–524
[38] Hermann BP, Wyler AR, Bush AJ, Tabatabai FR. Differential effects of left and right anterior temporal lobectomy on verbal learning and memory performance. Epilepsia 1992; 33: 289–297
[39] Hermann BP, Wyler AR, Somes G, Berry AD, Dohan FC. Pathological status of the mesial temporal lobe predicts memory outcome from left anterior temporal lobectomy. Neurosurgery 1992; 31: 652–656, discussion 656–657
[40] Arruda F, Cendes F, Andermann F, et al. Mesial atrophy and outcome after amygdalohippocampectomy or temporal lobe removal. Ann Neurol 1996; 40: 446–450
[41] Wieser HG, Yaşargil MG. Selective amygdalohippocampectomy as a surgical treatment of mesiobasal limbic epilepsy. Surg Neurol 1982; 17: 445–457
[42] Hori T, Yamane F, Ochiai T, et al. Selective subtemporal amygdalohippocampectomy for refractory temporal lobe epilepsy: operative and neuropsychological outcomes. J Neurosurg 2007; 106: 134–141
[43] Gleissner U, Helmstaedter C, Schramm J, Elger CE. Memory outcome after selective amygdalohippocampectomy in patients with temporal lobe epilepsy: one-year follow-up. Epilepsia 2004; 45: 960–962
[44] Engel J. Update on surgical treatment of the epilepsies: summary of the Second International Palm Desert Conference on the Surgical Treatment of the Epilepsies (1992). Neurology 1993; 43: 1612–1617
[45] Sherman EMS, Wiebe S, Fay-McClymont TB, et al. Neuropsychological outcomes after epilepsy surgery: systematic review and pooled estimates. Epilepsia 2011; 52: 857–869
[46] Pauli E, Pickel S, Schulemann H, Buchfelder M, Stefan H. Neuropsychologic findings depending on the type of the resection in temporal lobe epilepsy. Adv Neurol 1999; 81: 371–377
[47] Helmstaedter C, Richter S, Röske S, Oltmanns F, Schramm J, Lehmann TN. Differential effects of temporal pole resection with amygdalohippocampectomy versus selective amygdalohippocampectomy on material-specific memory in patients with mesial temporal lobe epilepsy. Epilepsia 2008; 49: 88–97
[48] Helmstaedter C, Van Roost D, Clusmann H, Urbach H, Elger CE, Schramm J. Collateral brain damage, a potential source of cognitive impairment after selective surgery for control of mesial temporal lobe epilepsy. J Neurol Neurosurg Psychiatry 2004; 75: 323–326
[49] Wolf RL, Ivnik RJ, Hirschorn KA, Sharbrough FW, Cascino GD, Marsh WR. Neurocognitive efficiency following left temporal lobectomy: standard versus limited resection. J Neurosurg 1993; 79: 76–83
[50] Lacruz ME, Alarcón G, Akanuma N, et al. Neuropsychological effects associated with temporal lobectomy and amygdalohippocampectomy depending on Wada test failure. J Neurol Neurosurg Psychiatry 2004; 75: 600–607
[51] Shin M-S, Lee S, Seol SH, et al. Changes in neuropsychological functioning following temporal lobectomy in patients with temporal lobe epilepsy. Neurol Res 2009; 31: 692–701
[52] Bartolomei F, Hayashi M, Tamura M, et al. Long-term efficacy of gamma knife radiosurgery in mesial temporal lobe epilepsy. Neurology 2008; 70: 1658–1663
[53] Barbaro NM, Quigg M, Broshek DK, et al. A multicenter, prospective pilot study of Gamma Knife radiosurgery for mesial temporal lobe epilepsy: seizure response, adverse events, and verbal memory. Ann Neurol 2009; 65: 167–175
[54] Quigg M, Rolston J, Barbaro NM. Radiosurgery for epilepsy: clinical experience and potential antiepileptic mechanisms. Epilepsia 2012; 53: 7–15
[55] Srikijvilaikul T, Najm I, Foldvary-Schaefer N, Lineweaver T, Suh JH, Bingaman WE. Failure of Gamma Knife radiosurgery for mesial temporal lobe epilepsy: report of five cases. Neurosurgery 2004; 54: 1395–1402, discussion 1402–1404
[56] Régis J, Rey M, Bartolomei F, et al. Gamma Knife surgery in mesial temporal lobe epilepsy: a prospective multicenter study. Epilepsia 2004; 45: 504–515
[57] Cmelak AJ, Abou-Khalil B, Konrad PE, Duggan D, Maciunas RJ. Low-dose stereotactic radiosurgery is inadequate for medically intractable mesial temporal lobe epilepsy: a case report. Seizure 2001; 10: 442–446
[58] Kawai K, Suzuki I, Kurita H, Shin M, Arai N, Kirino T. Failure of low-dose radiosurgery to control temporal lobe epilepsy. J Neurosurg 2001; 95: 883–887
[59] McDonald CR, Norman MA, Tecoma E, Alksne J, Iragui V. Neuropsychological change following Gamma Knife surgery in patients with left temporal lobe epilepsy: a review of three cases. Epilepsy Behav 2004; 5: 949–957
[60] Hoggard N, Wilkinson ID, Griffiths PD, Vaughan P, Kemeny AA, Rowe JG. The clinical course after stereotactic radiosurgical amygdalohippocampectomy with neuroradiological correlates. Neurosurgery 2008; 62: 336–344, discussion 344–346
[61] Vojtěch Z, Vladyka V, Kalina M, et al. The use of radiosurgery for the treatment of mesial temporal lobe epilepsy and long-term results. Epilepsia 2009; 50: 2061–2071
[62] Quigg M, Broshek DK, Barbaro NM, et al. Radiosurgery Epilepsy Study Group. Neuropsychological outcomes after Gamma Knife radiosurgery for mesial temporal lobe epilepsy: a prospective multicenter study. Epilepsia 2011; 52: 909–916
[63] Smith AP, Sani S, Kanner AM, et al. Medically intractable temporal lobe epilepsy in patients with normal MRI: surgical outcome in twenty-one consecutive patients. Seizure 2011; 20: 475–479
[64] Helmstaedter C, Petzold I, Bien CG. The cognitive consequence of resecting nonlesional tissues in epilepsy surgery—results from MRI- and histopathology-negative patients with temporal lobe epilepsy. Epilepsia 2011; 52: 1402–1408
[65] Choi H, Heiman GA, Munger Clary H, Etienne M, Resor SR, Hauser WA. Seizure remission in adults with long-standing intractable epilepsy: an extended follow-up. Epilepsy Res 2011; 93: 115–119
[66] Kwan P, Brodie MJ. Early identification of refractory epilepsy. N Engl J Med 2000; 342: 314–319
[67] Kwan P, Sperling MR. Refractory seizures: try additional antiepileptic drugs (after two have failed) or go directly to early surgery evaluation? Epilepsia 2009; 50 (Suppl 8): 57–62
[68] Engel J. Surgical treatment for epilepsy: too little, too late? JAMA 2008; 300: 2548–2550
[69] Helmstaedter C, Kockelmann E. Cognitive outcomes in patients with chronic temporal lobe epilepsy. Epilepsia 2006; 47 (Suppl 2): 96–98
[70] Wieser HG, Yaşargil MG. Selective amygdalohippocampectomy as a surgical treatment of mesiobasal limbic epilepsy. Surgical neurology 1982; 17: 445–57
[71] Choi H, Sell RL, Lenert L, et al. Epilepsy surgery for pharmacoresistant temporal lobe epilepsy: a decision analysis. JAMA 2008; 300: 2497–505

23 Radiosurgery for Temporal Lobe Epilepsy

Mark Quigg and Nicholas M. Barbaro

Introduction

Recently, the use of stereotactic radiosurgery (SRS) has expanded into the treatment of mesial temporal lobe epilepsy (MTLE). Studies show large variations in primary outcomes. In this chapter, we will outline the radiosurgical treatment of MTLE, discuss results in terms of protocols and mechanisms, and compare results between SRS and open surgery approaches. Also, the levels of evidence for major SRS and open surgery series are detailed in ▶ Table 23.1 and ▶ Table 23.2.

Why Consider Stereotactic Radiosurgery for Mesial Temporal Lobe Epilepsy?

Before discussing results and controversies, a reasonable question is "Why should SRS be used when standard techniques may be good enough?" For example, two randomized controlled trials of anterior temporal lobectomy (ATL) rigorously demonstrate that traditional surgery provides marked benefit in terms of seizure remission and quality of life compared to nonsurgical (or, more accurately, delayed surgical) controls.[1,2] However, ATL remains underutilized because of perceived risk, cost, and lack of willingness to seek specialized centers.[3,4] Patients and referring physicians may be reluctant to invoke invasive surgery, leading to delays of definitive treatment. Medical care costs, especially for open surgery requiring intensive care, are considerable. For example, the average cost per patient for treatment of arteriovenous malformation with open microsurgery is nearly 50% more than that with SRS.[5] A "noninvasive" alternative may increase access to and acceptance of epilepsy surgery. No study design yet has compared the merits of SRS to open surgery. At the time of this writing, a randomized controlled trial of open surgery—the Radiosurgery or Open Surgery for Epilepsy (ROSE) trial—is designed to provide this comparison. In this context, we present the results of human trials to date below.

Seizure Remission

The results of trials of SRS for MTLE vary widely in design and in the proportion of patients who achieve seizure remission (▶ Table 23.1). Variations in patient selection, presurgical localization, and targeting probably account more for the variation in primary outcome than any potential variance in biological response.

Stereotactic Radiosurgery

In 1995 Régis et al were the first to apply modern neuroimaging and SRS techniques for the treatment of MTLE.[6] They conducted a subsequent cohort treatment series of seven MTLE patients treated with the Gamma Knife (Elekta AB, Stockholm, Sweden).[7] In this cohort, a target comprising the parahippocampal gyrus, head and anterior body of the hippocampus, and amygdala, comprising an approximate volume of 6.5 mL within the 50% isodose volume, was treated with 25 Gy. Eighty-six percent of patients experienced seizure remission.

These results were countered by later single-center case series or prospective cohort reports.[8–12] With one exception,[11]

Table 23.1 Radiosurgery trials for mesial temporal lobe epilepsy

Study	No. patients	50% isodose (Gy)	Isodose volume (mL)	F/u duration	Rate of seizure remission (%)	Level of evidence
Régis et al[7]	7	25	6.25–6.9	24	86	II
Cmelak et al[8]	1	15	NS	12	0	IV
Kawai et al[9]	2	18	6.2–8.7	18	0	IV
McDonald et al[20]	5	20–24	4.3–5.2	27	0	IV
Srikijvilaikul et al[10]	5	20	6.1–8.7	24	0	II
Régis et al[13]	21	24	5.5–9.0	24	62	II
Prayson et al[12]	4	20	6.1–8.7	18–22	0	IV
Hoggard et al[11]	8	25	6.2 ± 0.7	24	37	II
Vojt ěch et al[15]	14	18–25	5.2–8.9	39	0	III
Barbaro et al[14]	17	20 low dose	5.5–7.0	36	59	I
	13	24 high dose	5.5–7.0	36	77	
Bartolomei et al[16]	15	24	5.5–9.0	60	60	III

Note: *Seizure remission rates defined as Engel class 1. Treatment dose and volumes are estimated at the 50% isodose limit. Follow-up duration is the lower limit or range of reported follow-up.*

* *Linear accelerator (LINAC), dose and volume at 57% isodose limit. Other SRS performed with the Gamma Knife.*

Abbreviations: *f/u, follow-up; NS, not specified; SRS, stereotactic radiosurgery.*

Table 23.2 Selected trials of open surgery for mesial temporal lobe epilepsy

Study	No. patients	Arm	F/u duration	Rate of seizure remission (%)	Level of evidence
Wiebe et al[1]	40	ATL	12	58	I
	40	Best medical	12	8	
Engel et al[2]	15	ATL	24	73	I
	23	Best medical	24	0	
Spencer et al[17]	312	ATL	12	77	II
Sperling et al[18]	89	ATL	60	70	II
Yasargil et al[19]	100	SAH	12	67	II

* *Seizure remission rates defined with Engel class 1.*
Abbreviations: *ATL, anterior temporal lobectomy; SAH, selected amygdala hippocampectomy.*

these trials used doses < 24 to 25 Gy, and rates of seizure remission were low or nil.

Two prospective, multicenter trials followed, including one European[13] and one US.[14] The European trial headed by Régis et al[13] demonstrated a 2-year postoperative seizure remission rate of 62% with the use of the group's published treatment protocol.

The US multicenter pilot study[14] was a prospective study that randomized 30 patients to a high (24 Gy, $n = 13$) or low dose (20 Gy, $n = 17$) delivered to the target as specified by Régis et al.[13] Fifty percent isodose volumes were restricted to 5.5 to 7.0 mL attained with two to six isocenters. Ten patients in each group were seizure free at 36 months' follow-up, resulting in a remission rate of 77% in the high-dose and 59% in the low-dose group, for an overall rate of 67%.

Vojtěch et al conducted a retrospective analysis of 14 patients with markedly different results.[15] Gamma Knife protocols were identical to that reported by Régis et al, and in fact, six of the patients overlapped with the European multicenter trial.[13] Doses decreased with experience; of the 14 patients in the report, the last 6 were treated with 18 Gy because of clinically significant "prominent radiosurgical responses" (large regions of radiation-induced changes) associated with 25 Gy. None of the 14 patients were seizure free after 39 months.

Finally, seizure remission rates were reported by Régis et al for a 15-patient sample with follow-up durations > 5 years.[16] It was not clear if any of these patients overlapped with earlier trials.[7,13] Nine of 15 (60%) remained seizure free, indicating that remission of the majority of patients treated with SRS was durable. Failure of remission was linked with extension of the "epileptic zone" (determined by intracranial electroencephalographic monitoring) beyond the restricted amygdala-hippocampal target.

Open Surgery

Open surgery for MTLE consists of either ATL or selective amygdalohippocampectomy (SAH). In two prospective, randomized trials of ATL compared to waiting list/nonsurgical "best medical management" controls, seizure remission rates after the first 2 years of ATL were 58%[1] and 73%,[2] compared to seizure remission without surgery of 0 to 8%. A sample of prospective cohort studies of ATL[17–19] show seizure remission rates between 70 and 77% (▶ Table 23.2).

In summary, published studies of treatment of SRS report seizure remission rates between 0 and 86%, with larger, multicenter studies reporting seizure remission rates between 62 and 67%. Therefore, seizure remission rates of larger SRS trials with the use of isodoses > 20 Gy are similar to those of standard open surgery. Factors accounting for variability are discussed below.

Secondary Outcomes

Stereotactic Radiosurgery

Neurocognitive and psychological outcomes have been measured at different points of the follow-up period after SRS for MTLE.

Two studies report neurocognitive changes during the period of development of the radiosurgical lesion. McDonald et al evaluated three patients treated on the language-dominant side. They found significant impairment in at least one measure of verbal memory with sparing of intelligence quotient (IQ), visual memory, and language.[20]

The US multicenter pilot study measured cognitive function at 12 months postoperatively (corresponding to the period of maximum radiosurgical edema).[21,22] Verbal memory had no consistent impairments, but tests of cognitive processing speed demonstrated trends of worsening in a dose-dependent fashion.[22] Impairment, however, was not reliably proportional to the volume of edema.[21]

The remainder of data is available for outcomes at 24 months postoperatively (when edema resolves in most patients, leaving atrophic residual tissue).[21] In the European multicenter trial, Régis et al noted no significant cognitive deficits.[13] In fact, 20% of patients experienced some degree of improvement. Only 1 patient out of a total of 21 worsened to a degree considered significant for that trial.

Similar findings were seen in the US multicenter pilot study.[14,22] Impairment occurred in one measure of verbal memory (Wechsler Memory Scale [WMS] or the California Verbal Learning Test [CVLT]) in 25% of patients treated on the language-dominant side when testing was measured in terms of relative change indices (significant score changes beyond that expected from test–retest variability). Conversely, 16% of language-dominant SRS patients experienced improvements.

One study evaluated longer-term secondary outcomes. Bartolomei et al reported that neuropsychological results were stable beyond 5 years (although the exact timing of testing in relationship to the follow-up course was not reported).[16]

Open Surgery

Cognitive outcomes of SRS compare favorably to those of open surgery. Between 10 and 60% of patients who undergo open surgery on the dominant hemisphere demonstrate impairments of verbal learning and memory,[23–26] whereas surgery on the nondominant hemisphere is associated with less consistent declines in visual memory.[27] A multicenter prospective epilepsy surgery trial reported an overall 38% prevalence of verbal memory decline after ATL, with the greatest predictor being side of surgery.[23] The researchers reported that, of dominant hemisphere surgery patients, 40% declined in one measure of verbal memory (either the WMS or CVLT), and another 20% declined in both measures for an overall prevalence of 60%.[23] In the US multicenter pilot study, comparable patients and methods showed a rate of impairment of 25%.[14] Therefore, in comparing studies, the estimated relative risk of verbal memory decline after ATL of the dominant hemisphere is ~ 2.4 times that of SRS. Furthermore, improvements in verbal memory are rare after ATL; for example, verbal memory improved in only 7 of 132 participants (5%).[23] In contrast, 3 of 26 (11%) showed significant improvements following SRS.[14]

One explanation for the preservation of verbal memory after SRS may be the "super-selective" nature of the SRS lesion. Accordingly, some studies show that the more anatomically limited resection (selective amygadalohippocampectomy or partial hippocampectomy) versus more widespread ATL leads to less impairment of verbal memory and other measures of dominant-hemisphere neuropsychological performance,[28,29] although other studies show no clear cognitive advantages with more restricted resection.[30–32]

In summary, SRS in MTLE promises to offer an advantage in cognitive morbidity over open surgery. Comparisons between SRS and open surgery, however, must be undertaken cautiously, as selection criteria, among other factors, make clear comparisons difficult. An ongoing, randomized trial of SRS versus open surgery—the ROSE trial—is designed to directly answer this question (see below).

Safety and Development of the Stereotactic Radiosurgery Lesion

The side effects of SRS for MTLE vary with the development of the radiosurgical lesion. The time course of the SRS lesion and associated symptoms has been well documented. MRI changes after SRS of mesial structures follow a predictable course (with the limitation that no study thus far has systematically obtained MRI from all patients at fixed intervals shorter than 1 year postoperatively). The most striking effects are the development of a dose-dependent T2 hyperintensity, contrast enhancement, and vasogenic edema with mass effect beginning 9 months postoperatively and peaking at 12 months. At 24 months, mass effects resolve, leaving atrophy of the radiosurgical target.[13,21]

Most studies report that the majority of patients experience an increase in the number of auras starting ~ 6 to 8 months and peaking between 9 and 12 months after SRS,[13,21] corresponding to development of MRI changes. The balance between auras (simple partial seizures) and complex partial seizures in duration and severity differs by dose. In studies with higher doses and greater proportions of seizure remission,[13,14] the number of complex partial seizures simultaneously drops with a transient increase in auras. Often, subjects have no complex partial seizures from the time they report the increase in auras. Vojtěch et al described an exacerbation of both auras and complex partial seizures, with auras predominating in lower dose protocols and complex partial seizures in higher dose protocols.[15]

New-onset headaches, occurring in 14%[13] to 70% of patients,[14] do not have predictable timing and can precede or follow changes in aura and seizure frequencies on MRI. They usually respond to steroid therapy.

Because SRS is a surgical technique, some chronic effects of SRS are similar to those of standard surgery. For example, typical "temporal lobe" homonymous visual field defects that are seen after ATL are present after SRS and occur in 43 to 50% of patients.[13,14]

Serious adverse events have also been reported with the use of SRS for MTLE.[10,12,14] One death reported by Prayson et al occurred 2 weeks postradiation, due to "persistent seizure complications." Because radiographic changes occur on the order of months, rather than days, it is unlikely that SRS contributed to this patient's outcome. An autopsy showing mesial temporal sclerosis, but no radiation-induced pathology, supports this interpretation.[12]

Srikijvilaikul et al described one death at 1 month and another at 1 year following SRS.[10] Both were attributed to complications of seizures, consistent with sudden unexplained death in epilepsy (SUDEP).

A protocol-defined severe event was reported by Barbaro et al.[14] Between 12 and 15 months after SRS at 24 Gy, one patient exhibited signs of increasing intracranial pressure (headaches, visual changes, and papilledema). Anterior temporal lobectomy was performed at 15 months, leading to seizure freedom and resolution of symptoms.

Although side effects and adverse events of SRS are important, they should be viewed in light of the rare (but real) complications of open surgery. For example, mortality and visual field changes have been reported in open surgery.[33] Complications include permanent hemiparesis (2%), bleeding requiring transfusion (2.3%), and infection (0.8%).[34,35] SUDEP may appear after open epilepsy surgery as well, although it is rare after seizure remission (as compared to surgery leading only to seizure reduction).[36]

Controversies in Stereotactic Radiosurgery

Trials of SRS for MTLE show a wide variation of clinical efficacies; therefore, differences in protocols and potential mechanisms require discussion.

Target

All studies of MTLE cited above target essentially the same anatomy: the amygdala, anterior hippocampus, and parahippocampal gyrus, regions corresponding to anatomical structures found important in seizure remission following resection.[37] However, those patients with "epileptogenic zones" that extend beyond those traditionally attributed to MTLE may not be good SRS candidates. For example, seizure remission is less in cases with extended epileptogenic zones because of the highly restricted field of SRS.[38] An analogue to this finding after SRS is proposed to account for the association between the volume of resected tissue after ATL and higher rates of seizure remission.[32]

Therefore, probably one factor accounting for variation of outcomes among studies is patient selection; the high selectivity of the SRS is best matched with a precisely defined target that has a restricted epileptic network. Classic MTLE without involvement of the epileptic zone outside the unilateral limbic target so far appears to be the only syndrome with well-documented response to SRS.

Isodose Centers

No data are available for determining the number of isodose centers ("shots") that best comprise the treatment volume for MTLE. Based on Régis et al's preliminary studies[6] (all of which were limited to two shots), Barbaro et al specified a range of two to six shots in the US multicenter pilot study.[14] In the ongoing randomized trial of SRS for MTLE (ROSE trial), restrictions on isocenter (i.e., shot number) have been lifted to promote conformal targeting.

Volume

The 50% isodose volumes of the radiosurgical target typically range between 6.0 and 8.5 mL. Régis et al in preliminary studies determined that there was a narrow window of ineffective anticonvulsant effect versus excessive toxicity in terms of volume of maximum radiation edema at 12 months postoperatively.[39] On this basis, Barbaro et al specified treatment volumes limited to 5.5 to 7.5 mL in their studies.[14]

Dose

Of the various parameters, dose appears to be best correlated to outcome and is the only variable studied by randomized control methods. In the US multicenter pilot study, patients randomized to 24 Gy had a higher proportion of seizure remission than those treated with 20 Gy (a finding tempered by the lack of statistical power).[14] As comparison across the studies in ▶ Table 23.1 suggests, 20 Gy appears to serve as a threshold at or over which seizure remission is most likely to occur.

Insufficient dose, probably greater or equal in importance to patient selection, may account not only for variation in seizure remission among trials, but also for severity of side effects. As discussed above, lower dose treatment plans are associated with greater durations and higher incidences of exacerbation of auras that typically arise in the second half of the first postoperative year.[14,15,21]

■ Mechanisms

A coherent mechanism has not been demonstrated that accounts for the anticonvulsant (and occasionally, proconvulsant) effects of SRS. Fundamental to SRS is the stripping of electrons (ionization) resulting in the alteration of chemical bonds or the production of free radicals.[40,41] Susceptibility to ionization is proportional to DNA synthesis. Neurons, therefore, are relatively radioresistant; actively proliferating cells, such as capillary cells, are radiosensitive. Furthermore, although animal models of epilepsy (usually rats) are helpful in evaluating mechanisms, rat brains are remarkably radioresistant, and "scaling up" directly to humans to predict dose is not straightforward.

Neuromodulation

Studies with rat models of limbic epilepsy emphasize that an anticonvulsant effect may arise from a nondestructive dose. For example, a dose-dependent reduction in seizures was shown in kainic acid–treated epileptic rats[42,43] and in electrical-stimulation epileptic rats,[44] despite the lack of gross neuronal injury. Cognitive functions are spared; for example, water maze performance is unimpaired after treatment.[42,43]

These nondestructive "neuromodulatory effects"[45,46] were further evaluated with SRS of normal rats. Fifty Gy isodoses induce different amplitudes and timing of changes in neuronal enzymes, raising the possibility of a differential susceptibility. Tsuchitani et al reported that, in hippocampi of normal rats treated with 40 Gy, the numbers of nonspecific neurons of the hippocampus remained unchanged, but both calbindin-staining interneurons (excitatory) and glutamic acid decarboxylase (GAD)–staining interneurons (inhibitory) were substantially decreased.[47]

Kindling experiments demonstrate that SRS may have different neuromodulatory effects, depending on whether normal or kindled circuitry is involved.[48] Three groups of rats were treated with hippocampal SRS at different times of a kindling protocol. Relative to controls, the occurrence of severe seizures is increased by irradiation before kindling, but it is unaffected by irradiation at midcourse and significantly is reduced by irradiation at the final stage of kindling. Thus, kindled epileptic tissue may lack plasticity and the ability to recover from irradiation. Other experiments with the use of more widespread radiation doses (analogous to traditional fractionated radiotherapy) support the hypothesis that irradiation causes defects in neurogenesis and plasticity. For example, Tan et al demonstrated that low doses (0.5–6 Gy) in normal rats induce an 80% decrement in neuronal precursor cells in the dentate gyrus.[49] Lower doses allow a compensatory proliferation of neuronal precursors during recovery, but higher doses completely block compensatory proliferation.

Neuromodulatory effects, however, may not be entirely beneficial. Sometimes proconvulsant effects are observed, as outlined in animal experiments noted above in which kindled seizures worsened in animals treated before kindling compared to those treated after kindling.[48] This point is emphasized by results of low-dose human protocols—perhaps designed to emulate nondestructive doses in animal models—that demonstrate transient exacerbations in auras or sometimes complex partial seizures.[15,21]

Neuronal Destruction

In contrast to neuromodulatory mechanisms, other data in both animal models and human epilepsy suggest that necrotic changes in the target zone better account for the anticonvulsant effects as seen in more successful protocols. MRI and mass spectroscopy[21] data from the US multicenter pilot study showed that the volume of contrast enhancement and T2 hyperintensity seen on MRI obtained 12 months after SRS correlated strongly with outcome. No patients with T2-weighted volumes of edema < 200 mL at 12 months went on to experience seizure remission between 24 and 36 months.[21] Furthermore, magnetic resonance spectroscopy (MRS) within the target zone shows evidence of frank ischemia; 1 year after SRS, lactate (evidence of anaerobic metabolism) appears, and choline, creatine, and *N*-acetylaspartate (NAA) levels (evidence of normal neuronal activity) are largely absent.[21] Similar findings of decreased markers of neuronal activity were observed with MRS > 1 year after SRS in a trial of six patients (without seizure responses results reported).[50]

Although animal models of epilepsy cited above do not demonstrate necrosis of tissue, one explanation is that they would have if followed for a sufficient duration after SRS. Hippocampi irradiated > 50 Gy in normal rats and followed for more than 6 months (longer than durations of Maesawa et al[42,43] or Chen et al[44]) show evidence of neuronal destruction.[51]

SRS probably causes necrosis through changes in vasculature rather than direct effects on neurons. Kamiryo et al[52] showed that rat brains treated with SRS at 75 Gy and examined 3 months later had, through the method of vascular casting, a markedly decreased vascular density. Electron microscopy demonstrated thickening of the vascular basement membrane. These vascular changes preceded development of necrosis within the radiosurgical target.

Human histology (as opposed to MRS data) is difficult to interpret because tissue is obtained from failed rather than successful SRS in the course of a "rescue" ATL. For example, patients who underwent open surgery after failed SRS demonstrated hippocampal sclerosis and "radiational changes" in operative samples.[10] In the US multicenter pilot study, the patient who underwent ATL for steroid-dependent symptoms (and who was seizure-free for ~ 3 months before open surgery) was found to have hippocampal sclerosis, as well as evidence of chronic infarcts with prominent hyalinization, thickening, and closure of small vessels. Similar findings—necrosis with evidence of vascular damage—were seen in four patients who had ATL between 18 and 22 months after SRS.[12] Therefore, limited data from human histopathology show that ischemic changes predominate after failed SRS.

Core and Penumbra: Combined Neuromodulatory and Destructive Effects

Clinical data suggest that the two mechanisms discussed above —neuromodulation and neuronal destruction—may not be mutually exclusive. For example, patients in the US multicenter pilot study were asked to describe the symptoms of their typical auras, which in turn were classified as originating from "mesial" or "nonmesial" structures, as validated by previous studies of auras recorded with intracranial monitoring.[53–55] At baseline, most patients had mesial auras. During the peak SRS effect at 12 months, corresponding to development of a penumbra of edema surrounding an ischemic core, mesial auras increased further. After resolution of the SRS lesion and simultaneous decrease in complex partial seizures, mesial auras decreased, and nonmesial auras increased. The inversion of proportion with mesial versus nonmesial auras, along with the decrease in complex partial seizures, suggests that successful SRS of the limbic system for MTLE causes a heterogeneous lesion: a core within the SRS target that includes destructive ischemia and a penumbra of tissue exposed to less intense, "neuromodulated" radiation. The "cockade" theory (after the concentric rosettes once fastened on military hats), originally proposed by Régis et al,[46] may be further characterized in ongoing trials of SRS.

Conclusion

Clinical trials of SRS for MTLE show mixed results. Protocols that depend on higher doses of SRS result in seizure remission rates within ranges reported for standard open surgery. Safety of SRS appears reasonable, tempered by exacerbations of auras or incomplete or delayed effects observed in low-dose protocols. SRS may yield postoperative cognitive sparing, a feature of a highly selective, small-volume, surgical lesion.

An ongoing multicenter trial, the ROSE trial, randomizes patients to either ATL or SRS and will compare seizure remission, cognitive outcomes, and cost. Not only will final outcomes (determined during the course of the last year of the 3-year follow-up period) be measured, but serial, interim measures in patient safety, quality of life, mood, and health care utilization will be compared between the two groups.

References

[1] Wiebe S, Blume WT, Girvin JP, Eliasziw M. Effectiveness and Efficiency of Surgery for Temporal Lobe Epilepsy Study Group. A randomized, controlled trial of surgery for temporal-lobe epilepsy. N Engl J Med 2001; 345: 311–318

[2] Engel J, McDermott MP, Wiebe S, et al. Early Randomized Surgical Epilepsy Trial (ERSET) Study Group. Early surgical therapy for drug-resistant temporal lobe epilepsy: a randomized trial. JAMA 2012; 307: 922–930

[3] Lhatoo SD, Solomon JK, McEvoy AW, Kitchen ND, Shorvon SD, Sander JW. A prospective study of the requirement for and the provision of epilepsy surgery in the United Kingdom. Epilepsia 2003; 44: 673–676

[4] Benbadis SR, Heriaud L, Tatum WO, Vale FL. Epilepsy surgery, delays and referral patterns: are all your epilepsy patients controlled? Seizure 2003; 12: 167–170

[5] Wellis G, Nagel R, Vollmar C, Steiger HJ. Direct costs of microsurgical management of radiosurgically amenable intracranial pathology in Germany: an analysis of meningiomas, acoustic neuromas, metastases and arteriovenous malformations of less than 3 cm in diameter. Acta Neurochir (Wien) 2003; 145: 249–255

[6] Régis J, Peragui JC, Rey M, et al. First selective amygdalohippocampal radiosurgery for 'mesial temporal lobe epilepsy'. Stereotact Funct Neurosurg 1995; 64 (Suppl 1): 193–201

[7] Régis J, Bartolomei F, Rey M, et al. Gamma Knife surgery for mesial temporal lobe epilepsy. Epilepsia 1999; 40: 1551–1556

[8] Cmelak AJ, Abou-Khalil B, Konrad PE, Duggan D, Maciunas RJ. Low-dose stereotactic radiosurgery is inadequate for medically intractable mesial temporal lobe epilepsy: a case report. Seizure 2001; 10: 442–446

[9] Kawai K, Suzuki I, Kurita H, Shin M, Arai N, Kirino T. Failure of low-dose radiosurgery to control temporal lobe epilepsy. J Neurosurg 2001; 95: 883–887

[10] Srikijvilaikul T, Najm I, Foldvary-Schaefer N, Lineweaver T, Suh JH, Bingaman WE. Failure of gamma knife radiosurgery for mesial temporal lobe epilepsy: report of five cases. Neurosurgery 2004; 54: 1395–1402, discussion 1402–1404

[11] Hoggard N, Wilkinson ID, Griffiths PD, Vaughan P, Kemeny AA, Rowe JG. The clinical course after stereotactic radiosurgical amygdalohippocampectomy with neuroradiological correlates. Neurosurgery 2008; 62: 336–344, discussion 344–346

[12] Prayson RA, Yoder BJ. Clinicopathologic findings in mesial temporal sclerosis treated with Gamma Knife radiotherapy. Ann Diagn Pathol 2007; 11: 22–26

[13] Régis J, Rey M, Bartolomei F, et al. Gamma Knife surgery in mesial temporal lobe epilepsy: a prospective multicenter study. Epilepsia 2004; 45: 504–515

[14] Barbaro NM, Quigg M, Broshek DK, et al. A multicenter, prospective pilot study of Gamma Knife radiosurgery for mesial temporal lobe epilepsy: seizure response, adverse events, and verbal memory. Ann Neurol 2009; 65: 167–175

[15] Vojtěch Z, Vladyka V, Kalina M, et al. The use of radiosurgery for the treatment of mesial temporal lobe epilepsy and long-term results. Epilepsia 2009; 50: 2061–2071

[16] Bartolomei F, Hayashi M, Tamura M, et al. Long-term efficacy of Gamma Knife radiosurgery in mesial temporal lobe epilepsy. Neurology 2008; 70: 1658–1663

[17] Spencer SS, Berg AT, Vickrey BG, et al. Multicenter Study of Epilepsy Surgery. Initial outcomes in the Multicenter Study of Epilepsy Surgery. Neurology 2003; 61: 1680–1685

[18] Sperling MR, O'Connor MJ, Saykin AJ, Plummer C. Temporal lobectomy for refractory epilepsy. JAMA 1996; 276: 470–475

[19] Yaşargil MG, Wieser HG, Valavanis A, von Ammon K, Roth P. Surgery and results of selective amygdala-hippocampectomy in one hundred patients with nonlesional limbic epilepsy. Neurosurg Clin N Am 1993; 4: 243–261

[20] McDonald CR, Norman MA, Tecoma E, Alksne J, Iragui V. Neuropsychological change following Gamma Knife surgery in patients with left temporal lobe epilepsy: a review of three cases. Epilepsy Behav 2004; 5: 949–957

[21] Chang EF, Quigg M, Oh MC, et al. Epilepsy Radiosurgery Study Group. Predictors of efficacy after stereotactic radiosurgery for medial temporal lobe epilepsy. Neurology 2010; 74: 165–172

[22] Quigg M, Broshek DK, Barbaro NM, et al. Radiosurgery Epilepsy Study Group. Neuropsychological outcomes after Gamma Knife radiosurgery for mesial temporal lobe epilepsy: a prospective multicenter study. Epilepsia 2011; 52: 909–916

[23] Stroup E, Langfitt J, Berg M, McDermott M, Pilcher W, Como P. Predicting verbal memory decline following anterior temporal lobectomy (ATL). Neurology 2003; 60: 1266–1273

[24] Hermann BP, Wyler AR, Bush AJ, Tabatabai FR. Differential effects of left and right anterior temporal lobectomy on verbal learning and memory performance. Epilepsia 1992; 33: 289–297

[25] Hermann BP, Seidenberg M, Dohan FC, et al. Reports by patients and their families of memory change after left anterior temporal lobectomy: relationship to degree of hippocampal sclerosis. Neurosurgery 1995; 36: 39–44, discussion 44–45

[26] Chelune GJ, Najm IM. Risk factors associated with postusurgical decrements in memory decline after anterior temporal lobectomy. In: Luders HO, Comair Y, eds. Epilepsy Surgery. 2nd ed. Philadelphia, PA: Raven; 2000:497–504

[27] Meador KJ. Cognitive outcomes and predictive factors in epilepsy. Neurology 2002; 58 (Suppl 5): S21–S26

[28] Clusmann H, Schramm J, Kral T, et al. Prognostic factors and outcome after different types of resection for temporal lobe epilepsy. J Neurosurg 2002; 97: 1131–1141

[29] Helmstaedter C, Kurthen M, Lux S, Reuber M, Elger CE. Chronic epilepsy and cognition: a longitudinal study in temporal lobe epilepsy. Ann Neurol 2003; 54: 425–432

[30] Jones-Gotman M, Zatorre RJ, Olivier A, et al. Learning and retention of words and designs following excision from medial or lateral temporal-lobe structures. Neuropsychologia 1997; 35: 963–973

[31] Wyler AR, Hermann BP, Somes G. Extent of medial temporal resection on outcome from anterior temporal lobectomy: a randomized prospective study. Neurosurgery 1995; 37: 982–990, discussion 990–991

[32] Shamim S, Wiggs E, Heiss J, et al. Temporal lobectomy: resection volume, neuropsychological effects, and seizure outcome. Epilepsy Behav 2009; 16: 311–314

[33] Engel JJ, Van Ness P, Rasmussen T. Outcome with respect to epileptic seizures. In: Engel JJ, ed. Surgical Treatment of the Epilepsies. 2nd ed. New York, NY: Raven Press; 1993:609–621

[34] Engel J. Update on surgical treatment of the epilepsies: summary of the Second International Palm Desert Conference on the Surgical Treatment of the Epilepsies (1992). Neurology 1993; 43: 1612–1617

[35] McClelland S, Guo H, Okuyemi KS. Population-based analysis of morbidity and mortality following surgery for intractable temporal lobe epilepsy in the United States. Arch Neurol 2011; 68: 725–729

[36] Sperling MR, Feldman H, Kinman J, Liporace JD, O'Connor MJ. Seizure control and mortality in epilepsy. Ann Neurol 1999; 46: 45–50

[37] Siegel AM, Wieser HG, Wichmann W, Yasargil GM. Relationships between MR-imaged total amount of tissue removed, resection scores of specific mediobasal limbic subcompartments and clinical outcome following selective amygdalohippocampectomy. Epilepsy Res 1990; 6: 56–65

[38] Rheims S, Fischer C, Ryvlin P, et al. Long-term outcome of Gamma Knife surgery in temporal lobe epilepsy. Epilepsy Res 2008; 80: 23–29

[39] Quigg M, Rolston J, Barbaro NM. Radiosurgery for epilepsy: clinical experience and potential antiepileptic mechanisms. Epilepsia 2012; 53: 7–15

[40] Khan FM. The Physics of Radiation Therapy. 4th ed. Philadelphia, PA: Lippincott Williams & Wilkins; 2010

[41] Haffty BG, Wilson LD, eds. Handbook of Radiation Oncology: Basic Principles and Clinical Protocols. Sudbury, MA: Jones & Bartlett; 2009

[42] Maesawa S, Kondziolka D, Balzer J, Fellows W, Dixon E, Lunsford LD. The behavioral and electroencephalographic effects of stereotactic radiosurgery for the treatment of epilepsy evaluated in the rat kainic acid model. Stereotact Funct Neurosurg 1999; 73: 115

[43] Maesawa S, Kondziolka D, Dixon CE, Balzer J, Fellows W, Lunsford LD. Subnecrotic stereotactic radiosurgery controlling epilepsy produced by kainic acid injection in rats. J Neurosurg 2000; 93: 1033–1040

[44] Chen ZF, Kamiryo T, Henson SL, et al. Anticonvulsant effects of Gamma surgery in a model of chronic spontaneous limbic epilepsy in rats. J Neurosurg 2001; 94: 270–280

[45] Régis J, Bartolomei F, Hayashi M, Chauvel P. Gamma Knife surgery, a neuromodulation therapy in epilepsy surgery! Acta Neurochir Suppl (Wien) 2002; 84: 37–47

[46] Régis J, Carron R, Park M. Is radiosurgery a neuromodulation therapy? A 2009 Fabrikant award lecture. J Neurooncol 2010; 98: 155–162

[47] Tsuchitani S, Drummond J, Kamiryo T, et al. Selective vulnerability of interneurons to low dosage radiosurgery [abstract]. Presented at the annual meeting of the Society for Neuroscience Annual Meeting; November 9–13 2003; New Orleans, LA

[48] Jenrow KA, Ratkewicz AE, Zalinski DN, Roszka KM, Lemke NW, Elisevich KV. Influence of ionizing radiation on the course of kindled epileptogenesis. Brain Res 2006; 1094: 207–216

[49] Tan YF, Rosenzweig S, Jaffray D, Wojtowicz JM. Depletion of new neurons by image guided irradiation. Front Neurosci 2011; 5: 59

[50] Hájek M, Dezortová M, Liscák R, Vymazal J, Vladyka V. 1 H MR spectroscopy of mesial temporal lobe epilepsies treated with Gamma Knife. Eur Radiol 2003; 13: 994–1000

[51] Liscák R, Vladyka V, Novotný J, et al. Leksell Gamma Knife lesioning of the rat hippocampus: the relationship between radiation dose and functional and structural damage. J Neurosurg 2002; 97 (Suppl): 666–673

[52] Kamiryo T, Lopes MB, Kassell NF, Steiner L, Lee KS. Radiosurgery-induced microvascular alterations precede necrosis of the brain neuropil. Neurosurgery 2001; 49: 409–414, discussion 414–415

[53] Maillard L, Vignal JP, Gavaret M, et al. Semiologic and electrophysiologic correlations in temporal lobe seizure subtypes. Epilepsia 2004; 45: 1590–1599

[54] Vignal JP, Maillard L, McGonigal A, Chauvel P. The dreamy state: hallucinations of autobiographic memory evoked by temporal lobe stimulations and seizures. Brain 2007; 130: 88–99

[55] Binder DK, Garcia PA, Elangovan GK, Barbaro NM. Characteristics of auras in patients undergoing temporal lobectomy. J Neurosurg 2009; 111: 1283–1289

Spinal Cord Tolerance

24 Preclinical Studies of Radiosurgical Tolerance of the Spinal Cord

Paul M. Medin, Ryan D. Foster, Timothy D. Solberg, and Arjun Sahgal

Introduction

Clinical implementation of spinal stereotactic body radiotherapy (SBRT) has increased rapidly in recent years.[1] Reports of clinical spinal cord toxicity following SBRT are rare but emerging. Recently, several cases of radiation-induced myelopathy have been reported with dosimetric analysis;[2,3] however, little is known regarding human normal tissue tolerance in the setting of SBRT. The sparse human toxicity data are confounded by the fact that the dose levels observed to cause spinal cord myelopathy are largely inconsistent with reports of patients who received much greater doses without toxicity,[4,5] emphasizing the need to determine risk-based probabilities of radiation myelopathy. We do not currently have these data to guide clinical practice.

Preclinical studies applicable to spine SBRT have been conducted since the 1970s, providing the overwhelming majority of data regarding spinal cord tolerance.[6] Despite the availability of preclinical data, the direct clinical application of the tolerance doses (and tolerance principles) derived from animal studies remains controversial. In this chapter, we review the literature regarding spinal cord tolerance in preclinical models as well as in humans for the purpose of evaluating the strength of correlation. Data regarding spinal cord tolerance to protracted (more than five fractions) irradiation regimens is beyond the scope of this chapter and has been excluded unless specifically identified.

Caveats of Preclinical Studies

Preclinical models provide an essential means for testing biological limits that carry a high risk of morbidity before clinical trials are developed. The relevance of a model to human biology and an understanding of the limitations of animal studies are crucial to the interpretation of their results. When a preclinical spinal cord tolerance study is evaluated for potential application to humans, the following questions need to be asked: (1) How many animals were studied?, (2) Was the follow-up period long enough?, (3) Do the animals have comorbidities?, (4) Did the animals receive additional or previous therapies?, (5) How were the study end points assessed?, and (6) Were the experimental conditions consistent with human clinical practice?

Preclinical studies are designed to minimize the number of animals involved while maintaining the reliability of results. Dose-response curves are commonly derived from four to seven dose groups with four or five subjects per group; thus, conclusions are drawn for a population from the response of a limited number of animals.[6] The reader is always compelled to consider the margin of error, which is usually reported as a 95% confidence interval (CI) or as standard error, in any study. Animal studies frequently employ a follow-up period that is either shorter than the possible latency of the morbidity or life expectancy of the corresponding human population. Exceptions exist, but most spinal cord tolerance studies include a follow-up period of 12 months or less, whereas latency for human myelopathy has been described with a bimodal distribution peaking at approximately 9 and 26 months.[7] Two distinct pathologies with differing latencies have also been noted in the rat model; white matter necrosis usually occurs in less than 8 months, whereas vascular injury can lead to paralysis between 8 and 18 months.[8] The authors of a pig study with 70- and 110-week follow-up reported that the latency for myelopathy was 7.5 to 16.0 weeks; however, two pigs experienced late myelopathy at 64.5 and 75.0 weeks postirradiation.[9] The only lesion found in the late-responding pigs was an 80% occlusion of the main ventral artery. In contrast, only a single phase of latencies has been observed for rhesus monkeys.[7]

Long-term follow-up is desirable for clinically oriented studies, but few investigators have been afforded the resources to make this possible. In contrast to the majority of patients who receive spine radiosurgery, preclinical spinal cord tolerance studies are performed in young, healthy animals without comorbidity or previous therapies. The effects of previous therapies on spinal cord tolerance are unknown but have been questioned in the human spine radiosurgery literature.[10] Preclinical studies of spinal cord tolerance commonly include functional and histopathologic end points. The assessment of functional response is limited compared to humans. Although methods to assess sensory neurologic deficits in animals have been reported,[11,12] practical challenges and the associated pitfalls limit their reliability; therefore, evaluation of function is commonly limited to motor neurologic changes as determined by observation of gait.

In contrast to clinical studies, histologic end points are readily evaluable in preclinical studies and could potentially have greater sensitivity than functional end points in animal models. The correlation of histologic and functional end points is variable. Gait change has been reported to correlate completely with the presence of histologic change in one pig study,[13] but studies in rats and pigs have reported a deviation between gait response and histologic response.[14,15] Finally, the similarity between preclinical and clinical experimental conditions should be questioned. For example, dose rate and anesthesia have been observed to modify spinal cord tolerance in preclinical studies. Scalliet et al observed that the median effective dose (ED_{50}) for paralysis in rats increased from 21.3 to > 45.0 Gy as the dose rate was reduced from 107.6 to 2.0 Gy/h.[16] The use of anesthesia in preclinical trials may also affect outcomes. Van der Kogel reported a decrease of 2.0 to 2.5 Gy in ED_{50} values for rats receiving single-dose irradiation with 1% halothane/99% O_2 versus intraperitoneal injection of sodium pentobarbital (60 mg/kg).[17]

Clinically Relevant Phenomena Discovered through Preclinical Studies

Preclinical studies have been performed to investigate many phenomena of spinal cord tolerance, including the influence of irradiated length, dose distribution, previous irradiation, irradiated region, dose rate, and irradiation of the adjacent spinal cord. The majority of preclinical studies have focused on the tolerance of the spinal cord to single-fraction irradiation, but multifraction regimens have also been studied, primarily in the setting of reirradiation. Irradiated length, dose distribution, and previous irradiation are summarized here.

Before a review of more complex spinal cord tolerance phenomena, animal response observed under simple experimental conditions requires discussion. A summary of spinal cord tolerance studies that have been performed under conditions of uniform irradiation to lengths ≥ 16 mm is presented in ▶ Table 24.1. The outcomes of studies that incorporate uniform irradiation are very consistent, spanning both multiple radiation modalities (X-rays, ^{60}Co, and protons) and multiple mammalian species (rat, guinea pig, mouse, and pig). The dose-response curves for rats, guinea pigs, mice, and pigs are all very steep and have similar ED_{50}'s clustered around 20 Gy. It should be noted that, although Scalliet et al[16] and van den Aardweg et al[18] reported ED_{50}'s that are significantly > 20 Gy, these animals were irradiated at low dose rates, which demonstrates that rats and pigs share a similar change in response as the dose rate is reduced. The radiation tolerance of the spinal cord has been observed to increase dramatically as the dose rate is decreased below the range typically delivered by current linear accelerators (LINACs).[6,16]

The influence of the length of the spinal cord irradiated on dose response is among the earliest and most broadly investigated phenomena,[19] with reports from three groups, including three radiation modalities and two animal models (▶ Table 24.2). Hopewell et al irradiated rat spinal cords with 250-kV X-rays to lengths of 0.4, 0.8, or 1.6 cm and observed a decrease in ED_{50} from 51.0 ± 2.3 Gy to 21.3 ± 0.3 Gy as the length increased.[20] Bijl et al irradiated rat spinal cords with 150- to 190-MeV protons to lengths ranging from 0.2 cm to 2.0 cm and observed that ED_{50} (95% CI) decreased from 87.8 Gy (80.4–96.4 Gy) to 20.4 Gy.[21] However, van den Aardweg et al irradiated pig spinal cords to lengths of 2.5, 5.0, and 10.0 cm

Table 24.1 Dose response for four species (uniform irradiation, length > 16 mm)

Study	Species	Dose rate (Gy/h)	Source	ED_{50} (Gy)
Lo et al.[36]	Mouse	155	250-kV X-ray	18.9 (17.8–19.9)*
Hopewell et al[20]	Rat	Not stated; radiation technique similar to Lo et al	250-kV X-rray	21.5 ± 0.3 SE
Wong et al[26]	Rat	148.8	100-kV X-ray	19.0 (18.5–19.3)*
Scalliet et al[16]	Rat	107.6	^{60}Co	21.3 (20.2–22.2)*
Scalliet et al[16]	Rat	14.7	^{60}Co	27.2 (26.2–28.2)*
Bijl et al[21]	Rat	600–900	150–190 MeV proton	20.4 (no error estimate)
Knowles[25,37]	Guinea pig	65.4	250-kV X-ray	20.5 (no error estimate)
Van den Aardweg et al[18]	Pig	12.6–18	^{60}Co	28.3 ± 0.8 SE
Medin et al[38]	Pig	228–378	6 MeV X-ray	20.2 Gy (19.1–25.8)*

* Ninety-five percent confidence interval.
Abbreviations: ^{60}Co, cobalt 60; ED_{50}, median effective dose; SE, standard error.
Source: Adapted from Medin PM, Boike TP. Spinal cord tolerance in the age of spinal radiosurgery: lessons from preclinical studies. Int J Radiat Oncol Biol Phys 2011;79(5):1302–1309, with permission.

Table 24.2 Longitudinally homogeneous dose response (length effect)

Study	Species	Location	Source	Length (cm)	ED_{50}
Bijl et al[21]	Rat	Cervical	150–190 MeV protons	0.2 0.4 0.8 2.0	87.8 (80.4–96.4)* 53.7 (49.2–61.9)* 24.9 (21.6–28.6)* 20.4
Hopewel, et al[20]	Rat	Cervical-thoracic	250 kV X-ray	0.4 0.8 1.6	50.98 (2.28) SE 30.11 (1.45) SE 21.5 (0.3) SE
Van den Aardweg et al[18]	Pig	Cervical	^{60}Co	2.5 5.0 10.0	28.28 (0.78) SE 27.68 (0.57) SE 27.02 (0.36) SE

* Ninety-five percent confidence interval.
Abbreviations: ^{60}Co, cobalt 60; ED_{50}, median effective dose; SE, standard error.
Source: From Medin PM, Boike TP. Spinal cord tolerance in the age of spinal radiosurgery: lessons from preclinical studies. Int J Radiat Oncol Biol Phys 2011;79(5):1302–1309, with permission.

using a cobalt 60 source and observed no appreciable change in response.[18] Independent confirmation of the "length effect" in these two rat studies and additional data for increased lengths in the pig provide convincing evidence that the length of spinal cord irradiated modifies the radiation response for lengths < 1.6 cm, whereas dose response is approximately constant for lengths > 1.6 cm.

The existence of a lateral dose-volume effect (modification of response by changing the dose distribution across the spinal cord in the lateral direction) remains a topic for continued debate. The lateral dose-volume effect has been studied in both rats and pigs with conflicting conclusions. Van Luijk et al used a 150-MeV proton beam to create an extremely steep dose gradient (100% to < 10% isodose) across the spinal cords of rats in the right/left direction.[22] An ED_{50} (95% CI) of 30 Gy (26.3–31.3 Gy) was observed for motor neurologic deficit compared to an ED_{50} of 20.4 Gy (19.6–21.1 Gy) for uniform cross-section irradiation. A more extensive follow-up study by the same group affirmed the lateral volume effect and demonstrated that the lateral white matter is much more radiosensitive than the central part of the white matter.[23] Medin et al (additional unpublished data under review for publication) sought to reproduce these rat studies in a pig model using a clinical 6-MV image-guided LINAC to determine if the physical dimensions of the spinal cord affect recovery from radiation damage.[13] A steep right/left dose gradient was created (95–10% isodose across the spinal cord) similar to van Luijk et al;[22] however, the diameter of the pig cervical spinal cord is ~ 3 × that of a rat (the spinal cord diameter is 8–11 mm for a pig vs 3.5 mm for a rat). No dose-volume effect was observed in pigs for the dose distributions studied; however, partial spinal cord irradiation resulted in less debilitating neurologic and histopathologic morbidity. The maximum point dose to the spinal cord was the parameter that best predicted the risk of motor neurologic deficit.

Spinal cord tolerance to reirradiation in the setting of SBRT has been investigated using rats, pigs, and guinea pigs in many different study designs, including (1) split dose, (2) single dose following conventional fractionation, (3) single dose following multifraction SBRT, and (4) various fractionation schemes following SBRT. Ruifrok et al performed split-dose studies in the cervical spines of 3-week-old rats.[24] Animals were irradiated by one of two schedules: (1) initial dose of 12 Gy, followed by reirradiation at 1, 3, or 6 months; or (2) initial dose of 14.9 Gy, followed by reirradiation at 1 day, 14 days, 1 month, 3 months, or 6 months. Over a follow-up period of 200 days, it was observed that the ED_{50} increased most quickly in the first month following irradiation and continued to increase up to 6 months. Reirradiation tolerance never fully recovered after 6 months with an ED_{50} of ~ 17 Gy compared to 21 Gy for nonirradiated spinal cord. It was observed in a companion study that 18-week-old rats experience significant recovery between 2 and 6 months and that the maximum extent of recovery is greater than that for the 3-week-old rats. Knowles investigated reirradiation tolerance using guinea pigs.[25] One-day-old guinea pigs received a single 10-Gy dose followed 1 year later by another single dose. The ED_{50} for paralysis for re-treated animals (19.5 Gy) was only slightly lower than animals treated de novo (20.5 Gy) at 1 year of age. Wong et al[26–28] used multiple study designs to investigate reirradiation tolerance involving SBRT dose schemes. In one study, rats were reirradiated with a single fraction 20 weeks after increasing numbers of 2.15-Gy fractions were delivered,[26] as presented in ▶ Table 24.3. Reirradiation tolerance decreased from 19.0 to 11.8 Gy as the total initial dose was increased from 0 to 77.4 Gy. In a second study, rats were reirradiated with a single fraction at various time points after an initial regimen of two or three large fractions,[28] as presented in ▶ Table 24.4. As observed in the first study, reirradiation tolerance decreased as the initial radiation dose increased, and the phenomenon of increasing recovery with increasing time to reirradiation was also demonstrated. In a third study, Wong et al reirradiated rats with various fractionation schemes 20 weeks after an initial regimen of 9 Gy × 3, as presented in ▶ Table 24.5.[27] Reirradiation tolerance was observed to increase from 14.0 to 47.8 Gy as the number of re-treatment fractions was increased from 1 to 20 fractions. Medin et al irradiated pigs with a single fraction 1 year following irradiation with 3 Gy × 10 fractions.[15] It was observed that pigs receiving spine radiosurgery 1 year following 30 Gy in 10 fractions are not at significantly higher risk of developing motor deficits than pigs that receive radiosurgery alone. Although none of the preclinical studies of spinal cord tolerance to reirradiation include identical study designs, and recovery estimates vary somewhat, all studies conclude that the spinal cord does indeed possess the ability to recover from radiation injury.

Table 24.3 Rat tolerance to single-fraction reirradiation 20 weeks after conventional fractionation

Initial dose	ED_{50} (Gy)*
Zero	19.0
2.15 Gy × 10	17.0
2.15 Gy × 20	15.7
2.15 Gy × 30	14.0
2.15 Gy × 36	11.8

* Ninety-five percent confidence intervals reported only in graph form.
Abbreviation: ED_{50}, median effective dose.
Source: Adapted from Wong CS, Poon JK, Hill RP. Re-irradiation tolerance in the rat spinal cord: influence of level of initial damage. Radiother Oncol 1993;26:132–138.

Caveats of Clinical Reports

Preclinical studies are performed on anesthetized animal subjects under controlled conditions, but human clinical practice is much less predictable. Doses reported in clinical case reports are derived from treatment plans and represent only the actual dose delivered under ideal conditions. Uncertainties in patient positioning, together with the potential for patient motion, result in uncertainty in reported doses. Slight shifts in patient position can result in large deviations from the planned spinal cord dose due to the steep dose gradients that are common in spinal SBRT treatment plans.[29] Dose uncertainties usually are not addressed in case reports. A comprehensive review of the factors that affect the spinal cord dose delivered during SBRT is provided in Chapter 26 of this book.

Table 24.4 Rat tolerance to single-fraction reirradiation after initial SBRT doses

Initial Tx	Time to Re-Tx	ED_{50} (95% confidence interval) (Gy)
9 Gy × 2	1 day	14.1 (12.5–15.6)
	8 weeks	14.8 (12.2–17.3)
	12 weeks	15.4 (14.9–15.8)
	20 weeks	16.3 (16.0–16.7)
	28 weeks	16.2 (15.8–16.7)
9 Gy × 3	1 day	10.0 (9.2–10.8)
	6 weeks	9.9 (9.4–10.4)
	8 weeks	9.8 (8.4–11.2)
	12 weeks	12.0 (11.5–12.6)
	20 weeks	13.9 (13.3-–14.5)
	28 weeks	14.6 (13.9–15.3)
	40 weeks	14.7 (14.3–15.2)
	52 weeks	15.5 (15.0–16.0)
10.25 Gy × 3	1 day	5.8 (5.2–6.4)
	8 weeks	6.1 (5.1–7.0)
	12 weeks	8.4 (7.5–9.4)
	20 weeks	10.6 (9.9–11.3)
	28 weeks	12.2 (11.6–12.8)
	40 weeks	13.3 (12.7–13.9)

Abbreviations: ED_{50}, median effective dose; Tx, irradiation.
Source: Adapted from Wong CS, Hao Y. Long-term recovery kinetics of radiation damage in rat spinal cord. Int J Radiat Oncol Biol Phys 1997; 37 (1):171–179, with permission.

Table 24.5 Rat tolerance to 9 Gy × 3 followed by reirradiation after 20 weeks

Reirradiation scheme	ED_{50} (95% CI) (Gy)
Single fraction	14.0 (13.3–14.2)
2 fractions	20.5 (19.9–21.2)
5 fractions	29.1 (28.0–30.1)
10 fractions	36.3 (35.1–37.4)
20 fractions	47.8 (46.2–48.3)

Abbreviations: CI, confidence interval; ED_{50}, median effective dose.
Source: Adapted from Wong CS, Minkin S, Hill RP. Re-irradiation tolerance of rat spinal cord to fractionated X-ray doses. Radiother Oncol 1993;28:197–202.

Large Single Doses to Human Spinal Cords without Neurologic Toxicity

When the spinal cord tolerance of humans and animals is compared, most attention is focused on the dose levels that resulted in myelopathy in human case reports. A review of doses that have been delivered safely should also be considered and is presented here. Yamada et al reported their experience treating a series of 103 spinal metastases in 93 patients with single-fraction SBRT.[30] The spinal cord was limited to a 14-Gy maximal point dose. After a median follow-up of 15 months, no case of myelopathy was observed. Macbeth et al reported a group of 114 patients who received a single 10-Gy spinal cord dose during treatment for non-small-cell lung cancer, and no myelopathy was observed.[31] Ryu et al treated 86 patients with single-fraction SBRT who survived at least 1 year.[4] The average maximum spinal cord dose was 12.2 ± 2.5 Gy, and one patient received a maximum spinal cord dose of 19.2 Gy without myelopathy. One case of myelopathy was observed in this series at a maximum spinal cord dose of 14.6 Gy and will be presented in detail later. Daly et al reported their experience treating 27 hemangioblastomas with SBRT (17 single fraction and 10 multifraction).[5] The median maximum single-fraction spinal cord dose was 22.7 Gy (range 17.8–30.9 Gy). The patient with the lowest single-fraction spinal cord dose (17.8 Gy) in the series was observed to have a grade 2 foot drop 5 months after irradiation. Two additional patients from this series reported new grade 1 sensory deficits (one following a single-fraction dose of 18 Gy and another after receiving 20 Gy in two fractions), but these cases are beyond the scope of this chapter. The authors are not aware of a preclinical spinal cord tolerance study in animals that has investigated sensory deficits. The report by Daly et al includes the largest known spinal cord doses to be delivered safely by SBRT.[5] Multiple factors, including irradiated length and axial dose gradient (as first defined by preclinical studies, presented above), may have contributed to the absence of myelopathy. Although the exact lengths of spinal cord treated in these patients were not reported, they were described as "short."[5] The ED_{50} for myelopathy in animals is ~ 20 Gy following uniform spinal cord irradiation to lengths > 1.6 cm (▶ Table 24.1), but tolerance increases markedly as irradiated length is decreased (▶ Table 24.2).

Comparison of Clinical Case Reports and Preclinical Myelopathy

In this section, we compare all individual reported clinical cases of motor neurologic deficit following spine radiosurgery with data from preclinical studies for the purpose of evaluating the strength of correlation.

SBRT de novo

As of May 2012, there were six clinical cases of motor neurologic deficit following de novo spine SBRT reported in the literature.[4,5,10] Sahgal et al have provided further analysis for five of these cases.[2] The number of fractions, maximum spinal cord dose, and latency to response for all cases are presented in ▶ Table 24.6. The four cases of motor deficit that have occurred following single-fraction SBRT have been plotted on the lower 95% confidence bound of a dose-response curve (▶ Fig. 24.1) from a study of spinal cord tolerance in pigs to uniform, single-fraction irradiation (unpublished data, under review for publication). This dose-response curve represents the probability of

Table 24.6 Cases of motor neurologic deficit in humans following de novo SBRT

Study	Fractions	Maximum cord dose (Gy)	Latency (months)
Daly et al[5]	1	17.8	5
Gibbs et al[10]	1	8.5	2
	1	10.0	5
	2	26.2	9
	3	29.9	9
Ryu et al[4]	1	14.6	13

motor neurologic deficits versus maximum point dose and is derived from pig cervical spinal cords that were irradiated to a length of ~ 5 cm and thus are not expected to exhibit any "length effect." Based on preclinical data, the probability estimate of a neurologic deficit is zero for patients who received doses of 8.5, 10.0, and 14.6 Gy; however, these doses are included within the lower bound of the 95% confidence limits and are associated with probabilities ranging from 7 to 20%. The probability of a deficit in the patient who received 17.8 Gy is < 1% or ~ 35% at the lower bound of the 95% confidence limit. Although preclinical data would predict that a neurologic deficit is very unlikely at the doses reported for these clinical cases, the statistical model allows for the possibility. The latency for neurologic deficits in humans is in good agreement with rats (5–10 months)[23,26] and pigs (2.5–9.0 months).[13]

Two of the six clinical cases of motor neurologic deficits following de novo spine SBRT involved multiple-dose fractions (► Table 24.6). No preclinical studies exactly match the fractionation schemes received by these patients, but we present the studies that match most closely in ► Table 24.7. A comparison between multifraction clinical and preclinical dose schemes could be made by converting to a single-fraction biologically effective dose (SFBED) using the linear-quadratic[32] or linear-quadratic-linear model.[33] Both models are subject to assumptions and uncertainties, and the conversion to SFBED has been left as an exercise for the reader. It should be noted that a direct comparison of these clinical and preclinical cases is confounded by differences in the dose distributions treated. The preclinical studies include uniform spinal cord irradiation, whereas common clinical practice is to have a heterogeneous dose distribution across the spinal cord. Data from a study using rats suggest a dose-volume effect for paralysis;[23] recent data from a study using pigs suggest that paralysis is correlated only with the

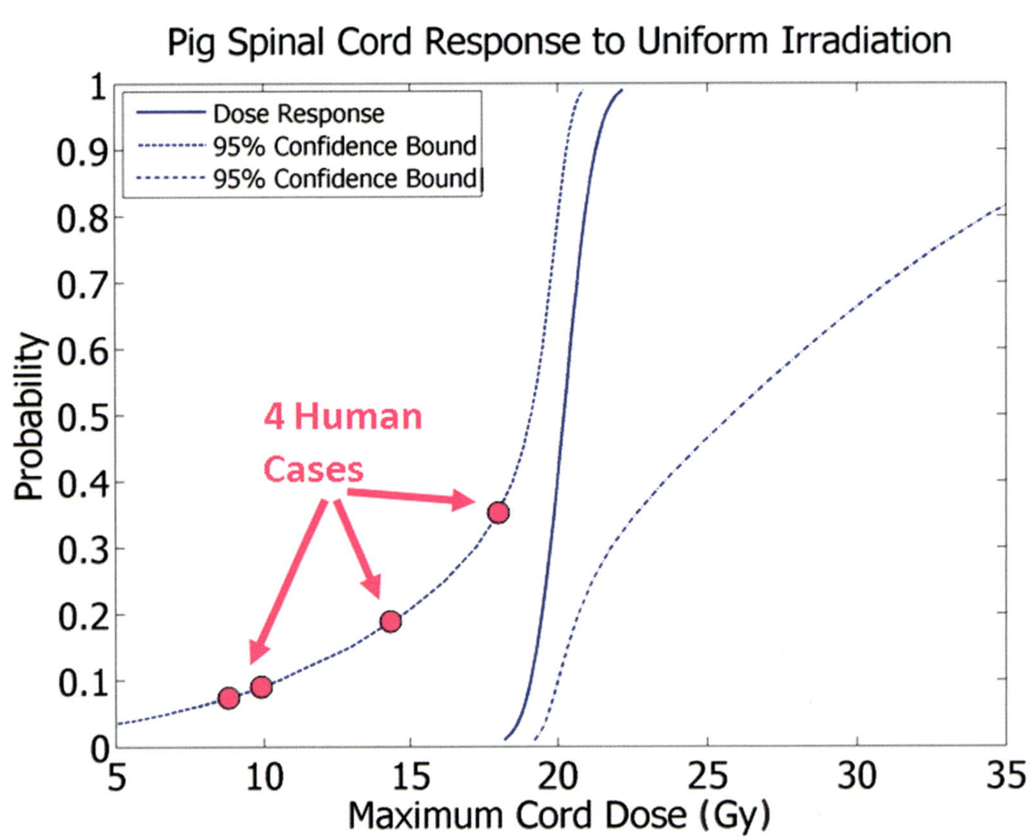

Fig. 24.1 Dose-response curve for single-fraction uniform irradiation of the pig spinal cord with human myelopathy cases superimposed.

Table 24.7 Motor neurologic deficit in humans and rats after de novo multifraction SBRT

Neurologic deficit reported	
Human cord dose	**Rat cord dose (95% CI) (Gy)**
13.1 Gy × 2[10]	If first dose = 12.0, and second dose is given next day, ED_{50} = 17.3 (range 15.6–19.2)[24]
	If first dose = 14.9, and the second dose is given 1 day later, ED_{50} = 14.5 (range 13.2–15.2)[24]
10 Gy × 3[10]	If the first two doses are 9 Gy, and a third dose is delivered 2 days later, ED_{50} = 14.1 (range 12.5 –15.6)[28]

maximum spinal cord dose[13] (additional unpublished data, under review for publication). The data presented in ▶ Table 24.7 suggest an approximate correlation between human and animal spinal cord response to multifraction SBRT.

Stereotactic Body Radiotherapy and Re-treatment

As of May 2012, five clinical cases of motor neurologic deficit involving reirradiation and spine SBRT were reported in the literature.[3,10,34] Sahgal et al[3] provided further analysis for all five cases. Study, previous spinal cord dose/fractionation, time interval before re-treatment, second spinal cord dose/fractionation, and latency to response for all cases are presented in ▶ Table 24.8. A comparison between clinical and preclinical retreatment tolerance is challenged by the wide range of doses and fractionation schemes involved. No preclinical studies exactly match the treatment regimens received by any of these patients. Patients A and B (▶ Table 24.8) received relatively modest spinal cord doses (25.2–40 Gy) by protracted fractionation schedules (22–28 fractions) and experienced long intervals (70.0–80.8 mo) between courses of radiation. For spinal cord tolerance to reirradiation, the longest interval between courses studied in a preclinical model is 36 months. Ang et al irradiated rhesus monkeys to 44 Gy in daily 2.2-Gy fractions and then reirradiated to doses of 57.2 Gy (2.2 Gy fractions) after 1- or 2-year intervals, or 66 Gy (2.2-Gy fractions) after 2- or 3-year intervals.[35] The early and late effects of their radiation treatment were observed for 2.0 to 2.5 years after reirradiation. Assuming all dose-response curves were parallel yielded recovery estimates of 33.6 Gy (76%), 37.6 Gy (85%), and 44.6 Gy (101%) of the initial dose after 1, 2, and 3 years, respectively. Using a model with more conservative assumptions resulted in an overall recovery equivalent of 26.8 Gy (61%).[35]

Patient A was reirradiated to a spinal cord dose of 19.2 Gy in two fractions, which is similar to the ED_{50} observed in rats 20 weeks following an initial dose of 27 Gy in three fractions (▶ Table 24.5). Also, the ED_{50} (95% CI) for single-dose reirradiation in pigs is 19.7 Gy (17.4–21.4 Gy) 1 year following a dose of 30 Gy in 10 fractions.[15] Patient B was reirradiated to 13.9 Gy in two fractions. The time interval between radiation courses for patients A and B is far beyond the longest interval ever studied in preclinical models, so a comparison is speculative. Guided by the general principle of increasing recovery over time that has been demonstrated in preclinical studies, one would expect significant recovery from the initial dose for these patients. The reirradiation dose for patient A is aggressive and close to the ED_{50} for rats that were reirradiated after a much shorter interval (20 wk) and different initial fractionation.[27] The initial and reirradiation doses for patient B are less aggressive and would probably not be predicted by preclinical models.

Patient C (▶ Table 24.8) received 51.9 Gy in 28 fractions, followed 18 months later by 32.9 Gy in 3 fractions. As described above, significant recovery is observed in all preclinical studies by 1 year. The extent of recovery, however, depends on the size of the initial radiation dose.[26,28] The reirradiation dose is aggressive; the tolerance dose (ED_{50}) for rats with no previous radiation is ~ 36 Gy in 3 fractions.[27] A fractionation scheme of 9 Gy + 9 Gy + 14.1 Gy (12.5–15.6, 95% CI) has been demonstrated to paralyze 50% of rats.[28] For patient C, clinical and preclinical outcomes appear to be in reasonable agreement. Patient D received 12.3 Gy in a single fraction, followed 11 months later by 21.2 Gy in five fractions (▶ Table 24.8). This patient is unique in the radiation toxicity literature because single-fraction SBRT was delivered first followed by fractionation. No preclinical study shares this irradiation paradigm. Ruifrok et al irradiated rats with a single dose of 12 Gy, followed by an additional single dose at fixed time points.[24] They observed that the ED_{50} (95%

Table 24.8 Cases of motor neurologic deficit in humans following reirradiation

Patient	Study	Prior radiation, maximum cord dose (Gy); fractions	Interval to re-treatment (months)	Second course, maximum cord dose (Gy); fractions	Latency to deficit (months)
A	Gibbs et al[10]	40; 22	80.8	19.2; 2	6
B	Gibbs et al[10]	25.2;* 28	70	13.9; 2	4
C	Gwak et al[34]	51.9;* 28	18	32.9; 3	8
D	Sahgal et al (with Cleveland Clinic)[3]	12.3;** 1	11	21.2; 5	3
E	Sahgal et al (with Thomas Jefferson University)[3]	43.2; 15	12	14.7;** 1	3

* Estimated by Sahgal et al.
** Dose reported to the thecal sac.

CI) for spinal cord response was 17.3 Gy (15.6–19.2 Gy) if the second dose was delivered 1 day after the first dose. The ED_{50} (95% CI) gradually increased to 19.8 Gy (19.0–20.6 Gy) as the interval increased to 6 months. Knowles irradiated guinea pigs with a single 10-Gy dose and reirradiated with a single dose 1 year later.[25] The resulting ED_{50} was 19.5 Gy, which was nearly the same as the ED_{50} for a single dose alone (20.5 Gy). Wong et al irradiated rats with five fractions, 20 weeks after an initial course of 27 Gy in three, and observed an ED_{50} (95% CI) of 29.1 (28.0–30.1).[27]

For patient D, preclinical data do not appear to predict the clinical outcome of this case. Patient E received 43.2 Gy in 15 fractions, followed by a single dose of 14.7 Gy 1 year later (▶ Table 24.8). Medin et al irradiated pigs with 30 Gy in 10 fractions, followed 1 year later by a single dose, and observed an ED_{50} (95% CI) of 19.7 Gy (17.4–21.4).[15] Wong et al irradiated rats with 43 Gy in 20 fractions, followed by a single dose 20 weeks later, and observed an ED_{50} of 15.7 Gy (▶ Table 24.3)[26]. Patient E falls between preclinical experience with pigs and rats. Pigs were observed to recover nearly 100% 1 year after 30 Gy in 10,[15] but patient E received a significantly larger initial dose (43.2 Gy in 15), and the extent of recovery depended on the size of the initial radiation dose.[26,28] Rats that received a less aggressive initial regimen (43 Gy in 20) had an ED_{50} (15.7 Gy) that was slightly greater than the dose delivered to the patient (14.7. Gy), but the reirradiation interval for the rats was only 20 weeks compared to 1 year for patient E. Compared to the preclinical data available, the dose delivered to patient E could be considered aggressive. The latency for neurologic deficits in humans (▶ Table 24.8) after reirradiation is in very close agreement with both rats (2.0–6.5 months)[26] and pigs (2.3–6.0 months).[15]

Discussion

Eleven cases of clinical motor neurologic deficit (6 from de novo irradiation and 5 from reirradiation) have been summarized for comparison with spinal cord tolerance data from preclinical studies. For some clinical cases, the correlation with preclinical data appears to be strong, whereas other cases cannot be explained. Series of patients who tolerated significantly greater spinal cord doses than those reported to cause myelopathy in others have also been presented. With limited clinical data that are not self-consistent, we are challenged to draw a firm conclusion regarding the correlation between humans and animals. The authors believe that current data favor the hypothesis that research animals provide a reasonable model to study spinal cord tolerance for humans. This belief is based on the following observations: (1) none of the cases of human myelopathy are "forbidden" by animal data, although a few cases are predicted to be unlikely; (2) several cases of human myelopathy are in reasonable agreement with animal data; (3) large numbers of patients have been irradiated safely with doses predicted to be safe by animal data; and (4) animal data are self-consistent between the species and modalities currently reported when irradiation conditions are similar. The authors have presented the use of preclinical data in a positive light, but preclinical data must be scrutinized for species and irradiation conditions appropriate to the clinical comparison being made. For example, dose-volume effects have been investigated in the spinal cords of rats[23] and pigs[13] (additional unpublished data, under review for publication) with much different conclusions, and uniform irradiation of both species resulted in similar outcomes.

Conclusion

Direct clinical application of spinal cord tolerance data derived from preclinical studies is controversial. Increased reliance on preclinical data will be necessary if dose escalation is indicated or if new applications arise for spine SBRT. Therefore, a thorough understanding of the available data is crucial. The volume of human data is still sparse but increasing steadily. The authors conclude that current data favor the hypothesis that research animals are reasonable models to study spinal cord tolerance for humans when the species and irradiation conditions are matched to the clinical phenomenon in question.

References

[1] Sahgal A, Bilsky M, Chang EL, et al. Stereotactic body radiotherapy for spinal metastases: current status, with a focus on its application in the postoperative patient. J Neurosurg Spine 2011; 14: 151–166

[2] Sahgal A, Ma L, Gibbs I, et al. Spinal cord tolerance for stereotactic body radiotherapy. Int J Radiat Oncol Biol Phys 2010; 77: 548–553

[3] Sahgal A, Ma L, Weinberg V, et al. Reirradiation human spinal cord tolerance for stereotactic body radiotherapy. Int J Radiat Oncol Biol Phys 2012; 82: 107–116

[4] Ryu S, Jin JY, Jin R, et al. Partial volume tolerance of the spinal cord and complications of single-dose radiosurgery. Cancer 2007; 109: 628–636

[5] Daly ME, Choi CY, Gibbs IC, et al. Tolerance of the spinal cord to stereotactic radiosurgery: insights from hemangioblastomas. Int J Radiat Oncol Biol Phys 2011; 80: 213–220

[6] Medin PM, Boike TP. Spinal cord tolerance in the age of spinal radiosurgery: lessons from preclinical studies. Int J Radiat Oncol Biol Phys 2011; 79: 1302–1309

[7] Schultheiss TE, Stephens LC. Invited review: permanent radiation myelopathy. Br J Radiol 1992; 65: 737–753

[8] van der Kogel A, ed. The Cellular Basis of Radiation-induced Damage to the Central Nervous System. Edinburgh, Scotland: Churchill Livingstone; 1983

[9] van den Aardweg GJ, Hopewell JW, Whitehouse EM, Calvo W. A new model of radiation-induced myelopathy: a comparison of the response of mature and immature pigs. Int J Radiat Oncol Biol Phys 1994; 29: 763–770

[10] Gibbs IC, Patil C, Gerszten PC, Adler JR, Burton SA. Delayed radiation-induced myelopathy after spinal radiosurgery. Neurosurgery 2009; 64 (Suppl): A67–A72

[11] Risdahl JM, Chao C, Murtaugh MP, Peterson PK, Molitor TW. Acute and chronic morphine administration in swine. Pharmacol Biochem Behav 1992; 43: 799–806

[12] Jarvis S, McLean KA, Chirnside J, et al. Opioid-mediated changes in nociceptive threshold during pregnancy and parturition in the sow. Pain 1997; 72: 153–159

[13] Medin PM, Foster RD, van der Kogel AJ, Sayre JW, McBride WH, Solberg TD. Spinal cord tolerance to single-fraction partial-volume irradiation: a swine model. Int J Radiat Oncol Biol Phys 2011; 79: 226–232

[14] Philippens ME, Pop LA, Visser AG, Peeters WJ, van der Kogel AJ. Bath and shower effect in spinal cord: the effect of time interval. Int J Radiat Oncol Biol Phys 2009; 73: 514–522

[15] Medin PM, Foster RD, van der Kogel AJ, Sayre JW, McBride WH, Solberg TD. Spinal cord tolerance to reirradiation with single-fraction radiosurgery: a swine model. Int J Radiat Oncol Biol Phys 2012; 83: 1031–1037

[16] Scalliet P, Landuyt W, van der Schueren E. Repair kinetics as a determining factor for late tolerance of central nervous system to low dose rate irradiation. Radiother Oncol 1989; 14: 345–353

[17] Van der Kogel A. Late Effects of Radiation on the Spinal Cord. Amsterdam, the Netherlands: University of Amsterdam; 1979:160

[18] van den Aardweg GJ, Hopewell JW, Whitehouse EM. The radiation response of the cervical spinal cord of the pig: effects of changing the irradiated volume. Int J Radiat Oncol Biol Phys 1995; 31: 51–55

[19] Hopewell JW, Wright EA. The effects of dose and field size on late radiation damage to the rat spinal cord. Int J Radiat Biol Relat Stud Phys Chem Med 1975; 28: 325–333

[20] Hopewell JW, Morris AD, Dixon-Brown A. The influence of field size on the late tolerance of the rat spinal cord to single doses of X rays. Br J Radiol 1987; 60: 1099–1108

[21] Bijl HP, van Luijk P, Coppes RP, Schippers JM, Konings AW, van der Kogel AJ. Dose-volume effects in the rat cervical spinal cord after proton irradiation. Int J Radiat Oncol Biol Phys 2002; 52: 205–211

[22] van Luijk P, Bijl HP, Coppes RP, et al. Techniques for precision irradiation of the lateral half of the rat cervical spinal cord using 150 MeV protons [corrected]. Phys Med Biol 2001; 46: 2857–2871

[23] Bijl HP, van Luijk P, Coppes RP, Schippers JM, Konings AW, van Der Kogel AJ. Regional differences in radiosensitivity across the rat cervical spinal cord. Int J Radiat Oncol Biol Phys 2005; 61: 543–551

[24] Ruifrok AC, Kleiboer BJ, van der Kogel AJ. Reirradiation tolerance of the immature rat spinal cord. Radiother Oncol 1992; 23: 249–256

[25] Knowles JF. The radiosensitivity of the guinea-pig spinal cord to X-rays: the effect of retreatment at one year and the effect of age at the time of irradiation. Int J Radiat Biol Relat Stud Phys Chem Med 1983; 44: 433–442

[26] Wong CS, Poon JK, Hill RP. Re-irradiation tolerance in the rat spinal cord: influence of level of initial damage. Radiother Oncol 1993; 26: 132–138

[27] Wong CS, Minkin S, Hill RP. Re-irradiation tolerance of rat spinal cord to fractionated X-ray doses. Radiother Oncol 1993; 28: 197–202

[28] Wong CS, Hao Y. Long-term recovery kinetics of radiation damage in rat spinal cord. Int J Radiat Oncol Biol Phys 1997; 37: 171–179

[29] Chuang C, Sahgal A, Lee L, et al. Effects of residual target motion for image-tracked spine radiosurgery. Med Phys 2007; 34: 4484–4490

[30] Yamada Y, Bilsky MH, Lovelock DM, et al. High-dose, single-fraction image-guided intensity-modulated radiotherapy for metastatic spinal lesions. Int J Radiat Oncol Biol Phys 2008; 71: 484–490

[31] Macbeth FR, Wheldon TE, Girling DJ, et al. The Medical Research Council Lung Cancer Working Party. Radiation myelopathy: estimates of risk in 1048 patients in three randomized trials of palliative radiotherapy for non-small cell lung cancer. Clin Oncol (R Coll Radiol) 1996; 8: 176–181

[32] Douglas BG, Fowler JF. The effect of multiple small doses of x rays on skin reactions in the mouse and a basic interpretation. Radiat Res 1976; 66: 401–426

[33] Park C, Papiez L, Zhang S, Story M, Timmerman RD. Universal survival curve and single fraction equivalent dose: useful tools in understanding potency of ablative radiotherapy. Int J Radiat Oncol Biol Phys 2008; 70: 847–852

[34] Gwak HS, Yoo HJ, Youn SM, et al. Hypofractionated stereotactic radiation therapy for skull base and upper cervical chordoma and chondrosarcoma: preliminary results. Stereotact Funct Neurosurg 2005; 83: 233–243

[35] Ang KK, Jiang GL, Feng Y, Stephens LC, Tucker SL, Price RE. Extent and kinetics of recovery of occult spinal cord injury. Int J Radiat Oncol Biol Phys 2001; 50: 1013–1020

[36] Lo YC, McBride WH, Withers HR. The effect of single doses of radiation on mouse spinal cord. Int J Radiat Oncol Biol Phys 1992; 22: 57–63

[37] Knowles JF. The effects of single dose X-irradiation on the guinea-pig spinal cord. Int J Radiat Biol Relat Stud Phys Chem Med 1981; 40: 265–275

[38] Medin PM, Foster RD, van der Kogel AJ, Sayre JW, McBride WH, Solberg TD. Spinal cord tolerance to single-session uniform irradiation in pigs: implications for a dose-volume effect. Radiother Oncol 2013; 106: 101–105

25 Spinal Cord Tolerance Up to 10 Gy

Samuel T. Chao and John H. Suh

Introduction

The development of spine stereotactic body radiotherapy (sSBRT) has allowed physicians to escalate the dose to treat symptomatic spinal metastases. Before the development of sSBRT, spinal metastases were treated with conventional radiation, typically with 30 Gy in 10 fractions, 20 Gy in 5 fractions, or 8 Gy in a single fraction. As such, the use of single-fraction radiation for bone metastases, including those in the spine, is not a novel concept. Although a single fraction is used frequently in the setting of sSBRT as a typical dose-fractionation scheme, its use in conventional radiation was found to be as effective as multiple fractions of radiation in terms of pain control.[1] The advantages of single-fraction radiation include convenience, cost, and less impact on the timing of systemic therapies. The spinal cord, which is a critical structure in the treatment of spine metastases, is included in the radiation field and receives essentially the same dose that is targeted to the disease if conventional radiation techniques are used. Conversely, sSBRT attempts to minimize the dose to the spinal cord while delivering a higher dose to the spine metastasis. In this chapter, we review the use of conventional radiation therapy to safely deliver radiation to the spine using up to 10 Gy, including re-treatment of the spine.

Single-Fraction Radiation Doses

Various single-fraction doses have been investigated prospectively in several studies. Hoskin et al studied the dose-response relationship in the treatment of metastatic bone pain, specifically, 4 Gy versus 8 Gy in a single fraction.[2] This was based on a dose deescalation pilot study of 4 Gy at the Royal Marsden Hospital, which, interestingly, showed a 43% rate of pain relief.[3] The higher dose followed a previous study showing equivalent outcomes of 8 Gy in 1 fraction and 30 Gy in 10 fractions as well, which will be discussed later.[4] Two-hundred seventy patients were randomized between groups receiving 4 and 8 Gy. Although all bony sites were included, 37% of cases treated the spine, with the prescription dose being delivered to a 5-cm depth. Median survival was 8 months in both arms. At 4 weeks, there was a higher rate of pain response with 8 Gy of 69% versus only 44% of patients who received 4 Gy ($p < 0.001$). However, there was no difference in complete response or duration of response. During the 12-week study period, 20% of the patients randomized to 4 Gy were re-treated due to a recurrence of symptoms compared to 9% of those randomized to 8 Gy. Although this study showed the superiority of 8 Gy with ***level I evidence***, 4 Gy may also be considered as an acceptable palliative dose for symptomatic bony metastases when higher doses may be difficult to deliver.

In the Netherlands, the use of 6 Gy delivered in a single fraction was investigated prospectively.[5] Of the 170 patients in the study, 49% involved treatment to the spine. Like the study by Hoskin et al, the dose was delivered to a 5-cm depth for spine treatment. In 88% of the patients, either a partial or a complete response to pain was noted. Of those treated to the spine, 9% later developed spinal cord compression. Re-treatment was delivered in 11% of patients. A dose of 6 Gy was found to be an effective palliative dose with ***level II evidence***, with outcomes very similar to those seen in the 8-Gy arm of the study by Hoskin et al.

Like Hoskin et al, Jeremic et al performed a study, randomizing 327 patients with painful bony metastases to groups of 4 Gy versus 6 Gy versus 8 Gy, all delivered in a single fraction.[6] Dose was also delivered to a 5-cm depth. Of these patients, 49% were treated to the spine. Approximately 80% had moderate to severe pain at presentation. They found that the 6- and 8-Gy groups had quicker and higher rates of pain response compared to the lower dose group. At 8 weeks, those receiving 8 Gy had a response rate of 78% compared to 73% in the 6 Gy arm and 59% in the 4 Gy arm. Time to pain relief was significantly faster in the 8 Gy arm compared to the 4 Gy arm ($p = 0.012$). There was no difference between 4 and 6 Gy, and 6 and 8 Gy. Also, there was no difference in the duration of response and re-treatment rate between the various arms. As a result of this study with ***level I evidence***, 8 Gy has been considered to be the standard dose for single-fraction radiation for bone metastases, although arguably 6 Gy can be considered, given the similar outcomes. None of these studies reported myelopathy. ▶ Table 25.1 summarizes the data.

Barak et al retrospectively compared 6, 8, and 10 Gy in 114 patients, 53% of whom had treatment to the spine, providing ***level III evidence***.[7] In the study, 70% received 8 Gy. Response to radiation was 71% and lasted up to 6 months in 37% of patients.

Table 25.1 Pain relief in various single-fraction doses

Study	Outcome	4 Gy (%)	6 Gy (%)	8 Gy (%)	*p* value
Hoskin et al[2]	Pain relief	44	NA	69	< 0.001
	Re-treatment	20	NA	9	NA
Uppelschoten et al[5]	Pain relief	NA	88	NA	NA
	Re-treatment	NA	10.6	NA	NA
Jeremic et al[6]	Pain relief	59	73	78	0.012
	Re-treatment	38	44	42	0.71

Abbreviation: *NA, Not applicable.*

Most of the patients who achieved pain relief did so in the first week after radiation. No mention was made of long-term toxicities, including myelopathy. In addition, there have been several historic retrospective studies that have used 15 Gy and 18 Gy with a 90% response rate (***level III evidence***).[8,9] In the study by Penn, 59% had treatment to the spine.[9] There did not appear to be any benefit beyond 10 Gy in this study. Of note, one patient developed transient myelopathy at 12 Gy. Although these were older, retrospective studies with ***level III evidence***, it is important to note that, based on these studies, doses up to 10 Gy can be delivered safely to the spine and spinal cord, noting that the overall survival of these patients may have been relatively short.

Multiple versus Single Fraction

A number of trials have investigated single fraction versus multiple fractions of radiation, focusing on bone metastases in general. In the United Kingdom, Price et al randomized 288 patients between two very common fractionation schemes, 30 Gy in 10 fractions versus 8 Gy in a single fraction.[4] Half of these patients were treated for spine metastases. Direct fields were used to treat the vertebral column. Doses were prescribed to a depth of 5 cm for the spine. No difference in survival was noted between the two arms with ***level I evidence***. This study also demonstrated no difference in pain control or duration of response between the two dose-fractionation schemes with ***level I evidence***. At 1 year, 57% and 59% of those who responded to a single fraction and multiple fractions, respectively, continued to respond. However, reirradiation was more frequent in the single-fraction regimen. Those treated with single-fraction radiation were more likely to be offered repeat radiation, whereas those treated with multiple fractions were more likely to be managed with analgesics alone.

The Edinburgh study, reported by Gaze et al, used a slightly higher dose of 10 Gy in the single-fraction arm and compared this to 22.5 Gy in five fractions.[10] Prescription depth was not specified in this study. The overall response rate (83.7% for single fraction vs 89.2% for five fractions), complete response rate (38.8% for single fraction vs 42.3% for five fractions), and duration of pain control (13.5 wk for single fraction vs 14 wk for five fractions) did not differ significantly between the two arms. No late toxicities were noted in either arm. As such, with ***level I evidence***, 10 Gy should be considered an efficacious dose, equivalent to multiple-fraction radiation.

Subsequently, similar studies, including several meta-analyses, have been conducted comparing conventional fractionated radiation therapy versus single-fraction radiation therapy, despite good existing phase III data, thus providing further ***level I*** data. The data from these studies ranged from improved pain outcomes with higher dose-fractionated regimens to no dose-response relationship.[1,11] The criticisms of these studies included the use of physician assessment of pain in these studies, the variety of primary sites and histologies, and the fact that narcotic relief and the incidence of re-treatment were not considered in many of these studies.

In contrast, Radiation Therapy Oncology Group (RTOG) 9714 evaluated a more homogeneous population (patients with breast and prostate cancer) and assessed outcomes using validated quality of life and pain instruments.[12] Patients were randomized to 8 Gy in 1 fraction versus 30 Gy in 10 fractions. A total of 949 patients were enrolled, 898 of whom were eligible for randomization. The number of patients with spine metastases was not specified, although they were included in the study as a non-weight-bearing site. The overall median survival was the same in both arms at 9 months. No significant difference in the rate of response and use of nonnarcotic and narcotic analgesics was noted. Complete and partial responses were 15% and 50%, respectively, in the 8-Gy arm, compared to 18% and 48%, respectively, in the 30-Gy-in-10-fractions arm. Grade 2 to 4 acute toxicities were higher in the 30-Gy arm at 17% versus only 10% in the 8-Gy arm. The re-treatment rate was higher in the 8-Gy arm at 18% versus 9% in the 30-Gy arm. This confirms the results of the aforementioned studies with more ***level I evidence***.

A large meta-analysis of 16 randomized trials was performed by Chow et al.[1] Based on their findings using ***level I evidence***, there was no difference in overall response rate, complete response rate, subsequent spinal cord compression rate, or pathological fracture rate. A difference in re-treatment rates favoring multiple fractions was demonstrated, keeping in mind that some patients may not survive long enough to see the benefit of multiple fractions.

▶ Table 25.2 summarizes various studies looking at single-fraction versus multiple-fraction radiation.

Table 25.2 Pain relief for single-fraction radiation versus multiple-fraction radiation

Study	Outcome	Single fraction (%)	Multiple fraction (%)	*p* Value
Price et al[4] (8 Gy/1 fx vs 30 Gy/10 fx)	Pain relief	82 for severe initial pain, 58 for mild/moderate	88 for severe initial pain, 69 for mild/moderate	>0.1 for onset of pain relief
	Re-treatment	10	3	NA
Gaze et al[10] (10 Gy/1 fx vs 22.5 Gy/5 fx)	Pain relief	83.7	89.2	NA
Hartsell et al[12] (8 Gy/1 fx vs 30 Gy/10 fx)	Pain relief	65	66	0.6
	Re-treatment	18	9	0.001
Chow et al[1] (meta-analysis)	Pain relief	58	59	0.6
	Re-treatment	20	8	<0.00001

Abbreviations: *fx, fraction(s); NA, Not applicable.*

Specifically assessing spinal cord compression, a retrospective review was conducted involving a total of 1,304 patients.[13] Schedules of 1 fraction of 8 Gy, 5 fractions of 4 Gy, 10 fractions of 3 Gy, 15 fractions of 2.5 Gy, and 20 fractions of 2 Gy were compared. Posttreatment ambulatory rates were similar, ranging from 63 to 74%. Factors associated with functional outcome included age, performance status, primary tumor, number of involved vertebrae, interval from cancer diagnosis to spinal cord compression, pretreatment ambulatory status, and time to developing motor deficits prior to radiation. The radiation schedule did not influence functional outcome. The in-field recurrence rate was higher in the shortened schedules of 8 Gy in one fraction and 20 Gy in five fractions over the more protracted regimens ($p < 0.001$). The authors concluded with ***level III evidence*** that 8 Gy in a single fraction should be considered the standard dose, and the more protracted regimen of 30 Gy in 10 fractions should be reserved for patients with longer predicted survival.

Consequently, there have been editorials emphasizing the equivalence of single-fraction radiation, resulting in a recommendation grade of 1A for single-fraction palliative radiation.[14,15] This global practice, however, does not reflect the results of 25 randomized phase III studies. This is believed to be secondary to higher reimbursement with multiple-fraction regimens. Changes in reimbursement patterns may result in greater adoption of single-fraction radiation.

Prescription

A component of the prescription that is often overlooked is how the dose is being delivered. When using a single field of radiation, a depth is chosen that determines the dose prescription. This affects the coverage of that radiation to the metastasis, with underdosing of disease beyond that depth. Barton et al performed a survey on palliation for vertebral metastases, asking questions regarding dose and depth of the prescription in comparison to location.[16] The most common prescriptions were to D_{max} (maximum depth of a particular photon energy) and 5 cm. Some physicians varied the prescription with the spinal level, using a higher depth for the lumbar spine, as it tends to be deeper to the skin. Only 7 out of the 91 respondents actually measured the depth of the prescription based on lateral screening at the time of simulation, which tailors the radiation based on the patient's anatomy rather than using a presumed standard depth for all patients large or small. The authors proceeded to measure the dose distribution of 8 Gy in a single fraction depending on depth, as the vertebral structures vary based on the location. This dose can vary tremendously, which is minimized using a parallel opposed, anteroposterior/posteroanterior (AP/PA) field technique, particularly for the lumbar spine. Varying photon energy also has an effect, with the least variation seen for 10 MV photons, as the dose fall-off tends to be less steep with higher energies. For deep metastases, as seen in the lumbar vertebrae, significant dose variation is seen when a lower energy source, such as Cobalt 60, is used when depth is varied, as this has a higher dose fall-off compared to higher energy photons. As such, for lumbar vertebral metastases, higher energy and/or AP/PA fields should be considered.

▶ Fig. 25.1 and ▶ Fig. 25.2 show how the prescribed depth can affect coverage.

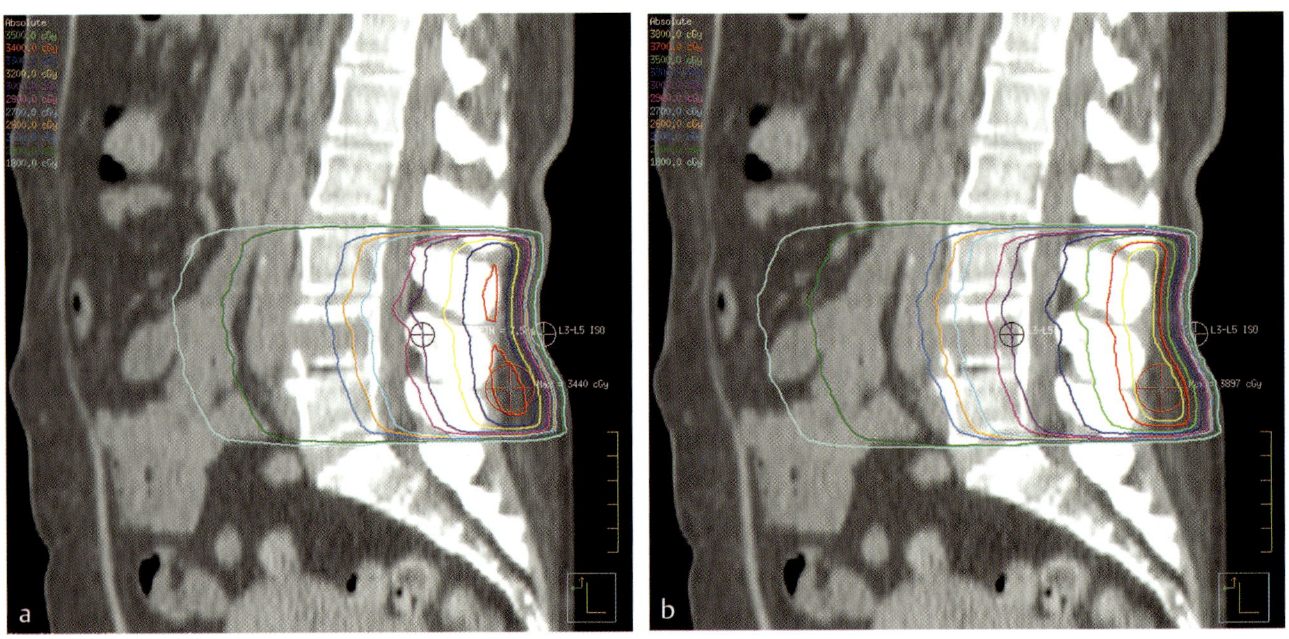

Fig. 25.1 (a) Dose distribution for 30 Gy in 10 fractions prescribed to a depth of 5 cm. The prescription dose is shown in *violet*. Note that this dose does not reach the thecal sac. Only half of the affected L4 vertebral body received 25 Gy. (b) Dose distribution for 30 Gy in 10 fractions prescribed to the anterior spinal canal. The prescription dose is shown in *violet*. The prescription dose covers the spinal canal and would cover epidural disease. Most of the affected L4 vertebral body received 26 Gy.

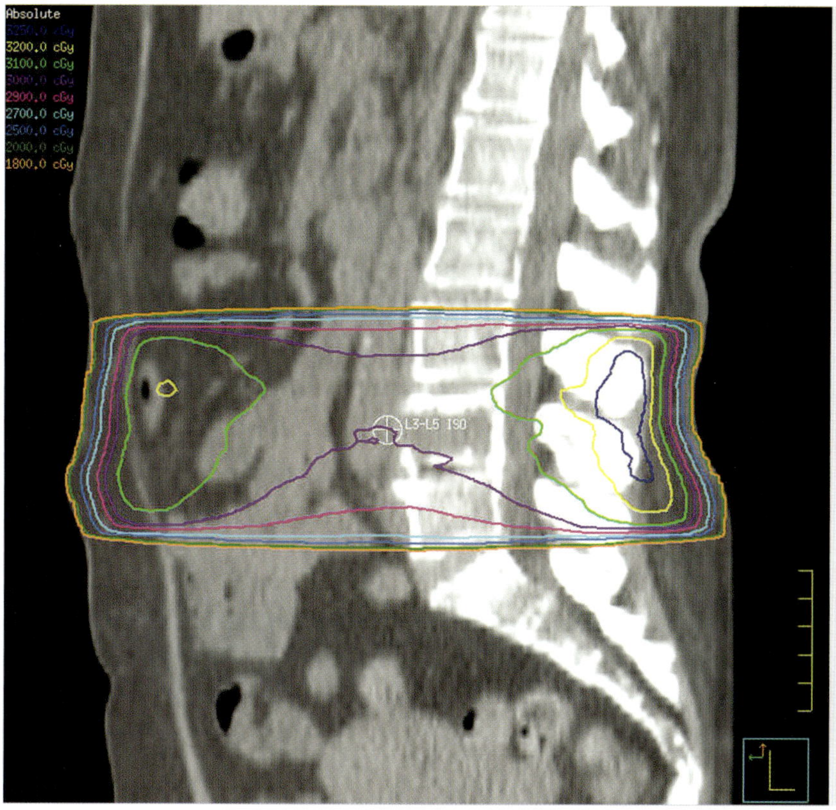

Fig. 25.2 Dose distribution for 30 Gy in 10 fractions using anteroposterior/posteroanterior fields delivered to the midplane. The prescription dose is shown in *violet*. Unlike in ► Fig. 25.1, the prescription dose of 30 Gy covers most of the affected L4 vertebral body.

Are Higher Doses Safe?

Although higher doses may be needed to improve disease control, the use of higher doses has been limited by concerns regarding spinal cord tolerance. As reviewed above, 10 Gy has been demonstrated to be safe with respect to late toxicities, namely, radiation-induced myelopathy (RIM).

As previously discussed, fractionated radiation does result in less re-treatment, suggesting a benefit to higher doses even when accounting for fractionation. It remains unclear what is the true tolerance dose of the spinal cord. Animal studies have been performed to gain insight into this question, the most recent being by Medin and colleagues using a pig model.[17] They demonstrated that, based on a pig model, a dose of 17.4 Gy in a single fraction results in a 1% probability of myelopathy. This curve is very steep, as a dose of 20 Gy results in a 50% probability of myelopathy. As such, higher doses may be possible beyond 10 Gy, although there is a higher safety margin with sSBRT.

Maranzano et al performed a clinical trial that prescribed 16 Gy in two fractions, each fraction separated by 1 week for spinal cord compression patients with a poor performance status or prognosis.[18] Pain relief was achieved in 67% of patients. Improvement in motor function was seen in 63%. Overall median survival was 5 months. Better survival was seen in patients who were ambulatory before and/or after radiation therapy. No late toxicities were reported. Based on this study, it may be safe to deliver higher doses using non-SBRT conventional techniques with ***level II evidence***. It also suggests that if 8 Gy had been given previously, 8 Gy as a re-treatment dose is safe as well. This will be discussed later in this chapter.

Biologically Effective Dose

The linear-quadratic equation is derived from the classical cell survival curve and allows for the comparison of different dose-fractionation schemes. The biologically effective dose (BED) can be calculated based on dose and number of fractions for a particular effect. Although this tends to work for multifractionated schemes, it does a poor job of estimating the BED for a single fraction, particularly for higher doses beyond 10 Gy. The reason for this is that beyond 10 Gy, additional cell kill is achieved by vascular effects on the tumor (and normal tissue).[19] Endothelial cells undergo apoptosis mediated by the sphingomyelin pathway.[20] This peaks within 6 hours after radiation and causes microvascular dysfunction, which acutely disrupts tumor perfusion. This pathway does not take place until 10 Gy.

One way to account for the additional cell kill from higher single-fraction doses is to define a single transition dose (D_T) at which the linear-quadratic equation transitions to the terminal asymptote of the multitarget model.[21] This is known as the "universal survival curve." For the H460 non–small-cell cancer cell line, this D_T was found to be 6.2 Gy. Beyond this dose, the traditional linear-quadratic equation falls apart, and another equation that accounts multiple targets that result in cell ablation and loss of clonogenicity is used instead. Although studies discussed later in this chapter may use the traditional BED equation even for single-fraction radiation, it is important to note this issue. At this time, however, the traditional BED equation, even for single-fraction radiation, is the most widely employed due to the lack of a simple, universal equation.

Reirradiation of Recurrent Spine Metastases

Although single-fraction radiation is demonstrated to be safe, there has been concern regarding the spinal cord tolerance after "full" dose radiation has been given to that region. With sSBRT, the spinal cord dose is minimized relative to the dose to the tumor. However, the dose received by the spinal cord may still be ≥ 10 Gy. Maranzano et al evaluated reirradiation using conventional radiation following the results of two randomized trials (***level III evidence***).[22] From these trials, 24 patients had an in-field recurrence, and 12 of these patients underwent reirradiation. Initial radiation dosing included 8 Gy in one fraction and 16 Gy in two fractions separated by 1 week apart. Time to reirradiation ranged from 2 to 31 months. Six patients received 8 Gy in one fraction, and the remaining patients received 15 Gy in three fractions, 20 Gy in five fractions, 16 Gy in two fractions, and 4 Gy in one fraction. The cumulative BED ranged from 80 Gy_2 to 120 Gy_2. Six out of seven patients retained their ability to walk. The median duration of response was 4.5 months. No RIM was observed.

Neider et al used a collection of 38 patients with RIM to calculate the risk of RIM based on the total BED.[23] A BED of 120 Gy_2 is safe, whereas with higher doses of 120.1 to 135.5 Gy_2, this risk is small when the interval is not shorter than 6 months, and the dose of each course is ≤ 98 Gy_2. Single-fraction radiation was not specifically investigated in this study, and the actual spinal cord dose could not be verified, as the data incorporated that of other institutions. However, they are the best data available to date that provide risk stratification based on dose specifically for conventional radiation. Data from Sahgal et al provide similar data specifically for sSBRT and are presented in the subsequent chapter.[24]

Conclusion

Radiation doses up to 10 Gy have been shown prospectively to be both safe and effective, even for single-fraction delivery (recommendation grade 1A). It is important to note that, specifically for the spine, the prescriptions used were not necessarily optimized, sometimes resulting in an underdosage to the vertebral body metastasis. Perhaps with optimization of the treatment plan based on depth of the specific metastasis, better pain and local control may be obtained even with single-fraction radiation.

As patients survive longer from their metastatic disease, further improvement in local pain control may result from the higher doses provided by sSBRT. RTOG 0631 is a phase II/III trial randomizing patients with one or two vertebral level involvement and allows up to three separate sites. The randomization is 8 Gy in one fraction delivered conventionally versus 16 to 18 Gy in one fraction delivered via sSBRT. For sSBRT, the dose to the spinal cord is limited to 10 Gy to the 10% of the partial spinal cord volume defined as 5 to 6 mm above and below the target. The absolute maximum dose to the spinal cord is 14 Gy for a volume of 0.03 cm^3. The primary end point of this study is local pain control.

In many cases, due to the proximity of disease to the spinal cord, urgency in starting radiation as soon as possible due to spinal cord compression, or poor prognosis of the patient, sSBRT may not be ideal. In such cases, single-fraction conventional radiotherapy may be the best approach for these patients.

Reirradiation can also be safely delivered in a single fraction, as long as the previous dose and time from previous treatment have been taken into account (recommendation grade 1C). Although the equation for BED may be somewhat inaccurate for single-fraction sSBRT, the proposed universal survival curve has yet to be confirmed for different histologies. Additional research is needed to better define a more accurate BED equation for single-fraction radiation.

References

[1] Chow E, Harris K, Fan G, Tsao M, Sze WM. Palliative radiotherapy trials for bone metastases: a systematic review. J Clin Oncol 2007; 25: 1423–1436

[2] Hoskin PJ, Price P, Easton D, et al. A prospective randomised trial of 4 Gy or 8 Gy single doses in the treatment of metastatic bone pain. Radiother Oncol 1992; 23: 74–78

[3] Price P, Hoskin PJ, Easton D, Austin D, Palmer S, Yarnold JR. Low dose single fraction radiotherapy in the treatment of metastatic bone pain: a pilot study. Radiother Oncol 1988; 12: 297–300

[4] Price P, Hoskin PJ, Easton D, Austin D, Palmer SG, Yarnold JR. Prospective randomised trial of single and multifraction radiotherapy schedules in the treatment of painful bony metastases. Radiother Oncol 1986; 6: 247–255

[5] Uppelschoten JM, Wanders SL, de Jong JM. Single-dose radiotherapy (6 Gy): palliation in painful bone metastases. Radiother Oncol 1995; 36: 198–202

[6] Jeremic B, Shibamoto Y, Acimovic L, et al. A randomized trial of three single-dose radiation therapy regimens in the treatment of metastatic bone pain. Int J Radiat Oncol Biol Phys 1998; 42: 161–167

[7] Barak F, Werner A, Walach N, Horn Y. The palliative efficacy of a single high dose of radiation in treatment of symptomatic osseous metastases. Int J Radiat Oncol Biol Phys 1987; 13: 1233–1235

[8] Vargha ZO, Glicksman AS, Boland J. Single-dose radiation therapy in the palliation of metastatic disease. Radiology 1969; 93: 1181–1184

[9] Penn CR. Single dose and fractionated palliative irradiation for osseous metastases. Clin Radiol 1976; 27: 405–408

[10] Gaze MN, Kelly CG, Kerr GR, et al. Pain relief and quality of life following radiotherapy for bone metastases: a randomised trial of two fractionation schedules. Radiother Oncol 1997; 45: 109–116

[11] Ratanatharathorn V, Powers WE, Moss WT, Perez CA. Bone metastasis: review and critical analysis of random allocation trials of local field treatment. Int J Radiat Oncol Biol Phys 1999; 44: 1–18

[12] Hartsell WF, Scott CB, Bruner DW, et al. Randomized trial of short- versus long-course radiotherapy for palliation of painful bone metastases. J Natl Cancer Inst 2005; 97: 798–804

[13] Rades D, Stalpers LJ, Veninga T, et al. Evaluation of five radiation schedules and prognostic factors for metastatic spinal cord compression. J Clin Oncol 2005; 23: 3366–3375

[14] Hartsell WF, Konski AA, Lo SS, Hayman JA. Single fraction radiotherapy for bone metastases: clinically effective, time efficient, cost conscious and still underutilized in the United States? Clin Oncol (R Coll Radiol) 2009; 21: 652–654

[15] Chow E, Hahn CA, Lutz ST. Global reluctance to practice evidence-based medicine continues in the treatment of uncomplicated painful bone metastases despite level 1 evidence and practice guidelines. Int J Radiat Oncol Biol Phys 2012; 83: 1–2

[16] Barton R, Robinson G, Gutierrez E, Kirkbride P, McLean M. Palliative radiation for vertebral metastases: the effect of variation in prescription parameters on the dose received at depth. Int J Radiat Oncol Biol Phys 2002; 52: 1083–1091

[17] Medin PM, Foster RD, van der Kogel AJ, Sayre JW, McBride WH, Solberg TD. Spinal cord tolerance to single-fraction partial-volume irradiation: a swine model. Int J Radiat Oncol Biol Phys 2011; 79: 226–232

[18] Maranzano E, Latini P, Perrucci E, Beneventi S, Lupattelli M, Corgna E. Short-course radiotherapy (8 Gy 2) in metastatic spinal cord compression: an effective and feasible treatment. Int J Radiat Oncol Biol Phys 1997; 38: 1037–1044

[19] Garcia-Barros M, Paris F, Cordon-Cardo C, et al. Tumor response to radiotherapy regulated by endothelial cell apoptosis. Science 2003; 300: 1155–1159

[20] Gulbins E, Kolesnick R. Raft ceramide in molecular medicine. Oncogene 2003; 22: 7070–7077

[21] Park C, Papiez L, Zhang S, Story M, Timmerman RD. Universal survival curve and single fraction equivalent dose: useful tools in understanding potency of ablative radiotherapy. Int J Radiat Oncol Biol Phys 2008; 70: 847–852

[22] Maranzano E, Trippa F, Casale M, Anselmo P, Rossi R. Reirradiation of metastatic spinal cord compression: definitive results of two randomized trials. Radiother Oncol 2011; 98: 234–237

[23] Nieder C, Grosu AL, Andratschke NH, Molls M. Update of human spinal cord reirradiation tolerance based on additional data from 38 patients. Int J Radiat Oncol Biol Phys 2006; 66: 1446–1449

[24] Sahgal A, Ma L, Weinberg V, et al. Reirradiation human spinal cord tolerance for stereotactic body radiotherapy. Int J Radiat Oncol Biol Phys 2012; 82: 107–116

26 Spinal Cord Tolerance Greater than 10 Gy

Arjun Sahgal, Eric L. Chang, Simon S. Lo, Paul M. Medin, David A. Larson, and Lijun Ma

Introduction

Spine stereotactic body radiotherapy (sSBRT) is a powerful treatment modality, and clinical data support a high rate of efficacy.[1,2] However, it is also directly responsible for the reemergence of the rare and devastating toxicity of radiation-induced myelopathy (RIM).[3,4] The diagnosis of RIM is a diagnosis of exclusion and defined as neurologic signs and symptoms consistent with radiation damage in the form of necrosis to the segment of the spinal cord irradiated, without imaging-based evidence of recurrent or progressive tumor affecting the spinal cord.[5] The clinical consequences of RIM to the patient are major, as the patient may be left paralyzed and can die if it occurs in the cervical spinal cord. Therefore, determining the spinal cord tolerance to high dose per fraction radiation is one of the most important areas of development for safe sSBRT practice.

It is important to understand that if one simply optimizes a radiation therapy plan to keep the spinal cord dose very low, such as 5 Gy in a single fraction, then one can maintain a negligible risk of RIM. However, the surrounding cancerous tissue will be underdosed and will not be treated effectively. Therefore, one explanation of why progression of disease within the epidural space is the most common pattern of failure following sSBRT[1,6] is the relative underdosing that occurs within the epidural space to keep the spinal cord dose safe. Therefore, the challenge of safe sSBRT practice is to maintain the dose to the spinal cord just at tolerance, neither above nor below. Before it is possible to determine if the threshold spinal cord dose should be 10 Gy in a single fraction, some fundamental principles of spinal cord tolerance specific to spine SBRT must be considered.

Contouring Practice

Contouring of the spinal cord must be performed on magnetic resonance imaging (MRI) fused to the treatment planning computed tomography (CT) or directly on a planning CT myelogram.[1,7] MR images optimally should be acquired using volumetric T1 and T2 sequences, and one or two vertebrae rostral and caudal to the target segment,[8,9] for fusion. Some clinicians advocate the practice of contouring the thecal sac, which would be contoured according to the MRI or CT myelogram.[8] The thecal sac has the advantage of also being visualized directly on the treatment planning CT, which facilitates operator consistency among practices.

On which Contoured Structure should you Base the Spinal Cord Dose Limit?

One controversy lies in whether to base the dose limit on the contoured spinal cord itself or on a margin beyond the spinal cord.[10] An international clinical practice survey specific to sSBRT highlighted the variability in practice.[7] It was reported that dose limits have been applied to the spinal cord itself, a spinal cord planning organ-at-risk volume (PRV, typically a margin of 1.5 mm beyond the true cord), the thecal sac, or the spinal canal. Those who advocate applying the dose limit to the spinal cord plus a margin argue that it is a safer practice because you cannot assume that the dose stated by the treatment planning system is that truly delivered. The potential dose discrepancy is due to several factors:

1. The spinal cord is not a static organ. A recent investigation reported that motion linked with the respiratory cycle is on average ~ 0.5 mm in the axial plane.[11]
2. The patient moves during treatment. Even when technology is applied to its fullest extent for sSBRT treatments[12] (i.e., near-rigid body immobilization, kilovoltage cone-beam CT [CBCT] image guidance, and six degree of freedom [6-DOF] patient-positioning corrections using a robotic couch), there is still intrafraction motion of ~ 1.2 mm and 1.0 degree.[12] This level of precision is also consistent with robotic linear accelerator (LINAC)–based systems.[13]
3. Tumor location and the immobilization system employed can both affect the level of precision in treatment delivery. It has been reported that cervical locations are more susceptible to intrafraction motions as compared to thoracic and lumbar locations.[14] This observation was based on the cervical spine immobilized in a thermoplastic head and shoulder mask, and thoracic and lumbar targets immobilized in a vacuum suctionned body immobilization cushion (vac-loc) system. However, the target position was verified with intrafraction stereoscopic imaging every 30 to 45 seconds with near-real-time corrections of the LINAC itself in all six degrees of freedom via a robotic arm (CyberKnife, Accuray Inc., Sunnyvale, CA). In this analysis, thoracic tumors were shown to be the least likely to be affected by intrafraction motions; this is probably due to the physiologic stability gained by the attached ribs.[14] A study by researchers at the University of Toronto failed to determine any difference in intrafraction motion between thoracic and lumbar tumors, suggesting a stabilizing effect on the lumbar spine by using a near-rigid body immobilization system (BodyFIX, Elekta AB).[12] The use of a near-rigid body immobilization system has also been shown to be more robust in minimizing intrafraction motions as compared to a simple vac-loc system,[15] and it can reduce uncertainty margins by 1 mm. Overall, these studies point to intrinsic site-dependent target motions, and they reinforce the use of a rigid external immobilization device for fixating the patient's torso. However, proper immobilization may counter only certain aspects of motions; this is why an applied margin of 1 to 2 mm as a planning target volume (PTV) beyond the gross spinal target volume cannot be avoided. A similar argument has been made with respect to applying a cord PRV.
4. Intrafraction imaging is required to ensure that the patient remains in the intended position during treatment.[12,14] This is necessary due to the relatively long treatment times associated with high-dose sSBRT, which can range from 45 to 90 minutes. For example, the University of Toronto study concluded that, in order to maintain delivery precision within 1.2 mm and 1 degree using LINAC-based stereotactic

radiosurgery (SRS) coupled with CBCT image guidance and a 6-DOF robotic couch (Elekta Axesse, Crawley, UK), the target position must be imaged every 15 to 20 minutes with a threshold for patient repositioning set at 1 mm and 1 degree[12]. With stereoscopic imaging coupled to near-real-time robotic LINAC positioning adjustments (CyberKnife), the optimal imaging frequency was reported as approximately every 5 minutes to maintain a 1-mm and 1-degree precision based on patients immobilized in a less robust body immobilization device (vac-loc).[14] The point here is that without intrafraction imaging of a sufficient frequency, the position of the target will systematically drift, creating a large directionally biased margin on the target volume that may affect the actual dose delivered to the spinal cord[14].

The requirement for intrafractional imaging is highly dependent on treatment time,[12] and it will likely be rendered unnecessary in the future due to the advent of volumetric modulated arc therapy (VMAT). VMAT reduces treatment times for a single-fraction 24-Gy dose to ~ 10 to 20 minutes. Furthermore, when VMAT technology is coupled to new ultra-high monitor unit output LINAC systems, a single fraction of 24 Gy can be delivered in as fast as 3 minutes. These new technologies may negate the need for intrafraction imaging, but patient setup and stability will continue to be of utmost importance, as a small positional shift could result in a major dosing error to the spinal cord.

5. There are several other factors in the overall sSBRT process to consider with respect to precision of delivery. For example, there are uncertainties associated with the MR-CT image fusion, as well as those inherent to the image guidance system, treatment-planning calculation algorithms, and treatment couch motions.

Although these sources of uncertainties are small (millimeter to submillimeter) in magnitude, their impact is compounded if independence among the individual processes is assumed. The steepest dose gradient is at the target-spinal cord interface, which makes it dosimetrically susceptible to minor motions.[13,16,17] This is the reason why the technique of applying the dose limit to a PRV margin of ~ 1.5 mm beyond the true spinal cord (or to the thecal sac) is felt to be a safer practice.[8] The following question is then raised.

What is the Dosimetric Effect of these Very Small Intra- and Interfractional Errors on the True Spinal Cord Dose?

This question can be answered by the study reported by Chuang et al.[13] Based on CyberKnife treatments, with intrafraction positional data obtained every 30 to 45 seconds, minor motions were observed. Typically, the targets were stable to within 1 mm and 1 degree; however, sporadic 2-mm and 2-degree motions were also observed. The dosimetric impact of these intrafraction motions was then modeled for the spinal cord. The delivered dose was potentially 4.5% greater than expected based on the treatment plan. Therefore, if the spinal cord is believed to be exposed to 10 Gy, but it actually received 10.5 Gy, then that individual patient would have been exposed to some greater degree of risk for RIM than otherwise expected. The degree of increased dose was found to be highly dependent on individual treatment plans.

Ultimately, if one applies the dose limit to the true spinal cord, then one runs the risk of assuming the dosimetric effect of these sources of inaccuracies can be compensated by simply lowering, raising, or maintaining a certain dose level. However, without patient-specific spinal cord motion and setup data, the decision to lower, increase, or maintain a dose limit is highly subjective, as noted in the preceding study. A more consistent practice is achieved by applying the dose limit thought applicable to the true spinal cord to the spinal cord PRV (a margin of 1.5 mm) or to the thecal sac itself.[7,8] Alternatively, the spinal cord constraint can be based according to data generated from the thecal sac or spinal cord PRV and not the true spinal cord itself. It is important to note that the thecal sac essentially refers to an anatomical margin beyond the spinal cord and, typically, equivalent to a 1.5-mm spinal cord PRV margin. Either way, the true spinal cord dose is less than the spinal cord PRV, and the worst case dosimetric scenario has been taken into account.

Human Spinal Cord Dose Limits Specific to Spine Stereotactic Body Radiotherapy

Patients with no Prior Radiation

In 2010 Sahgal et al reported an initial dosimetric analysis for RIM specific to sSBRT[4] (***level III evidence***). This analysis was based on 5 cases of RIM following sSBRT and 19 sSBRT controls. All spinal cords were contoured based on the thecal sac as an anatomical margin beyond the true cord. Based on the specific thecal sac volumes analyzed, which consisted of the maximum point (P_{max}) volume, 0.1-, 1.0-, 2.0-, and 5-cm^3, a significant difference in the doses was observed only at the P_{max} volume. This led to the conclusion that the human spinal cord behaves as a serial organ, and that small volumes of spinal cord irradiated to higher doses than otherwise thought tolerant does indeed matter. There has been debate on this specific conclusion, as recent rat spinal cord data supported the potential for a partial volume effect;[18] however, recent experiments in pigs failed to render a similar conclusion.[19]

From the analysis by Sahgal et al, it was concluded that a single-fraction thecal sac dose of 10 Gy within a P_{max} volume is safe; this corresponds to a normalized biologically effective dose (nBED, i.e., an equivalent dose in 2 Gy/d fractions) of 30 $Gy_{2/2}$ ($Gy_{2/2}$ refers to the nBED calculated using an alpha beta ratio of 2).[4] This conclusion was driven by one case of RIM that was observed at a thecal sac dose of 10.6 Gy in a single fraction. However, for two- to five-fraction sSBRT, the dose limit increased to an nBED of 35 $Gy_{2/2}$, which reflects the protective effect of fractionation. This nBED translates to a dose limit of 14.5 Gy in two fractions, 17.5 Gy in three fractions, 20.0 Gy in four fractions, and 22.0 Gy in five fractions. These thresholds were not based on risk probability, but simply where RIM was not observed and the doses within the control group.

An updated analysis of the initial report was presented at the American Society of Therapeutic Radiation Oncology meeting[20] in 2011 (***level III evidence***). With 9 cases of RIM and 66 controls, Sahgal et al were able to perform a logistic regression analysis to generate risk profiles.[20] They also performed a more extensive dose-volume histogram (DVH) analysis comparing the doses within the P_{max}, 0.1- to 1.0-cm^3 volumes in increments of 0.1 cm^3, and 2-cm^3 volumes between the RIM cases and controls. A significant difference was observed only up to the 0.8-cm^3 volume, with the most significant difference observed at the P_{max} volume, supporting the previous observation that the dose within small volumes of the spinal cord does indeed predict for toxicity. One to 5% risk profiles according to the P_{max} volume for one- to five-fraction SBRT have been presented to date. A ≤ 5% risk of RIM was predicted for thecal sac P_{max} volume doses of 12.4 Gy in one fraction, 17.0 Gy in two fractions, 20.3 Gy in three fractions, 23.0 Gy in four fractions, and 25.3 Gy in five fractions.

Re-treatment Spinal Cord Tolerance

The literature on spinal cord tolerance in the re-treatment scenario has been extremely limited until recently. Sahgal et al reported a DVH analysis of 5 cases of retreatment RIM following sSBRT and compared these cases to 16 re-treatment sSBRT controls[3] (***level III evidence***). All spinal cords were contoured based on the thecal sac. Given that these were re-treatment cases, the analysis was based on consideration of the first course of conventional radiation and the re-treatment SBRT course separately, then the cumulative total doses.

The authors first concluded that the recommendations are applicable to an initial conventional radiotherapy course such that the thecal sac nBED ranges from 30 to 50 $Gy_{2/2}$. Accordingly, the cumulative thecal sac P_{max} nBED should not exceed 70 $Gy_{2/2}$. This total dose is based on the provision that the SBRT thecal sac re-treatment P_{max} nBED does not exceed 25 $Gy_{2/2}$, and the thecal sac SBRT P_{max} nBED/total P_{max} nBED ratio does not exceed 0.5. The authors also recommended a minimum 5-month time interval to reirradiation; this was consistent with previous recommendations based on conventional reirradiation practice.[21] Practical dose limits are summarized in Table 6 of the referenced study.[3] As an example, for a patient initially treated with 30 Gy in 10 fractions to a vertebral body tumor, the re-treatment SBRT should be planned such that the thecal sac dose does not exceed 9 Gy in a single fraction, 12.2 Gy in 2 fractions, 14.5 Gy in 3 fractions, 16.5 Gy in 4 fractions, or 18 Gy in 5 fractions.

■ Authors' Practice

The corresponding authors led the international collaborative studies defining spinal cord tolerance specific to spine SBRT.[3,20] Currently, our center is very comfortable with applying the published thecal sac dose limits to the cord plus 1.5-mm PRV margin, as we are confident in the precision of our LINAC, the image fusion process, and the near-rigid immobilization system used. We have published our technical results with respect to treatment delivery and report a precision of 1.2 mm and 1 degree with 95% confidence.[8,12] In situations where the spinal cord is not visible to the degree that we are confident (e.g., in postoperative cases) and we need to assume a worst case scenario, we contour the thecal sac itself and apply the dose limit to that structure. Alternatively, we perform CT myelography and base the limits on the thecal sac or cord PRV depending on the image quality.

■ Future Directions

In the event that additional cases of post-SBRT RIM do occur, we will be able to improve upon the robustness of the logistic model and provide more accurate estimates of the percent probabilities associated with spinal cord toxicity. We anticipate that RIM cases will become less frequent in the future as a respect for dosing small volumes of the spinal cord has been learned and adopted; the majority of RIM cases occurred as a result of P_{max} doses that would traditionally be considered unsafe. Phase 1 dose escalation studies would be one way in which to determine if the estimates are correct. However, such studies are not likely to be feasible, as large patient numbers would be required per dose level, and, as RIM is a late toxicity, the duration of follow-up before one could move to the next spinal cord dose level would be quite lengthy. Furthermore, there are ethical issues in conducting such a study, and patient participation would be an issue, given that the clinical consequences of RIM are so severe.

One area for improvement is to more accurately model the BED for high single-fraction doses.[22] This is an active area of research[23,24] and may alter the published thresholds. Some work has been done already to model the nonuniformity of the dose distribution into the BED calculation.[23]

With respect to reirradiation spinal cord tolerance, we know that the cord has a significant ability to repair radiation damage and subsequently to tolerate a second course of radiation.[3,5,21,25] However, more refined models are needed to predict acceptable cumulative doses as a function of the time interval between courses.

■ Conclusion

The initial question posed in this chapter was whether or not the spinal cord tolerance for single-fraction sSBRT is > 10 Gy. The answer is yes; however, this is specific to patients with no history of prior irradiation to the involved level, single-fraction sSBRT, and comes at a cost of a greater possibility for RIM. For single-fraction sSBRT, the current data suggest a probability of ≤ 3% when the thecal sac dose is 10 Gy, and < 5% when the dose is 12.4 Gy. For re-treatment, the current data support a thecal sac dose of 9 Gy in a single fraction within a limited range of previous radiation exposure.[3] When the dose is fractionated, whether in the setting of prior radiation or not, the dose limit is > 10 Gy as a result of the protective effect of fractionation on the spinal cord. These guidelines for safe practice have been published and summarized in ▶ Table 26.1.[3,4,20]

Table 26.1 Suggested doses to the thecal sac P_{max} volume for spine stereotactic body radiotherapy

Prior conventional radiotherapy (nBED)	One-fraction SBRT P_{max} (Gy)	Two-fraction SBRT P_{max} (Gy)	Three-fraction SBRT P_{max} (Gy)	Four-fraction SBRT P_{max} (Gy)	Five-fraction SBRT P_{max} (Gy)
0*	10	14.5	17	20	22
20 Gy in 5–30 Gy in 10 fx (30.0–37.5 $Gy_{2/2}$)	9	12.2	14.5	16.5	18
37.5 Gy in 15–45 Gy in 25 fx (40–43 $Gy_{2/2}$)	NA	12.2	14.5	16.2	18
50 Gy in 25 fx (50 $Gy_{2/2}$)	NA	11	12.5	14	15.5

Abbreviations: fx, fraction(s); NA, Not Applicable; nBED, normalized biologically effective dose; P_{max}, maximum point; SBRT, stereotactic body radiotherapy.
** These numbers are based on our initial analysis,[4] and the updated analysis in abstract form qualify these doses to suggest a ≤ 3% risk of radiation-induced myelopathy, according to Sahgal et al.[20] Re-treat dose limits are not risk-based estimates but where we found the dose to be safe, according to Sahgal et al.[3]*
Source: Adapted from Sahgal A, Ma L, Weinberg V, et al. Reirradiation human spinal cord tolerance for stereotactic body radiotherapy. Int J Radiat Oncol Biol Phys 2012;82(1):107–116, with permission.

References

[1] Sahgal A, Bilsky M, Chang EL, et al. Stereotactic body radiotherapy for spinal metastases: current status, with a focus on its application in the postoperative patient. J Neurosurg Spine 2011; 14: 151–166

[2] Sahgal A, Larson DA, Chang EL. Stereotactic body radiosurgery for spinal metastases: a critical review. Int J Radiat Oncol Biol Phys 2008; 71: 652–665

[3] Sahgal A, Ma L, Weinberg V, et al. Reirradiation human spinal cord tolerance for stereotactic body radiotherapy. Int J Radiat Oncol Biol Phys 2012; 82: 107–116

[4] Sahgal A, Ma L, Gibbs I, et al. Spinal cord tolerance for stereotactic body radiotherapy. Int J Radiat Oncol Biol Phys 2010; 77: 548–553

[5] Wong CS, Van Dyk J, Milosevic M, Laperriere NJ. Radiation myelopathy following single courses of radiotherapy and retreatment. Int J Radiat Oncol Biol Phys 1994; 30: 575–581

[6] Chang EL, Shiu AS, Mendel E, et al. Phase I/II study of stereotactic body radiotherapy for spinal metastasis and its pattern of failure. J Neurosurg Spine 2007; 7: 151–160

[7] Guckenberger M, Sweeney RA, Flickinger JC, et al. Clinical practice of image-guided spine radiosurgery—results from an international research consortium. Radiat Oncol 2011 Dec 15; 6: 172

[8] Foote M, Letourneau D, Hyde D, et al. Technique for stereotactic body radiotherapy for spinal metastases. J Clin Neurosci 2011; 18: 276–279

[9] Sohn MJ, Lee DJ, Yoon SW, Lee HR, Hwang YJ. The effective application of segmental image fusion in spinal radiosurgery for improved targeting of spinal tumours. Acta Neurochir (Wien) 2009; 151: 231–238, discussion 238

[10] Lo SS, Wang JZ, Radawski JD, Mayr NA. Reporting of true spinal cord dose is encouraged for stereotactic body radiation therapy for spinal tumors. In regard to Sahgal et al. (Int J Radiat Oncol Biol Phys 2010;77:548–553). Int J Radiat Oncol Biol Phys 2010; 78: 314

[11] Cai J, Sheng K, Sheehan JP, Benedict SH, Larner JM, Read PW. Evaluation of thoracic spinal cord motion using dynamic MRI. Radiother Oncol 2007; 84: 279–282

[12] Hyde D, Lochray F, Korol R, et al. Spine stereotactic body radiotherapy utilizing cone-beam CT image-guidance with a robotic couch: intrafraction motion analysis accounting for all six degrees of freedom. Int J Radiat Oncol Biol Phys 2012; 82: e555–e562

[13] Chuang C, Sahgal A, Lee L, et al. Effects of residual target motion for image-tracked spine radiosurgery. Med Phys 2007; 34: 4484–4490

[14] Ma L, Sahgal A, Hossain S, et al. Nonrandom intrafraction target motions and general strategy for correction of spine stereotactic body radiotherapy. Int J Radiat Oncol Biol Phys 2009; 75: 1261–1265

[15] Li W, Sahgal A, Foote M, et al. Impact of immobilization on intra-fraction motion for spine stereotactic body radiotherapy (SBRT) using cone beam computed tomography (CBCT). Int J Radiat Oncol Biol Phys 2012; 78: S285

[16] Wang H, Shiu A, Wang C, et al. Dosimetric effect of translational and rotational errors for patients undergoing image-guided stereotactic body radiotherapy for spinal metastases. Int J Radiat Oncol Biol Phys 2008; 71: 1261–1271

[17] Gutfeld O, Kretzler AE, Kashani R, Tatro D, Balter JM. Influence of rotations on dose distributions in spinal stereotactic body radiotherapy (SBRT). Int J Radiat Oncol Biol Phys 2009; 73: 1596–1601

[18] Bijl HP, van Luijk P, Coppes RP, Schippers JM, Konings AW, van der Kogel AJ. Unexpected changes of rat cervical spinal cord tolerance caused by inhomogeneous dose distributions. Int J Radiat Oncol Biol Phys 2003; 57: 274–281

[19] Medin PM, Foster RD, van der Kogel AJ, Sayre JW, McBride WH, Solberg TD. Spinal cord tolerance to single-fraction partial-volume irradiation: a swine model. Int J Radiat Oncol Biol Phys 2011; 79: 226–232

[20] Sahgal A, Ma L, Weinberg V, et al. Stereotactic body radiotherapy (SBRT) spinal cord tolerance. Int J Radiat Oncol Biol Phys 2012; 82: 107–116

[21] Nieder C, Grosu AL, Andratschke NH, Molls M. Proposal of human spinal cord reirradiation dose based on collection of data from 40 patients. Int J Radiat Oncol Biol Phys 2005; 61: 851–855

[22] Park C, Papiez L, Zhang S, Story M, Timmerman RD. Universal survival curve and single fraction equivalent dose: useful tools in understanding potency of ablative radiotherapy. Int J Radiat Oncol Biol Phys 2008; 70: 847–852

[23] Sahgal A, Ma L, Fowler J, et al. Impact of dose hot spots on spinal cord tolerance following stereotactic body radiotherapy: a generalized biological effective dose analysis. Technol Cancer Res Treat 2012; 11: 35–40

[24] Daly ME, Luxton G, Choi CY, et al. Normal tissue complication probability estimation by the Lyman-Kutcher-Burman method does not accurately predict spinal cord tolerance to stereotactic radiosurgery. Int J Radiat Oncol Biol Phys 2012; 82: 2025–2032

[25] Nieder C, Grosu AL, Andratschke NH, Molls M. Update of human spinal cord reirradiation tolerance based on additional data from 38 patients. Int J Radiat Oncol Biol Phys 2006; 66: 1446–1449

27 Spinal Radiosurgery after Radiation Therapy XRT or Radiosurgery

Matthias Guckenberger and Reinhart A. Sweeney

Introduction

About one third of all cancer patients will develop bone metastases during their history of malignant disease.[1] Of these patients, ~ 70% will have metastases involving the vertebral column, most commonly the thoracic and lumbar spine. Radiotherapy plays an important role in the treatment of symptomatic vertebral metastases, including palliation of pain, control or prevention of neurologic symptoms, and prevention of pathologic fractures. Randomized trials and meta-analyses have reported reasonable rates of pain and motor function improvement despite the use of moderate to low irradiation doses in these palliative settings.[2,3] However, these radiotherapy treatments show limited long-term efficacy, with median duration of pain control of only 3 to 6 months[2] and maintenance of ambulatory status for only a few weeks.[4]

Reirradiation of patients with recurring pain or metastatic spinal cord compression appears effective but is practiced in only a few patients.[5] Simultaneously, it is hoped that improvements of systemic treatment options will further prolong overall survival of cancer patients, which makes the need for a safe and effective re-treatment option even more essential.

With conventional radiotherapy techniques, the potential to perform reirradiation is mainly limited by the tolerance of the human spinal cord. Because of the devastating consequences of radiation-induced myelopathy (RIM), radiation oncologists have been particularly cautious. Within the past several years, however, sophisticated radiotherapy technologies—intensity-modulated radiotherapy (IMRT) for generation of highly conformal dose distributions and image-guided radiation therapy (IGRT) for precise treatment delivery—have become available that allow for the reirradiation of vertebral lesions while sparing the spinal cord from potentially toxic irradiation doses. This radiosurgical reirradiation is performed as hypofractionated or even single-fraction treatment, and a steep dose gradient is frequently located within the spinal cord.

This fundamental difference in fractionation and dose distribution makes the direct transfer of experiences from reirradiation using conventional concepts and technologies highly questionable. It is therefore the aim of this chapter to summarize, evaluate, and discuss the current knowledge of spinal cord reirradiation tolerance with a particular focus on recent experiences with stereotactic radiosurgical concepts. A clinical case example is described in ▶ Fig. 27.1.

Spinal Cord Tolerance in Preclinical Animal Models

Animal models have been used for systematic evaluation of spinal cord reirradiation tolerance for many decades and generated highly valuable insights into the radiobiology of radiation-induced spinal cord damage and recovery. Despite the fact that all animal studies attempt to mimic human patient treatment as close as possible, an understanding of their limitations is important for the correct interpretation of these studies.[6] The number of animal tests is relatively small in all studies, causing large error margins of the results. These uncertainties need to be considered, and the error margin representing the worst case scenario should form the basis for transfer of the preclinical results to the human context. Animal numbers are especially too small to accurately model the flat regions of the dose-response curves, of which the low-incidence region of RIM is of highest relevance in human radiotherapy. The end point of the animal studies is most frequently paralysis, with gait changes as a clinical consequence; more subtle endpoints cannot be evaluated in animal studies but may be of high importance for our patients. Comorbidities as well as previous therapies may influence the spinal cord tolerance, and such parameters are not modeled in these animal studies. Finally, follow-up periods in all animal studies are somewhat shorter than the time frame for the development of late RIM in humans.

All animal studies using rodents, guinea pigs, and rhesus monkeys agree that there is substantial recovery of the spinal cord from previous radiotherapy. This close agreement among different species supports the applicability of animal studies for clinical practice in humans. The recovery of the spinal cord was observed in the cervical,[7,8] thoracic,[9] and lumbar spine regions[10,11] without obvious differences between the spinal cord levels. Repair of the subclinical damage seems to be similar for fractionated[8,11] and single-fraction radiotherapy[7] at the first irradiation course. Full recovery is not reported by the majority of the studies, with two main factors influencing the amount of recovery and residual damage: intensity of the initial radiotherapy course and time interval between the two radiotherapy courses.

The intensity of the first irradiation series was shown to have a strong influence on the recovery of the spinal cord. When doses < 50% of the ED_{50} (the median effective dose, or the dose with 50% complication rate) are delivered in the first radiotherapy course, an almost complete recovery of the spinal cord has been observed.[7,9,11] The radiation tolerance at the second radiotherapy course was almost as high as at the first course. For doses between 50 and 75% of the ED_{50}, spinal cord recovery was still substantial, but the spinal cord showed more damage.[7,12] When doses close to the tolerance level were given in the first course, almost no recovery was observed.[11]

The interval between the first and second irradiation course influences the recovery of the spinal cord. In a rat model, the majority of the recovery occurred within 6 months after the first radiotherapy course. Differences in the exact time frame of recovery have been reported between younger and adult rats, but recovery seems to plateau after 6 months for both age groups.[7]

Two animal studies will be presented in more detail. The first study, by Ang et al, simulated a scenario in which the spinal cord is irradiated with conventionally fractionated radiotherapy at the first and re-treatment courses.[9] The study

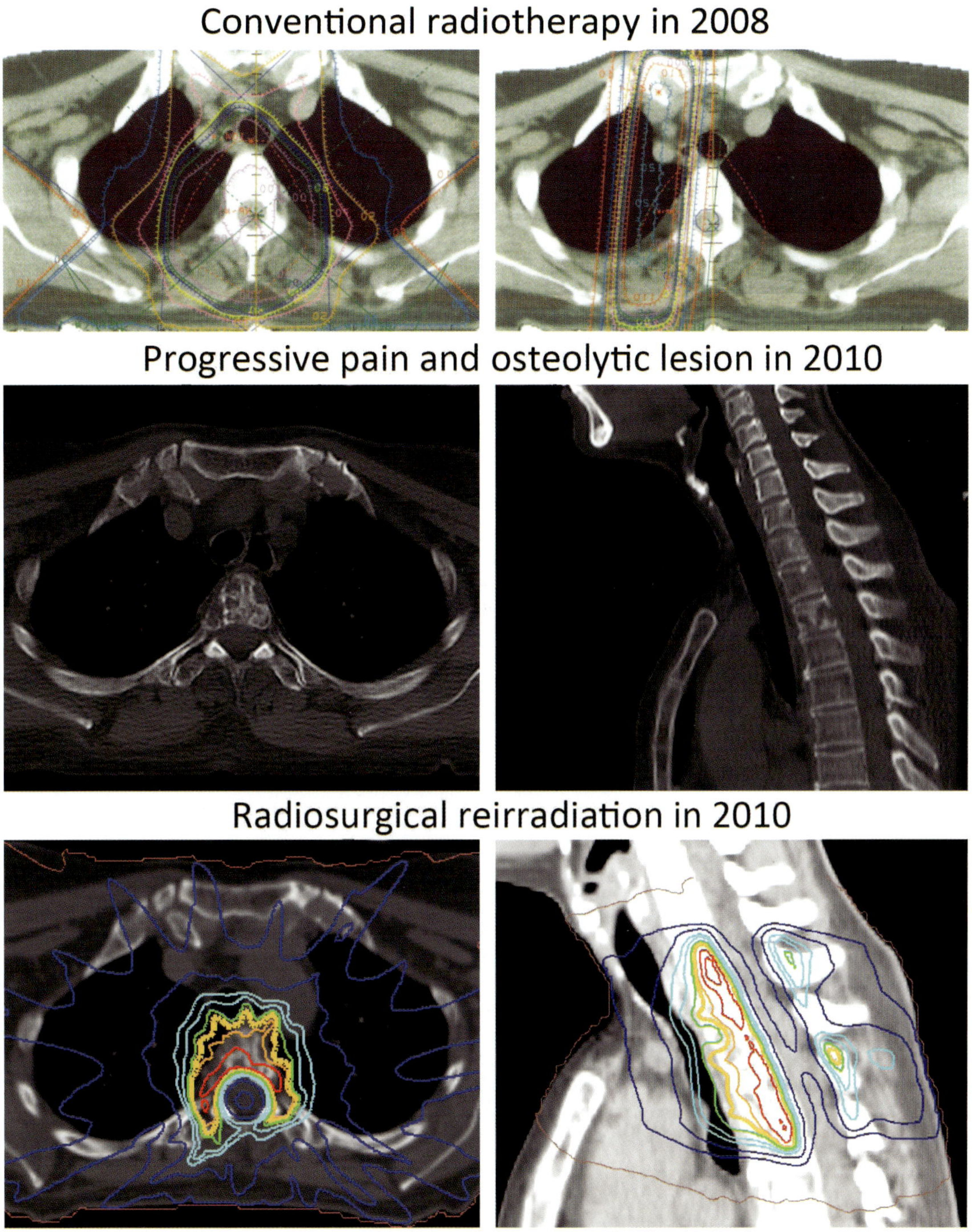

Fig. 27.1 A 50-year-old woman with a history of papillary thyroid cancer in 1979 was treated with iodine 131, followed by external beam radiotherapy consisting of 40-Gy photon radiotherapy and 20-Gy electron radiotherapy. Details of radiotherapy techniques and doses to organs at risk were unknown. The patient developed breast cancer in 2002 and bone metastases in 2007. In 2008 palliative radiotherapy of thoracic vertebrae 2 to 4 was performed with a total dose of 40 Gy: 20 Gy delivered using posterior wedged fields and 20 Gy using anteroposterior/posteroanterior fields with sparing of the spinal cord. In 2010 the patient suffered from recurrent pain in these vertebrae, and computed tomographic (CT) imaging showed progressive osteolytic metastases. Reirradiation was offered to the patient using intensity-modulated radiation therapy treatment planning and daily cone-beam CT–based image guidance. A dose of 40 Gy was delivered in 15 fractions to the involved vertebrae, while the maximum dose to the spinal cord was limited to 20 Gy. At the last follow-up 18 months after treatment, pain in the thoracic spine was controlled, irradiated vertebrae were sclerotic in CT imaging, and the patient described no neurologic symptoms indicating myelopathy.

was conducted in rhesus monkeys, which should make results more clinically applicable compared to rodent experiments. A group of 56 rhesus monkeys was irradiated at the cervical and upper thoracic level with a total dose of 44 Gy in 2.2-Gy single fractions. The animals were reirradiated with 57.2 Gy in 1- and 2-year intervals or with 66 Gy in 2- and 3-year intervals. Despite accumulated doses between 101.2 and 110.0 Gy, only 4 of 45 animals developed myeloparesis, which was the primary end point of the study. Data were fitted to different models, and no model was statistically superior to another. The "optimistic" model described substantial spinal cord recovery within the first year (76%) and further recovery after 2 years (85%) and 3 years (101%). The most conservative model described a 61% recovery after 1 year with no further recovery.

The second study, by Medin et al, simulated a scenario of hypofractionated irradiation, followed by re-treatment with single-fraction radiosurgery.[13] Using a swine model, the cervical and upper thoracic spine levels of 23 animals were irradiated with a homogeneous dose of 10 fractions of 3 Gy, and radiosurgical re-treatment was performed 1 year later with single-fraction doses between 24 and 14 Gy (90% isodose line). The radiosurgical target volume was placed laterally to the spinal cord, resulting in a dose distribution with the 90% and 10% isodose lines traversing the ipsilateral and contralateral spinal cord, respectively. The ED_{50} was 19.7 Gy in that study, which was identical to single-fraction radiosurgery in the primary situation, indicating full recovery of 10×3 Gy within the 1-year interval.[14] It has been hypothesized that the partial sparing of the spinal cord in the axial direction as practiced in radiosurgery may actually improve recovery by migration of remyelinating cells into the high-dose region. However, the ED_{50} in the Medin "radiosurgery" study was no different than studies where the whole axial diameter of the spinal cord was homogeneously irradiated.[49] Consequently, partial sparing of the spinal cord in the axial direction did not improve radiation tolerance.

This absence of a partial volume effect is in contrast to proton experiments in rats by Bijl et al, where the ED_{50} was 20.4, 33.4, and 71.9 Gy (single fraction irradiation doses) when the full diameter, lateral or central portions of the spinal cord were irradiated.[15] Additionally, the ED_{50} increased from 20.4 to 87.8 Gy when 20-mm versus 2-mm segments were irradiated,[50] indicating improved recovery when irradiated volumes are very small in longitudinal direction.

From animal studies, the following conclusions can be drawn for human clinical practice:

1. Substantial recovery of the spinal cord seems highly likely based on strong agreement between different studies, as well as across species.
2. If the irradiation dose of the first course is < 50 to 75% of the ED_{50}, spinal cord damage seems to be reparable.
3. Recovery happens mostly within 6 months after radiotherapy, with uncertain further recovery after 1 year and later.
4. Reirradiation with meaningful doses appears feasible based on conclusions 2 and 3.
5. The beneficial effect of sparing parts of the spinal cord in axial directions remains controversial and unknown at this time.

Reirradiation Spinal Cord Tolerance Using Conventional Fractionation

Unfortunately, there is no high level of evidence (***level I*** or ***II*** studies) with a dedicated focus on spinal cord tolerance or toxicity. Consequently, all data regarding the safety of spinal cord reirradiation and tolerance are based on retrospective studies with well-known limitations.

Wong et al identified 24 and 11 patients with a diagnosis of RIM after single-course radiotherapy and reirradiation, respectively. All patients treated at the Princess Margaret Hospital, Toronto, between 1955 and 1985 were the basis for this study, confirming the low incidence of RIM in radiotherapy practice.[17] Radiotherapy doses were converted to biologically effective doses (BEDs) for comparison of different fractionation protocols, and an α/β value of 2 Gy was used for the spinal cord. BEDs need to be divided by a factor of 2 for calculation of 2-Gy-equivalent doses (EQD2) if an α/β value of 2 Gy is used. Myelopathy following reirradiation developed after a median of 11.4 months, and the cumulative BED of the spinal cord was 148 Gy_2 (BED using α/β of 2 Gy) on average. This dose was significantly higher compared to the average BED of 121 Gy_2 in patients who developed myelopathy after single-course radiotherapy. When spinal cord recovery of 10 and 25% was assumed within 14 months and later than 14 months after the first radiotherapy course, respectively, this difference between single-course radiotherapy and reirradiation lost statistical significance. The authors acknowledged that this was a crude estimation of spinal cord recovery without precise knowledge of the magnitude and kinetics of long-term recovery.

Nieder et al performed a comprehensive analysis of human spinal cord reirradiation tolerance with conventional fractionation.[18,19] Detailed data of 78 patients were collected from studies in the literature in which reirradiation of the spinal cord had been performed. Irradiation doses were converted to BED using α/β values of 2 Gy for the cervical and thoracic cord and 4 Gy for the lumbar region. The interval between the radiotherapy courses, as well as the length of overlap, was included in the analysis. The median BED of the first radiotherapy course was 80 Gy_2 (range 34–124 Gy_2), and after a median interval of 24 months (2–152 mo), a second course of median BED 46 Gy_2 (range 4.7–108 Gy_2) was delivered to the spinal cord.

Eleven patients developed myelopathy after irradiation with cumulative BED of 145 Gy_2 (range 128.5–171 Gy_2) and an interval of median 19 months (range 2–71 mo) between the radiotherapy courses; 10 of 11 cases of myelopathy were taken from the study by Wong et al.[17] Myelopathy was seen only when one of the radiation courses was at least BED 102 Gy_2 or the interval between the radiation courses was very short, within 2 months. A scoring system was proposed for generation of three risk groups based on cumulative BED, dose of the highest radiotherapy course, and interval between the treatment courses. This scoring system differentiated between low (1/30), intermediate (2/8), and high risk (9/10) for the development of RIM. The risk of myelopathy is low if the accumulated BED is a maximum of 150 Gy_2, no radiotherapy course delivered a BED $\geq$ 102 Gy_2, and the interval is $\geq$ 6 months. This accumulated BED of 150 Gy_2 is higher than the accepted spinal cord tolerance doses of single-course radiotherapy. Consequently, the results of this study confirm experiences from animal studies that spinal cord recovery occurs within the first months after radiotherapy unless the irradiation dose is close to the tolerance dose.

Multiple studies have reported on the feasibility of reirradiation, especially for head and neck cancer, lung cancer, and palliative treatment of vertebral metastases. However, the majority of the studies limited the lifetime cumulative spinal cord dose to EQD 50 Gy_2, which is well within the spinal cord tolerance, assuming no recovery at all. Only a few studies assumed spinal cord recovery and allowed cumulative doses above the accepted tolerance dose of one radiotherapy course. Sulman et al defined a spinal cord lifetime tolerance of EQD 50 Gy_2 and assumed 50% spinal cord recovery if reirradiation was performed after an interval of at least 12 months between treatment courses; no myelopathy was reported in 78 patients with recurrent head and neck tumors after a median follow-up of 25 months.[20] A similar protocol was reported by Duprez et al. A spinal cord tolerance of EQD 50 Gy_2 was used, and 50% spinal cord recovery was assumed with a minimum 12 months between the radiotherapy courses.[21] After a median follow-up of 10 months, no case of myelopathy was observed in 84 patients; however, the concept of spinal cord recovery was used in an unknown proportion of all patients. Wu et al performed reirradiation in 23 patients with recurrent lung cancer, and a maximum cord dose of 25 Gy was allowed at re-treatment irrespective of the prior radiotherapy course.[22] Again, no myelopathy was described after a median follow-up of 15 months. Rades et al reported a large multicenter series of reirradiation for metastatic spinal cord compression, and 30 patients were treated with a cumulative BED of > 100 Gy_2, maximum 146 Gy_2.[23] After a median follow-up of 11 months for living patients, no case of myelopathy was described.

Based on a search in ClinicalTrials.gov using the keyword *reirradiation* (performed April 2012), no active phase III study was detected. Several active phase II trials regarding reirradiation, especially in the head and neck region, were found, but all study protocols limited the cumulative spinal cord dose to EQD2 doses of 50 to 60 Gy, which is within the accepted spinal cord tolerance assuming no spinal cord recovery.

The following conclusions can be drawn from studies on reirradiation using conventionally fractionated radiotherapy:

1. No high ***level of evidence*** defining spinal cord recovery is available.
2. Myelopathy is extremely rare after reirradiation using conventional fractionation schemes.
3. Retrospective studies support the hypothesis of spinal cord recovery with the interval between the radiotherapy courses, the cumulative dose, and the highest dose of one single radiotherapy course influencing the risk of myelopathy.
4. Conservative estimations indicate that spinal cord recovery in humans is lower than in animals.

Spinal Cord Tolerance in Radiosurgery

In this section, we will summarize and compare experiences of single-course radiosurgery to conventionally fractionated radiotherapy. Again, no high ***level of evidence*** is available, and all data and recommendations of spinal cord tolerance in single-fraction and fractionated radiosurgery are based on retrospective analyses.

There are essentially four different recommendations of spinal cord tolerance in radiosurgery. Gibbs et al pooled 1,075 patients treated using the CyberKnife (Accuray Inc., Sunnyvale, CA) at two institutions and reported six cases of myelopathy after a mean interval of 6 months.[24] Patients were treated with one to three fractions. Maximum physical doses and BEDs of the spinal cord ranged from 8.5 to 29.9 Gy and 44.6 to 197.8 Gy_2, respectively. The authors recommended limiting the volume of the spinal cord exposed to 8 Gy. This recommendation is difficult to understand, considering that single-fraction doses of 8 to10 Gy are safe using conventional radiotherapy, where the whole spinal cord diameter is exposed to these doses.[25] Inter- or intrafractional patient motion with the consequence of higher than intended doses to the spinal cord[26] could possibly explain the three cases where myelopathy developed after radiosurgery treatment with doses that are considered safe.

Ryu et al suggested that the partial volume tolerance of the human spinal cord is at least 10 Gy to 10% of the spinal cord volume, defined as 6 mm above and below the radiosurgery target.[27] This recommendation is based on 177 patients treated with single-fraction radiosurgery, and 10 Gy to 10 % of the spinal cord was the average dose in the cohort of patients treated at the highest dose level of 18 Gy. This recommendation is based on only one patient with a myelopathy, and 10% of the cord volume received only 9.6 Gy, which is below the recommendation.

A comprehensive analysis of spinal cord tolerance in single-fraction and fractionated radiosurgery was performed by Sahgal et al, who collected 5 cases of myelopathy and compared them to 19 cases without myelopathy.[28] This small number of control patients, where patient and treatment characteristics were not matched to the myelopathy cases, is a limitation of the study. Doses were converted to 2-Gy equivalent doses using an α/β ratio of 2 Gy, and the thecal sac instead of the actual spinal cord was delineated as organ at risk. Differences between myelopathy patients and controls were significant for the maximum dose to the thecal sac, and the authors recommended a dose threshold of 10 Gy in a single fraction and 2-Gy equivalent doses of 30 to 35 Gy for up to five fractions.

The QUANTEC recommendation of spinal cord tolerance using spinal radiosurgery, where only parts of the spinal cord are exposed to maximum doses, is a maximum cord dose of 13 and 20 Gy in one fraction and three fractions, respectively, for a risk of myelopathy < 1%.[29] Unfortunately, the methodology used to determine how these radiosurgical dose thresholds were obtained was not fully explained.

Recent studies based on radiosurgery of mostly intramedullary hemangioblastomas suggest a somewhat higher partial volume tolerance of the spinal cord.[30,31] The majority of the lesions were treated with single-fraction radiosurgery of median 20 Gy, resulting in small volumes of the spinal cord exposed to doses > 20 Gy. Neurologic toxicity was low: one patient developed grade 2 unilateral foot drop at 5 months, and 2 patients developed grade 1 sensory deficits. However, the median tumor volume was only 0.16 cm^3, which limits the applicability of these results for more frequent indications, such as much larger bony vertebral metastases. Nevertheless, these data confirm the animal studies by Bijl et al,[15,16] which are discussed above.

A note of caution should be considered when models are used for estimating spinal cord toxicity or for comparing different fractionation protocols. The mechanisms of spinal cord damage and repair are poorly understood, which makes modeling of toxicity difficult. In general, the applicability of the linear-quadratic model seems to be uncertain when single-fraction doses ≥ 10 Gy are used.[32] For modeling of spinal cord toxicity, both animal studies[33,34] and human data[31] found that currently available normal tissue complication probability (NTCP) models fail to precisely describe spinal cord toxicity, mostly because of the volume effect observed in these studies.

The available data allow for the following conclusions:

1. A spinal cord tolerance dose of 10 Gy—as the maximum dose to the thecal sac or 10% of the spinal cord volume—is currently the most valid recommendation for single-fraction radiosurgery based on the available literature.
2. Very small volumes of the spinal cord appear to tolerate substantially higher doses of ~ 20 Gy.
3. These recommendations of the spinal cord tolerance dose in radiosurgery are based on retrospective studies, small patient and event numbers, studies using different methodology, and relatively short follow-up.
4. Prospective trials and/or large cooperative studies are required for refinement of the accepted human spinal cord tolerance.

Reirradiation Spinal Cord Tolerance Using Radiosurgery

An increasing number of studies have evaluated the feasibility, safety, and efficacy of single- and multifraction radiosurgical reirradiation for vertebral metastases. These studies are summarized in ▶ Table 27.1. All studies agree that the risk of myelopathy is remarkably low: only 3 cases of myelopathy are described in more than 1,000 cases of radiosurgical reirradiation. Additionally, few cases with toxicity to the nerve roots are described. This is most likely at least partially explained by sophisticated radiotherapy treatment planning and delivery: all studies used some form of IMRT planning and highly accurate image-guided treatment delivery. Consequently, these two technologies are prerequisites for the safe practice of radiosurgical reirradiation.

However, these promising results need to be interpreted with caution. Patient numbers are still small in most of the studies, and follow-up is usually in the range of only 12 months, in some studies even shorter. Therefore, a large proportion of the patients with metastatic disease in these studies died before being at risk for developing RIM. Most importantly, essential information about the methodology of radiosurgical reirradiation is missing in many studies. In the following section, key findings from these studies are summarized and discussed.

The median dose of the first radiotherapy course was most frequently in the range of 30 to 40 Gy, with single-fraction doses of 1.8 to 3.0 Gy. The interval to reirradiation was usually between 1 and 2 years. Consequently, the majority of patients in these studies fulfill the criteria by Nieder et al for low risk of myelopathy.[19] Only one study reported 20 patients being treated with two courses of radiosurgery, and no case of myelopathy was reported in that study;[35] however, detailed information about this patient cohort study is missing. A large variability of fractionations was used for radiosurgical reirradiation, but the majority of the studies performed multisession radiosurgery with three to five fractions and total doses of 20 to 30 Gy; single-fraction radiosurgery as the preferred fractionation was practiced by only two institutions.[36,37] Two German studies performed conventionally fractionated reirradiation using radiosurgical technology.[38,39]

Interestingly, almost one half of the studies did not describe their definition of spinal cord tolerance, information that is crucial for treatment planning. Three different concepts of spinal cord tolerance were identified: (1) Most studies defined a fixed dose threshold for the spinal cord irrespective of the prior irradiation series;[37,38,40–42] volume and dose thresholds varied considerably between studies. (2) One study chose a conservative approach, assuming no spinal cord recovery and no partial volume effect, and limited the cumulative spinal cord EQD2 dose to < 50 Gy_2.[43] (3) The most sophisticated concept was described by Nelson et al, where experiences from animal studies discussed above were transferred to clinical practice.[44] The spinal cord tolerance was set at EQD2 50 Gy_3, and spinal cord recovery of 25%, 33%, and 50% at 6 months, 1 year, and 2 years was assumed.

Unfortunately, the cumulative doses of the first radiotherapy course and radiosurgical reirradiation were not provided by the majority of these published studies. Three studies reported cumulative EQD2 doses of 50 to 60 Gy_2, which is within accepted limits.[39,40,43] Higher cumulative doses were accepted by Choi et al, where the cumulative EQD2 dose ranged from 32 to 122 Gy_3, median 76 Gy_3;[45] however, 1 of 42 patients in that series developed myelopathy. A Korean study with 49 patients reported an average cumulative EQD2 dose of 83.4 Gy_2 with no case of myelopathy after a median follow-up of 17 months.

A detailed analysis of spinal cord tolerance for radiosurgical reirradiation was performed by Sahgal et al, who collected and compared 5 cases of myelopathy to 16 without myelopathy.[46] Like the previously described analysis of this group, the small number of controls and the lack of matched patient and treatment characteristics are limitations of this study. Importantly, the thecal sac was defined as the spinal cord organ at risk, and maximum doses were used for modeling of myelopathy. It was concluded that radiosurgical reirradiation is safe if the following criteria are met: (1) if the interval between the radiotherapy courses is at least 5 months, (2) if the reirradiation EQD is limited to 20 to 25 Gy_2, (3) if the cumulative dose stays below EQD 70 Gy_2, and (4) if the stereotactic body radiotherapy dose constitutes no more than ~ 50% of the total cumulative dose. No case of myelopathy was observed if all these criteria were met. This recommendation is in very good agreement with the analysis of Nieder et al using conventional fractionation for reirradiation.[19]

Conclusion

A growing experience of radiosurgery reirradiation of spine metastases is available in the literature, and rates of severe

Table 27.1 Studies describing clinical practice and outcome after radiosurgery for reirradiation of vertebral metastases

Study	Study type	No. patients/ cases	Dose on first RT course	Interval	Planning	Setup/ imaging	Fractions of reirradiation	Reirradiation dose	Spinal cord tolerance	Spinal cord reirradiation	Accumulated dose	Spinal cord OAR	Follow-up	Myelopathy
Studies with detailed analysis and/or description of radiosurgery for reirradiation of vertebral metastases														
Milker-Zabel et al[38]	Retrospective, single institution	18/19	Median 38 Gy (28–46 Gy) in CF	17.7 mo (range 6.2 −108.2 mo)	IMRT	Stereotactic	CF	39.6 Gy (range 24 −45) in CF	< 20 Gy in reirradiation	< 20 Gy in all patients	NS	Cord + 2 −3 mm	12.3 mo	0%
Mahan et al[43]	Retrospective, single institution	8/8	Median 30 Gy (range 3045 Gy) in CF	NS	Tomotherapy	Daily MVCT	Median 15 (range 10–17)	Median 30 Gy (20–34)	Cumulative max. cord dose < 50 Gy	Median 14 Gy (range 6 −20 Gy)	Median 48 Gy (range 37.0–50.1 Gy), 2-Gy equivalent; α/β = 2 Gy	Spinal canal	15.2 mo	0%
Sahgal et al[47]	Retrospective, single institution	25/37	Median 36 Gy in median 14 fx	Median 11 mo	CyberKnife	kV tracking	Median 3 (range 1–5)	Median 24 Gy (range 8 −30 Gy)	NS	Spinal cord: D_{max} median 12.8 Gy (range 5.4–24 Gy) cauda: D_{max} median 13 Gy (range 8–21 Gy)	NS	Thecal sac	7 mo	0%
Choi et al[45]	Retrospective, single institution	42/51	Median 40 Gy (range 24.2 −50.4 Gy) with median 2-Gy single-fraction dose (range 1.8 −3.0 Gy)	Median 19 months (2–219)	CyberKnife	kV tracking	Median 2 (range 1–5)	Median 20 Gy (range 10 −30 Gy)	NS	Spinal cord: D_{max} median 19.3 Gy (range 5.1 −31.3 Gy)	Median 76 Gy (32 −122 Gy), 2-Gy equivalent; α/β = 3 Gy	NS	7 mo	1 case with grade 4 myelopathy
Sterzing et al[39]	Retrospective, two institutions	36/36	Median 30 Gy (range 30 −54 Gy) in median 10 fx (range 30−4 fx)	Median 17.5 mo (range 6 −198 mo)	Tomotherapy	Daily MVCT	Median 10 (range 22 −4)	Median 30 Gy (range 30 −70 Gy)	NS	Spinal cord: D_{max} median 9.8 Gy (range 5.2 −21.8 Gy)	Median 45 Gy (max 59.2 Gy), 2-Gy equivalent; α/β = 2 Gy	NS	7.5 mo	0%
Damast et al[40]	Retrospective, single institution	94/97	Median 30 Gy (range 8 −66 Gy); 91% using single-fraction dose ≤ 3 Gy	NS	IMRT	Daily portal images or CBCT	4 × 4 Gy (*n* = 42) 5 × 6 Gy (*n* = 55)		Cord max: 14 Gy for cauda and 16 Gy for cord irrespective of previous RT	D_{max} 5 × 4 Gy:	Median 54.3 Gy; 2-Gy equivalent; α/β = 2 Gy for the cohort treated with 5 × 6 Gy	Cord	12.1 mo	0%

Table 27.1 continued

Study	Study type	No. patients/ cases	Dose on first RT course	Interval	Planning	Setup/ imaging	Fractions of reirradiation	Reirradiation dose	Spinal cord tolerance	Spinal cord reirradiation	Accumulated dose	Spinal cord OAR	Follow-up	Myelopathy
Garg et al[41]	Prospective, single institution	59/63	Median 30 Gy (range 7.5–42)	NS	IMRT	Daily CT on rails or CBCT	5 × 6 Gy (n = 8) 3 × 9 Gy (n = 50) 5 × 4 Gy n=1		Median cord dose: 9 Gy in 3 fx, 10 Gy in 5 fx	NS	NS	NS	13 mo	0%; 2 cases with grade 3 peripheral nerve injury
Mahadevan et al[42]	Retrospective, single institution	60/81	Median 30 Gy (range 8 –46 Gy) in median 10 fx (range 1–25 fx)	Median 20 mo (range 6 –74 mo)	CyberKnife	kV tracking	Tumors abutting the cord: 5 × 5–6 Gy (*n* = 35); otherwise 3 × 8 Gy (*n* = 46)		Maximum; prescribed dose limited to the surface of the spinal cord	NS	NS	NS	12 mo	0%; 3 cases of persistent radicular pain; 1 case of new lower extremity pain; weakness
Chang et al[48]	Retrospective, single institution	49/54	Average 39.2 Gy, 2-Gy equivalent; α/β = 2 Gy	Median 24.5 mo (range 3 –80 mo)	CyberKnife	kV tracking	Median 3	Median 27 Gy	NS	Spinal cord: D_{max} 46.2 ± 35.2 Gy, 2-Gy equivalent; α/β = 2 Gy	Average 83.4 Gy, 2-Gy equivalent; α/β = 2 Gy	Thecal sac	17.3 mo	0%
Studies with mixed patient collectives of radiosurgery for primary treatment and reirradiation if vertebral metastases														
Gerszten et al[36]	Retrospective, singles institution	NS/344	Range: 10 × 3 Gy to 14 × 2.5 Gy	NS	CyberKnife	kV tracking	1	Median 20 Gy (range 12.5 –25 Gy)	NS	NS	NS	NS	21 mo	0%
Amdur et al[37]	Prospective, singles institution	12/15	NS	NS	IMRT	Daily CBCT	1	Median 14 Gy (range 8 –16 Gy)	5 Gy to 0.5mL	NS	NS	NS	8 mo	0%
Gagnon et al[35]	Retrospective, singles institution	NS/125: median 35 Gy NS/20: CyberKnife		NS	CyberKnife	kV tracking	3	Average 21.05 Gy	NS	NS	NS	NS	10.5 mo	0%
Nelson et al[44]	Retrospective, singles institution	22/	Median 35 Gy (range 20.0 –50.4 Gy; 1.8 –3 Gy/fx)	Median 16 mo (range 4 –30)	IMRT	Daily CBCT	Median 3	Median 18 Gy (range 14 –30 Gy)	50 Gy cord tolerance 2 Gy equivalent; α/β = 3 Gy; recovery of 25%, 33%, and 50% at 6 mo, 1 y, and 2 y	NS	NS	Spinal canal	7 mo	0%

Abbreviations: *CBCT, cone-beam computed tomography; CF, conventional fractionation;* D_{max}, *maximum dose; CT, computed tomography; fx, fraction(s); IMRT, intensity-modulated radiation therapy; MVCT, megavoltage computed tomography; NS, not stated; OAR, organ at risk; RT, radiotherapy.*

toxicity, especially RIM, are consistently low. However, small patient numbers, short follow-up, and substantial variation in the practice of reirradiation need to be considered, which precludes strong recommendations regarding the routine clinical practice of reirradiation of spine metastases with radiosurgery. Patients should be treated within prospective clinical trials, of which few are currently open.

Despite the fact that spinal cord recovery is consistently demonstrated in animal studies after radiotherapy, the majority of the reirradiation studies limited the spinal cord tolerance to EQD2 doses of 50 to 60 Gy_2, assuming no recovery of the spinal cord. Few studies with small patient numbers transferred the concept of spinal cord recovery into patient treatment, and no increased risk of myelopathy was observed in these studies. Therefore, it seems justified to discuss this more aggressive approach with the patient if traditional spinal cord tolerance cannot be realized and if no other treatment options are available. Despite the fact that a 50% rate of spinal cord recovery is used in some studies, based on the rhesus monkey experiences by Ang et al,[9] a more conservative recommendation appears appropriate, considering the limited clinical experiences: a spinal cord recovery of one fourth to one third can be assumed within an interval of 1 year and with none of the irradiation series delivering > 75% of total spinal cord tolerance.

There is no consensus in the literature regarding fractionation. The majority of the reirradiation studies used fractionated regimens with 3 to 10 fractions; single-fraction regimens are therefore not recommended in the reirradiation situation unless there is a reasonable distance between the spinal cord and the recurrent tumor, and doses to the spinal cord are low. More specific recommendations are not possible based on current evidence. Considering the low α/β value of the spinal cord, more fractionated regimens may increase the therapeutic ratio. However, the duration of the radiotherapy treatment needs to be balanced with the individual patient situation, considering life expectancy, performance status, and palliative versus curative indications for reirradiation.

There is no clear proof in the literature that the spinal cord can tolerate higher doses in the reirradiation situation if the dose is limited to small volumes of the spinal cord. Therefore, the maximum dose to the spinal cord should be considered as highly relevant for calculation of the tolerance dose. It is further recommended that a safety margin around the spinal cord should be established, or the thecal sac or spinal canal should be delineated as an organ at risk. Although daily image guidance will achieve highly accurate patient setup for the precise delivery of planned dose distributions, other uncertainties, such as registration between the planning CT and magnetic resonance imaging, delineation variability, and especially intrafractional patient motion, all need to be considered.

It is hoped that these recommendations will contribute to minimizing the risk of myelopathy. Future studies should further refine the spinal cord tolerance and the practice of reirradiation in general. It is important that all cases of myelopathy be reported in the literature; detailed clinical and dosimetric information of a larger number of myelopathy cases is essential for a better understanding of spinal cord reirradiation tolerance.

References

[1] Wong DA, Fornasier VL, MacNab I. Spinal metastases: the obvious, the occult, and the impostors. Spine 1990; 15: 1–4

[2] Chow E, Harris K, Fan G, Tsao M, Sze WM. Palliative radiotherapy trials for bone metastases: a systematic review. J Clin Oncol 2007; 25: 1423–1436

[3] Rades D, Stalpers LJ, Veninga T, et al. Evaluation of five radiation schedules and prognostic factors for metastatic spinal cord compression. J Clin Oncol 2005; 23: 3366–3375

[4] Patchell RA, Tibbs PA, Regine WF, et al. Direct decompressive surgical resection in the treatment of spinal cord compression caused by metastatic cancer: a randomised trial. Lancet 2005; 366: 643–648

[5] van der Linden YM, Lok JJ, Steenland E, et al. Dutch Bone Metastasis Study Group. Single fraction radiotherapy is efficacious: a further analysis of the Dutch Bone Metastasis Study controlling for the influence of retreatment. Int J Radiat Oncol Biol Phys 2004; 59: 528–537

[6] Medin PM, Boike TP. Spinal cord tolerance in the age of spinal radiosurgery: lessons from preclinical studies. Int J Radiat Oncol Biol Phys 2011; 79: 1302–1309

[7] Ruifrok AC, Kleiboer BJ, van der Kogel AJ. Reirradiation tolerance of the immature rat spinal cord. Radiother Oncol 1992; 23: 249–256

[8] Wong CS, Poon JK, Hill RP. Re-irradiation tolerance in the rat spinal cord: influence of level of initial damage. Radiother Oncol 1993; 26: 132–138

[9] Ang KK, Jiang GL, Feng Y, Stephens LC, Tucker SL, Price RE. Extent and kinetics of recovery of occult spinal cord injury. Int J Radiat Oncol Biol Phys 2001; 50: 1013–1020

[10] Knowles JF. The radiosensitivity of the guinea-pig spinal cord to X-rays: the effect of retreatment at one year and the effect of age at the time of irradiation. Int J Radiat Biol Relat Stud Phys Chem Med 1983; 44: 433–442

[11] Mason KA, Withers HR, Chiang CS. Late effects of radiation on the lumbar spinal cord of guinea pigs: re-treatment tolerance. Int J Radiat Oncol Biol Phys 1993; 26: 643–648

[12] Hornsey S, Myers R, Warren P. Residual injury in the spinal cord after treatment with X rays or neutrons. Br J Radiol 1982; 55: 516–519

[13] Medin PM, Foster RD, van der Kogel AJ, Sayre JW, McBride WH, Solberg TD. Spinal cord tolerance to reirradiation with single-fraction radiosurgery: a swine model. Int J Radiat Oncol Biol Phys 2012; 83: 1031–1037

[14] Medin PM, Foster RD, van der Kogel AJ, Sayre JW, McBride WH, Solberg TD. Spinal cord tolerance to single-fraction partial-volume irradiation: a swine model. Int J Radiat Oncol Biol Phys 2011; 79: 226–232

[15] Bijl HP, van Luijk P, Coppes RP, Schippers JM, Konings AW, van Der Kogel AJ. Regional differences in radiosensitivity across the rat cervical spinal cord. Int J Radiat Oncol Biol Phys 2005; 61: 543–551

[16] Bijl HP, van Luijk P, Coppes RP, Schippers JM, Konings AW, van der Kogel AJ. Unexpected changes of rat cervical spinal cord tolerance caused by inhomogeneous dose distributions. Int J Radiat Oncol Biol Phys 2003; 57: 274–281

[17] Wong CS, Van Dyk J, Milosevic M, Laperriere NJ. Radiation myelopathy following single courses of radiotherapy and retreatment. Int J Radiat Oncol Biol Phys 1994; 30: 575–581

[18] Nieder C, Grosu AL, Andratschke NH, Molls M. Proposal of human spinal cord reirradiation dose based on collection of data from 40 patients. Int J Radiat Oncol Biol Phys 2005; 61: 851–855

[19] Nieder C, Grosu AL, Andratschke NH, Molls M. Update of human spinal cord reirradiation tolerance based on additional data from 38 patients. Int J Radiat Oncol Biol Phys 2006; 66: 1446–1449

[20] Sulman EP, Schwartz DL, Le TT, et al. IMRT reirradiation of head and neck cancer-disease control and morbidity outcomes. Int J Radiat Oncol Biol Phys 2009; 73: 399–409

[21] Duprez F, Madani I, Bonte K, et al. Intensity-modulated radiotherapy for recurrent and second primary head and neck cancer in previously irradiated territory. Radiother Oncol 2009; 93: 563–569

[22] Wu KL, Jiang GL, Qian H, et al. Three-dimensional conformal radiotherapy for locoregionally recurrent lung carcinoma after external beam irradiation: a prospective phase I-II clinical trial. Int J Radiat Oncol Biol Phys 2003; 57: 1345–1350

[23] Rades D, Rudat V, Veninga T, Stalpers LJ, Hoskin PJ, Schild SE. Prognostic factors for functional outcome and survival after reirradiation for in-field recurrences of metastatic spinal cord compression. Cancer 2008; 113: 1090–1096

[24] Gibbs IC, Patil C, Gerszten PC, Adler JR, Burton SA. Delayed radiation-induced myelopathy after spinal radiosurgery. Neurosurgery 2009; 64 (Suppl): A67–A72

[25] Macbeth FR, Wheldon TE, Girling DJ, et al. The Medical Research Council Lung Cancer Working Party. Radiation myelopathy: estimates of risk in 1048 patients in three randomized trials of palliative radiotherapy for non-small cell lung cancer. Clin Oncol (R Coll Radiol) 1996; 8: 176–181

[26] Guckenberger M, Meyer J, Wilbert J, et al. Precision required for dose-escalated treatment of spinal metastases and implications for image-guided radiation therapy (IGRT). Radiother Oncol 2007; 84: 56–63

[27] Ryu S, Jin JY, Jin R, et al. Partial volume tolerance of the spinal cord and complications of single-dose radiosurgery. Cancer 2007; 109: 628–636

[28] Sahgal A, Ma L, Gibbs I, et al. Spinal cord tolerance for stereotactic body radiotherapy. Int J Radiat Oncol Biol Phys 2010; 77: 548–553

[29] Kirkpatrick JP, van der Kogel AJ, Schultheiss TE. Radiation dose-volume effects in the spinal cord. Int J Radiat Oncol Biol Phys 2010; 76 (Suppl): S42–S49

[30] Daly ME, Choi CY, Gibbs IC, et al. Tolerance of the spinal cord to stereotactic radiosurgery: insights from hemangioblastomas. Int J Radiat Oncol Biol Phys 2011; 80: 213–220

[31] Daly ME, Luxton G, Choi CY, et al. Normal tissue complication probability estimation by the Lyman-Kutcher-Burman method does not accurately predict spinal cord tolerance to stereotactic radiosurgery. Int J Radiat Oncol Biol Phys 2012; 82: 2025–2032

[32] Kirkpatrick JP, Meyer JJ, Marks LB. The linear-quadratic model is inappropriate to model high dose per fraction effects in radiosurgery. Semin Radiat Oncol 2008; 18: 240–243

[33] Philippens ME, Pop LA, Visser AG, Schellekens SA, van der Kogel AJ. Dose-volume effects in rat thoracolumbar spinal cord: an evaluation of NTCP models. Int J Radiat Oncol Biol Phys 2004; 60: 578–590

[34] van Luijk P, Bijl HP, Konings AW, van der Kogel AJ, Schippers JM. Data on dose-volume effects in the rat spinal cord do not support existing NTCP models. Int J Radiat Oncol Biol Phys 2005; 61: 892–900

[35] Gagnon GJ, Nasr NM, Liao JJ, et al. Treatment of spinal tumors using cyberknife fractionated stereotactic radiosurgery: pain and quality-of-life assessment after treatment in 200 patients. Neurosurgery 2009; 64: 297–306, discussion 306–307

[36] Gerszten PC, Burton SA, Ozhasoglu C, Welch WC. Radiosurgery for spinal metastases: clinical experience in 500 cases from a single institution. Spine 2007; 32: 193–199

[37] Amdur RJ, Bennett J, Olivier K, et al. A prospective, phase II study demonstrating the potential value and limitation of radiosurgery for spine metastases. Am J Clin Oncol 2009; 32: 515–520

[38] Milker-Zabel S, Zabel A, Thilmann C, Schlegel W, Wannenmacher M, Debus J. Clinical results of retreatment of vertebral bone metastases by stereotactic conformal radiotherapy and intensity-modulated radiotherapy. Int J Radiat Oncol Biol Phys 2003; 55: 162–167

[39] Sterzing F, Hauswald H, Uhl M, et al. Spinal cord sparing reirradiation with helical tomotherapy. Cancer 2010; 116: 3961–3968

[40] Damast S, Wright J, Bilsky M, et al. Impact of dose on local failure rates after image-guided reirradiation of recurrent paraspinal metastases. Int J Radiat Oncol Biol Phys 2011; 81: 819–826

[41] Garg AK, Wang XS, Shiu AS, et al. Prospective evaluation of spinal reirradiation by using stereotactic body radiation therapy: the University of Texas MD Anderson Cancer Center experience. Cancer 2011; 117: 3509–3516

[42] Mahadevan A, Floyd S, Wong E, Jeyapalan S, Groff M, Kasper E. Stereotactic body radiotherapy reirradiation for recurrent epidural spinal metastases. Int J Radiat Oncol Biol Phys 2011; 81: 1500–1505

[43] Mahan SL, Ramsey CR, Scaperoth DD, Chase DJ, Byrne TE. Evaluation of image-guided helical tomotherapy for the retreatment of spinal metastasis. Int J Radiat Oncol Biol Phys 2005; 63: 1576–1583

[44] Nelson JW, Yoo DS, Sampson JH, et al. Stereotactic body radiotherapy for lesions of the spine and paraspinal regions. Int J Radiat Oncol Biol Phys 2009; 73: 1369–1375

[45] Choi CY, Adler JR, Gibbs IC, et al. Stereotactic radiosurgery for treatment of spinal metastases recurring in close proximity to previously irradiated spinal cord. Int J Radiat Oncol Biol Phys 2010; 78: 499–506

[46] Sahgal A, Ma L, Weinberg V, et al. Reirradiation human spinal cord tolerance for stereotactic body radiotherapy. Int J Radiat Oncol Biol Phys 2012; 82: 107–116

[47] Sahgal A, Ames C, Chou D, et al. Stereotactic body radiotherapy is effective salvage therapy for patients with prior radiation of spinal metastases. Int J Radiat Oncol Biol Phys 2009; 74: 723–731

[48] Chang UK, Cho WI, Kim MS, Cho CK, Lee DH, Rhee CH. Local tumor control after retreatment of spinal metastasis using stereotactic body radiotherapy; comparison with initial treatment group. Acta Oncol 2012; 51: 589–595

[49] Medin PM, Foster RD, van der Kogel AJ, Sayre JW, McBride WH, Solberg TD. Spinal cord tolerance to single-session uniform irradiation in pigs: implications for a dose-volume effect. Radiother Oncol 2013; 106: 101–105

[50] Bijl HP, van Luijk P, Coppes RP, Schippers JM, Konings AW, van der Kogel AJ. Dose-volume effects in the rat cervical spinal cord after proton irradiation. Int J Radiat Oncol Biol Phys 2002; 52: 205–211

Fractionation and Complications of Spine Radiosurgery

28 Multisession Spinal Radiosurgery

Peter C. Gerszten, John C. Flickinger, and Mubina Quader

Introduction

Malignancy involving the spine is an important clinical problem in oncology. Secondary malignancy of the spinal column is extremely common. In a study of 2,000 patients with bony metastases, nearly 70% were found to have vertebral body metastases.[1] There are over 180,000 new cases of spinal metastases diagnosed in North America each year, with 20,000 clinical cases of spinal cord compression.[2–4] Furthermore, the incidence and prevalence of spine tumors are expected to rise in the future.

The role of radiation therapy in the treatment of metastatic tumors of the spine is well established and is often the initial treatment modality.[5–11] The goals of local radiation therapy in the treatment of spinal tumors have been palliation of pain, prevention of local disease progression and subsequent pathologic fractures, and halting progression or reversing of neurologic compromise.[12] Patients with metastatic spine tumors are often debilitated and at high risk for surgical morbidity.[13] For patients with limited life expectancies from their underlying disease, the impact of surgical complications with subsequent decrease in quality of life is not ideal. External beam radiotherapy theoretically avoids the morbidity associated with open surgical intervention.

The primary factor that limits radiation dose for local vertebral body and paraspinal tumor control with conventional radiotherapy is the relatively low tolerance of the spinal cord to radiation. Conventional external beam radiotherapy lacks the precision to deliver large single-fraction doses of radiation to vertebral tumors near radiosensitive structures, such as the spinal cord. It is the low tolerance of the spinal cord to radiation that often limits the treatment dose to a level that is far below the optimal therapeutic dose.[5,14,15]

Radiosurgery is currently widely employed as an effective means for spine metastases. Hamilton et al[16] first described the possibility of linear-accelerator (LINAC)–based spinal stereotactic radiosurgery in 1995 using a frame-based technique. Since that pioneering work, multiple centers have pursued large fraction conformal radiation delivery to spinal lesions using a variety of frameless technologies.[4,15,17–32] The ability to deliver a tumoricidal dose has improved responses of metastatic spine tumors previously considered resistant to conventional external beam radiation. The adoption of radiosurgery to the multimodality treatment of metastatic spine disease has translated into a significant improvement in the following areas of clinical outcomes for this patient population:[33–35]

- Pain
- Primary treatment modality
- Prevention of tumor progression
- Radiation boost for radioresistant tumors
- Progressive neurologic deficit
- Treatment of residual tumor after surgery
- Postsurgical tumor progression

Although there is general consensus regarding the efficacy of spine radiosurgery, there is little consensus and continued controversy regarding the ideal delivery schedule.

The Rationale for Radiosurgery for Spinal Metastases

Conventional external beam radiotherapy remains a commonly employed adjuvant therapy for spine metastases and offers significant short-term and, in some cases, long-term palliation. Thirty Gy delivered in 10 fractions is the most frequently employed fractionation schedule, but other schemes have been reported.[36,37]

One of the most significant applications of radiosurgery to date for metastatic spine disease has been as definitive local treatment.[15,18,19,38,54] In most series, the use of radiosurgery has been restricted to tumors that involve the vertebrae alone or with minimal epidural abutment. Tumors with high-grade spinal cord compression have been considered a relative contraindication to radiosurgery. Although radiosensitive tumors (e.g., hematologic malignancies) can be treated with hypofractionated regimens, the greatest utility of radiosurgery is the improved response of radioresistant tumors, even in the setting of prior conventional fractionated radiotherapy. The response rates for radiation-resistant tumors (e.g., renal cell and melanoma) using conventional radiotherapy regimens are poor, and many patients demonstrated tumor progression.[33,56] Large series reporting outcomes after conventional radiotherapy for spine metastases without stratifying for radiosensitivity of the tumors often reported excellent results only because of the large numbers of hematologic malignancies, breast, prostate, and neuroendocrine tumors.[33] When stratified by radiosensitivity to conventional external beam radiation, marked differences are seen in tumoral responses.[38–45] In one large series, Maranzano and Latini reported that radioresistant tumors such as hepatocellular carcinoma demonstrated only a 20% response rate with a durability of 1 to 3 months. Favorable, or radiosensitive, tumors showed an 80% response at 16 months.[39]

Although multiple studies have demonstrated success in treating spine metastases with radiosurgery, the ideal dose and other treatment parameters have yet to be determined. One of the more controversial topics has been the decision to perform spine radiosurgery in either a single or multiple sessions. The utilization of a single-session versus a multisession technique has previously been determined more by institutional preference than by quality comparative data or specific clinical criteria. We will attempt to explain the rationale for multisession radiosurgery in a variety of different clinical situations.

Rationale for the Use of Multisession Radiosurgery for Spinal Metastases

Historically, frame-based intracranial radiosurgery necessitated the use of single-fraction radiosurgery for the treatment of intracranial metastases due to the impracticality of multisession frame-based treatment. With the advent of frameless radiosurgery technology that led to the ability to perform spine radiosurgery, two different "camps" emerged. Neurosurgeons and some radiation oncologists with a strong background and comfort with frame-based intracranial radiosurgery preferred to directly translate doses and single-session fractionation schedules from the treatment of intracranial metastases to spine radiosurgery. In distinction, many radiation oncologists with training in non-image-guided conventional radiotherapy preferred a hypofractionated (or multisession) paradigm using higher and more conformal doses of radiation that could be achieved with the newer image-guided radiotherapy technology. The primary reason for employing a multisession technique is to increase the overall dose that can be delivered to the target volume, and thereby achieve a better clinical outcome while theoretically decreasing the possibility of spinal cord toxicity.

The radiobiological reasons for fractionation are well known, and the therapeutic gains are achieved by increasing the tolerance of the dose-limiting adjacent normal tissue and increasing the sensitivity of the target tissue.[46] Staging treatments exploit the differential repair between normal tissue and tumor (normal cells undergo more efficient DNA repair) and allow redistribution of cells within the cell cycle (irradiated cells are held up in the G2 and mitosis phases and are thus more susceptible to further irradiation), and reoxygenation (tumors become hyperemic after the first irradiation; the subsequent increase in oxygenation of tumor cells confers increased sensitivity to irradiation).

A large body of literature supports the benefits of fractionation, including the use of multisession therapy even in the setting of highly conformal image-guided radiosurgery. Although single large doses may overwhelm repair, reoxygenation, and reassortment effects, multisession radiosurgery combines surgically ablative radiation doses with modest fractionation to improve the sparing of adjacent normal tissues.[46] This allows for radiosurgery to be employed in certain clinical situations, especially in the setting of previously irradiated sites, large tumor volumes, and lesions that are particularly close to critical structures, such as the spinal cord.

■ Literature Supporting Multisession Radiosurgery for Spinal Metastases

A systematic literature review of radiosurgery for metastatic disease employing the GRADE criteria set out by Guyatt et al[47] specifically asked the question What are the current fractionation schedules for radiosurgery for metastatic spine disease?[33] From an analysis of 27 single-institution manuscripts published through 2009, no consensus on dose or fractionation could be determined in regard to symptomatic response, toxicity, or radiographic tumor control. Significant toxicity did not appear to be associated with any hypofractionation schedule (4 Gy × 4, 6 Gy × 5, 8 Gy × 3, 9 Gy × 3) or single dose (16–24 Gy × 1).

A more recent systematic literature review by Sohn and Chung[48] analyzed 31 studies on radiosurgery for spinal metastases. No large-scale study has yet developed an optimal dose or fractionation schedule for spine radiosurgery. The prescribed dose and fractionation are determined based on tumor histology, spinal cord or cauda equina tolerance, and previous radiation dosage to normal tissue, especially the spinal cord. Dose and fractionation schedules vary by institution. Currently, there is no evidence to support one regimen over the other. There is a tendency to employ multisession radiosurgery in the setting of previous irradiation to the target volume and for lesions that are close to the spinal cord. Previously irradiated lesions that were treated in multiple sessions were prescribed a median dose of 20 Gy in five fractions (range 20–30 Gy),[49] and a median dose of 20 Gy (range 10–30 Gy) in one to five fractions (median two fractions).

Gagnon et al published a prospective study of 151 spine metastases treated with multisession radiosurgery.[46] Pain and quality-of-life assessments were recorded for all patients. Treatment doses depended on histology but ranged from 21 to 24 Gy in three fractions and up to 37.5 Gy in five fractions. Mean pain scores decreased significantly ($p < 0.001$) and continued to decrease over a 4-year follow-up period ($p < 0.05$). The Mental Component scores of the SF-12 survey were significantly higher after treatment ($p < 0.01$), representing a quality-of-life improvement. The treatment was extremely well tolerated in all patients, and no late radiation toxicity was observed. Gagnon et al[50] also published a matched-pair analysis in a series of patients with breast cancer metastases using a multisession radiosurgery technique that demonstrated the benefit of radiosurgery compared to similarly matched control cases treated with conventional radiotherapy.

Yamada et al[49] reported a series of 21 patients with spine metastases who all underwent multisession radiosurgery with or without previous radiation. The tumors were prescribed 20 Gy in five fractions. Pain improvement occurred in > 90% of patients, and local radiographic control was achieved in 75%. Once again, using this multisession technique, no case of radiation-induced myelopathy or radiculopathy occurred in this series with a median follow-up of 11 months.

Nelson et al[51] reported a series of 32 spine metastases treated with radiosurgery using a median number of three fractions and total dose delivered of 18 Gy (range 14–30 Gy). Thirteen patients reported complete and 17 patients reported partial pain relief within 1 month of treatment. There were no treatment-related neurologic side effects. The majority of patients in this series had undergone conventional fractionated radiotherapy to the index lesion, and the authors emphasized the minimization of spinal cord toxicity, especially in the setting of reirradiation, for their dose and fractionation selection.

Chang et al[52] reported a phase I/II study of radiosurgery in a series of 63 patients with spinal metastases representing ***level III evidence***. The median survival time was 24 months from the time of enrollment. The first 32 patients were treated with five 6-Gy fractions to a total dose of 30 Gy. Because of the lengthy treatment duration, the subsequent patients received three 9-Gy fractions to a total dose of 27 Gy. No neuropathy or myelopathy was observed during a median follow-up period of 21 months. There was also no subacute or late grade 3 or 4 toxicity. The actuarial 1-year tumor progression-free incidence was 84% for all tumors. A careful analysis of the patterns of failure in 17 cases revealed two primary mechanisms: (1) tumor recurrence in the bone adjacent to the site of treatment, especially in the pedicles and posterior elements, and (2) tumor recurrence in the epidural space adjacent to the spinal cord. The employment of a multisession radiosurgical technique that avoided lower doses to tumor adjacent to the spinal cord because of fear of radiation-induced toxicity would likely translate to an overall higher local tumor control in this clinical setting.

This same group reported a more recent analysis of 55 renal cell carcinoma spinal metastases treated with 27 Gy delivered in three fractions or 30 Gy delivered in five fractions (eight cases were treated with 24 Gy delivered in a single fraction).[53] The actuarial 1-year spine tumor progression-free survival was 82%. No grade 3 or 4 neurologic toxicity occurred with a median follow-up time of 13 months. Once again, the majority of failures in this series occurred in the epidural space, and the failure was most likely due to the limited radiation dose to the tumor constrained by the dose to the spinal cord.

Multisession Radiosurgery in the Setting of Prior Open Surgery

The rationale for using radiosurgery as opposed to conventional radiotherapy as an adjuvant to surgical decompression is the predicted improvement in tumor control based on radioresponsiveness. Klekamp and Samii reviewed the local control rates for 106 spinal metastasis cases undergoing decompression followed by conventional radiotherapy.[54] The overall local recurrence rates as determined by the Kaplan-Meier method were 58% after 6 months, 69% after 1 year, and 96% after 4 years. If patients lived long enough, the tumor recurred locally in essentially all patients. Among the most important predictors of local tumor recurrence was tumor histology.

The poor local control rates using conventional radiotherapy for solid spine metastases have led investigators to explore the use of radiosurgery as a postoperative adjuvant therapy.[55] The ability to deliver cytotoxic doses to even gross residual tumor has radically changed the aggressiveness of tumor resection during surgery. Prior to the ability to perform radiosurgery and with adjuvant radiotherapy alone, the goal of surgery was to gross totally resect even metastatic tumors due to the high probability of tumor progression and recurrence. With improved rates of tumor control provided by radiosurgery, the principle surgical goal is epidural tumor decompression and instrumented stabilization. Large paraspinal tumors and even vertebral body tumors can be controlled with radiosurgery, rather than gross total tumor resection, often requiring anterior and posterior decompression and fixation.

If a tumor is only partially resected during an open surgery, radiosurgery may be used to treat the residual tumor at a later date. The spinal tumors can be removed away from neural structures, allowing for immediate decompression, the spine can be instrumented if necessary, and the residual tumor can be safely treated at a later date with radiosurgery, thus further decreasing surgical morbidity. Given the steep falloff gradient of the target dose with negligible skin dose, such treatments can be given early in the postoperative period as opposed to the usual significant delay before standard external beam irradiation is permitted. Rock et al[55] specifically evaluated the combination of open surgical procedure followed by adjuvant radiosurgery. They found this to be a successful treatment paradigm that was associated with a significant chance of stabilizing or improving neurologic function. Local control was 94%. The technique was well tolerated and associated with little to no morbidity.

Saghal et al[56] also analyzed the use of spine radiosurgery for its application in the postoperative patient. In this cohort, spine radiosurgery in patients with prior conventional radiotherapy resulted in equivalent local and pain control when compared to spine radiosurgery in patients with no history of prior radiation. The major consideration critical to the safety of spine radiosurgery is the need to avoid doses that exceed the tolerance of the spinal cord. With spine radiosurgery, the area of tumor adjacent to the spinal cord is most at risk for local failure, given that the principle of spine radiosurgery is to treat the target region and avoid the uninvolved normal structures. The interface between the tumor and the spinal cord is frequently underdosed relative to the target to keep the dose to the spinal cord within a safe limit. This is especially true in cases of repeat irradiation. Therefore, there is potential for microscopic epidural tumor to be exposed to a subtherapeutic dose; this is certainly also true of gross epidural tumor when it directly abuts the spinal cord.[56] The consequence of failure at this interface is disease progression and tumor recurrence.

Once again, this underdosing at the tumor–spinal cord interface could be avoided by employing a multisession radiosurgery technique, as previously described. Furthermore, multisession radiosurgery theoretically would decrease the potential for adverse effects to the normal healing postsurgical tissue, as well as permit a larger planned tumor volume that would allow for treatment uncertainty within the postsurgical tumor bed.

To further underscore the importance of this point, Saghal et al[57] reported local failure in a series of 8 of 60 patients undergoing spine radiosurgery and analyzed the potential for treatment failure as the tumor approached the thecal sac. A trend was found when the minimum distance between the target and the thecal sac was < 1 mm, and there was a significant risk of failure for tumors essentially touching the thecal sac.[58]

Multisession Radiosurgery in the Setting of Reirradiation

Choi et al reported on a series of 51 spine metastases treated with radiosurgery that had recurred in close proximity to previously irradiated spinal cord.[59] Forty-one (80%) of the lesions were treated using a multisession technique in two to five fractions with a median marginal target dose of 20 Gy. Of the 13 failures in this series, 5 recurrences were associated with the epidural space and potentially resulted from target underdosing out of concern for spinal toxicity. One patient treated in two sessions experienced grade 4 spinal cord toxicity 6 months after receiving radiosurgery. The authors concluded that, unless the location of the tumor is sufficiently far from the spinal cord, multisession radiosurgery should be employed. Furthermore, patients should be treated in multiple sessions when the single-session plan would have exposed the spinal cord to > 70% of the prescription dose. Once again, interfraction tumor reoxygenation and cell reassortment may increase tumor kill by minimizing hypoxia-associated radiation resistance and cell cycle–specific radiation sensitivity, respectively.[59]

Mahadevan et al[60] also reported on a series of 81 lesions in 60 consecutive patients who were treated with radiosurgery for progressive epidural involvement after previous radiation for spine metastases. Patients were treated with 3 × 8 Gy (24 Gy) when the tumor did not touch the spinal cord or 5 × 5 to 6 Gy (25–30 Gy) when the tumor abutted the spinal cord. The cord surface received up to the prescription dose with no hot spots within the spinal cord itself. Overall, 93% of patients had stable or improved disease. There was no significant spinal cord toxicity demonstrated. Multisession radiosurgery was demonstrated to be a highly safe and effective technique for this difficult and high-risk clinical scenario.

Damast et al[61] specifically evaluated the causes of local failure (i.e., "in-field recurrence") after radiosurgery for recurrent spine metastases in a series of 92 patients. Patients were treated with either five 4-Gy or five 6-Gy fractions. Forty-eight percent of patients were treated after surgery to decompress epidural disease. Of all treatment characteristics examined, only the total dose had a significant impact on actuarial local failure incidence. There was no incidence of myelopathy in this group. Therefore, a significant decrease in local failure with a higher total dose was observed without increased risk of myelopathy.

Garg et al[62] published a series of 63 spine tumors that were reirradiated with multisession radiosurgery. Doses included 30 Gy in five fractions or 27 Gy in three fractions. Actuarial 1-year radiographic local control for all patients was 76%. Of the tumors that progressed after radiosurgery, 81% were within 5 mm of the spinal cord, thus translating into a failure at the tumor–spinal cord interface. Multisession radiosurgery allows for a higher dose of radiation that translates into greater long-term local tumor control while avoiding the risk of spinal cord toxicity through fractionation.

Direct Evidence in Favor of Multisession Radiosurgery for Spine Metastases

To date, only one study has attempted to compare single- and multisession radiosurgery for spine metastases.[63] In this study, 195 metastatic spine lesions were treated at the University of Pittsburgh using a single-session technique versus 153 lesions treated at Georgetown University Medical Center using a multisession technique. Eligible patients had a primary diagnosis of melanoma, lung, renal cell, breast, colon, prostate, multiple myeloma, or thyroid cancer metastatic to the spine. The primary end point was pain relief. Secondary end points included local tumor control, median survival time, treatment toxicity, and neurologic improvement. All cases were contoured, and the radiosurgical treatment plan was designed in a similar manner based on tumor geometry, proximity to the spinal cord, and location. In each case, the gross tumor volume (GTV) was the tumor discernible on imaging, and the clinical treatment volume (CTV) included the GTV and a margin of tissue at risk for microscopic extension. Patients receiving three to five fractions were treated daily (▶ Fig. 28.1).

The median follow-up for the entire cohort was 360 days. Both groups were balanced based on tumor histology, age, and patient gender. The mean tumor volume was larger in the multisession arm compared to the single-session arm (81 vs 35 cm^3, $p < 0.01$). Patients in the single-session group were more likely to receive radiosurgery as primary therapy compared to the multisession group (36% vs 5%, $p < 0.001$). The mean prescription dose in the multisession group was 21 Gy delivered in three fractions, 24 Gy in four fractions, and 25 Gy in five fractions. In the single-session group, the mean prescription dose was 16 Gy. The mean maximum dose to the spinal cord was 12 Gy for three fractions, 11 Gy for four fractions, and 16 Gy for five fractions in the multisession group, and 10 Gy in the single-session group.

The long-term pain relief was not significantly different between the two groups (73% vs 71%, $p = 0.617$). For those patients with neurologic deficits at the time of radiosurgery, patients in both groups were equally likely to experience improved neurologic function at each evaluated time point up to 2 years (71% of patients in the single-session group and 79% of patients in the multisession group). The remaining patients had stabilized symptoms, and no patients in either group were found to have progression of neurologic symptoms. This remained the case when the biological effective dose (BED) was taken into account.

The major difference between the two groups was found in the tumor control rates. At 2, 4, 6, 12, and 24 months, tumor control was superior in the multisession group. At 2 years, tumor control probability in the multisession group was 96% versus 70% in the single-session group ($p = 0.001$). The greater tumor control observed in the multisession group remained significant when the initial volume of the tumor was adjusted for both groups.

The need for re-treatment was also different between the two groups. The need for re-treatment is an important assessment parameter of the overall durability of the radiosurgery treatment. In the single-session group, 13% of patients required retreatment with radiosurgery versus 1% in the multisession group ($p < 0.001$). The median overall survival for the entire cohort was 13 months (11 mo in the single-session group and 18 mo in the multisession group). In the single-session group, the 1-year overall survival was 46% compared to 63% in the multisession group ($p = 0.002$).

Finally, the overall rate of any adverse event was similar in both groups (4.6% vs 5.9%) using the National Cancer Institute's Common Toxicity Criteria. There was a single grade 3 complication in the single-session group but no grade 2 or 3 complications in the multisession group. Of note is that pain control was significantly higher in the single-session group compared to the multisession group for all measured time points (100% vs 88%, $p = 0.003$).

Thus, ***level III evidence*** demonstrated that long-term local tumor control was significantly better with multisession treatment. Furthermore, the re-treatment rate was significantly lower when multisession radiosurgery was used. Failure to achieve long-term local tumor control may translate into costly further interventions. Despite the fact that most proponents of multisession radiosurgery emphasize the theoretical decrease in toxicity associated with fractionation, there was no statistically significant difference in complications between the two groups. The calculated BED (using an α/β ratio of 2.2 for the spinal cord) demonstrated that the maximum dose to the spinal

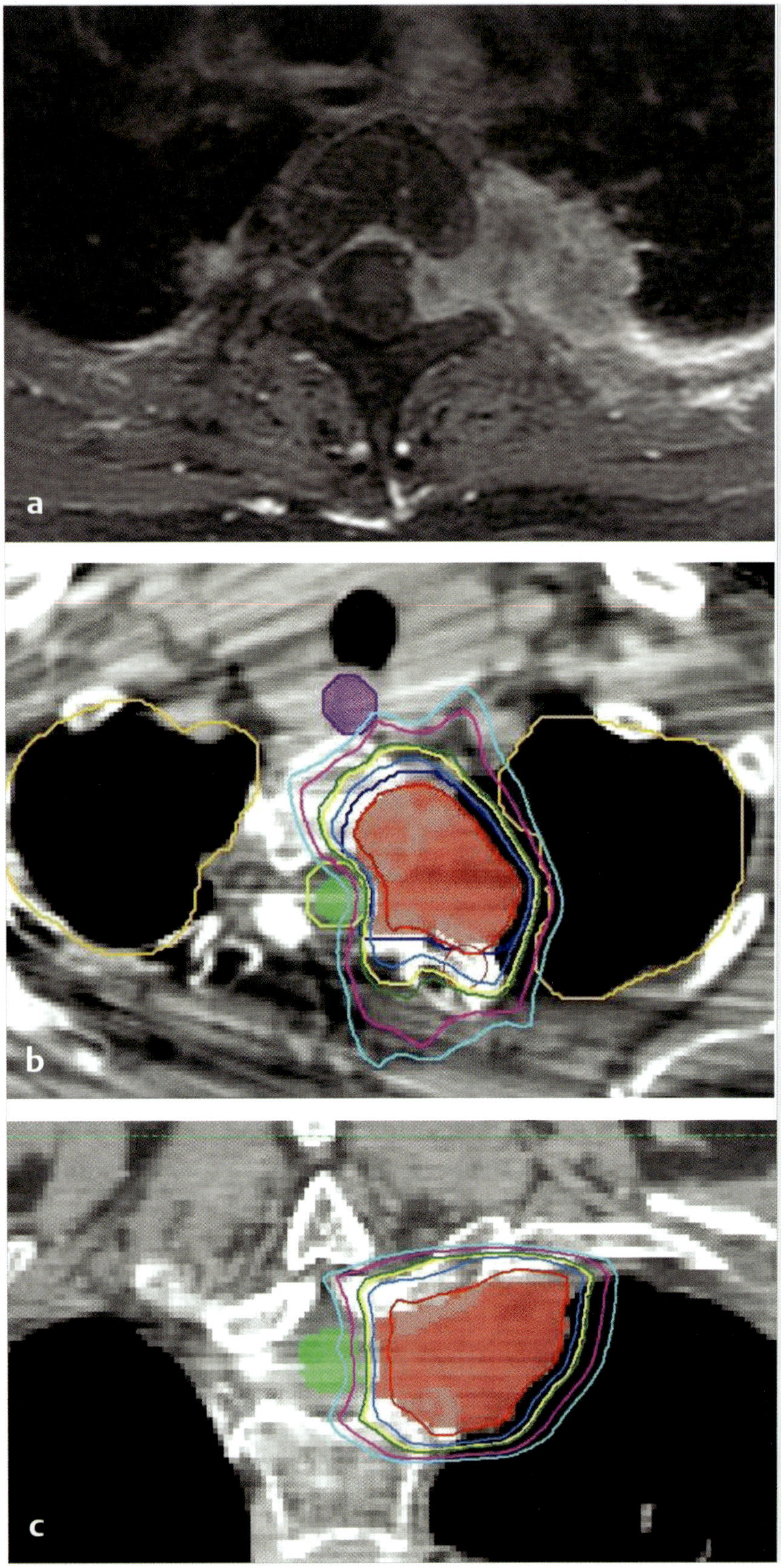

Fig. 28.1 Representative case of a 79-year-old woman with a symptomatic left T2-level renal cell carcinoma oligometastasis. Despite treatment with prior conventional fractionated radiotherapy, the lesion continued to increase in size on serial imaging, resulting in a left T2 radiculopathy. (a) Axial T1-weighted gadolinium-enhanced magnetic resonance image demonstrating the tumor encroaching upon the spinal cord. (b) Axial and (c) coronal computed tomographic scans showing the isodose lines of the treatment plan. The prescription dose was 9 Gy to the gross tumor volume delivered in three sessions.

cord was greater in the single-session than in the multisession group (57.5 Gy for the single-session group vs 30.9 Gy for the multisession group).

To reinforce this point, Lovelock et al conducted a failure analysis of single-fraction radiosurgery patients.[64] All tumor progression occurred in tumors that received < 15 Gy to some portion of the planning target volume, most often at the dural margin. The spinal cord tolerance constraint used in this study was a maximum spinal cord dose of 14 Gy. Any significant degree of spinal cord abutment or compression therefore effectively precludes effective therapy. Lowering the dose at the margin of the spinal cord risks progression of tumor and compression where the greatest measure of control is required, that is, adjacent to the spinal cord. However, treating to a cytotoxic dose introduces the risk of spinal cord injury. Hypofractionated radiotherapy (27 Gy in three fractions) may offer effective therapy for cases of spinal cord compression with less risk of toxicity to the spinal cord, but this remains unproven.[34] Furthermore, radiosurgery to such radioresistant tumors does not create immediate decompression of the spinal cord, often requiring months to demonstrate a radiographic response.

Summary of the Optimization of Tumor Control and Toxicity through Multisession Radiosurgery

The employment of multisession versus single-session radiosurgery for the treatment of spine metastases has been determined more by the preferences and personal biases of the treating physicians than by peer-reviewed published data favoring one technique over the other. Most single-institution published series have described one technique or the other, but none have compared them directly in a randomized fashion. In many instances, experienced institutions have moved over time from a multisession to a single-session technique as they have acquired confidence in the safety and low incidence of toxicity associated with spine radiosurgery.

There is sufficient ***level III*** and ***IV evidence*** to support the use of multisession radiosurgery for the treatment of spine metastases. There is no ***level I*** or ***II evidence*** that compares the use of single- versus multisession spine radiosurgery for the treatment of spine metastases. In the foreseeable future, there is little likelihood of a randomized clinical trial that would directly compare single- versus multisession spine radiosurgery. Most physicians appear comfortable with reserving multisession radiosurgery for specific clinical indications that have a higher risk of poor tumor control by either underdosing tumor in close proximity to the spinal cord or overdosing the spinal cord, especially in the setting of prior conventional fractionated radiotherapy.

A single retrospective study was performed specifically to compare the outcomes and toxicities of a large series of patients treated at two different institutions using each of the two fractionation schedules. Overall radiation-related toxicity was equally low in both treatment groups. However, this study found long-term survivors who were treated with a multisession technique achieved greater tumor control and had less need for re-treatment than those patients who were treated with a single-session technique.

At our institution, we favor the use of multisession radiosurgery in the setting of intradural tumors with spinal cord impingement or epidural tumors associated with significant spinal canal compromise, especially in the setting of prior irradiation:

- Prior fractionated radiotherapy to the target level
- Significant spinal cord or cauda canal compromise
- Significant amount of epidural tumor, especially over a long segment of the spinal cord
- Patients with an expected long survival
- Residual tumor after surgery adjacent to critical structures
- Inability to clearly define residual tumor after open surgical decompression
- Intradural metastases at the level of the spinal cord

Such use of multisession radiosurgery has allowed us to achieve an extremely high clinical response while avoiding spinal cord or cauda equina radiation-induced toxicity. It is perhaps best for centers that are just beginning a spine radiosurgery program and are still becoming familiar with their specific radiosurgery delivery technology to begin with multisession radiosurgery to err on the side of safety before transitioning to a single-session radiosurgery technique.

Conclusion

Radiosurgery represents a great advance in the treatment of spinal metastases. The ability to deliver cytotoxic doses to the tumor while sparing normal tissue tolerance offers a better chance at significant palliation and durable tumor control for metastatic patients. Radiosurgery is safe and effective with durable symptomatic response and local control for even radioresistant histologies, regardless of prior fractionated radiotherapy. Radiosurgery may be considered over conventional fractionated radiotherapy for the treatment of solid tumor spine metastases, particularly in the setting of oligometastatic disease and radioresistant histology. Due to a paucity of data, controversy remains regarding the indication and relative benefit for single- versus multisession radiosurgery.

Multisession radiosurgery for spine metastases is perhaps safer and achieves long-term radiographic response compared to single-session radiosurgery. There appears to be less toxicity associated with multisession radiosurgery, especially grade 3 toxicity. Perhaps increasing the single-session dose would negate this efficacy but might also translate into higher radiation-induced toxicity to normal tissue. Multisession radiosurgery is preferable for those centers that are uncomfortable with the treatment setup and radiation delivery of their system. These are intermediate-strength recommendations; the best actions may differ depending on the specific clinical circumstances of the individual patient.

References

[1] Clain A. Secondary malignant disease of bone. Br J Cancer 1965; 19: 15–29

[2] Black P. Spinal metastasis: current status and recommended guidelines for management. Neurosurgery 1979; 5: 726–746

[3] Gokaslan ZL, York JE, Walsh GL, et al. Transthoracic vertebrectomy for metastatic spinal tumors. J Neurosurg 1998; 89: 599–609

[4] Yamada Y, Lovelock DM, Bilsky MH. A review of image-guided intensity-modulated radiotherapy for spinal tumors. Neurosurgery 2007; 61: 226–235, discussion 235

[5] Faul CM, Flickinger JC. The use of radiation in the management of spinal metastases. J Neurooncol 1995; 23: 149–161

[6] Kim YH, Fayos JV. Radiation tolerance of the cervical spinal cord. Radiology 1981; 139: 473–478

[7] Markoe AM, Schwade JG. The role of radiation therapy in the management of spine and spinal cord tumors. In: Rea GL, ed. Spine Tumors. Rolling Meadows, IL: American Association of Neurological Surgeons; 1994: 23–35

[8] Shapiro W, Posner JB. Medical vs surgical treatment of metastatic spinal cord tumors. In: Thompson R, Green J, eds. Controversies in Neurology. New York, NY: Raven Press; 1983: 57–65

[9] Sundaresan N, Krol G, Digiacinto CV, Hughes JEO. Metastatic tumors of the spine. In: Sundaresan B, Schmidek H, Schiller A, Rosenthal D, eds. Tumors of the Spine. Philadelphia, PA: WB Saunders; 1990: 279–304

[10] Sundaresan N, Digiacinto GV, Hughes JEO, Cafferty M, Vallejo A. Treatment of neoplastic spinal cord compression: results of a prospective study. Neurosurgery 1991; 29: 645–650

[11] Gerszten PC, Welch WC. Current surgical management of metastatic spinal disease. Oncology (Williston Park) 2000; 14: 1013–1024, discussion 1024, 1029–1030

[12] Lu C, Stomper PC, Drislane FW, et al. Suspected spinal cord compression in breast cancer patients: a multidisciplinary risk assessment. Breast Cancer Res Treat 1998; 51: 121–131

[13] Vitaz TW, Oishi M, Welch WC, Gerszten PC, Disa JJ, Bilsky MH. Rotational and transpositional flaps for the treatment of spinal wound dehiscence and infections in patient populations with degenerative and oncological disease. J Neurosurg 2004; 100 (Suppl Spine): 46–51

[14] Loblaw DA, Laperriere NJ. Emergency treatment of malignant extradural spinal cord compression: an evidence-based guideline. J Clin Oncol 1998; 16: 1613–1624

[15] Ryu SI, Chang SD, Kim DH, et al. Image-guided hypo-fractionated stereotactic radiosurgery to spinal lesions. Neurosurgery 2001; 49: 838–846

[16] Hamilton AJ, Lulu BA, Fosmire H, Stea B, Cassady JR. Preliminary clinical experience with linear accelerator-based spinal stereotactic radiosurgery. Neurosurgery 1995; 36: 311–319

[17] Baisden JM, Benedict SH, Sheng K, Read PW, Larner JM. Helical tomotherapy in the treatment of central nervous system metastasis. Neurosurg Focus 2007; 22: E8

[18] Benzil DL, Saboori M, Mogilner AY, Rocchio R, Moorthy CR. Safety and efficacy of stereotactic radiosurgery for tumors of the spine. J Neurosurg 2004; 101 (Suppl 3): 413–418

[19] Bilsky MH, Yamada Y, Yenice KM, et al. Intensity-modulated stereotactic radiotherapy of paraspinal tumors: a preliminary report. Neurosurgery 2004; 54: 823–830, discussion 830–831

[20] Chang SD, Adler JR. Current status and optimal use of radiosurgery. Oncology (Williston Park) 2001; 15: 209–216, discussion 219–221

[21] De Salles AA, Pedroso AG, Medin P, et al. Spinal lesions treated with Novalis shaped beam intensity-modulated radiosurgery and stereotactic radiotherapy. J Neurosurg 2004; 101 (Suppl 3): 435–440

[22] Gerszten PC, Welch WC. CyberKnife radiosurgery for metastatic spine tumors. Neurosurg Clin N Am 2004; 15: 491–501

[23] Medin PM, Solberg TD, De Salles AA, et al. Investigations of a minimally invasive method for treatment of spinal malignancies with LINAC stereotactic radiation therapy: accuracy and animal studies. Int J Radiat Oncol Biol Phys 2002; 52: 1111–1122

[24] Milker-Zabel S, Zabel A, Thilmann C, Schlegel W, Wannenmacher M, Debus J. Clinical results of retreatment of vertebral bone metastases by stereotactic conformal radiotherapy and intensity-modulated radiotherapy. Int J Radiat Oncol Biol Phys 2003; 55: 162–167

[25] Ryu S, Rock J, Rosenblum M, Kim JH. Patterns of failure after single-dose radiosurgery for spinal metastasis. J Neurosurg 2004; 101 (Suppl 3): 402–405

[26] Ryu S, Fang Yin F, Rock J, et al. Image-guided and intensity-modulated radiosurgery for patients with spinal metastasis. Cancer 2003; 97: 2013–2018

[27] Yin FF, Ryu S, Ajlouni M, et al. Image-guided procedures for intensity-modulated spinal radiosurgery. Technical note. J Neurosurg 2004; 101 (Suppl 3): 419–424

[28] Chang EL, Shiu AS, Lii M-F, et al. Phase I clinical evaluation of near-simultaneous computed tomographic image-guided stereotactic body radiotherapy for spinal metastases. Int J Radiat Oncol Biol Phys 2004; 59: 1288–1294

[29] Colombo F, Pozza F, Chierego G, Casentini L, De Luca G, Francescon P. Linear accelerator radiosurgery of cerebral arteriovenous malformations: an update. Neurosurgery 1994; 34: 14–20, discussion 20–21

[30] Hitchcock E, Kitchen G, Dalton E, Pope B. Stereotactic LINAC radiosurgery. Br J Neurosurg 1989; 3: 305–312

[31] Pirzkall A, Lohr F, Rhein B, et al. Conformal radiotherapy of challenging paraspinal tumors using a multiple arc segment technique. Int J Radiat Oncol Biol Phys 2000; 48: 1197–1204

[32] Gerszten PC, Burton SA, Ozhasoglu C, Welch WC. Radiosurgery for spinal metastases: clinical experience in 500 cases from a single institution. Spine 2007; 32: 193–199

[33] Gerszten PC, Mendel E, Yamada Y. Radiotherapy and radiosurgery for metastatic spine disease: what are the options, indications, and outcomes? Spine 2009; 34 (Suppl): S78–S92

[34] Bilsky M, Angelov L, Rock J. Spinal radiosurgery: a neurosurgical perspective. J Radiosurg SBRT. 2011; 1: 47–54

[35] Martin AG, Cowley IR, Taylor BA, Cassoni AM, Landau DB, Plowman PN. (Stereotactic) radiosurgery XIX: spinal radiosurgery—two year experience in a UK centre. Br J Neurosurg 2012; 26: 53–58

[36] Hartsell WF, Scott CB, Bruner DW, et al. Randomized trial of short- versus long-course radiotherapy for palliation of painful bone metastases. J Natl Cancer Inst 2005; 97: 798–804

[37] Tong D, Gillick L, Hendrickson FR. The palliation of symptomatic osseous metastases: final results of the Study by the Radiation Therapy Oncology Group. Cancer 1982; 50: 893–899

[38] Katagiri H, Takahashi M, Inagaki J, et al. Clinical results of nonsurgical treatment for spinal metastases. Int J Radiat Oncol Biol Phys 1998; 42: 1127–1132

[39] Maranzano E, Latini P. Effectiveness of radiation therapy without surgery in metastatic spinal cord compression: final results from a prospective trial. Int J Radiat Oncol Biol Phys 1995; 32: 959–967

[40] Maranzano E, Bellavita R, Rossi R, et al. Short-course versus split-course radiotherapy in metastatic spinal cord compression: results of a phase III, randomized, multicenter trial. J Clin Oncol 2005; 23: 3358–3365

[41] Rades D, Fehlauer F, Stalpers LJ, et al. A prospective evaluation of two radiotherapy schedules with 10 versus 20 fractions for the treatment of metastatic spinal cord compression: final results of a multicenter study. Cancer 2004; 101: 2687–2692

[42] Rades D, Stalpers LJ, Hulshof MC, Zschenker O, Alberti W, Koning CC. Effectiveness and toxicity of single-fraction radiotherapy with 1 8 Gy for metastatic spinal cord compression. Radiother Oncol 2005; 75: 70–73

[43] Rades D, Fehlauer F, Schulte R, et al. Prognostic factors for local control and survival after radiotherapy of metastatic spinal cord compression. J Clin Oncol 2006; 24: 3388–3393

[44] Maranzano E, Latini P, Perrucci E, Beneventi S, Lupattelli M, Corgna E. Short-course radiotherapy (8 Gy 2) in metastatic spinal cord compression: an effective and feasible treatment. Int J Radiat Oncol Biol Phys 1997; 38: 1037–1044

[45] Rades D, Karstens JH, Alberti W. Role of radiotherapy in the treatment of motor dysfunction due to metastatic spinal cord compression: comparison of three different fractionation schedules. Int J Radiat Oncol Biol Phys 2002; 54: 1160–1164

[46] Gagnon GJ, Nasr NM, Liao JJ, et al. Treatment of spinal tumors using cyber-Knife fractionated stereotactic radiosurgery: pain and quality-of-life assessment after treatment in 200 patients. Neurosurgery 2009; 64: 297–306, discussion 306–307

[47] Guyatt G, Walter S, Norman G. Measuring change over time: assessing the usefulness of evaluative instruments. J Chronic Dis 1987; 40: 171–178

[48] Sohn S, Chung CK. The role of stereotactic radiosurgery in metastasis to the spine. J Korean Neurosurg Soc 2012; 51: 1–7

[49] Yamada Y, Lovelock DM, Yenice KM, et al. Multifractionated image-guided and stereotactic intensity-modulated radiotherapy of paraspinal tumors: a preliminary report. Int J Radiat Oncol Biol Phys 2005; 62: 53–61

[50] Gagnon GJ, Henderson FC, Gehan EA, et al. CyberKnife radiosurgery for breast cancer spine metastases: a matched-pair analysis. Cancer 2007; 110: 1796–1802

[51] Nelson JW, Yoo DS, Sampson JH, et al. Stereotactic body radiotherapy for lesions of the spine and paraspinal regions. Int J Radiat Oncol Biol Phys 2009; 73: 1369–1375

[52] Chang EL, Shiu AS, Mendel E, et al. Phase I/II study of stereotactic body radiotherapy for spinal metastasis and its pattern of failure. J Neurosurg Spine 2007; 7: 151–160

[53] Nguyen Q-N, Shiu AS, Rhines LD, et al. Management of spinal metastases from renal cell carcinoma using stereotactic body radiotherapy. Int J Radiat Oncol Biol Phys 2010; 76: 1185–1192

[54] Klekamp J, Samii H. Surgical results for spinal metastases. Acta Neurochir (Wien) 1998; 140: 957–967

[55] Rock JP, Ryu S, Shukairy MS, et al. Postoperative radiosurgery for malignant spinal tumors. Neurosurgery 2006; 58: 891–898, discussion 891–898

[56] Sahgal AMD, Bilsky M, Chang EL, et al. Stereotactic body radiotherapy for spinal metastases: current status, with a focus on its application in the postoperative patient. J Neurosurg Spine 2011; 14: 151–166

[57] Sahgal A, Ames C, Chou D, et al. Stereotactic body radiotherapy is effective salvage therapy for patients with prior radiation of spinal metastases. Int J Radiat Oncol Biol Phys 2009; 74: 723–731

[58] Masucci GL, Yu E, Ma L, et al. Stereotactic body radiotherapy is an effective treatment in reirradiating spinal metastases: current status and practical considerations for safe practice. Expert Rev Anticancer Ther 2011; 11: 1923–1933

[59] Choi CYH, Adler JR, Gibbs IC, et al. Stereotactic radiosurgery for treatment of spinal metastases recurring in close proximity to previously irradiated spinal cord. Int J Radiat Oncol Biol Phys 2010; 78: 499–506

[60] Mahadevan A, Floyd S, Wong E, Jeyapalan S, Groff M, Kasper E. Stereotactic body radiotherapy reirradiation for recurrent epidural spinal metastases. Int J Radiat Oncol Biol Phys 2011; 81: 1500–1505

[61] Damast S, Wright J, Bilsky M, et al. Impact of dose on local failure rates after image-guided reirradiation of recurrent paraspinal metastases. Int J Radiat Oncol Biol Phys 2011; 81: 819–826

[62] Garg AK, Wang X-S, Shiu AS, et al. Prospective evaluation of spinal reirradiation by using stereotactic body radiation therapy: the University of Texas MD Anderson Cancer Center experience. Cancer 2011; 117: 3509–3516

[63] Heron DE, Stone B, Burton S, et al. Single- vs. multi-session CyberKnife radiosurgery for spine metastases: the Georgetown and University of Pittsburgh experience. J Neurosurg Spine 2012; 17(1): 11–18

[64] Lovelock DM, Zhang Z, Jackson A, et al. Correlation of local failure with measures of dose insufficiency in the high-dose single-fraction treatment of bony metastases. Int J Radiat Oncol Biol Phys 2010; 77: 1282–1287

29 Single-Session Spinal Radiosurgery

Simon S. Lo, Arjun Sahgal, Jason Sohn, Samuel T. Chao, Nina A. Mayr, Mitchell Machtay, and Eric L. Chang

Introduction

Lars Leksell from the Karolinska Institute, Sweden, pioneered the concept of stereotaxy and the use of stereotactic radiosurgery (SRS) based on the Gamma Knife (Elekta AB, Stockholm Sweden) for intracranial lesions. Intracranial SRS entails the delivery of a single high dose of radiation to a brain lesion and has been proven to be effective in the management of skull base tumors, brain metastases, and various benign disorders, such as arteriovenous malformations (AVMs) and trigeminal neuralgia.[1] Rigid immobilization is typically achieved with the use of a head frame or, less commonly, a frameless system.

Building on the experience with Gamma Knife–based SRS, investigators from the Karolinska Institute extended the concept of SRS to extracranial sites and pioneered the use of stereotactic body radiation therapy (SBRT) in lung and liver tumors.[1,2] Hamilton et al from the University of Arizona applied the concept of intracranial SRS to patients with recurrent spinal tumors and treated them with single-fraction SBRT using rigid fixation of the spine, achieving promising results.[3] Subsequently, colleagues from the University of Pittsburgh Medical Center (UPMC),[4] Stanford University,[5] Memorial Sloan-Kettering Cancer Center (MSKCC),[6,7] MD Anderson Cancer Center (MDACC),[8–11] and the Henry Ford Hospital[12–17] also started their spinal SBRT program using different systems, with the CyberKnife system (Accuray Inc., Sunnyvale, CA) used at UPMC and Stanford University, a linear accelerator (LINAC)–based system used at MSKCC and MDACC, and the Novalis system (Brainlab AG, Munich, Germany) used at the Henry Ford Hospital. The number of fractions used ranged from one to five. In the past 5 years, many other centers have also adopted this treatment modality for spinal tumors.[18] This chapter discusses various aspects of single-session spinal radiosurgery (single-fraction spinal SBRT). The rationale for spinal radiosurgery has been covered in Chapter 28 and will not be repeated here.

Radiation and Cancer Biology of Radiosurgery

Traditionally, the linear-quadratic (LQ) model is used to describe the relationship between cell kill and radiation dose in a conventional fractionation setting. Although it adequately estimates the effect of conventionally fractionated radiotherapy, the LQ model overestimates the radiation effect in the ablative dose range as used in radiosurgery or SBRT. Park et al from the University of Texas Southwestern Medical Center constructed a Universal Survival Curve (USC) model that provides a better approximation in the ablative dose range.[19] However, the model does not allow extrapolation from conventional fractionation to the ablative dose range. Wang et al from the Ohio State University proposed a generalized LQ model that allows for a good approximation in the ablative dose range and extrapolation throughout the dose range.[20]

Investigators from MSKCC have suggested that the actual mechanism of tumor killing with ablative radiotherapy may be different from that of conventionally fractionated radiotherapy. Rapid endothelial apoptosis was observed 1 to 6 hours after the delivery of a single dose of radiation of 15 to 20 Gy to mouse fibrosarcoma and melanoma cells with 15 to 20 Gy. This was followed by the death of cells that appeared to be intact for 2 or 3 days.[2,21,22] The acid sphingomyelinase (ASMase) pathway has been implicated in this process. Interestingly, this mechanism of tumor killing was not observed in mice treated with conventionally fractionated radiotherapy. Investigators from the University of Chicago discovered that CD8 + T cells are responsible for the therapeutic effects of ablative radiation in that the delivery of an ablative dose of radiation of 15 to 25 Gy was found to lead to a significant increase in T-cell priming in draining lymphoid tissue, resulting in the reduction or eradication of the primary tumor or distant metastasis in a CD8 + T-cell–dependent fashion in an animal model.[23]

Retrospective Studies of Single-Session Spinal Radiosurgery

There are numerous retrospective studies examining the outcomes of single-fraction SBRT for spinal metastasis. Treatments were given in different settings, including as primary treatment, as postoperative treatment, or for reirradiation. In one of the largest series from UPMC, 393 patients with 500 spinal metastases were treated with single-fraction CyberKnife-based SBRT to a median dose of 20 Gy.[4] Long-term pain improvement was achieved in 86% of the patients and long-term local control in 90% of lesions treated as a primary treatment modality and in 88% of lesions treated for radiographic tumor progression. For patients with progressive neurologic deficits before SBRT, at least some clinical improvement was observed in 84% of the patients.[4] However, these data were not evaluated in an actuarial manner. Other studies from UPMC looking at histology-specific spinal metastases showed similar results. In a study in which 48 patients with 60 renal cell carcinoma (RCC) spinal metastases were treated with single-fraction SBRT to a dose of 17.5 to 25.0 Gy (median 20 Gy), at a median follow-up of 37 months, 34 (89%) of 38 patients who were treated primarily for pain reported improvement for axial and radicular pain. Seven of eight patients treated primarily for radiographically documented tumor progression achieved tumor control.[24] Eventually, six patients required open surgical intervention for tumor progression causing neurologic dysfunction after SBRT. Of note, 42 of 60 treated lesions had prior external beam radiotherapy. No neurologic toxicities were noted.

In another study from UPMC, 36 melanoma spine metastases were treated with a single-fraction SBRT to a dose of 17.5 to 25.0 Gy (median 21.7 Gy). Twenty-three of the 36 lesions had received prior external beam radiotherapy. At a median follow-up of 13 months, 27 of 28 patients (96%) who were treated primarily for pain achieved improvement of axial and radicular pain. Long-term tumor control was achieved in three (75%) of four patients treated primarily for radiographic tumor progression.[25] Two patients required surgical intervention for tumor progression that led to neurologic deterioration. Again, no neurologic toxicity was observed. Two other histology-specific studies were reported from UPMC. In a study on single-fraction SBRT for breast cancer spinal metastases, 50 patients with 68 spinal metastases were treated. Prescribed dose was 19 Gy (range 15.0–22.5 Gy). At a median follow-up time of 16 months, long-term axial and radicular pain improvement was achieved in 55 of 57 (96%) patients who were treated primarily for pain, and long-term radiographic tumor control was observed in all patients who underwent SBRT as their primary treatment modality, for radiographic tumor progression, or as a postoperative treatment.[26] No radiation-induced toxicity was observed. In the other study on single-fraction SBRT for lung cancer spinal metastases, 77 patients with 87 spinal metastases were treated to a dose of 20 Gy (range 15–25 Gy). Long-term axial and radicular pain improvement was achieved in 65 of 73 patients (89%) who were treated for pain, and long-term radiographic tumor control was observed in all patients who underwent SBRT as their primary treatment modality or for radiographic tumor progression at a median follow-up of 12 months. No radiation-induced toxicity was observed.[27]

Postkyphoplasty single-fraction SBRT (16–20 Gy, mean 18 Gy) was offered to 26 patients with pathologic fractures from spinal metastases at UPMC, At a median follow-up of 16 months, axial pain improved in 24 (92%) of 26 patients.[28] In another study from UPMC, single-fraction CyberKnife-based SBRT after balloon kyphoplasty was offered to 11 patients with symptomatic vertebral body metastases causing moderate spinal canal compromise (≤ 50%) but with no associated myelopathy or neurologic deficits. The mean dose was 19 Gy. All patients achieved long-term pain and tumor control. No complications were observed.[29] It is important to note that these data are not actuarial and can only provide a crude estimate indicative of efficacy.

Colleagues from the Henry Ford Hospital also reported their experience with single-fraction SBRT for spinal metastases as a boost, as postoperative treatment, as primary treatment, and in the setting of spinal cord compression. In a study of 18 patients (4 had conventional radiotherapy with SBRT as a boost) who received postoperative single-fraction SBRT with spinal tumors (10 with spinal metastases), the crude local control rate was 94%.[12] The prescribed dose ranged from 6 to 16 Gy (mean 11.6 Gy). Among the patients initially presenting with neurologic deficits, 92% either remained neurologically stable or improved. In another study, of 49 patients with 61 solitary spinal metastases, single-fraction SBRT to a dose of 10 to 16 Gy was given. Complete and partial pain relief was achieved in 85% of the lesions treated.[13] The overall rate of pain control was 84%. In a recent study from the Henry Ford Hospital, 124 patients with 165 spinal metastases were treated with single - fraction SBRT to a dose of 18 Gy, and 92% of patients achieved local control.[30]

In regard to the use of SBRT for spinal cord compression, the first study from the Henry Ford Hospital analyzed the outcomes of 18 patients, 10 with extremity weakness from spinal cord compression prior to decompression surgery and 10 with spinal metastases, who received postoperative SBRT for spinal tumors. The mean SBRT dose was 11.4 Gy (range 6–16 Gy) in one fraction. Neurologic improvement was observed in 62% of patients.[12] One patient developed neurologic progression caused by rapidly progressive tumor. In the second study, SBRT was used as the primary treatment for metastatic epidural spinal cord compression from myeloma in 24 patients with 31 lesions. All patients were treated with single-fraction SBRT to a dose of 16 Gy (range 10–18 Gy). At a median follow-up of 11.2 months, complete and partial pain relief was achieved in 54 and 32% of patients, respectively. Five (71%) of seven patients who presented with neurologic deficits had improved or normalized neurologic function after SBRT. Complete radiologic response rate was 81.2% in the 16 evaluable patients.[16] There were no neurologic toxicities observed. In the third study, 62 patients with 85 spinal metastases causing epidural compression from nonradiosensitive tumors were treated with single-fraction SBRT as primary treatment. The median dose was 16 Gy (range 12–20 Gy). All patients in this study had motor power of ≥ 4 of 5. At a median follow-up time of 11.5 months, the reduction of mean epidural tumor volume was 65% at 2 months after treatment.[17] Eighty-one percent of the patients noticed improvement of neurologic function. Again, there were no neurologic toxicities observed.

The use of single-fraction SBRT for spinal metastasis has also been reported from MSKCC. Researchers there reported a series of 93 patients with 103 spinal metastases treated with single-fraction SBRT, and the prescribed dose ranged from 18 to 24 Gy. A local control rate of 90% was reported at a median follow-up of 15 months. Median overall survival was 15 months.[6] A radiation dose response was observed for local control with doses > 20 Gy. No radiation radiculopathy or myelopathy was reported. The MSKCC team also reported their experience with single-fraction SBRT in 21 patients treated with surgical decompression and instrumentation for epidural spinal cord compression from spinal metastasis. The prescribed dose ranged from 18 to 24 Gy. The crude local control rate was 81%, and the median survival was 10.3 months. A dose response was demonstrated in those patients receiving 24 Gy having a local control rate of 93.8% compared to 40% in those receiving 18 or 21 Gy.[31] It is important to note that this analysis is limited to a small sample size and retrospective uncontrolled comparison. Significant radiation-related complication was observed in one patient.

Prospective Clinical Trials of Single-Session Spinal Radiosurgery

There are a limited number of prospective trials on the use of single-session SBRT for spinal metastasis. Amdur et al from the University of Florida reported the results of their phase II trial of single-fraction SBRT for spinal metastasis. The protocol dose was 15 Gy in one fraction, limiting the spinal cord dose to 12 and 5 Gy in previously unirradiated and previously irradiated patients, respectively. The crude local control rate was 96%, and pain relief was achieved in 43% of patients.[32] In a phase I/II trial from MD Anderson Cancer Center, 61 patients with 63 spinal metastases were treated with a single session to a marginal dose of 16 to 24 Gy in one fraction. A higher prescribed dose was used for spinal metastases from renal cell carcinoma. At a mean follow-up of 20 months, the actuarial 18-month imaging local control and overall survival rates were 88 and 64%, respectively.[9] The median survival was 30 months. There was no difference observed with regard to tumor histology or SBRT dose. Grade 3 or higher radiation adverse events were observed in two patients. The actuarial rate of 18-month freedom from neurologic deterioration from any cause was 82%. One patient whose T1 spinal metastasis was treated developed hemicord syndrome 11 months after SBRT and required a wheelchair for ambulation. Another patient developed right foot drop from radiculopathy 9 months after SBRT for a renal cell carcinoma metastasis at L5.[9]

Direct Comparison of Single- and Multiple-Session Spinal Radiosurgery

In the two successive trials of spinal SBRT from MDACC, a three- or five-fraction regimen and a single-fraction regimen were used, respectively. Similar treatment planning and delivery techniques were used for both trials. When examining the local tumor control rates for single- and multiple-fraction SBRT, the former seemed to yield a slightly higher local control rate, although the follow-up was longer for the multiple-session cohort.[9,11]

Colleagues from the University of Pittsburgh Medical Center (UPMC) and Georgetown University pooled their patients with spinal metastases treated with SBRT using either a single- or multiple-session regimen. There were a total of 228 patients with 348 spinal metastases, with 195 lesions treated with single-session SBRT to a mean dose of 16.3 Gy and 153 lesions treated with mean doses of 20.6 Gy in three fractions, 23.8 Gy in four fractions, and 24.5 Gy in five fractions. With regard to pain control, single-session SBRT yielded better outcomes in that the 1-year post-SBRT pain control rate was 100% compared to 88% for multiple-session regimens ($p = 0.003$).[31] The rates of toxicity and neurologic deficit improvement were not different statistically. However, the local control was 96% for multiple-session SBRT, which was better than a local control rate of 70% for single-session SBRT ($p = 0.001$) up to 2 years post-SBRT.[31] The need for re-treatment was significantly lower for patients receiving multiple-session SBRT (1% vs 13% for single-session SBRT, $p < 0.001$). The 1-year overall survival rate was significantly higher for patients receiving multiple-session SBRT compared to those receiving single-session SBRT (63% vs 46%, $p = 0.002$).

Spinal Cord Tolerance to Spinal Radiosurgery

Within spine SBRT practice, we have observed cases of radiation myelopathy emerge, which is a major devastating late effect of this treatment. It has been unique to spine SBRT, as a spinal tumor by its location is intimate with the cord to be spared, and the aim is to keep the dose to the spinal cord at what we consider safe to minimize the degree of underdosing at the critical spinal cord–tumor interface.[33] This is unlike other SBRT sites, where the principle to keep the spinal cord dose as low as possible is readily achievable, as tumor tends to be far removed from the spinal canal. Recently, Sahgal et al reported probabilities of radiation myelopathy specific to one- to five-fraction SBRT based on 9 cases of radiation myelopathy in patients with no prior radiation, as compared to 66 controls, and a logistic regression analysis.[30] For a ≤ 5% toxicity probability and limits based on the point maximum volume dose to the thecal sac and/or a cord 1.5-mm planning organ at risk volume (PRV), it was suggested the point maximum dose be kept under 12.4 Gy in one fraction, 17 Gy in two fractions, 20.3 Gy in three fractions, 23 Gy in four fractions, and 25.3 Gy in five fractions. In a recent study of single-fraction SBRT for spinal metastases (18 Gy) from the Henry Ford Hospital, maximum cord dose of 14 Gy and $D_{0.35}$ (dose to 0.35 cc of spinal cord) of 10 Gy were observed to be safe dose constraints.[34]

For the patient with previous radiation exposure, the application of a second course of radiation is often limited by the cumulative spinal cord tolerance. This has been an area with little data to guide safe practice and, in particular, no specific data for hypofractionated re-treatment cord tolerance had yet to be reported. Again, within spine SBRT practice, we are observing re-treatment radiation myelopathy cases emerge. Sahgal et al performed an analysis of five cases of re-treatment radiation myelopathy and compared to controls to generate doses that can be considered as safe.[35] Specific percent probabilities were not determinable due to the limited numbers of events, but absolute dose limits for safe practice for one to five fraction practice, and according to the amount of prior radiation exposure were proposed. For example, for the patient previously irradiated with 20 Gy in five fractions, a point maximum cord dose (contoured per the thecal sac and/or cord + 1.5-mm PRV margin) of 9 Gy in one fraction, 12.2 Gy in two fractions, 14.5 Gy in three fractions, 16.5 Gy in four fractions, and 18 Gy in five fractions were proposed as safe.

Esophageal Toxicity from Single-Session Spinal Radiosurgery

Recently, researchers at MSKCC published their esophageal dose-volume histogram analysis specific to spine SBRT practice.[36] Based on 204 spinal metastases treated with a median tumor dose of 24 Gy in a single fraction, Cox et al reported on 12% of patients experiencing a late grade ≥ 3 esophageal complication. The analysis suggested that the esophagus maximum point volume dose should be < 22 Gy, and Cox and colleagues extrapolated other dose-volume parameters as significant predictors. One factor they highlighted is the dose to 2.5 cm^3 of contoured esophagus; they suggested this volume be constrained to < 14 Gy. For this organ at risk (OAR), which can be considered a mixed radiobiologically organized OAR, the complement of maximum point volume dose constraints in conjunction with other volumetric parameters may be a sensible approach; however, this is unlike the spinal cord, which is a serial organ where dose to small volumes (point maximum) have been shown to be causal and crucial. Interestingly, Cox et al also reported that those with grade 4 toxicity were associated with radiation recall reactions after doxorubicin or gemcitabine chemotherapy or iatrogenic manipulation of the esophagus. In a recent study of single-fraction SBRT for spinal metastases from the Henry Ford Hospital, the use of V_{10} (cord volume receiving 10 Gy) of 3 cm^3 and V_{15} of 1 cm^3 as constraints for esophagus was observed to be safe.[34]

Vertebral Bone Fractures

Historically, the risk of vertebral compression fracture (VCF) following palliative low-dose radiation has been regarded as low, or ~ 5%.[37] Specific hypofractionated treatments had not been widely adopted to the bone until the emergence of spine SBRT. The potential for bone damage had not been considered as a major risk, but now with mature data we are observing high rates of VCF. The postulated mechanism is radiation necrosis of the bone/tumor tissue itself that destabilizes the vertebrae and ultimately results in VCF. The rates of VCF vary in the literature, and crude rates of 39,[38] 20,[39] and 11%[40] have been reported by the MSKCC, MDACC, and University of Toronto (UT), respectively. Single-fraction SBRT was used in the MSKCC study, whereas one to five fractions were used in the MDACC study. The analysis of risk of fracture for one versus three or five fractions was not performed in the MDACC study. The UT group analyzed predictors of VCF and importantly identified a dose per fraction of ≥ 20 Gy, which is used in single-fraction SBRT, as predictive of VCF.[40]

In Support of Single-Session Spinal Radiosurgery

Single-session spinal radiosurgery or single-fraction SBRT has been shown in multiple studies, including two prospective trials,[9,32] to yield excellent local control of spinal metastases in various settings, including as primary treatment, as postoperative treatment, and in the setting of spinal cord compression with a low risk of radiation myelopathy and other serious complications (***level III evidence***).[30,41] It offers a significant advantage in that the radiation dose is delivered on 1 day. This is particularly advantageous for patients living in rural areas who need to travel a long distance to a tertiary center for treatment (***level V evidence***). Radioresistant spinal metastases may respond better to single-fraction SBRT than to multiple-session SBRT (***level III evidence***). Colleagues from UPMC showed that single-dose SBRT for spinal metastases from renal cell carcinoma and melanoma yielded local control rates of 96[24] and 89%,[25] respectively, which apparently were better than the 1-year spine tumor progression-free survival rate of 82.1% in the MDACC series of SBRT for renal cell carcinoma spinal metastases, where one, three, or five fractions (mostly three and five fractions) were used.[42] However, the methods of target volume delineation, method of statistical analyses, and median follow-up times were different; therefore, a meaningful comparison cannot be made. There is no ***level II*** or higher evidence to support this notion. In terms of pain control, it appears that single-fraction SBRT yields better pain control (***level III evidence***) compared to multiple-session SBRT for spinal metastasis.[43]

Case against Single-Session Spinal Radiosurgery

A direct comparative study showed that multiple-session SBRT yielded better local control of spinal metastasis up to 2 years post-SBRT and lower rate of re-treatment compared to single-session SBRT (***level III evidence***).[31] Single-dose SBRT to a dose of 18 to 24 Gy (median 24 Gy) has been shown by colleagues from MSKCC to carry a rate of fracture progression of 39% (***level III evidence***).[38] Treatment with a single dose of 20 Gy or higher has been shown by colleagues from UT to be associated with a higher risk of vertebral compression fracture (***level III evidence***).[40] Among the nine patients who developed radiation myelopathy after SBRT for previously unirradiated spinal metastases, seven of them received SBRT delivered in a single fraction to doses ranging from 14 to 25 Gy (***level III evidence***).[30] For those patients receiving single-fraction SBRT, the maximum point dose to the thecal sac, a surrogate for the spinal cord, ranged from 10.6 to 16.5 Gy (***level III evidence***).[30]

Should Single-Session Spinal Radiosurgery Be Offered?

Based on the data in the literature, there is no ***level II*** or higher evidence to confirm whether single-fraction SBRT is better or worse than multiple-session SBRT for spinal metastases in terms of local control. There is ***level III evidence*** to suggest that short-term pain control may be better with single-fraction SBRT.[43] In terms of toxicities, there is ***level III evidence*** to suggest that among those never irradiated patients who have radiation myelopathy after SBRT, most of them had single-session treatment,[30] and the risk of VCF may be higher with single-fraction SBRT if a dose > 20 Gy is given.[40]

Similar to intracranial SRS for brain metastases, single-fraction SBRT for spinal metastases is a very attractive treatment option because of the convenience of a single treatment, especially for patients living very far away from the treatment center, and when rapid pain relief is desired. In a national health care setting, single-fraction SBRT can significantly decrease the machine load in a very busy radiation oncology department. In theory, there may be an advantage to using single-fraction SBRT for spinal metastases from radioresistant histologies.[24] However, this theoretical advantage has not been confirmed in any of the studies.

Compared to multiple-session SBRT, single-fraction SBRT for spinal metastases has higher technical requirements because in the single-fraction dose range, even a small shift of 2 to 3 mm can result in a steeper increase in the biologically effective dose (BED) delivered to the spinal cord, resulting in a very significantly elevated risk of radiation myelopathy (***level V evidence***).[18] Therefore, for low-volume centers or centers just starting SBRT, it seems to be reasonable to use multiple-session SBRT, which may be a safer approach.

For spinal metastases with epidural involvement, especially when there is spinal cord compression, there is very little or no gap between the gross tumor volume (GTV) and the spinal cord. To spare the spinal cord from radiation injury, the portion of the GTV close to or abutting the spinal cord will need to be significantly underdosed if a single fraction is used for SBRT.[18] Colleagues from MSKCC observed no local failures if the minimum dose to the GTV was > 15 Gy (***level III evidence***).[44] Data in the literature also suggest that half of the recurrences after SBRT for spinal metastases occurs in the epidural space, which is most likely due to underdosing of microscopic disease while attempting to spare the spinal cord (***level III evidence***).[8,43] If an attempt is made to improve the coverage of the GTV to improve local control, the risk of radiation myelopathy will be significantly elevated as a result of a higher maximum spinal cord point dose. This is especially true for patients undergoing reirradiation of spinal metastases with SBRT. Multiple-session SBRT allows for delivery of a higher BED to the portion of the GTV immediately adjacent to the spinal cord, which would still be able to spare the latter.

Given the lack of ***level II*** or higher evidence whether single- or multiple-session SBRT is a more cost-effective treatment for newly diagnosed spinal metastases, single-session SBRT can be offered as one of the SBRT regimens under the following conditions (recommendation grade 2C):

1. If there is an at least 2- to 3-mm gap between the GTV and spinal cord[18,41] (▶ Fig. 29.1) or if the spinal segment is below the spinal cord (▶ Fig. 29.2)

2. If there are no risk factors predisposing the patient to VCF as outlined by investigators from MSKCC, MDACC, and UT[38–40]

3. If the treatment team and facility have the technical capability, expertise, and experience with planning and delivery of single-fraction SBRT[45]

In patients with newly diagnosed spinal metastases from a radioresistant histology such as renal cell carcinoma, melanoma, or sarcoma, albeit the lack of evidence that any of the SBRT regimens is superior to others, if the above three criteria are fulfilled, single-fraction SBRT may be recommended (recommendation grade 2C). It is also appropriate to offer single-fraction SBRT in patients with transportation issues or patients coming from faraway locations.

For patients with a life expectancy that is < 1 year, it may also be reasonable to offer single-fraction SBRT, as pain control is likely the most important goal of treatment. Single-fraction SBRT provides better short pain control compared to multiple-session SBRT. At Vrije Universiteit (VU), Netherlands, the fractionation regimen offered for spinal SBRT is based on life expectancy. For patients with a life expectancy < 12 months, a single fraction of

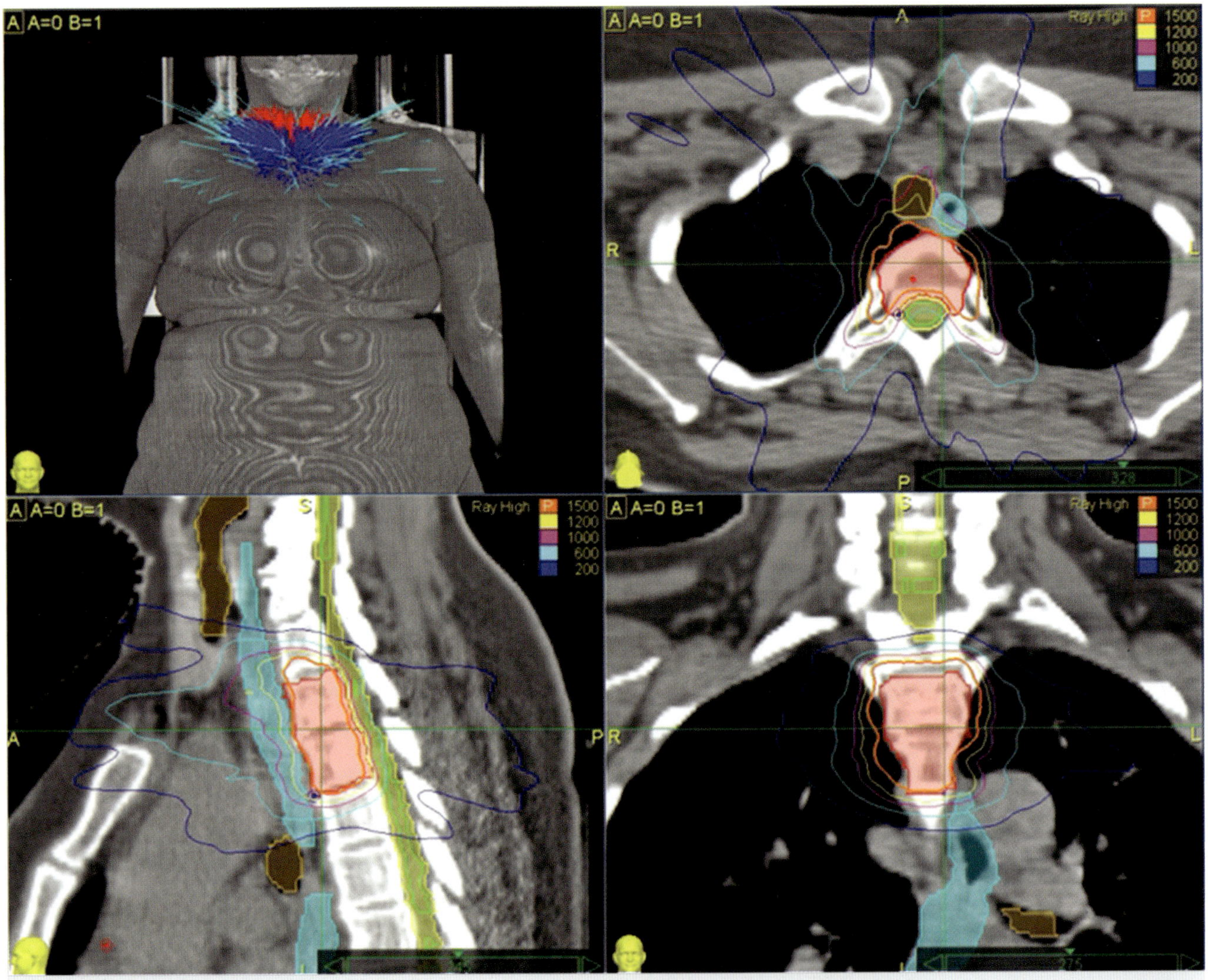

Fig. 29.1 A 53-year-old woman with oligometastatic lesions at T2, T3, L3, and L5 from breast cancer, status postsystemic therapy. She received CyberKnife-based single-fraction stereotactic body radiotherapy (SBRT) to those lesions. The picture shows the plan for the treatment to T2 and T3. A dose of 15 Gy was prescribed at 80%. The plan for treatment to L3 and L5 is not shown. The patient had no progression of disease in the spine and extraspinal sites 6 months after SBRT.

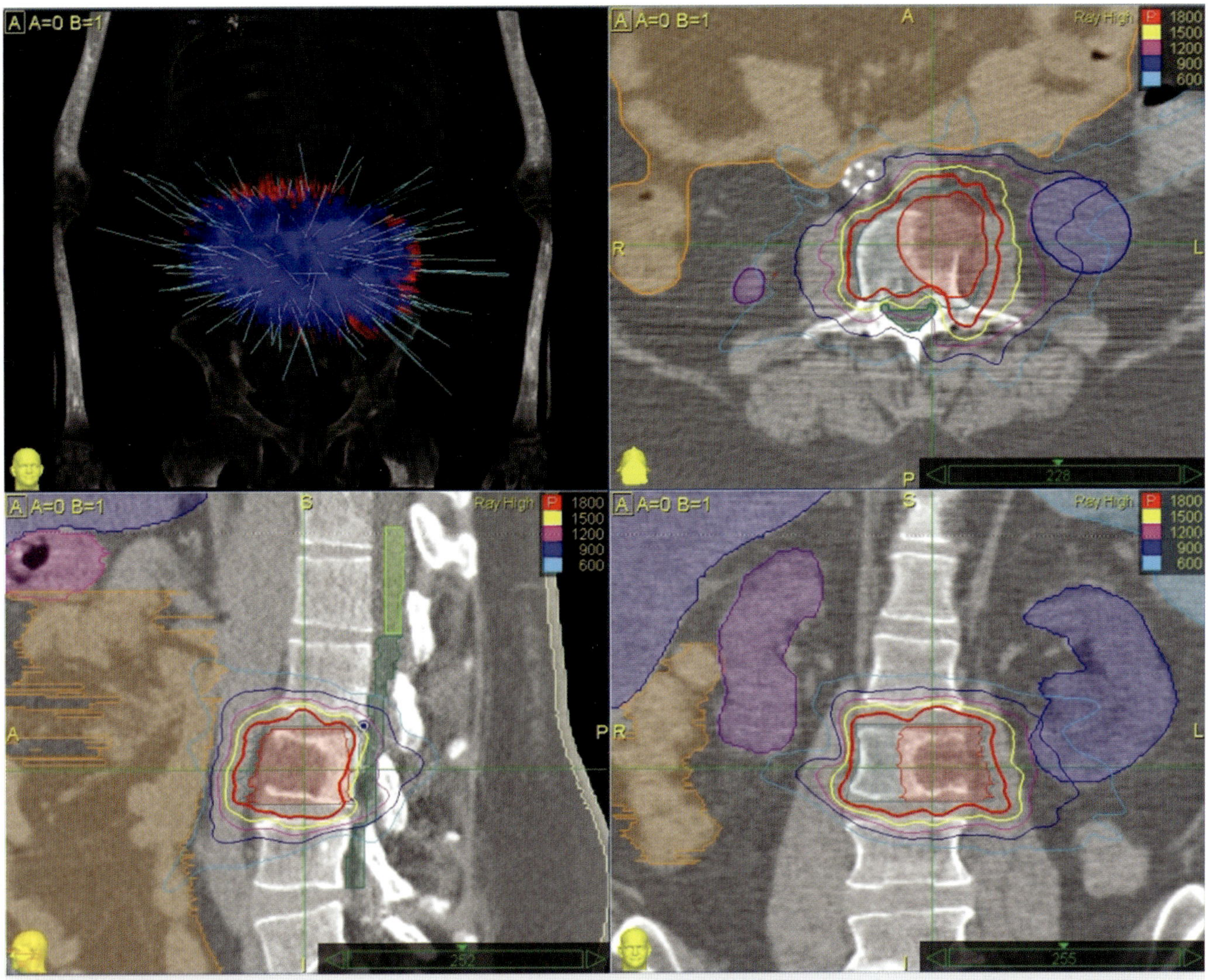

Fig. 29.2 A 56-year-old man with metastatic non–small-cell lung cancer to L3, causing severe lower back pain for which CyberKnife-based single-fraction SBRT was given. A dose of 18 Gy was prescribed to the 81% isodose line. Pain relief was achieved within 24 hours of treatment. The patient also developed radiation-induced bilateral L3 radiculopathy, mainly in the form of shooting sensation in an L3 dermatome, which gradually resolved over the next 3 months.

16 Gy will be offered, and the maximum cord dose is limited to 10 Gy. For patients with a life expectancy of > 12 months, a dose of 27 Gy in three fractions will be offered, and the maximum cord dose is limited to 18 Gy.[46]

On the contrary, for patients who have received prior radiotherapy to the index spinal segments, there are concerns about an elevated risk of radiation myelopathy from reirradiation with SBRT.[34] The constraints for spinal cord for reirradiation with SBRT were estimated by Sahgal et al for one to five fractions based on human data.[34] Based on these data, the GTV will have to be very significantly underdosed to limit the spinal cord dose to below the estimated tolerance should a single-fraction regimen be used. Surgical intervention to clear any epidural disease can potentially increase the gap between the GTV and spinal cord,[33] but the remaining BED that can be delivered is still limited by prior radiotherapy to the same region. In this situation, multiple-fraction SBRT is recommended, as a higher BED can be delivered while maintaining a low risk of radiation myelopathy (recommendation grade 2C).

Conclusion

Controversies exist as to whether single- or multiple-fraction SBRT has a better therapeutic ratio in the management of patients with newly diagnosed spinal metastases without epidural involvement or risk factors for VCF. Both approaches seem to yield similar local control, although one direct comparative study[43] shows that short-term pain control is better with single-fraction SBRT, and long-term local control is better with multiple-fraction SBRT. It would be appropriate to offer single-fraction SBRT as one of the options for the above-mentioned group of patients. Single-fraction SBRT may be favored in patients with spinal metastases from radioresistant histologies and without epidural involvement or risk factors for

VCF or patients who have short life expectancy or transportation issues. For patients who have epidural involvement resulting in a very small or no gap between the spinal cord and GTV, who have risks factors predisposing to VCF, or who undergo reirradiation for recurrent spinal metastasis, single-fraction SBRT is not recommended.

References

[1] Timmerman RD, Kavanagh BD. Stereotactic body radiation therapy. Curr Probl Cancer 2005; 29: 120–157

[2] Lo SS, Fakiris AJ, Chang EL, et al. Stereotactic body radiation therapy: a novel treatment modality. Nat Rev Clin Oncol 2010; 7: 44–54

[3] Hamilton AJ, Lulu BA, Fosmire H, Stea B, Cassady JR. Preliminary clinical experience with linear accelerator-based spinal stereotactic radiosurgery. Neurosurgery 1995; 36: 311–319

[4] Gerszten PC, Burton SA, Ozhasoglu C, Welch WC. Radiosurgery for spinal metastases: clinical experience in 500 cases from a single institution. Spine 2007; 32: 193–199

[5] Gibbs IC, Kamnerdsupaphon P, Ryu MR, et al. Image-guided robotic radiosurgery for spinal metastases. Radiother Oncol 2007; 82: 185–190

[6] Yamada Y, Bilsky MH, Lovelock DM, et al. High-dose, single-fraction image-guided intensity-modulated radiotherapy for metastatic spinal lesions. Int J Radiat Oncol Biol Phys 2008; 71: 484–490

[7] Yamada Y, Lovelock DM, Yenice KM, et al. Multifractionated image-guided and stereotactic intensity-modulated radiotherapy of paraspinal tumors: a preliminary report. Int J Radiat Oncol Biol Phys 2005; 62: 53–61

[8] Chang EL, Shiu AS, Mendel E, et al. Phase I/II study of stereotactic body radiotherapy for spinal metastasis and its pattern of failure. J Neurosurg Spine 2007; 7: 151–160

[9] Garg AK, Shiu AS, Yang J, et al. Phase 1/2 trial of single-session stereotactic body radiotherapy for previously unirradiated spinal metastases. Cancer 2012; 118: 5069–5077

[10] Garg AK, Wang XS, Shiu AS, et al. Prospective evaluation of spinal reirradiation by using stereotactic body radiation therapy: the University of Texas MD Anderson Cancer Center experience. Cancer 2011; 117: 3509–3516

[11] Wang XS, Rhines LD, Shiu AS, et al. Stereotactic body radiation therapy for management of spinal metastases in patients without spinal cord compression: a phase 1–2 trial. Lancet Oncol 2012; 13: 395–402

[12] Rock JP, Ryu S, Shukairy MS, et al. Postoperative radiosurgery for malignant spinal tumors. Neurosurgery 2006; 58: 891–898, discussion 891–898

[13] Ryu S, Rock J, Rosenblum M, Kim JH. Patterns of failure after single-dose radiosurgery for spinal metastasis. J Neurosurg 2004; 101 (Suppl 3): 402–405

[14] Ryu S, Fang Yin F, Rock J, et al. Image-guided and intensity-modulated radiosurgery for patients with spinal metastasis. Cancer 2003; 97: 2013–2018

[15] Ryu S, Jin JY, Jin R, et al. Partial volume tolerance of the spinal cord and complications of single-dose radiosurgery. Cancer 2007; 109: 628–636

[16] Jin R, Rock J, Jin JY, et al. Single fraction spine radiosurgery for myeloma epidural spinal cord compression. J Exp Ther Oncol 2009; 8: 35–41

[17] Ryu S, Rock J, Jain R, et al. Radiosurgical decompression of metastatic epidural compression. Cancer 2010; 116: 2250–2257

[18] Lo SS, Sahgal A, Wang JZ, et al. Stereotactic body radiation therapy for spinal metastases. Discov Med 2010; 9: 289–296

[19] Park C, Papiez L, Zhang S, Story M, Timmerman RD. Universal survival curve and single fraction equivalent dose: useful tools in understanding potency of ablative radiotherapy. Int J Radiat Oncol Biol Phys 2008; 70: 847–852

[20] Wang JZ, Huang Z, Lo SS, Yuh WT, Mayr NA. A generalized linear-quadratic model for radiosurgery, stereotactic body radiation therapy, and high-dose rate brachytherapy. Sci Transl Med 2010; 2: 39ra48

[21] Fuks Z, Kolesnick R. Engaging the vascular component of the tumor response. Cancer Cell 2005; 8: 89–91

[22] Garcia-Barros M, Paris F, Cordon-Cardo C, et al. Tumor response to radiotherapy regulated by endothelial cell apoptosis. Science 2003; 300: 1155–1159

[23] Lee Y, Auh SL, Wang Y, et al. Therapeutic effects of ablative radiation on local tumor require CD8+T cells: changing strategies for cancer treatment. Blood 2009; 114: 589–595

[24] Gerszten PC, Burton SA, Ozhasoglu C, et al. Stereotactic radiosurgery for spinal metastases from renal cell carcinoma. J Neurosurg Spine 2005; 3: 288–295

[25] Gerszten PC, Burton SA, Quinn AE, Agarwala SS, Kirkwood JM. Radiosurgery for the treatment of spinal melanoma metastases. Stereotact Funct Neurosurg 2005; 83: 213–221

[26] Gerszten PC, Burton SA, Welch WC, et al. Single-fraction radiosurgery for the treatment of spinal breast metastases. Cancer 2005; 104: 2244–2254

[27] Gerszten PC, Burton SA, Belani CP, et al. Radiosurgery for the treatment of spinal lung metastases. Cancer 2006; 107: 2653–2661

[28] Gerszten PC, Germanwala A, Burton SA, Welch WC, Ozhasoglu C, Vogel WJ. Combination kyphoplasty and spinal radiosurgery: a new treatment paradigm for pathological fractures. J Neurosurg Spine 2005; 3: 296–301

[29] Gerszten PC, Monaco EA. Complete percutaneous treatment of vertebral body tumors causing spinal canal compromise using a transpedicular cavitation, cement augmentation, and radiosurgical technique. Neurosurg Focus 2009; 27: E9

[30] Sahgal A, Weinberg V, Ma L, et al. Probabilities of radiation myelopathy specific to stereotactic body radiation therapy to guide safe practice. Int J Radiat Oncol Biol Phys 2013: 341–347

[31] Moulding HD, Elder JB, Lis E, et al. Local disease control after decompressive surgery and adjuvant high-dose single-fraction radiosurgery for spine metastases. J Neurosurg Spine 2010; 13: 87–93

[32] Amdur RJ, Bennett J, Olivier K, et al. A prospective, phase II study demonstrating the potential value and limitation of radiosurgery for spine metastases. Am J Clin Oncol 2009; 32: 515–520

[33] Masucci GL, Yu E, Ma L, et al. Stereotactic body radiotherapy is an effective treatment in reirradiating spinal metastases: current status and practical considerations for safe practice. Expert Rev Anticancer Ther 2011; 11: 1923–1933

[34] Schipani S, Wen W, Jin JY, Kim JK, Ryu S. Spine radiosurgery: a dosimetric analysis in 124 patients who received 18 Gy. Int J Radiat Oncol Biol Phys 2012; 84: e571–e576

[35] Sahgal A, Ma L, Weinberg V, et al. Reirradiation human spinal cord tolerance for stereotactic body radiotherapy. Int J Radiat Oncol Biol Phys 2012; 82: 107–116

[36] Cox BW, Jackson A, Hunt M, Bilsky M, Yamada Y. Esophageal toxicity from high-dose, single-fraction paraspinal stereotactic radiosurgery. Int J Radiat Oncol Biol Phys 2012: 7–13

[37] Chow E, Harris K, Fan G, Tsao M, Sze WM. Palliative radiotherapy trials for bone metastases: a systematic review. J Clin Oncol 2007; 25: 1423–1436

[38] Rose PS, Laufer I, Boland PJ, et al. Risk of fracture after single fraction image-guided intensity-modulated radiation therapy to spinal metastases. J Clin Oncol 2009; 27: 5075–5079

[39] Boehling NS, Grosshans DR, Allen PK, et al. Vertebral compression fracture risk after stereotactic body radiotherapy for spinal metastases. J Neurosurg Spine 2012; 16: 379–386

[40] Cunha MV, Al-Omair A, Atenafu EG, et al. Vertebral compression fracture (VCF) after spine stereotactic body radiation therapy (SBRT): analysis of predictive factors. Int J Radiat Oncol Biol Phys 2012; 84: e343–e349

[41] Sahgal A, Larson DA, Chang EL. Stereotactic body radiosurgery for spinal metastases: a critical review. Int J Radiat Oncol Biol Phys 2008; 71: 652–665

[42] Nguyen QN, Shiu AS, Rhines LD, et al. Management of spinal metastases from renal cell carcinoma using stereotactic body radiotherapy. Int J Radiat Oncol Biol Phys 2010; 76: 1185–1192

[43] Heron DE, Rajagopalan MS, Stone B, et al. Single-session and multisession CyberKnife radiosurgery for spine metastases: University of Pittsburgh and Georgetown University experience. J Neurosurg Spine 2012; 17: 11–18

[44] Lovelock DM, Zhang Z, Jackson A, et al. Correlation of local failure with measures of dose insufficiency in the high-dose single-fraction treatment of bony metastases. Int J Radiat Oncol Biol Phys 2010; 77: 1282–1287

[45] Potters L, Kavanagh B, Galvin JM, et al. American Society for Therapeutic Radiology and Oncology. American College of Radiology. American Society for Therapeutic Radiology and Oncology (ASTRO) and American College of Radiology (ACR) practice guideline for the performance of stereotactic body radiation therapy. Int J Radiat Oncol Biol Phys 2010; 76: 326–332

[46] Lo, Sahgal, Ma et al. Normal tissue constraints. In: Stereotactic body radiation therapy (Eds: Lo, Teh, Lu, Schefter); 393–410. Springer 2012

30 Vertebral Compression Fractures Are High Risk after Radiosurgery

John Cuaron, Ilya Laufer, Eric Lis, Mark H. Bilsky, and Yoshiya Yamada

Introduction

Spine radiosurgery is rapidly gaining traction as an effective method of treating solid tumor spine metastases, providing excellent rates of durable tumor control in the order of 85 to 90%[1,2] and minimal serious complications, such as spinal cord injury[3,4] or esophageal complications.[5] As follow-up has matured, an increasingly common sequela is weakening of bone integrity as a consequence of delivery of ablative treatment to tumors housed within the spine, resulting in vertebral body fractures.[6]

The negative impact of radiation on bone integrity is well documented. Sarcomas, which are typically irradiated to doses > 6,000 cGy, are known to be at increased risk for fracture when the bone undergoes radiation therapy. When conformal intensity modulated radiation was used to minimize radiation dose to the bone in those at highest risk for fracture (bone stripping or bone resection during tumor resection prior to radiation therapy), only 4% of patients actually experienced a fracture.[7] Patients who undergo pelvic radiation for cervical cancer have been noted to have a cumulative incidence of pelvic insufficiency fractures of 45%.[8] Increased risk of rib fractures has been noted in patients who received higher doses of breast radiation.[9]

The Risk of Vertebral Body Fracture with Spine Radiosurgery

Vertebral body fracture risk after spine radiosurgery was first reported by the Spine Service at Memorial Sloan-Kettering Cancer Center (MSKCC) in 2008.[6] Sixty-two patients were treated with high-dose spine radiosurgery (1,800–2,400 cGy, median 2,400 cGy) at 71 sites. These patients received a full dose to the entire vertebral body. Serial computed tomography (CT) or magnetic resonance imaging (MRI), obtained in three or four monthly follow-up intervals, was reviewed by a team of surgeons and neuroradiologists to assess the rate of posttreatment fractures (Fig. 30.1). Fracture progression was noted in 27 patients, with a gross fracture rate of 39%, and the median time to fracture was 25 months. In multivariate analysis, CT appearance (lytic vs mixed or sclerotic), lesion location, and percent of tumor replacement of the vertebral body were independent predictors of fracture progression. In this analysis, it was found that lesions between T10 and the sacrum were 4.6 times more likely to fracture than lesions above T10. Lytic lesions were 6.8 times more likely to fracture than their nonlytic counterparts. The risk of fracture increased with greater vertebral body replacement with tumor, but in this regard, there was no group with a zero risk of fracture. Even in the smallest tumors occupying < 20% of the vertebral body at the time of treatment, if followed long enough, patients would eventually experience fracture. Obesity, local kyphosis, bisphosphonate use, and the radiation dose were not found to be significantly associated with fracture risk. Patients who experienced radiographic evidence of fracture also had lower Karnofsky performance scale (KPS) scores and had higher narcotic requirements. This suggests that, in this cohort, vertebral body fractures were clinically significant.

Sheehan et al[10] reported the results of 110 spine metastases that underwent radiosurgery to a median dose of 1,730 cGy (range 1,000–2,400 cGy); kyphosis was found to be the most common sequela of successful treatment. The mean follow-up was 12.3 months (range 4–32 months). Progression of kyphosis at the site of treatment was found in 73% of patients alive ($N = 16$) at 12 months. The mean increase of kyphosis was 7.3 ± 4.5 degrees. Similar to the MSKCC study, there was an association between the degree of kyphosis and worsening Visual Analogue Scale (VAS) scores and Oswestry Disability Index (ODI) scores. Lesions in the junctional zones of the spine were more likely to undergo a more pronounced kyphosis.

Boehling et al[11] reported the rates of vertebral body fracture in 123 lesions treated in 93 patients. The median follow-up was 15 months (range 1–71 months). Twenty patients had received prior radiation therapy. Thirty-one patients received single-fraction radiosurgery (median dose 1,800 cGy), and the rest were treated with either three (median dose 2,700 cGy) or five fractions (median dose 3,000 cGy) of treatment. Twenty-five new or progressing fractures were noted (20%) with a median time to progression of 3 months. In multivariate analysis, age > 55 years, presence of a preexisting fracture, and higher baseline pain scores were significant predictive factors for fracture. Larger, lytic lesions were at greater risk for fracture. The location (below or above T10) and the use of bisphosphonates were not associated with fracture risk, whereas obesity was found to have a protective effect. Perhaps because of small numbers, the impact of radiation dose on fracture risk was not included in this report; neither is there mention of the effect of prior radiation on fracture risk.

A recent report of 167 lesions treated in 90 patients found an 87% chance of freedom from fracture after spine radiosurgery at 1 year.[12] Patients were treated with 800 to 2,400 cGy in a single fraction, 1,800 to 2,400 cGy in two fractions, 2,000 to 2,700 cGy in three fractions, 3,000 Gy in four fractions, or 2,500 to 3,000 cGy in five fractions. The median follow-up was 7.4 months, and 19 fractures were noted (11%). In this study, the mean time to fracture was 3.3 months (0.5–21.6 mo). Multivariate analysis found that the dose of radiation > 2,000 cGy resulted in a greater likelihood of fracture. Interestingly, hepatocellular carcinoma and lung cancer metastases were more likely to fracture.

Although the available literature reports outcomes at different time intervals, it is clear that the risk of fracture is not insignificant. It appears that with longer follow-up, the risk of fracture increases. Patients with spine metastases are at increased risk of fracture due to frequent steroid use, exposure to cytotoxic chemotherapy, prior radiation therapy, poor nutrition, and hormonal therapy that may threaten bone health.

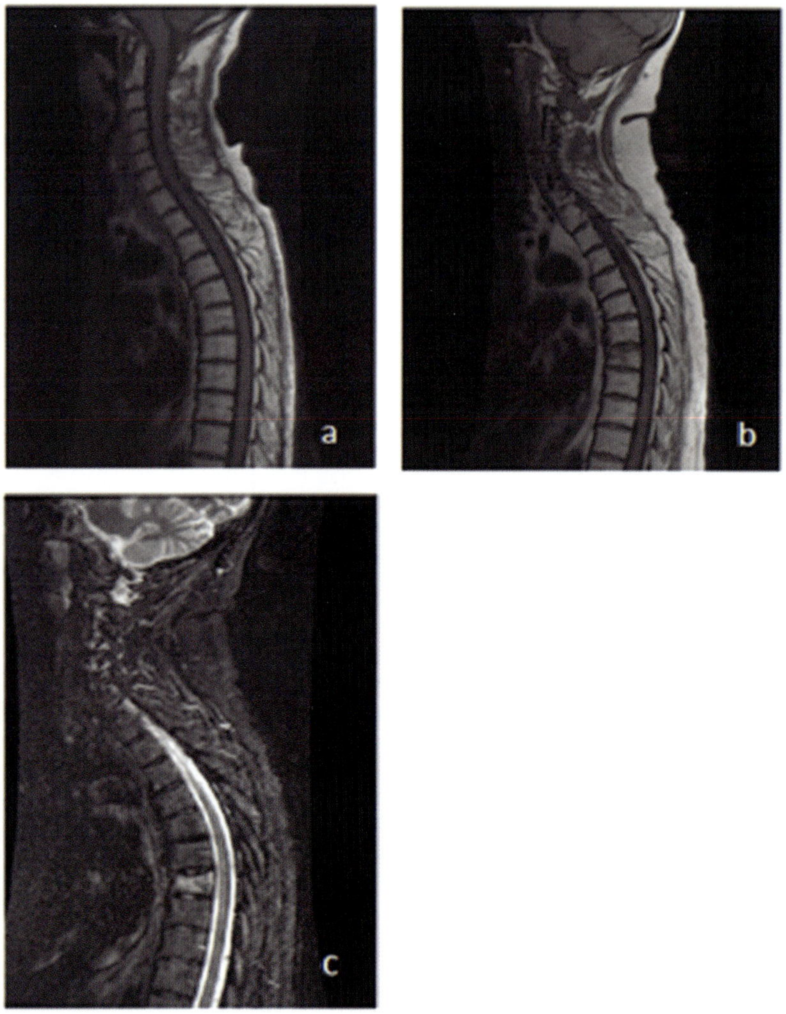

Fig. 30.1 Progressive fracture at T5 after 2,400 cGy × 1. (a) T1 prior to treatment. (b) T1 6 months after treatment. (c) T2 fat suppressed 6 months after treatment.

Spine radiosurgery patients typically experience fractures in the absence of active tumor, suggesting that radiation may play a role in the development of a fracture. In a preliminary survey of biopsies of 20 consecutive patients who underwent kyphoplasty for vertebral body fracture after spine radiosurgery without evidence of tumor progression, 80% of the specimens were found to be acellular fibrosis without any evidence of intact bone. These findings suggest that high-dose radiosurgery not only is ablative for tumor but also has similar effects on bone included in the target volume. Observations that end plate infractions in adjacent vertebral bodies without tumor that were included in the high-dose volume of the neighboring diseased vertebral body also suggest that radiation plays an important role in the development of vertebral body fracture. Risk factors for vertebral compression factors after SBRT are shown in ▶ Table 30.1.

Management of Fractures

Pain, especially pain that worsens with movement and in particular is made worse with axial load bearing, is the hallmark symptom associated with vertebral body fractures after spine radiosurgery. When the fracture involves the neural foramen or displaces bone fragments into the neural foramen, positional radiculopathy is also present. Anti-inflammatory drugs, both steroidal and nonsteroidal, reduce the inflammation that often accompanies vertebral body fractures and are effective ways to manage such pain. Narcotics are also often prescribed to help alleviate pain and are often used in conjunction with anti-inflammatory drugs. In cases of radiculopathy, nerve stabilizers are also effective agents. Muscle relaxants can help with muscle spasm pain that may result from spinal instability. Judicious use of botulin toxin injections has been helpful in relieving back spasm pain.

Radiographic studies, in particular MRI and CT imaging, are used in diagnosing vertebral body fracture. Vertebral bodies typically demonstrate loss of vertebral body height and/or loss of superior or inferior end plate integrity. Acute fractures will typically be associated with increased bone edema, usually well demonstrated on fat-suppressed MRI sequences. Often imaging will demonstrate progressive worsening over time.

Radiographic evidence of progressive fracture is accompanied by progressive symptoms in the majority of cases. Symptomatic management includes careful and appropriate use of

Table 30.1 Multivariate analyses of risk factors for vertebral compression factures after SBRT

	Rose et al[6]	Boehling et al[11]	Cunha et al[12]
Number of patients	62	93	90
Number of lesions	71	123	167
Median dose	24 Gy	27 Gy	NR
Median follow-up (mo)	13	14.9	7.4
Rate of vertebral compression fracture	39%	20%	11%
Age	NR	< 0.05	NR
Karnofsky performance scale	NR	NS	NR
Location (T10–sacrum vs other spine)	< 0.05	NS	NS
Type of lesion (lytic vs other)	< 0.05	< 0.05	0.007
Abnormal alignment (kyphosis or scoliosis)	NS	NR	0.0003
Preexisting pain	NR	< 0.05	NS
Preexisting fracture or vertebral body Collapse	NR	< 0.05	NS
Amount of vertebral body involved	< 0.05*	NS	NR
Lung histology	NR	NR	0.03
Hepatocellular carcinoma histology	NR	NR	< 0.0001
Dose > 20 Gy	NS	NR	0.004
Obesity	NS	< 0.05**	NR
Bisphosphonate use	NS	NS	NR

* *Lesions occupying 41 to 60% of vertebral body were associated with significant risk of vertebral compression fracture on MVA.*
** *Obesity was protective with hazard ration 0.02.*
Abbreviations: *NR, not reported; NS, nonsignificant.*

analgesic medications. Pain is often the predominant complaint associated with vertebral body fractures. Care should be taken to differentiate between pain from tumor progression (tumor pain) and pain that results from mechanical failure in the spine. The Spine Instability Neoplastic Score (SINS) developed by the Spine Oncology Study Group (SOSG)[13] is an instrument designed to designate a spine as mechanically stable, potentially unstable, or mechanically unstable based on a scoring criteria that assigns points based on the location of the lesion within the spine, CT appearance, nature of pain, degree of vertebral body and posterior element involvement, and the presence of subluxation. Using this classification, Cunha et al found that 5% of lesions deemed stable underwent fracture, and 19% of potentially unstable lesions experienced fracture.[12] No patients met the criteria for mechanically unstable, as these patients typically underwent surgical fixation and were excluded from the analysis. Mechanically unstable spines cannot be adequately palliated with radiotherapy, and some type of intervention, such as vertebral body augmentation or surgical fixation to bolster the mechanical integrity of the spine, will be necessary.

Gerszten et al first described the use of kyphoplasty in 26 patients with pathologic vertebral body fractures in the setting of spine radiosurgery.[14] These patients underwent tumor debulking with a radiofrequency ablative device, followed by kyphoplasty. This was done to minimize the risk of extravasation of tumor into the spinal canal during kyphoplasty. These patients then had adjuvant radiotherapy. The patients reported pain relief in the range of 80 to 100%.

Vertebral body augmentation for vertebral body fracture has become a controversial topic. A multicenter, randomized trial suggested that kyphoplasty provided a benefit in terms of earlier improvement in pain and functional status at 1 month. However, this study has been criticized because it was nonblinded and was industry sponsored.[15] Two randomized, double-blinded, placebo-controlled trials have been recently reported that question the utility of percutaneous vertebral body augmentation in the setting of osteoporotic fractures. Buchbinder et al[16] found no benefit in the use of vertebroplasty versus a sham procedure in terms of pain, physical functioning, or quality of life in 78 patients at 1 week, 1 month, 3 months, or 6 months after treatment. Kallmes et al[17] reported the results of vertebroplasty versus a sham procedure in 131 patients. Patient pain and functional disability were assessed at 3, 14, 30, and 90 days. A trend toward improved pain at 1 month in patients who underwent vertebroplasty was not statistically significant. It should be noted that these trials were conducted in noncancer patients, in particular, patients who had never been irradiated. Thus, given their patient population, these trials differed from those studies involving patients who underwent spine radiosurgery, and the results are not likely transferable to the spine radiosurgery population. Nonetheless, in the setting of asymptomatic radiographic fractures, kyphoplasty may not provide added benefit. In the cancer population, uncontrolled back pain can have a significant impact on performance status, and vertebral body augmentation should be considered for patients with vertebral body fracture who suffer from instability pain.

In cases of nerve root impingement as a result of vertebral body compression, kyphoplasty is generally unable to adequately relieve nerve root compression. Particularly in the case of lumbar radiculopathy, these patients may be best palliated with surgical fixation,[18] either with minimally invasive percutaneous posterior fixation or, in more severe cases of wedging of the nerve root, open surgical decompression of the nerve root. In rare cases of bone fragment–induced spinal cord compression, surgical decompression is the best management option.

Conclusion

Progressive vertebral body fracture after spine radiosurgery has been reported in 11 to 39% of cases. It appears that the risk of fracture increases with longer follow-up. The majority of fractures are symptomatic and in cases of mechanical instability will require interventions beyond medical management.

References

[1] Gerszten PC, Burton SA, Ozhasoglu C, Welch WC. Radiosurgery for spinal metastases: clinical experience in 500 cases from a single institution. Spine 2007; 32: 193–199

[2] Yamada Y, Bilsky MH, Lovelock DM, et al. High-dose, single-fraction image-guided intensity-modulated radiotherapy for metastatic spinal lesions. Int J Radiat Oncol Biol Phys 2008; 71: 484–490

[3] Gibbs IC, Patil C, Gerszten PC, Adler JR, Burton SA. Delayed radiation-induced myelopathy after spinal radiosurgery. Neurosurgery 2009; 64 (Suppl): A67–A72

[4] Sahgal A, Ma L, Gibbs I, et al. Spinal cord tolerance for stereotactic body radiotherapy. Int J Radiat Oncol Biol Phys 2010; 77: 548–553

[5] Cox BW, Jackson A, Hunt M, Bilsky M, Yamada Y. Esophageal toxicity from high-dose, single-fraction paraspinal stereotactic radiosurgery. Int J Radiat Oncol Biol Phys 2012; 83: e661–e667

[6] Rose PS, Laufer I, Boland PJ, et al. Risk of fracture after single fraction image-guided intensity-modulated radiation therapy to spinal metastases. J Clin Oncol 2009; 27: 5075–5079

[7] Alektiar KM, Brennan MF, Healey JH, Singer S. Impact of intensity-modulated radiation therapy on local control in primary soft-tissue sarcoma of the extremity. J Clin Oncol 2008; 26: 3440–3444

[8] Kwon JW, Huh SJ, Yoon YC, et al. Pelvic bone complications after radiation therapy of uterine cervical cancer: evaluation with MRI. AJR Am J Roentgenol 2008; 191: 987–994

[9] Pierce SM, Recht A, Lingos TI, et al. Long-term radiation complications following conservative surgery (CS) and radiation therapy (RT) in patients with early stage breast cancer. Int J Radiat Oncol Biol Phys 1992; 23: 915–923

[10] Sheehan JP, Shaffrey CI, Schlesinger D, Williams BJ, Arlet V, Larner J. Radiosurgery in the treatment of spinal metastases: tumor control, survival, and quality of life after helical tomotherapy. Neurosurgery 2009; 65: 1052–1061, discussion 1061–1062

[11] Boehling NS, Grosshans DR, Allen PK, et al. Vertebral compression fracture risk after stereotactic body radiotherapy for spinal metastases. J Neurosurg Spine 2012; 16: 379–386

[12] Cunha MV, Al-Omair A, Atenafu EG, et al. Vertebral compression fracture (VCF) after spine stereotactic body radiation therapy (SBRT): analysis of predictive factors. Int J Radiat Oncol Biol Phys 2012; 84: e343–e349

[13] Fourney DR, Frangou EM, Ryken TC, et al. Spinal instability neoplastic score: an analysis of reliability and validity from the spine oncology study group. J Clin Oncol 2011; 29: 3072–3077

[14] Gerszten PC, Germanwala A, Burton SA, Welch WC, Ozhasoglu C, Vogel WJ. Combination kyphoplasty and spinal radiosurgery: a new treatment paradigm for pathological fractures. J Neurosurg Spine 2005; 3: 296–301

[15] Wardlaw D, Cummings SR, Van Meirhaeghe J, et al. Efficacy and safety of balloon kyphoplasty compared with non-surgical care for vertebral compression fracture (FREE): a randomised controlled trial. Lancet 2009; 373: 1016–1024

[16] Buchbinder R, Osborne RH, Ebeling PR, et al. A randomized trial of vertebroplasty for painful osteoporotic vertebral fractures. N Engl J Med 2009; 361: 557–568

[17] Kallmes DF, Comstock BA, Heagerty PJ, et al. A randomized trial of vertebroplasty for osteoporotic spinal fractures. N Engl J Med 2009; 361: 569–579

[18] Bilsky M, Smith M. Surgical approach to epidural spinal cord compression. Hematol Oncol Clin North Am 2006; 20: 1307–1317

31 Vertebral Compression Fractures Are Low Risk after Radiosurgery

Jason A. Weaver, Gabriel H. Phillips, Matthew A. VanLandingham, and Kyle S. Gabrick

Introduction

Radiation therapy has a well-established role in the multimodal approach to treating spinal metastases. The earliest application of radiation therapy for the treatment of spinal metastases, at doses of 25 to 40 Gy over 10 to14 fractions, resulted in modest improvements to patients' pain and length of continued ambulation at rates comparable to those associated with open surgical decompression via laminectomy.[1–6] As the methods and indications for radiation therapy have evolved within the management paradigm of metastatic spinal disease, patients have experienced improved outcomes. However, conventional radiotherapy delivers a wide-field beam to the target, and dosing is limited by the tolerance of surrounding normal tissues. Consequently, the tumor may not receive a cytotoxic dose, especially in cases of relatively radioresistant histologies. Stereotactic, image-guided radiotherapy allows multiple beams to converge on the target structure while sparing the surrounding healthy, normal tissues, particularly the spinal cord, from toxic doses. As a result, the tumor itself can receive much higher biologic equivalent doses than allowed with conventional external beam radiotherapy. Radiosurgery as the primary treatment modality affords excellent radiographic control, pain control, and preservation of neurologic function, even for historically described radioresistant tumors.[7–12] As an adjunct to open surgery, radiosurgery has shown promising results for durable local control, while decreasing the morbidity of radical tumor resection followed by an anterior spinal column reconstruction.[13]

As the use of spine radiosurgery has become more widespread in the management of spinal tumors, some authors have reported an association with progressive or new vertebral compression fractures (VCFs).[14–16] Because compression fractures are a significant source of pain and may lead to spinal deformity and compromise of neurologic structures, this potential drawback of stereotactic radiosurgery (SRS) must be considered and addressed. The overall frequency for vertebral body fractures following spine radiosurgery and identifiable risk factors should be accounted for in order to provide the greatest symptom relief and durability of response for patients. No prospective, randomized study exists to compare the natural prevalence and progression of VCFs in the setting of spinal metastases to those tumors treated with radiosurgery. Without such a study, assigning relative risk to fracture after radiosurgery is somewhat speculative because the natural prevalence of VCF in the setting of metastatic disease is quite high. However, an analysis of the available data may allow us to stratify risk to identify subsets of patients who might benefit from prophylactic vertebral augmentation or spinal instrumentation prior to spine radiosurgery delivery.

Radiotherapy and Vertebral Compression Fractures

Radiation therapy is known to predispose patients to the spontaneous development of bony fractures in a dose-dependent manner,[17,18] and osseous structures already compromised by metastatic disease or exposed to increased axial loads may display an even higher tendency to fracture. Femur fractures are significantly more common after removal of soft tissue sarcomas followed by adjuvant radiation.[19,20] Direct evidence concerning VCFs after radiation to adjacent structures is limited to a single case report. Rodriguez-Ruiz et al[15] reported a T7–T8 compression fracture after administration of intensity-modulated radiation therapy (IMRT) to the lung for primary lung cancer. In their patient, the vertebral bodies were included in the margins of the radiation field.

By the time spinal metastases come to medical attention, many patients already have pathologic compression fractures. This delay in presentation makes the natural history of spinal metastases difficult to determine because patients present at different points in their disease progression. The best approximation of the incidence of VCFs in untreated spinal metastases is the prevalence at the initiation of treatment. Depending on the method of patient recruitment for initiation of treatment, reported VCF prevalence can be highly variable. Furthermore, although the stated primary goal of radiosurgery is the prevention of tumor progression and subsequent fracture, many clinical cohort studies have failed to document the precise incidence of pre- and posttreatment VCFs.[10]

Because the risk of fractures appears to be dose-dependent, larger doses of radiation such as those given in stereotactic treatment of spinal metastases may reasonably be hypothesized to produce a higher incidence of posttreatment vertebral collapse than conventionally delivered radiotherapy. Boehling et al[14] found a 20% incidence of either new or progressing vertebral body fractures after treatment with 18 to 30 Gy, with a median time to fracture of 3 months. Rose et al[16] reported a 39% incidence of progressive VCFs after treatment with18 to 24 Gy, with a median time to fracture of 25 months. The results in these studies were not stratified by dose; therefore, no conclusions can be drawn regarding dose and VCFs. Temporally, these two studies suggest different pathological processes, given the median time to the development of a fracture (3 vs 25 mo).

Vertebral Compression Fractures after Radiosurgery Are Low Risk

Although some studies suggest that VCFs occur or progress at a rate of possibly 20 to 39% after treatment with spine SRS,[14,16] the degree to which these fractures can be attributed to radiation treatment remains unclear. A pathophysiological basis for increased fracture risk in irradiated bone has been established for other osseous structures, but the applicability of these results to the spine is merely speculative. A multifactorial model may be a better explanation for VCFs in the clinical setting of metastatic spinal disease.

Defining the Natural Prevalence of VCF in the Setting of Metastatic Spinal Disease

Although SRS has been a component of the treatment of spinal metastases for over a decade, very few studies have specifically examined VCFs occurring after treatment. Looking back even further, the literature concerning VCFs that occur after the lower doses of conventional radiotherapy is similarly sparse. The two studies[14,16] currently available that provide data on the incidence of VCFs lack a control group and cannot establish causation.

Without an adequate control group for comparison, it cannot be determined whether the incidence of VCFs after radiosurgery differs from the natural history of metastatic spinal disease. Overall, the prevalence of pathologic fracture is quite high. In an epidemiologic study looking at 44,120 Medicare beneficiaries with an International Classification of Diseases, ninth revision (ICD-9) diagnosis code of fracture, 48% of VCFs were found to be pathologic. Twenty-five percent of these had a possible association with a cancer diagnosis.[21] Furthermore, the prevalence of VCFs in most cohorts of patients with spinal metastases ranges from 28% to 38% (▶ Table 31.1). In a study retrospectively reviewing 407 cancer patients at a tertiary cancer center, 1,156 fractures were identified, with an average of 2.8 fractures per patient.[22] Progression of systemic metastatic disease with subsequent decreased nutritional status, decreased mobility, and increased corticosteroid use may independently or collectively reduce bone quality and increase fracture risk. Tumor infiltration into vertebral structures, especially lytic metastases, increases the risk of vertebral body collapse even in the setting of no prior radiotherapy.[23]

A review of the literature concerning the prevalence of VCFs in patients with metastatic disease ranges widely, from 28 to 75% (▶ Table 31.1).[24–26] Biomechanical studies and prospective analyses suggest that anatomical location, degree of metastatic involvement, and tumor histology in part predict compression fractures.[27] As Rose et al[16] indicated, there is a lack of evidence in the literature relating compression fractures to radiotherapy, either conventional fractionated radiotherapy or SRS. Nonetheless, compression fractures are frequent in metastatic disease in the presence or absence of radiation. Therefore, the incidence of new or progressive fractures after radiosurgery could merely be a reflection of the natural history of the disease.

▶ Table 31.1 attempts to define the prevalence of VCFs in the setting of metastatic spinal disease and to identify factors that

Table 31.1 Natural prevalence of vertebral compression fracture in the setting of metastatic spinal disease

Study	Prevalence in patients	Factors that increase risk	Level of evidence	Recommendation grade
Maranzano et al[28]	31%	N/A	II	1B
Taneichi et al[29]	75% (50% of infiltrated VBs)	- % of VB occupied with tumor -% destruction of the pedicle - % destruction of costovertebral joint	III	2B
Shah et al[23]	34% (7.4% of infiltrated VBs)	- 80% infiltration or > (4 × risk) - undifferentiated histology - upper lumbar spine	III	1C +
Chaichana et al[30]	32%	N/A	III	1C
Chaichana et al[24]	37%	- 4 × increased risk in breast carcinoma - 3–4 × increased risk in anterior disease - 3–4 × increased risk in thoracic spine - 2 × increased risk after chemo	III	1C
Patchell et al[25]	38%	N/A	I	1A
Rose et al[16]	28%	- T10–S1 location - Lytic lesions with > 40% VB involvement - No correlation to histology	III	1C +
Boehling et al[14]	29% (28% of treated VBs)	- Age > 55 y - Preexisting fracture - Baseline pain	III	1C +

Abbreviations: *N/A, not applicable; VB, vertebral body; VCF, vertebral compression fracture.*

predispose a tumor-laden vertebral body to fracture. Maranzano et al[28] investigated 275 consecutive patients with VCFs. The authors reported that of the 209 patients that entered their treatment protocol, 31% had pathologic vertebral body fractures. Taneichi et al[29] specifically attempted to define the factors that increased risk of fracture in metastases of the thoracic and lumbar spine. The authors identified 100 thoracic and lumbar vertebral bodies infiltrated with tumor in 53 patients, 48 of whom had back pain. The prevalence of a fracture in tumor-involved vertebral bodies was 50%. Significant risk factors associated with collapse were costovertebral joint destruction, size of tumor (defined as a percentage of infiltration within the vertebral body), and pedicle involvement. The most important risk factor for VCF in the thoracic and lumbar spine was percentage of tumor infiltration within the vertebral body. Although the authors did not study the effect of radiotherapy on fracture risk, they proposed that if radiation could prevent progression within the affected vertebral body, it might indeed lower fracture risk. The authors then attempted to stratify risk of fracture through multivariate analysis to determine when prophylactic intervention would be beneficial. This study was retrospective and, by admission of the authors, largely depended on obtaining measurements of destruction after a fracture had occurred. Furthermore, because of selection criteria and the high incidence of back pain at inclusion, it can be argued that prevalence of fractures was relatively high for this particular study.

Similarly, Shah et al[23] attempted to identify risk factors associated with VCF in the setting of metastatic disease. Also retrospective in design, this study included randomly selected patients from a large and varied population of patients with known metastatic spinal tumors. The authors analyzed 756 vertebrae in 53 patients. Thirty-four percent of patients had a fracture. The authors identified 253 vertebrae infiltrated with tumor; of these, 7.4% were fractured. Fracture risk was greatest for tumor-infiltrated bodies in the upper lumbar spine and for undifferentiated tumors. A fourfold increased risk of fracture was observed if > 80% of the vertebral body was infiltrated by tumor.

Chaichana et al[30] reviewed all patients undergoing surgery for metastatic epidural spinal cord compression from 1995 to 2005 at a tertiary center. Of those patients, they identified a fracture prevalence of 32%. Similarly, in a later study including 162 patients presenting with epidural cord compression, the same authors identified a fracture in 60 (37%) patients with a total of 73 pathologic fractures. In this particular study, factors that increased risk of fracture were a histology of breast cancer (fourfold increase), tumors located anteriorly and involving the thoracic spine (three- to fourfold increase), and prior treatment with chemotherapy (twofold increase risk). Importantly, this study did not demonstrate an increased risk of fracture after radiotherapy.[28] In a prospective, randomized trial, also looking at patients presenting with epidural spinal cord compression, Patchell et al[25] found that 38% entered the study with unstable spines, suggesting at least some degree of fracture. It is also important to note that this study was exclusively for patients with a single area of disease that could include several segments. Because metastatic disease of the spine frequently involves multiple vertebral segments, admittedly the prevalence of fracture among infiltrated vertebral bodies is likely lower, perhaps more on the order of 7.4%, as demonstrated by Shah et al,[23] as described above.

It is known that the prevalence of VCF in the setting of metastatic spinal disease falls within a range of 28 to 38% of patients (▸ Table 31.1). Some studies have shown an even higher prevalence in select populations (i.e., symptomatic patients presenting with back pain). Because of this high prevalence, it is difficult to assign a true relative risk to radiosurgery and the subsequent development or progression of VCF. Comparing the natural prevalence of fracture to the incidence of new or progressive fracture after radiosurgery may provide a better analysis.

Defining Fracture Incidence or Progression after Radiosurgery

Two studies have specifically looked at the risk of vertebral body fracture after radiosurgery. Rose et al[16] enrolled 62 patients with 71 treated lesions, including 20 (28%) patients with a preexisting fracture at the treatment site (12 with end plate only, 8 with mild compression fractures). The main outcome measure was the development of new fractures or progression of an existing fracture. New or progressive VCF was noted in 27 of 71 patients (39%). In this study, the presence of a preexisting fracture was not predictive for progression of the fracture when compared with other vertebral bodies. Of the 27 new or progressive fractures, only one was directly related to tumor progression. Risk factors included location from T10 to S1, percentage of tumor involvement within the vertebral body, and lytic lesions. Tumor histology, obesity, local kyphosis, and radiation dose were not related to new or progressive VCFs. In their population, 11 of13 patients with lytic lesions involving > 40% of the vertebral body had progression or development of new fractures. Patients who underwent surgery or had prior radiation were excluded from the analyses.[16] It is unclear how many of these fractures are directly related to radiosurgery versus the natural history of metastatic disease to the spine. The lack of a control group for this cohort makes definitive conclusions difficult. Also, the rate of new fracture without the appearance of tumor progression or infiltration has not been duplicated in other studies.

Boehling et al[14] also looked at both new and progressive fractures in their cohort. Exclusion criteria included patients with unstable spines and those who underwent an operation. Of the potential 209 patients who had received SRS, 93 were included in the analysis. The median time to progression or fracture was 3 months. In this study, Boehling et al[14] noted that 27 of 93 patients (29%) already had pre-existing fractures. More specifically, of the 123 tumor-laden vertebral bodies treated with radiosurgery, 34 (28%) had preexisting fractures. Progression of a preexisting fracture occurred in 11 of 34 (32%) vertebral bodies. Overall, a new or progressive fracture after radiosurgery occurred in 25 of 123 (20%) treated segments. Looking at tumor histology, specifically renal cell carcinoma, 10 of 36 treated vertebral bodies developed a new fracture or fracture progression. Tumor progression was noted in all 10 incidences. The rate of fracture therefore may have as much to do with tumor progression as it does with the SRS treatment itself. Risk factors for fractures in this study included age greater than 55, preexisting fracture, and baseline pain. Obesity was interestingly found to be a protective factor.[14]

A similar retrospective review of patients treated at our institution with SRS for spinal metastases from 2007 to 2011. ▶ Table 31.2 provides a point of comparison to the studies of Rose et al[16] and Boehling et al.[14] Seventy-one patients directly referred to our department have been managed with SRS for oligometastatic disease of the spine. Of the 52 patients with available follow-up imaging, 46% had preexisting fractures. This prevalence is slightly higher than the rates reported by Rose et al[6] and Boehling et al,[14] but our referral pattern tends to favor patients that require open surgical intervention. Excluding patients treated with open surgery, the overall incidence of new or progressive fractures was 37%, which is similar to that rate reported by Rose et al.[16]

Table 31.2 Characteristics of patients ($n = 52$) entering treatment with stereotactic radiosurgery to treat spinal metastasis

Characteristic	No. patients with compression fractures	Patients without compression fractures
Age (years)	62.7±16	64.3±12
Sex		
Male	12/24 (50%)	10/28 (35.7%)
Female	12/24 (50%)	18/28 (64.3%)
Tumor histology		
Lung	0/24 (0%)	5/28 (17.9%)
Thyroid	0/24 (0%)	1/28 (7.1%)
Colon	0/24 (0%)	0/28 (0%)
Breast	7/24 (29.2%)	7/28 (25%)
Prostate	1/24 (4/2%)	2/28 (7/1%)
Renal	7/24 (29.1%)	9/28 (32.1%)
Other	9/24 (37.5%)	4/28 (14.3%)
Prior treatment		
Surgical resection/stabilization	14/25 (56%)	11/25 (44%)
Radiation	11/24 (45.8%)	11/28 (39.2)
Chemotherapy	15/24 (62.5%)	15/28 (53%)

A Closer Analysis: the Distinction Between New and Progressive Vertebral Compression Fracture after Radiosurgery

Although Rose et al[16] and Boehling et al[14] concluded that the overall incidence of new or progressive fracture after radiosurgery was 39 and 20%, respectively, as noted above, a distinction should be made between a new fracture and progression of a preexisting fracture ▶ Table 31.3. Although Rose et al[16] did not specifically point out the difference in rate, Boehling et al[14] showed that 11 out of the 25 fractures after radiosurgery were due to fracture progression of preexisting VCF. It could even be argued that this is the natural progression of a pathologic fracture, especially in segments with the associated risk factors as they reported. In addition, the study by Boehling et al[14] demonstrated new fracture development in 14 of 123 vertebral bodies at a rate of 19%. Our analysis demonstrated a new fracture rate of 26% in those segments treated with radiosurgery alone. This is in fact lower than the natural prevalence of VCF in the setting of metastatic spinal disease.

Clinical Significance of Vertebral Compression Fracture after Radiosurgery and the Shift in Management Paradigm

An analysis of our patient population referred for neurosurgical consultation shows a higher rate of patients with preexisting fracture, namely 46%. This difference may be due to the referral pattern seen in a neurosurgical practice versus that seen in the cancer center model of the other studies. Accordingly, about half of our patients (25 of 52) were taken to surgery for instrumented stabilization followed with adjuvant SRS. As ▶ Table 31.3 illustrates, stabilization provides a degree of protection against the development of new or progressive fracture after radiosurgery. With the emerging evidence of long-term local tumor control with radiosurgery, a shift in strategy has been demonstrated at some institutions to offer less radical resection of the tumor and to provide spinal stabilization followed with adjuvant radiosurgery.[13] This has been our approach for oligometastatic disease with high-grade epidural compression or mechanical instability associated with fracture, or both. Elimination of the biomechanical forces on the treated segment

Table 31.3 Analysis of new versus progressive fractures after radiosurgery

Study	Pretreatment prevalence of VCF (no. and % of patients)	New fracture after radiosurgery N, [% of patients]	Progressive fracture after radiosurgery [no. and % of patients]	New or progressive fracture [no. and % of patients]	Median f/u (months)
Rose et al[16]	20/62 (32%)	N/A	N/A	27/71 (39%)	19
Boehling et al[14]	27/93 (29%)	14/123 (11%)	11/34 (32%)	25/123 (20%)	14.9
Weaver* (radiosurgery only)	10/27 (37%)	7/27 (26%)	3/10 (30%)	10/27 (37%)	N/A
Weaver* (surgery + radiosurgery	14/25 (56%)	3/25 (12%)	1/14 (7%)	4/25 (16%)	N/A
Weaver* (total)	24/52 (46%)	10/52 (19%)	4/24 (17%)	14/52 (27%)	10

Abbreviations: *N/A, not applicable; VCF, vertebral compression fracture.*
* unpublished data

appears to reduce the radiographic appearance of fracture progression. In our analysis, of the 4 of 25 patients who showed new or progressive fracture after surgery and radiosurgery, none required any additional intervention.

Boehling et al[14] found that 10 of the 25 new or progressive VCFs after radiosurgery were then treated with kyphoplasty or vertebroplasty. Fracture progression led to surgery in two patients and kyphoplasty in one in the study by Rose et al.[16] Therefore, the vast majority of these patients required no intervention. However, as the authors point out, patients with fracture progression were 1.7 times more likely to require narcotic pain medication and showed a twofold greater decrease in the Karnofsky performance scale (KPS) score. Therefore, the identification of risk factors is an important consideration in determining which patients may benefit from prophylactic spinal stabilization or percutaneous cement augmentation.[31] Although identifying significant factors in a group with a wide range of variance is quite difficult, some common variables do stand out. The percentage of tumor infiltration within the vertebral body is proportional to the risk of fracture. Both Shah et al[23] and Boehling et al[14] found statistically significant higher rates of fracture if > 80% of the vertebral body was involved by a lytic tumor. Although Rose et al[16] demonstrated a proportional increase in fracture risk with increased tumor infiltration of the vertebral body, statistical significance was not reached at > 80% tumor infiltration because of low patient numbers. In addition to the percentage of vertebral body involved, other risk factors for VCFs after radiosurgery were lytic lesions, age > 55 years, location from T10 to S1, a preexisting fracture, and the degree of baseline pain.[4,14,16,29,32] Tumor histology was not a predicting factor for development of new or progressive fractures after radiosurgery in these studies.

Conclusion

Although it seems reasonable to assume that SRS of the spine provides some risk for the subsequent development of compression fractures, the attributable risk associated with radiosurgery may be overstated in the literature, mainly because of the uncertainty regarding the natural history of metastatic spinal disease. A number of variables exist, such as tumor location in the spinal column, degree of infiltration into the vertebral body, overall disease status, patient comorbidities, and performance status, all of which make a cohesive analysis difficult. Without an existing prospective, controlled clinical study, one is left to compare retrospective patient cohorts in order to draw a conclusion about fracture risk after radiosurgery. New or progressive fractures may occur in 20 to 39% of treated segments after SRS.[14,16] The prevalence of VCFs in vertebral bodies involved with tumor, regardless of prior radiation treatment, ranges from 7[23] to > 50% in patients at high risk.[29] Furthermore, the prevalence in patient populations ranges mainly from 28 to 38%[14,16,23–25,28,30] but has been reported as to be as high as 75% in patients with known spinal disease presenting with significant back pain.[29] In the current analysis of the available data, we simply cannot conclude that fracture risk, either new or progressive, represents a significantly higher risk than what is seen naturally in the setting of metastatic disease of the spine.

Nonetheless, a subset of patients at higher risk for the development of symptomatic VCF after radiosurgery may benefit from prophylactic instrumented stabilization or percutaneous cement augmentation. Identification of such patient populations, with subsequent intervention, may ultimately decrease the morbidity associated with VCF after radiosurgery. In addition, new surgical strategies such as open decompression and surgical stabilization followed by adjuvant SRS[13] mark a new era in treatment that may minimize the clinical relevance of new and progressive fractures within the treatment field. Until a prospective randomized trial is completed, the true role of SRS in causing new or progressive VCF will remain uncertain.

References

[1] Gilbert RW, Kim JH, Posner JB. Epidural spinal cord compression from metastatic tumor: diagnosis and treatment. Ann Neurol 1978; 3: 40–51

[2] Khan FR, Glicksman AS, Chu FC, Nickson JJ. Treatment by radiotherapy of spinal cord compression due to extradural metastases. Radiology 1967; 89: 495–500

[3] Klimo P, Schmidt MH. Surgical management of spinal metastases. Oncologist 2004; 9: 188–196

[4] Sciubba DM, Petteys RJ, Dekutoski MB, et al. Diagnosis and management of metastatic spine disease. J Neurosurg Spine 2010; 13: 94–108

[5] Vieth RG, Odom GL. Extradural spinal metastases and their neurosurgical treatment. J Neurosurg 1965; 23: 501–508

[6] Young RF, Post EM, King GA. Treatment of spinal epidural metastases: randomized prospective comparison of laminectomy and radiotherapy. J Neurosurg 1980; 53: 741–748

[7] Chang EL, Shiu AS, Mendel E, et al. Phase I/II study of stereotactic body radiotherapy for spinal metastasis and its pattern of failure. J Neurosurg Spine 2007; 7: 151–160

[8] Degen JW, Gagnon GJ, Voyadzis JM, et al. CyberKnife stereotactic radiosurgical treatment of spinal tumors for pain control and quality of life. J Neurosurg Spine 2005; 2: 540–549

[9] Gerszten PC, Burton SA, Ozhasoglu C, et al. Stereotactic radiosurgery for spinal metastases from renal cell carcinoma. J Neurosurg Spine 2005; 3: 288–295

[10] Gerszten PC, Burton SA, Ozhasoglu C, Welch WC. Radiosurgery for spinal metastases: clinical experience in 500 cases from a single institution. Spine 2007; 32: 193–199

[11] Gerszten PC, Ozhasoglu C, Burton SA, et al. CyberKnife frameless stereotactic radiosurgery for spinal lesions: clinical experience in 125 cases. Neurosurgery 2004; 55: 89–98, discussion 98–99

[12] Gerszten PC, Ozhasoglu C, Burton SA, et al. CyberKnife frameless single-fraction stereotactic radiosurgery for tumors of the sacrum. Neurosurg Focus 2003; 15: E7

[13] Moulding HD, Elder JB, Lis E, et al. Local disease control after decompressive surgery and adjuvant high-dose single-fraction radiosurgery for spine metastases. J Neurosurg Spine 2010; 13: 87–93

[14] Boehling NS, Grosshans DR, Allen PK, et al. Vertebral compression fracture risk after stereotactic body radiotherapy for spinal metastases. J Neurosurg Spine 2012; 16: 379–386

[15] Rodríguez-Ruiz ME, San Miguel I, Gil-Bazo I, et al. Pathological vertebral fracture after stereotactic body radiation therapy for lung metastases: case report and literature review. Radiat Oncol 2012; 7: 50

[16] Rose PS, Laufer I, Boland PJ, et al. Risk of fracture after single fraction image-guided intensity-modulated radiation therapy to spinal metastases. J Clin Oncol 2009; 27: 5075–5079

[17] Overgaard M. Spontaneous radiation-induced rib fractures in breast cancer patients treated with postmastectomy irradiation: a clinical radiobiological analysis of the influence of fraction size and dose-response relationships on late bone damage. Acta Oncol 1988; 27: 117–122

[18] Pettersson N, Nyman J, Johansson KA. Radiation-induced rib fractures after hypofractionated stereotactic body radiation therapy of non-small cell lung cancer: a dose- and volume-response analysis. Radiother Oncol 2009; 91: 360–368

[19] Fuchs B, Valenzuela RG, Inwards C, Sim FH, Rock MG. Complications in long-term survivors of Ewing sarcoma. Cancer 2003; 98: 2687–2692

[20] Lin PP, Schupak KD, Boland PJ, Brennan MF, Healey JH. Pathologic femoral fracture after periosteal excision and radiation for the treatment of soft tissue sarcoma. Cancer 1998; 82: 2356–2365

[21] Curtis JR, Taylor AJ, Matthews RS, et al. "Pathologic" fractures: should these be included in epidemiologic studies of osteoporotic fractures? Osteoporos Int 2009; 20: 1969–1972

[22] Burton AW, Mendoza T, Gebhardt R, et al. Vertebral compression fracture treatment with vertebroplasty and kyphoplasty: experience in 407 patients with 1,156 fractures in a tertiary cancer center. Pain Med 2011; 12: 1750–1757

[23] Shah AN, Pietrobon R, Richardson WJ, Myers BS. Patterns of tumor spread and risk of fracture and epidural impingement in metastatic vertebrae. J Spinal Disord Tech 2003; 16: 83–89

[24] Chaichana KL, Pendleton C, Wolinsky JP, Gokaslan ZL, Sciubba DM. Vertebral compression fractures in patients presenting with metastatic epidural spinal cord compression. Neurosurgery 2009; 65: 267–274, discussion 274–275

[25] Patchell RA, Tibbs PA, Regine WF, et al. Direct decompressive surgical resection in the treatment of spinal cord compression caused by metastatic cancer: a randomised trial. Lancet 2005; 366: 643–648

[26] Vogel MN, Weisel K, Maksimovic O, et al. Pathologic fractures in patients with multiple myeloma undergoing bisphosphonate therapy: incidence and correlation with course of disease. AJR Am J Roentgenol 2009; 193: 656–661

[27] Fisher CG, DiPaola CP, Ryken TC, et al. A novel classification system for spinal instability in neoplastic disease: an evidence-based approach and expert consensus from the Spine Oncology Study Group. Spine 2010; 35: E1221–E1229

[28] Maranzano E, Latini P. Effectiveness of radiation therapy without surgery in metastatic spinal cord compression: final results from a prospective trial. Int J Radiat Oncol Biol Phys 1995; 32: 959–967

[29] Taneichi H, Kaneda K, Takeda N, Abumi K, Satoh S. Risk factors and probability of vertebral body collapse in metastases of the thoracic and lumbar spine. Spine 1997; 22: 239–245

[30] Chaichana KL, Woodworth GF, Sciubba DM, et al. Predictors of ambulatory function after decompressive surgery for metastatic epidural spinal cord compression. Neurosurgery 2008; 62: 683–692, discussion 683–692

[31] Gerszten PC, Germanwala A, Burton SA, Welch WC, Ozhasoglu C, Vogel WJ. Combination kyphoplasty and spinal radiosurgery: a new treatment paradigm for pathological fractures. Neurosurg Focus 2005; 18: e8

[32] Meyer SA, Singh H, Jenkins AL. Surgical treatment of metastatic spinal tumors. Mt Sinai J Med 2010; 77: 124–129

Malignant Spine Tumors

32 En Bloc Resection of Spinal Tumors

Ali A. Baaj, Jean-Paul Wolinsky, and Ziya L. Gokaslan

Introduction

En bloc resection is a surgical technique aimed at maximizing local control and potentially offering a cure in cases of primary spinal vertebral body tumors. As aggressive local recurrence directly affects survival, and as many primary spinal tumors are radioresistant, en bloc resection provides the best surgical option and should be offered in the correct clinical setting.

There are three types of en bloc resections: wide (resection completely outside the tumor and includes negative margins), marginal (dissection along the pseudocapsule but without violation of the tumor), and intralesional/contaminated (the tumor capsule is violated during resection). The principles of en bloc resection in the spine are based on the Enneking classification of musculoskeletal tumors.[1] This staging system is based on grade, site, and metastasis of bone and soft tissue tumors. However, because tumors may invade the dura and critical neural structures, wide en bloc resections are not always feasible in the case of spinal tumors. In addition, this technique is surgically demanding, can be associated with high perioperative risks, and often requires a multidisciplinary team to implement. In this chapter, we review the published literature on en bloc resection of spinal tumors, with a focus on chordomas, and provide our personal experience with treating this disease entity.

Review of the Literature

Ever since its introduction and refinement by Stener and Roy-Camille,[2–5] en bloc spondylectomy has gained popularity as the treatment of choice for malignant primary bone tumors. Several early clinical studies confirmed that wide en bloc resection of spinal tumors, with negative margins, correlated with decreased tumor recurrence[6–8] (***level III evidence***).

In a retrospective study reviewing 40 years of experience with sacral chordomas, York et al[6] demonstrated better local control and increased survival with radical versus intralesional resection. The procedures were classified as either radical resection (en bloc with wide margins) or subtotal excision (en bloc with wide margins or intralesional). The overall recurrence rate was 70%, and the rate of recurrence was 5 times higher for patients who underwent subtotal excision than for patients who underwent radical resection. The median time to recurrence after first surgical procedure was 3.37 years for radical resection versus 8 months for subtotal excision.

Fuchs et al[9] retrospectively reviewed their case series of 52 patients with sacral chordomas treated surgically between 1980 and 2001. Wide en bloc resection was successfully achieved in only 21 patients. Their reported rate of recurrence-free survival was 59% at 5 years and 46% at 10 years. The overall survival rates were 74, 52, and 47% at 5, 10, and 15 years, respectively. The wide margin group had significantly decreased recurrence and increased survival rates. The authors thus concluded that the most important factor in survival and recurrence is obtaining a disease-free wide margin.

Another large series reviewing the surgical resection of primary spinal tumors is from Boriani et al.[10] Spinal chordomas were treated as follows: (1) radiation with or without palliative surgery, (2) Intralesional excision, (3) intralesional excision plus radiotherapy, (4) en bloc resection with contamination, or (5) wide/marginal en bloc resection. This study confirmed that the only treatment associated with "continuously disease-free" at follow-up longer than 5 years is wide en bloc resection (***level III evidence***).

Hsieh et al[11] retrospectively reviewed 20 consecutive patients with sacral chordomas or chondrosarcomas treated surgically at one institution. Wide or marginal en bloc resection was achieved in 14 patients and contaminated/intralesional resection in the other 6 patients. The mean disease-free survival for patients with wide or marginal en bloc tumor excisions was 51 months, but only 17.5 months for patients who had contaminated/intralesional resections (***level III evidence***).

The role of adjuvant radiation therapy for these tumors remains unclear, as chordomas tend to be relatively resistant. Possible indications for radiotherapy include known contamination or intralesional resection and recurrence after surgical resection.[9,12–14] Although several modalities have been used, including conventional radiotherapy, stereotactic radiosurgery, and proton beam radiation, the clinical efficacy of radiotherapy has been marginal at best. Chemotherapy and radiation therapy play an adjuvant role, but no single modality, other than radical resection, has been shown to decrease recurrence and increase survival.[12–15]

Personal Experience

The best available evidence in the literature (primarily ***level III evidence***), including our own clinical experience,[11,15] supports the technique of en bloc resection for primary spinal tumors. Our patients who present with primary tumors (most commonly chordomas and chondrosarcomas) and who have no evidence of systemic disease are offered en bloc excision as the primary treatment of choice.

We have devised a systematic approach when considering en bloc resections of spinal tumors. The first step must always involve determining the precise biology via a computed tomographically guided trochar biopsy. Once a primary tumor is confirmed, the perioperative risks, including wound infections and thromboembolic events, are thoroughly discussed with the patient. We do believe that a multidisciplinary team is often needed to successfully implement these procedures, including plastic surgery (particularly when vascularized flaps are needed), general surgery, and vascular surgery, in addition to the primary spinal surgical team (▶ Fig. 32.1).

A useful paradigm for surgical planning is the Weinstein, Boriani, and Biagini (WBB) classification system.[16] This model divides the vertebrae into 12 segments in a clockwise fashion and also considers the neural tissue involvement and the number of contiguous segments affected. Surgical approach, for example, can be guided by location of pathology (dorsal vs ventral).

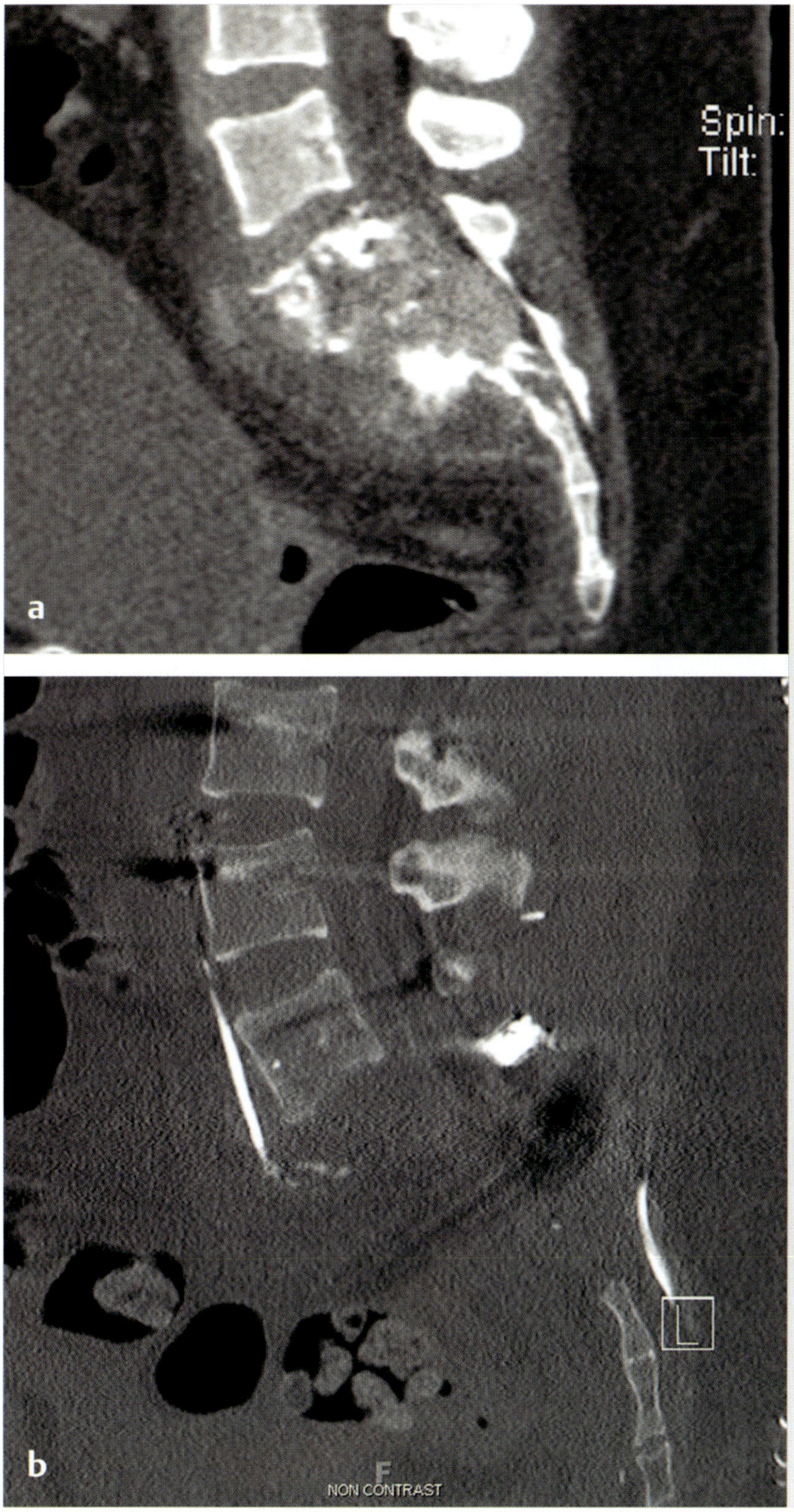

Fig. 32.1 (a) Sagittal computed tomography (CT) image demonstrating S1–S3 chordoma. (b) Postoperative sagittal CT image demonstrating resection cavity.

Furthermore, the feasibility of wide or marginal resection can be assessed depending on the extent of neural tissue encroachment or involvement.

The surgical steps have been previously described, but the general goals include (1) creating a negative margin around the tumor when possible, (2) developing a plane between critical neurovascular and visceral structures and the mass, (3) delivering the mass, and (4) spinal reconstruction when necessary. En bloc spondylectomy in the mobile spine always necessitates circumferential instrumented fusion, whereas resections that do

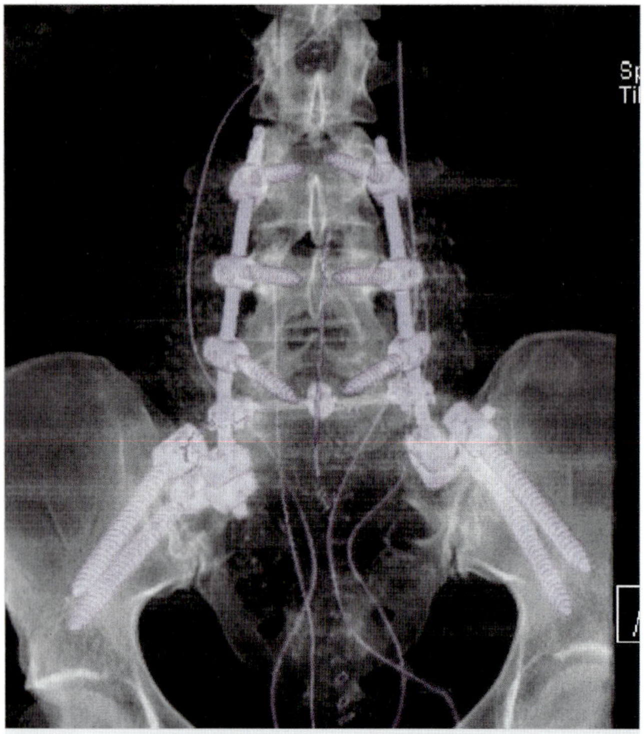

Fig. 32.2 Posteroanterior radiograph demonstrating an example of lumboiliac fixation.

not significantly disturb the sacroiliac joint in the sacrum rarely require reconstruction (▶ Fig. 32.2). Adjuvant fractionated radiation therapy is used in cases where there was known contamination or in cases of recurrence after surgery. Neoadjuvant proton beam radiation is sometimes employed when it is preoperatively determined that violation of the tumor capsule may be required in order to complete the en bloc resection.

Conclusion

En bloc resection affords the patient with primary spinal column tumors the best chance of local control and a potential for cure. This approach is technically demanding, and the perioperative risks must be thoroughly discussed with the patient. The benefits of successful wide resection typically outweigh the risks when performed by an experienced, multidisciplinary team.

References

[1] Enneking WF, Spanier SS, Goodman MA. Current concepts review: the surgical staging of musculoskeletal sarcoma. J Bone Joint Surg Am 1980; 62: 1027–1030

[2] Stener B. Total spondylectomy in chondrosarcoma arising from the seventh thoracic vertebra. J Bone Joint Surg Br 1971; 53: 288–295

[3] Roy-Camille R, Mazel Ch, Sailant G, et al. Treatment of malignant tumors of the spine with posterior instrumentation. In: Sundaresan N, Schmidek HH, Schiller AL, et al, eds. Tumors of the Spine: Diagnosis and Clinical Management. Philadelphia, PA: WB Saunders; 1990: 473–487

[4] Roy-Camille R, Mazel Ch. Vertebrectomy through an enlarged posterior approach for tumors and malunions. In: Bridwell KH, Wald RL, eds. The Textbook of Spinal Surgery. Philadelphia, PA: Lippincott; 1991: 1245–1256

[5] Roy-Camille R, Saillant G, Mazel CH, Monpierre H. Total vertebrectomy as treatment of malignant tumors of the spine. C hir Organi Mov 1990; 75 (Suppl): 94–96

[6] York JE, Kaczaraj A, Abi-Said D, et al. Sacral chordoma: 40-year experience at a major cancer center. Neurosurgery 1999; 44: 74–79, discussion 79–80

[7] Sundaresan N, Huvos AG, Krol G, Lane JM, Brennan M. Surgical treatment of spinal chordomas. Arch Surg 1987; 122: 1479–1482

[8] Kaiser TE, Pritchard DJ, Unni KK. Clinicopathologic study of sacrococcygeal chordoma. Cancer 1984; 53: 2574–2578

[9] Fuchs B, Dickey ID, Yaszemski MJ, Inwards CY, Sim FH. Operative management of sacral chordoma. J Bone Joint Surg Am 2005; 87: 2211–2216

[10] Boriani S, Bandiera S, Biagini R, et al. Chordoma of the mobile spine: fifty years of experience. Spine 2006; 31: 493–503

[11] Hsieh PC, Xu R, Sciubba DM, et al. Long-term clinical outcomes following en bloc resections for sacral chordomas and chondrosarcomas: a series of twenty consecutive patients. Spine 2009; 34: 2233–2239

[12] Park L, Delaney TF, Liebsch NJ, et al. Sacral chordomas: Impact of high-dose proton/photon-beam radiation therapy combined with or without surgery for primary versus recurrent tumor. Int J Radiat Oncol Biol Phys 2006; 65: 1514–1521

[13] Catton C, O'Sullivan B, Bell R, et al. Chordoma: long-term follow-up after radical photon irradiation. Radiother Oncol 1996; 41: 67–72

[14] Cummings BJ, Hodson DI, Bush RS. Chordoma: the results of megavoltage radiation therapy. Int J Radiat Oncol Biol Phys 1983; 9: 633–642

[15] Fourney DR, Gokaslan ZL. Current management of sacral chordoma. Neurosurg Focus 2003; 15: E9

[16] Boriani S, Weinstein JN, Biagini R. Primary bone tumors of the spine: terminology and surgical staging. Spine 1997; 22: 1036–1044

33 Stereotactic Radiosurgery for Spinal Tumors

Ilya Laufer, Yoshiya Yamada, and Mark H. Bilsky

Introduction

Stereotactic radiosurgery (SRS) represents an integral component of modern paradigms for the treatment of primary and metastatic tumors. Numerous studies have reported outstanding tumor control rates with radiosurgery in patients with metastases to the spine. Importantly, the majority of these studies documented low tumor recurrence risks regardless of tumor histology, size, and location. These results have led to the exploration of the role of SRS in the treatment of primary spinal tumors, which have largely been resistant to conventional radiation treatment. Data suggest that SRS provides effective tumor control in the treatment of primary spinal tumors.

Historically, tumors have been classified as radiosensitive or radioresistant based on their response to conventional external beam radiotherapy (cEBRT), administered as fractionated photon therapy.[1] Ewing sarcoma, hematologic malignancies, seminoma, small cell lung, breast, and prostate carcinomas generally exhibit durable response to cEBRT.[1–7] On the other hand, the majority of primary and metastatic solid tumors in the spine exhibit a relative resistance to cEBRT, and if any tumor control is achieved, it is generally brief.[2,6] Thus, primary and metastatic solid tumors of the spine, with the exception of metastatic breast and prostate carcinoma, have been classified as radioresistant to cEBRT.

Increasingly, laboratory and clinical findings suggest that high-dose radiation employs tumor control pathways that differ from the ones used by low-dose per fraction radiation. Clinically, this is largely supported by the fact that the linear-quadratic (LQ) model, which was developed to describe tumor response to cEBRT, fails to accurately predict the effect of SRS.[8,9] Single-fraction SRS achieves tumor control at doses much lower than the ones predicted by the LQ model. This is partially ascribed to the fact that the LQ model was largely developed based on the DNA damage/repair observed in tumors and surrounding tissues in response to cEBRT.[10] However, laboratory data indicate that treatment with high-dose radiation acts to kill tumor cells by several additional mechanisms. Xenograft experiments showed that doses > 10 Gy per fraction activated microvascular endothelial apoptosis.[11] Furthermore, data indicate that stem cells exhibit radioresistance at doses < 17 Gy.[12] Thus, if tumor stem cells play a role in clonogenic expansion, eradication of the tumor requires high-dose fractions.

These data are starting to provide the justification for the hope that the increasing understanding and implementation of radiosurgery may render the concept of radioresistance obsolete. Multiple publications have reported that spinal SRS provides excellent local tumor control rates in histologies that do not respond to cEBRT. Experience with SRS in the treatment of primary spinal tumors is also starting to provide promising results.

Metastatic Tumors

Palliation represents the primary treatment goal of spinal metastatic tumors. Interventions are mainly undertaken to control pain and prevent or halt the development of neurologic deficits. Surgery has been shown to be beneficial in patients with spinal cord compression secondary to solid metastases[13] and mechanical instability. Radiation may be used as the primary treatment in patients who do not require surgery or as an adjuvant treatment in order to provide postoperative tumor control. The low recurrence rate of spinal metastases after SRS has been documented in multiple studies. Gerszten et al reported excellent tumor control rates for renal cell,[14] melanoma,[15] and lung[16] metastases to the spine, without radiation-induced toxicity in any of the cases. The aggregate experience of this group was reported for 500 spinal metastases located in the mobile spine and sacrum.[17] The most commonly treated histologies in this series included renal cell, breast, lung, and melanoma, with median follow-up of 21 months and tumor volume range from 0.2 to 264.0 cm^3. The researchers reported 86% overall pain improvement and 88% radiographic control. This was confirmed by Yamada et al, who prospectively followed 362 consecutive patients with 413 treated spinal metastases.[18] They noted a 2.4% risk of recurrence at 3 years after treatment, when death was accounted as a competing risk to recurrence. Furthermore, excellent tumor control rates were achieved in all of the histologies, with 3-year local control rates of 89% for renal cell, 90% for melanoma, 92% for thyroid, 96% for sarcoma, and 98% for breast, lung, prostate, and colorectal. In agreement with these data, low risk of tumor progression and recurrence was reported by multiple oncology centers, with low risk of toxicity and excellent rates of pain resolution.[19–24]

The majority of studies reported that the local control is independent of tumor size or histology, with radioresistant tumors exhibiting tumor control rates comparable to the rates in radiosensitive tumors. Several studies have documented an inverse association between radiation dose and local recurrence risk, with patients receiving 24-Gy single-fraction SRS exhibiting significantly lower recurrence risk than patients with lower-dose treatments.[25,26] The Spine Oncology Study Group (SOSG) performed a systematic review of the literature summarizing the experience with spinal radiosurgery up to 2009.[1] They concluded that radiosurgery provides durable symptomatic and radiographic tumor control irrespective of histology or prior radiation and that, while the available quality of evidence is low, they were able to make a strong recommendation that radiosurgery should be used in the treatment of oligometastatic or radioresistant solid metastases to the spine (▸ Table 33.1).

In addition to being an effective primary treatment of spinal metastases that do not require open surgery, SRS has been shown to be very useful as a postoperative adjuvant treatment to provide local tumor control. Rock et al[63] administered single-fraction SRS to 18 patients as a postoperative treatment with a median follow-up of 7 months. Ninety-two percent of the patients remained neurologically stable or improved, while one patient deteriorated due to rapid tumor progression. Moulding et al treated 21 patients with single-fraction SRS, resulting in a 1-year recurrence risk of 9.5%. Patients who received 24 Gy had significantly better local control with a 1-year recurrence risk of 6.3%. This patient group was included in the larger analysis of

Table 33.1 Surgery and radiation in the treatment of primary and metastatic tumors of the spine

Tumor type	Treatment	Result	Recommendation grade	Level of evidence
Metastases	Surgery	Improves outcome in patients with spinal cord compression secondary to solid metastatic tumors	1B	II
	cEBRT	Reduces pain and maintains ambulation in patients with radiosensitive spinal metastases	1C+	III
	SRS	Reduces pain and maintains ambulation in patients with radioresistant spinal metastases	1C+	III
Primary osseous malignant tumors	Surgery	En bloc resection decreases risk of local recurrence and mortality	1C+	III
	cEBRT	Adjuvant treatment after incomplete resection or intralesional margin	2C	III
	SRS	Prevents tumor progression/recurrence when used as primary, adjuvant or neoadjuvant treatment	2C	IV

Abbreviations: *cEBRT, conventional external beam radiotherapy; SRS, stereotactic radiosurgery.*

186 patients who underwent surgery followed by single-fraction or hypofractionated post-operative radiation.[27] The 1-year recurrence risk was 16.4%, with patients receiving high-dose hypofractionated radiation having a 1-year recurrence risk of 4.1%, which was significantly lower than after low-dose hypofractionated radiation. The 1-year recurrence rate after single-fraction SRS was 9.0%. Furthermore, hypofractionated SRS may be safely employed in previously irradiated patients.[28,29] The durable tumor control rates in the postoperative setting allow the surgeon to minimize the extent of tumor resection, in order to perform surgery in a safer manner. Because postoperative tumor control is reliably achieved by SRS, irrespective of tumor histology, size, or location, extensive tumor resection and vertebrectomy are no longer necessary. The operation may be limited to spinal stabilization and spinal cord decompression to safely administer postoperative SRS without the risk of spinal cord toxicity, obviating the need for extensive anterior reconstruction and complex approaches.

Primary Tumors

The goals of treatment in patients with primary spinal tumors may range from cure to palliation, depending on the histology and the stage of the tumor. If the tumor is amenable to total excision, surgery may provide a definitive cure. Depending on the degree of aggressive behavior typical to the specific histology, neoadjuvant or adjuvant chemotherapy or radiation may be required. Within the individual tumor histologies, there is also a range of degree of aggressive behavior. For example, although the majority of osteoblastomas are low-grade tumors with low propensity for recurrence after total excision, an "aggressive" subtype has also been described.[30] The SOSG has critically evaluated the evidence for surgery, chemotherapy and radiation for the majority of primary tumors that arise in the spine. The authors concluded that surgery represents the primary treatment modality for local control of osteoblastoma, aneurysmal bone cyst, giant cell tumors, chordoma, chondrosarcoma, Ewing sarcoma, and osteosarcoma.[31–33] At the time of the review, very little data were available about the results of SRS in the treatment of primary spinal tumors, and the review of the efficacy of cEBRT as an adjuvant treatment confirmed the limited utility of fractionated radiation.

The Enneking system of staging musculoskeletal neoplasms recommends intracapsular or marginal excision of benign tumors and wide excision of malignant tumors.[34] Intracapsular or intralesional procedures involve piecemeal tumor excision, whereas en bloc excisions remove the tumor without violating the tumor capsule. At the completion of the excision, residual tumor may remain, or complete tumor excision may be carried out through the marginal reactive zone or through normal tissue, providing a wide margin. The Weinstein, Boriani, and Biagini (WBB) system was devised to adapt the principles of the Enneking system specifically to the spine.[35] The vexing problems of tumor excision in the spine are the importance of neural function preservation and epidural extension. Although in the appendicular skeleton loss of limb function or amputation may be acceptable surgical outcomes in order to achieve tumor cure, in the axial skeleton, amputation is considered an acceptable option only in the sacrum. Tumor control at the cost of spinal cord or cauda equina injury is generally not undertaken. Furthermore, spinal tumors with extraosseous extension generally extend into the epidural compartment, putting the entire epidural space at risk for malignant seeding. Thus, in patients with tumor extension into the epidural space of the mobile spine, only a marginal excision is possible, whereas in the sacrum, a wide margin may be achieved with nerve root sacrifice.

The results of primary tumor excision in the mobile spine and sacrum have been thoroughly documented. The recurrence risk of benign tumors after complete excision is generally quite low, and a wide margin is not advocated.[32] However, in patients with chordoma, chondrosarcoma, and osteosarcoma, wide margin has been consistently shown to decrease the risk of recurrence.[33,36–45] Unfortunately, many of these tumors are

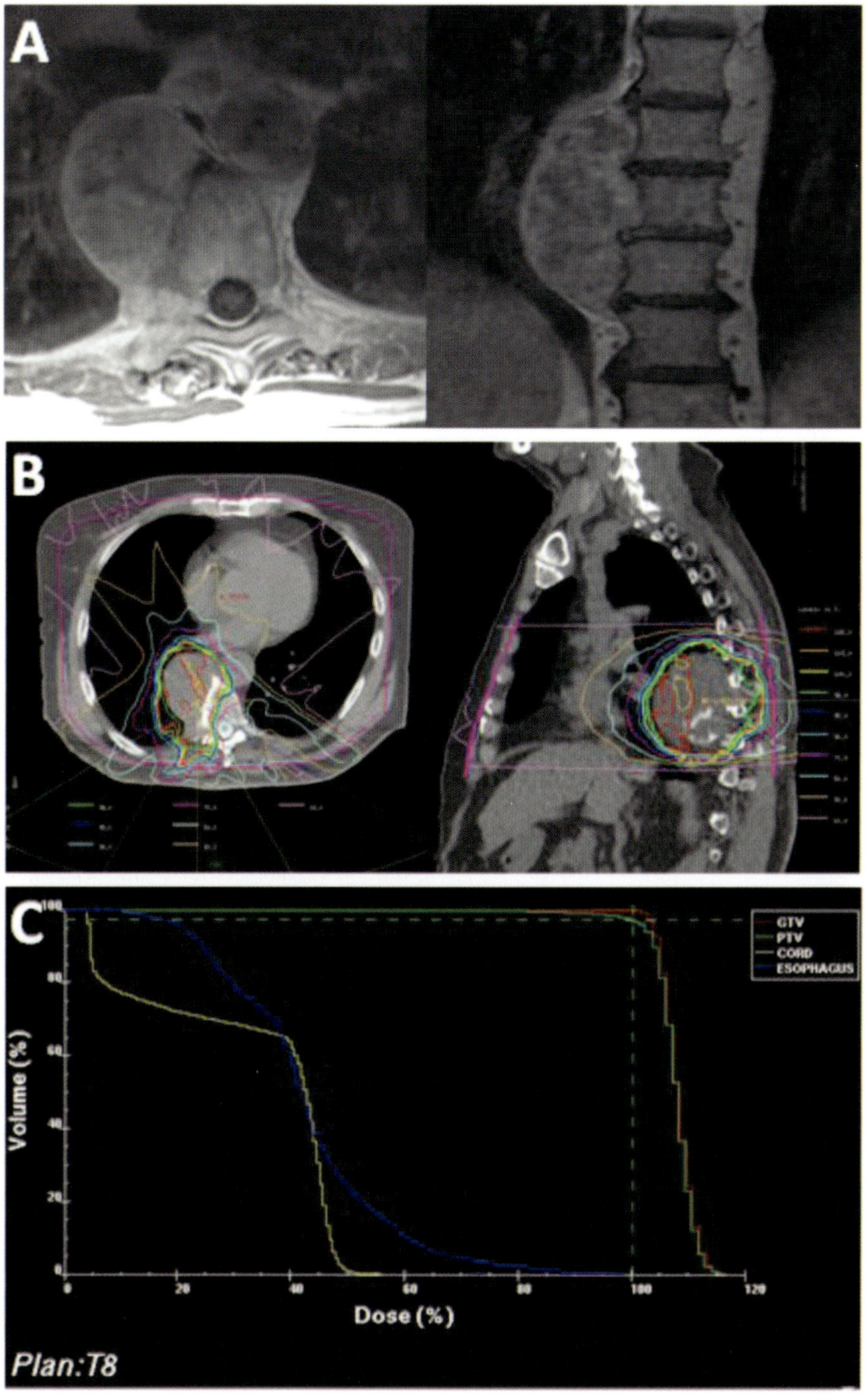

Fig. 33.1 (a) A 79-year-old man with an incidentally diagnosed 7-cm T7–T9 right paraspinal chordoma with extension into the T8–T9 foramen. (b) The patient was treated with 24-Gy single-fraction stereotactic radiosurgery. To date, the tumor has remained stable on serial imaging with 51-month follow-up. (c) Dose-volume histogram for the T8 target.

not amenable to wide excision, with large surgical series reporting only 35 to 65% of patients undergoing a wide margin excision. The recurrence rates even after wide excision remain high, with overall reported recurrence rates ranging from 40 to 50%.[33,36–45] Furthermore, sacral amputations are associated with a high risk of infection and wound complications and may require nerve root sacrifice leading to bowel and bladder dysfunction or even lower extremity motor deficits.[46–49] Thus, although surgery represents the best chance of cure in select patients, it may be associated with significant morbidity and significant risk of recurrence, confirming that the search for a better tumor control modality must continue.

To date, chemotherapy and cEBRT have not provided significant improvement in tumor control. Imatinib shows some promise in the treatment of patients with platelet-derived growth factor (PDGF) β-expressing chordomas.[50] Chordoma, chondrosarcoma, and most osteosarcomas have proven to be resistant to fractionated photon radiation.[33] On the other hand, heavy particle irradiation with protons and carbon ions has yielded promising results. The combination of photon irradiation with surgery has yielded 5-year local control rates from 62 to 100%.[51–53] The results of fractionated carbon ion irradiation of large sacral chordomas have been even more promising, with two studies reporting local control rates of 94% in 34 patients with a mean 43-month follow-up and 100% in 7 patients with a mean 58-month follow-up.[54,55]

The efficacy of SRS in the treatment of spinal chordomas remains to be determined. Several studies have described the efficacy of SRS in the treatment of cranial chordomas.[56–59] Based on the cranial results and convincing evidence that SRS is able to provide durable tumor control in significantly radioresistant metastases, SRS has been used as a salvage strategy in inoperable and recurrent tumors and as planned postoperative adjuvant treatment. Henderson et al treated three sacral, eight mobile spine, and seven clival chordomas with CyberKnife (Accuray Inc., Sunnyvale, CA) in four or five fractions as a postoperative adjuvant treatment.[60] The 5-year actuarial control rate was 59% for the entire series. None of the patients with gross total resection of spinal chordomas who received at least 37.5 Gy to the tumor margin had a recurrence. Gerszten et al reported the use of single-fraction SRS in the treatment of two spinal chordomas.[61] Wu et al described the results of a pathologic examination of an L3 chordoma that was treated with 2,400-cGy single-fraction SRS.[62] The tumor was excised when the patient developed mechanical instability 14 weeks after SRS. Pathological analysis showed that nearly the entire tumor was necrotic with only a small focus of viable chordoma.

To date, 24 spinal chordomas were treated at our institution with single-fraction SRS, with a median dose of 24 Gy. The series includes primary, recurrent, and metastatic chordomas of the mobile spine and the sacrum, with a median follow-up of 24 months. Only one instance of local progression has been diagnosed, resulting in an actuarial local control rate of 95%. Initially, SRS was used only as a salvage strategy in patients with recurrent tumors or patients who were excluded from surgery due to medical comorbidities or the extensive nature of their tumors. The encouraging results with these patients led to the use of SRS as a neoadjuvant treatment in an attempt to reduce the risk of postoperative recurrence. Six patients underwent surgery after SRS, with three of them having > 90% tumor necrosis at the time of surgery and one with 50% necrosis. Six patients underwent SRS as an intended neoadjuvant treatment but based on the lack of tumor progression refused to have surgery and are being followed radiographically (▶ Fig. 33.1). Most of the patients experienced only grade I or II skin reactions or odynophagia. One patient developed a sciatic radiculopathy, and one developed partial vocal cord paralysis requiring vocal cord augmentation.

Conclusion

High-dose single-fraction SRS employs mechanisms of tumor control that differ from the ones activated by fractionated radiation. SRS provides durable local control as a definitive or adjuvant treatment of spinal metastatic tumors irrespective of histology or tumor size. The success of radiation has led to modification of the role of surgery in the treatment of spinal metastases. Extensive tumor resection is no longer necessary to achieve tumor control, and surgery can be limited to spinal stabilization and minimal tumor excision in order to decompress the spinal cord and to provide a small separation between the tumor and the spinal cord. The results of SRS in the treatment of radioresistant metastases, including metastatic chordoma and sarcoma, indicate that single-fraction SRS may have a role as a neoadjuvant or adjuvant treatment in patients undergoing surgery or even as the primary treatment to spare the patients the morbidity that may be associated with extensive resection or amputation. Long-term follow-up data are being collected to evaluate the results of SRS in the treatment of primary spinal malignancies.

References

[1] Gerszten PC, Mendel E, Yamada Y. Radiotherapy and radiosurgery for metastatic spine disease: what are the options, indications, and outcomes? Spine 2009; 34 (Suppl): S78–S92

[2] Maranzano E, Latini P. Effectiveness of radiation therapy without surgery in metastatic spinal cord compression: final results from a prospective trial. Int J Radiat Oncol Biol Phys 1995; 32: 959–967

[3] Katagiri H, Takahashi M, Inagaki J, et al. Clinical results of nonsurgical treatment for spinal metastases. Int J Radiat Oncol Biol Phys 1998; 42: 1127–1132

[4] Rades D, Fehlauer F, Schulte R, et al. Prognostic factors for local control and survival after radiotherapy of metastatic spinal cord compression. J Clin Oncol 2006; 24: 3388–3393

[5] Rades D, Fehlauer F, Stalpers LJ, et al. A prospective evaluation of two radiotherapy schedules with 10 versus 20 fractions for the treatment of metastatic spinal cord compression: final results of a multicenter study. Cancer 2004; 101: 2687–2692

[6] Mizumoto M, Harada H, Asakura H, et al. Radiotherapy for patients with metastases to the spinal column: a review of 603 patients at Shizuoka Cancer Center Hospital. Int J Radiat Oncol Biol Phys 2011; 79: 208–213

[7] Gilbert RW, Kim JH, Posner JB. Epidural spinal cord compression from metastatic tumor: diagnosis and treatment. Ann Neurol 1978; 3: 40–51

[8] Leith JT, Cook S, Chougule P, et al. Intrinsic and extrinsic characteristics of human tumors relevant to radiosurgery: comparative cellular radiosensitivity and hypoxic percentages. Acta neurochirurgica, Supplement. 1994; 62: 18–27

[9] Kocher M, Treuer H, Voges J, Hoevels M, Sturm V, Müller RP. Computer simulation of cytotoxic and vascular effects of radiosurgery in solid and necrotic brain metastases. Radiother Oncol 2000; 54: 149–156

[10] Kirkpatrick JP, Meyer JJ, Marks LB. The linear-quadratic model is inappropriate to model high dose per fraction effects in radiosurgery. Semin Radiat Oncol 2008; 18: 240–243

[11] Garcia-Barros M, Paris F, Cordon-Cardo C, et al. Tumor response to radiotherapy regulated by endothelial cell apoptosis. Science 2003; 300: 1155–1159

[12] Ch'ang H-J, Maj JG, Paris F, et al. ATM regulates target switching to escalating doses of radiation in the intestines. Nat Med 2005; 11: 484–490

[13] Patchell RA, Tibbs PA, Regine WF, et al. Direct decompressive surgical resection in the treatment of spinal cord compression caused by metastatic cancer: a randomised trial. Lancet 2005; 366: 643–648

[14] Gerszten PC, Burton SA, Ozhasoglu C, et al. Stereotactic radiosurgery for spinal metastases from renal cell carcinoma. J Neurosurg Spine 2005; 3: 288–295

[15] Gerszten PC, Burton SA, Quinn AE, Agarwala SS, Kirkwood JM. Radiosurgery for the treatment of spinal melanoma metastases. Stereotact Funct Neurosurg 2005; 83: 213–221

[16] Gerszten PC, Burton SA, Belani CP, et al. Radiosurgery for the treatment of spinal lung metastases. Cancer 2006; 107: 2653–2661

[17] Gerszten PC, Burton SA, Ozhasoglu C, Welch WC. Radiosurgery for spinal metastases: clinical experience in 500 cases from a single institution. Spine 2007; 32: 193–199

[18] Yamada Y, Cox BW, Zelefsky MJ, et al. An analysis of prognostic factors for local control of malignant spine tumors treated with spine radiosurgery. Int J Radiat Oncol Biol Phys 2011; 81: S132–S133

[19] Gibbs IC, Kamnerdsupaphon P, Ryu MR, et al. Image-guided robotic radiosurgery for spinal metastases. Radiother Oncol 2007; 82: 185–190

[20] Ryu S, Fang Yin F, Rock J, et al. Image-guided and intensity-modulated radiosurgery for patients with spinal metastasis. Cancer 2003; 97: 2013–2018

[21] Ryu S, Jin R, Jin JY, et al. Pain control by image-guided radiosurgery for solitary spinal metastasis. J Pain Symptom Manage 2008; 35: 292–298

[22] Chang EL, Shiu AS, Mendel E, et al. Phase I/II study of stereotactic body radiotherapy for spinal metastasis and its pattern of failure. J Neurosurg Spine 2007; 7: 151–160

[23] Gibbs IC, Chang SD. Radiosurgery and radiotherapy for sacral tumors. Neurosurg Focus 2003; 15: E8

[24] Gerszten PC, Ozhasoglu C, Burton SA, et al. CyberKnife frameless single-fraction stereotactic radiosurgery for tumors of the sacrum. Neurosurg Focus 2003; 15: E7

[25] Moulding HD, Elder JB, Lis E, et al. Local disease control after decompressive surgery and adjuvant high-dose single-fraction radiosurgery for spine metastases. J Neurosurg Spine 2010; 13: 87–93

[26] Lovelock DM, Zhang Z, Jackson A, et al. Correlation of local failure with measures of dose insufficiency in the high-dose single-fraction treatment of bony metastases. Int J Radiat Oncol Biol Phys 2010; 77: 1282–1287

[27] Laufer I, Iorgulescu B, Chapman T, et al. Local disease control for spinal metastases following separation surgery and adjuvant hypofractionated or high-dose single-fraction stereotactic radiation therapy: outcomes analysis in 186 patients. Neurosurgery 2012; 71: E557

[28] Damast S, Wright J, Bilsky M, et al. Impact of dose on local failure rates after image-guided reirradiation of recurrent paraspinal metastases. Int J Radiat Oncol Biol Phys 2011; 81: 819–826

[29] Garg AK, Wang XS, Shiu AS, et al. Prospective evaluation of spinal reirradiation by using stereotactic body radiation therapy: the University of Texas MD Anderson Cancer Center experience. Cancer 2011; 117: 3509–3516

[30] Schajowicz F, Lemos C. Malignant osteoblastoma. J Bone Joint Surg Br 1976; 58: 202–211

[31] Sciubba DM, Okuno SH, Dekutoski MB, Gokaslan ZL. Ewing and osteogenic sarcoma: evidence for multidisciplinary management. Spine 2009; 34 (Suppl): S58–S68

[32] Harrop JS, Schmidt MH, Boriani S, Shaffrey CI. Aggressive "benign" primary spine neoplasms: osteoblastoma, aneurysmal bone cyst, and giant cell tumor. Spine 2009; 34 (Suppl): S39–S47

[33] Boriani S, Saravanja D, Yamada Y, Varga PP, Biagini R, Fisher CG. Challenges of local recurrence and cure in low grade malignant tumors of the spine. Spine 2009; 34 (Suppl): S48–S57

[34] Enneking WF. A system of staging musculoskeletal neoplasms. Clin Orthop Relat Res 1986: 9–24

[35] Boriani S, Weinstein JN, Biagini R. Primary bone tumors of the spine. Terminology and surgical staging. Spine 1997; 22: 1036–1044

[36] Bergh P, Gunterberg B, Meis-Kindblom JM, Kindblom LG. Prognostic factors and outcome of pelvic, sacral, and spinal chondrosarcomas: a center-based study of 69 cases. Cancer 2001; 91: 1201–1212

[37] Boriani S, Bandiera S, Biagini R, et al. Chordoma of the mobile spine: fifty years of experience. Spine 2006; 31: 493–503

[38] Boriani S, De Iure F, Bandiera S, et al. Chondrosarcoma of the mobile spine: report on 22 cases. Spine 2000; 25: 804–812

[39] Fuchs B, Dickey ID, Yaszemski MJ, Inwards CY, Sim FH. Operative management of sacral chordoma. J Bone Joint Surg Am 2005; 87: 2211–2216

[40] Schwab J, Gasbarrini A, Bandiera S, et al. Osteosarcoma of the mobile spine. Spine 2012; 37: E381–E386

[41] Schwab JH, Healey JH, Rose P, Casas-Ganem J, Boland PJ. The surgical management of sacral chordomas. Spine 2009; 34: 2700–2704

[42] York JE, Berk RH, Fuller GN, et al. Chondrosarcoma of the spine: 1954 to 1997. J Neurosurg 1999; 90 (Suppl): 73–78

[43] York JE, Kaczaraj A, Abi-Said D, et al. Sacral chordoma: 40-year experience at a major cancer center. Neurosurgery 1999; 44: 74–79, discussion 79–80

[44] Ruggieri P, Angelini A, Ussia G, Montalti M, Mercuri M. Surgical margins and local control in resection of sacral chordomas. Clin Orthop Relat Res 2010; 468: 2939–2947

[45] Stacchiotti S, Casali PG, Lo Vullo S, et al. Chordoma of the mobile spine and sacrum: a retrospective analysis of a series of patients surgically treated at two referral centers. Ann Surg Oncol 2010; 17: 211–219

[46] Cheng EY, Ozerdemoglu RA, Transfeldt EE, Thompson RC. Lumbosacral chordoma. Prognostic factors and treatment. Spine 1999; 24: 1639–1645

[47] Fourney DR, Rhines LD, Hentschel SJ, et al. En bloc resection of primary sacral tumors: classification of surgical approaches and outcome. J Neurosurg Spine 2005; 3: 111–122

[48] Guo Y, Palmer JL, Shen L, et al. Bowel and bladder continence, wound healing, and functional outcomes in patients who underwent sacrectomy. J Neurosurg Spine 2005; 3: 106–110

[49] Sciubba DM, Nelson C, Gok B, et al. Evaluation of factors associated with postoperative infection following sacral tumor resection. J Neurosurg Spine 2008; 9: 593–599

[50] Stacchiotti S, Longhi A, Ferraresi V, et al. Phase II study of imatinib in advanced chordoma. J Clin Oncol 2012; 30: 914–920

[51] DeLaney TF, Liebsch NJ, Pedlow FX, et al. Phase II study of high-dose photon/proton radiotherapy in the management of spine sarcomas. Int J Radiat Oncol Biol Phys 2009; 74: 732–739

[52] Wagner TD, Kobayashi W, Dean S, et al. Combination short-course preoperative irradiation, surgical resection, and reduced-field high-dose postoperative irradiation in the treatment of tumors involving the bone. Int J Radiat Oncol Biol Phys 2009; 73: 259–266

[53] Staab A, Rutz HP, Ares C, et al. Spot-scanning-based proton therapy for extracranial chordoma. Int J Radiat Oncol Biol Phys 2011; 81: e489–e496

[54] Imai R, Kamada T, Tsuji H, et al. Working Group for Bone, Soft Tissue Sarcomas. Carbon ion radiotherapy for unresectable sacral chordomas. Clin Cancer Res 2004; 10: 5741–5746

[55] Serizawa I, Imai R, Kamada T, et al. Changes in tumor volume of sacral chordoma after carbon ion radiotherapy. J Comput Assist Tomogr 2009; 33: 795–798

[56] Kano H, Iqbal FO, Sheehan J, et al. Stereotactic radiosurgery for chordoma: a report from the North American Gamma Knife Consortium. Neurosurgery 2011; 68: 379–389

[57] Kato TA, Tsuda A, Uesaka M, et al. In vitro characterization of cells derived from chordoma cell line U-CH1 following treatment with X-rays, heavy ions and chemotherapeutic drugs. Radiat Oncol 2011; 6: 116

[58] Krishnan S, Foote RL, Brown PD, Pollock BE, Link MJ, Garces YI. Radiosurgery for cranial base chordomas and chondrosarcomas. Neurosurgery 2005; 56: 777–784

[59] Martin JJ, Niranjan A, Kondziolka D, Flickinger JC, Lozanne KA, Lunsford LD. Radiosurgery for chordomas and chondrosarcomas of the skull base. J Neurosurg 2007; 107: 758–764

[60] Henderson FC, McCool K, Seigle J, Jean W, Harter W, Gagnon GJ. Treatment of chordomas with CyberKnife: georgetown university experience and treatment recommendations. Neurosurgery 2009; 64 (Suppl): A44–A53

[61] Gerszten PC, Ozhasoglu C, Burton SA, et al. CyberKnife frameless single-fraction stereotactic radiosurgery for benign tumors of the spine. Neurosurg Focus 2003; 14: e16

[62] Wu AJ, Bilsky MH, Edgar MA, Yamada Y. Near-complete pathological response of chordoma to high-dose single-fraction radiotherapy: case report. Neurosurgery 2009; 64: E389–E390, discussion E390

[63] Rock JP, Ryu S, Shukairy MS, Yin FF, Sharif A, Schreiber F, et al. Postoperative radiosurgery for malignant spinal tumors. Neurosurgery 2006; 58: 891–898, discussion 891–898

34 Spinal Cord Decompression with Spinal Radiosurgery

Samuel Ryu, Ian Lee, and Jack Rock

Introduction

Metastatic spinal cord compression (MSCC) includes a spectrum of epidural tumor ranging from vertebral bone metastases with minimal spinal canal compromise to overt spinal cord compression. Spine metastases and MSCC are among the most debilitating and common complications of cancer. MSCC is reported to involve between 5 and 14% of all cancer patients, with an estimated annual incidence of more than 20,000 cases in the United States.[1,2] Early detection and treatment when the patient is still ambulatory result in the highest chance of neurologic preservation.[3,4] Once diagnosed with MSCC, immediate treatment intervention is required. Without treatment, MSCC can progress to cause paralysis, incontinence, and a significant decline in quality of life. Even with aggressive therapy, results can often be unsatisfactory. Patients with MSCC generally have other widespread metastases elsewhere, and this fact frequently poses an oncologic dilemma as to how the treatments should be coordinated. In contrast to the general perception of a short survival time of these patients, the median survival may be much longer in certain patients, with up to one third surviving beyond 1 year.[4–6] Therefore, optimal local therapy for MSCC is required to ultimately improve or maintain quality of life.

Detection and Evaluation

Symptoms and signs of MSCC vary, depending on the extent of spinal cord compression and the location of epidural tumor within the spinal canal or paraspinal area. Common presenting symptoms are back pain and mild sensory or motor changes of the extremities. The duration of symptoms may be gradual, but symptoms can progress rapidly, causing severe debilitation. Therefore, it is prudent to pay attention to back pain at the early stage. Furthermore, a careful neurologic examination may detect MSCC before it manifests as an overt spinal cord syndrome. Magnetic resonance imaging (MRI) provides anatomical information of paraspinal or epidural soft tissue extension, spinal cord compression, and the possible involvement of nerve roots. Myelograms can be used, but are largely replaced by MRI. Computed tomographic (CT) imaging is complementary and provides anatomical information about the integrity of vertebral bone, deformity, or pathological fracture. Imaging of the entire spinal column is recommended because of the multiple levels of involvement, and it may affect the choice of appropriate treatment. Bone scans and positron emission tomography (PET) scans can also help to determine the extent of disease but are not as important as a full spine MRI when treating MSCC.

Treatments and Outcome

The ultimate goal of treatment of MSCC is decompression of the spinal cord, thereby improving or preserving neurologic function. Because back pain is the most common presenting symptom, pain control is also an immediate goal of the treatment. The selection of treatment approach involves an informed decision based on a combination of overall oncologic disease status, imaging studies, and associated symptoms, including pain and neurologic status, presence of mechanical spinal instability, and overall general patient status. Common treatments include corticosteroid, external beam radiotherapy (EBRT), and open surgical resection.

Corticosteroid

Corticosteroid is immediately administered once MSCC is identified or when there is neurologic deficit. Steroid doses vary widely, and it is unclear if higher doses offer a therapeutic benefit.[7] In general practice, a moderate dexamethasone dose (8-16 mg/day) is commonly used. The dose can be tapered once neurologic improvement or epidural decompression has been achieved. It is advisable to limit the duration of steroid treatment, as it can cause long-term wasting symptoms.

External Beam Radiotherapy

EBRT has been the main treatment of MSCC for palliation of symptoms. Radiation dose and fractionation scheme are usually weighed against the performance status and expected survival of the patient, which may explain the wide range of radiation regimens reported in the literature. The common regimen used is either a total dose of 30 Gy in 10 fractions with 3-Gy daily dose (in the United States) or a shorter course of 8 Gy in a single fraction or 20 Gy in four or five fractions (in Europe). Regardless of the regimen, EBRT resulted in consistent pain control, and ~ 30% to 50% of patients were able to walk.[8–13]

The need to deliver an optimal radiation dose to the tumor for adequate palliation must be balanced with the necessity of avoiding undue toxicity, the most serious of which is radiation-induced myelopathy (RIM). Even though the radiation dose escalation may be planned, the limiting factor of EBRT is that the radiation dose necessary for tumor control cannot be given due to concern of developing RIM. It is even more so when it comes to a larger fraction dose or single-fraction radiosurgery. For example, let us assume hypothetically that the necessary dose for epidural tumor control to be 60 Gy given in 2-Gy fractions for 6 weeks. One can also calculate the biological effective dose as at least 45 Gy in 3-Gy hypofractionation to make the treatment duration shorter, or a single radiosurgery dose of 18 to 20 Gy. Any of these regimens are beyond the acceptable tolerance dose of the spinal cord and thus will require more sophisticated techniques or radiation planning and delivery, more so with extreme hypofractionated or single doses. It may also be worthwhile to reduce the length of treatments, especially in patients with limited performance status and/or other sites of metastatic diseases to not delay systemic therapy.

Decompression Surgery and External Beam Radiotherapy

Surgical treatment of MSCC ranges from a simple laminectomy to direct decompressive surgery (DDS) with removal of tumor via corpectomy and reconstruction of the spine for immediate stabilization. Before the 1980s, surgery for MSCC typically consisted of a simple decompressive laminectomy, which resulted in poor rates of neurologic preservation no better than fractionated EBRT. Because of this, there was a generally nihilistic attitude toward surgical decompression. Recently, surgical techniques evolved to include anterolateral approaches to the spine, which provided avenues for direct tumor extirpation, along with improved spinal instrumentation for stabilization purposes. As such, enthusiasm for surgical management of MSCC increased.

Given the rising popularity of these new surgical techniques, Patchell and colleagues reported, in 2005, a phase III randomized trial testing the impact of DDS followed by EBRT in patients with MSCC.[14] This study compared the standard EBRT of 30 Gy in 3-Gy daily fractions to the combined treatment with DDS followed by the same EBRT. The trial was terminated early at interim analysis when early-stopping rules were met. The primary end point was ambulatory rate, which was defined as at least two steps with each foot (four steps total), with or without the aid of a cane or walker. Overall, the ambulatory rate was 84% in the combined group versus 57% after EBRT ($p < 0.001$). The combined treatment had a median ambulation time of 122 days, compared to 13 days for radiotherapy alone ($p = 0.003$). For ambulatory patients, the ambulatory rate was 94% versus 74% ($p < 0.024$) in favor of surgery. For nonambulatory patients, the combined treatment had a significantly higher chance of regaining the ability to walk (62% vs 19%, $p = 0.01$). The duration of ambulation was longer in the surgery group. The need for corticosteroid and opioid analgesics was reduced in the combined surgery and radiation group. The primary end point of ambulatory rate is summarized in ▶ Table 34.1. The results provide ***level I evidence*** on the role of DDS in the management of MSCC.

One significant problem with DDS is that many patients with MSCC are not candidates for such an extensive surgery. Many patients often present with poor performance status and prolonged/complete paraplegia, or the patient and/or family wish to pursue conservative nonsurgical treatment. The ambulatory rate in patients who were previously nonambulatory was only 62% despite the extensive surgery. Although this rate is still significantly better than the radiation-alone group, it highlights the importance of developing a more efficacious, noninvasive treatment that is readily available for this group of patients.

Rationale of Radiosurgery for Epidural Compression

The results of EBRT indicate that some degree of epidural tumor control may be achieved,[8,9,15,16] even though the treatment was given for pure palliation with suboptimal radiation dose for tumor control. Recent technical progress in radiosurgical treatment delivery in conjunction with frameless stereotactic targeting of extracranial body sites made it possible to deliver a high radiation dose to the spine, in particular, the epidural area.[17–23] For treatment of MSCC with radiosurgery, the target volume includes only the involved vertebral body segment and its epidural soft tissue tumor while minimizing the dose to the spinal cord or other adjacent normal tissues. The clinical experiences accumulated knowledge of partial volume tolerance of the spinal cord following SRS.[5,24] Therefore, it was hypothesized that SRS could control or shrink the epidural tumor and thus achieve epidural decompression, as shown in ▶ Fig. 34.1. The radiation dose to the epidural tumor may be slightly compromized because of the intimate anatomical relationship of the epidural tumor and the spinal cord. It is arguable that this underdosed area of epidural lesion can recur and cause epidural compression again. It was therefore hypothesized that even partial, if not complete, reduction of the epidural lesion may provide sufficient decompression of the spinal cord.

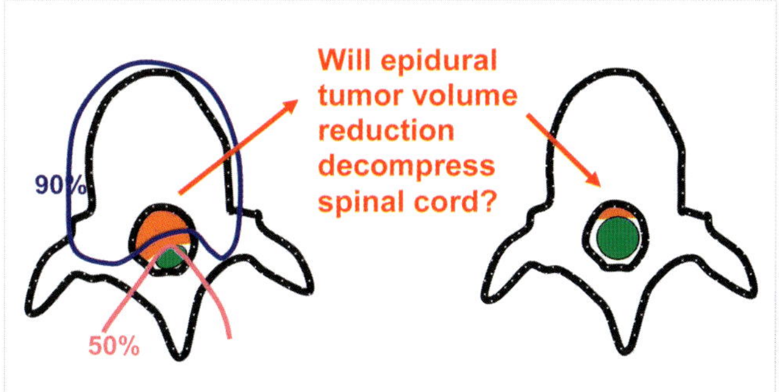

Fig. 34.1 Schematic illustration of hypothesis of radiosurgical decompression of radiosurgery.

Table 34.1 Results of phase III trial of surgery and radiation for metastatic spinal cord compression

	Surgery + RT group	RT-alone group	*p* Value
Overall ambulatory rate	84% (42/50)	57% (29/51)	0.001
Duration of ambulation (median)	122 days	13 days	0.003
Ambulatory rate in ambulatory patients	94% (32/34)	74% (26/35)	0.024
Ambulatory rate in nonambulatory patients	62% (10/16)	19% (3/16)	0.01

Abbreviation: *RT, radiotherapy.*
Source: *From Patchell RA, Tibbs PA, Regine WF, et al. Direct decompressive surgical resection in the treatment of spinal cord compression caused by metastatic cancer: a randomised trial. Lancet 2005;366(9486):643–648.*

Evidence for Radiosurgery

A prospective phase II study was performed to demonstrate the feasibility of epidural decompression employing radiosurgery for MSCC. Ryu et al reported, in 2010, the phase II results of spinal cord decompression after radiosurgery of MSCC.[25] The purpose of the study was to determine quantitatively the magnitude of SRS decompression of epidural tumor. This study enrolled 62 patients with previously untreated MSCC with or without neurologic deficit. Patients with progressive systemic tumors with documented widespread metastases and with poor performance status and limited expected life expectancy were also included. This patient population was included because the investigators felt that a single session of SRS could achieve a rapid control of spine metastasis with less morbidity to the sick patient than open surgery. Therefore, no stopping rules were applied. Radioresistant tumors, such as melanoma, renal cell carcinoma, and chordoma, were also included in this study. The radiosurgery doses ranged from 14 to 20 Gy (median 16 Gy) according to a dose escalation scheme. For the spinal cord tolerance, the study used the partial volume spinal cord tolerance of 10 Gy to 10% of the spinal cord volume, which was defined as 6 mm above and below the radiosurgery target.[5]

The results of radiographic epidural tumor control and spinal cord decompression were found to be promising. Tumor response was measured using gadolinium contrast-enhanced T1-weighted MR images at 2 months after radiosurgery. Overall epidural tumor response rate was 80% (complete response 27%, partial response 30%, and minimal response 23%). Radiographic tumor progression was seen in only 6% of cases. The rate of overall epidural tumor volume reduction in all patients was 65 ± 14% at 2 months after radiosurgery. At the level of the most significant spinal cord compression, the epidural tumor was 0.82 ± 0.08 cm^2 before radiosurgery, and the tumor was reduced to 0.41 ± 0.06 cm^2 at 2 months after radiosurgery ($p < 0.001$). To demonstrate epidural decompression by SRS, a measurement of the thecal sac area was determined using T2-weighted MR axial imaging. The thecal sac area improved (i.e., increased) from 1.05 ± 0.11 cm^2 to 1.35 ± 0.11 cm^2 ($p < 0.001$). Ultimately, the thecal sac patency increased from 55 ± 4% to 76 ± 3% by SRS ($p < 0.01$). These findings are summarized in ▶ Table 34.2.

Neurologic outcome was also documented in this trial. With a median clinical follow-up of 11.5 months for 62 patients, overall 85% (53/62) remained intact or ambulatory after radiosurgery, whereas 15% deteriorated neurologically. The neurologic status remained intact in 88% (31/35) of patients who were intact before radiosurgery. Among the 27 patients who presented with neurologic deficit, 59% (16/27) had complete recovery to normal, 11% (3/27) improved, and 11% (3/27) remained stable.

The results of this clinical study provide a ***level II evidence*** for radiosurgical epidural decompression and serve well in challenging the current status achieved with EBRT alone or in combination with surgery in the management of MSCC. The results of this clinical trial indicate the potential value of epidural decompression by radiosurgery for the end points of both radiographic and neurologic outcomes. Overall, > 80% of the patients with MSCC and minimal neurologic signs improved or remained intact. Indeed, the majority of the patients in this clinical trial included patients with no neurologic deficits, and 94% of them remained intact after radiosurgery.

It is a provoking concept that ambulatory patients with minimal neurologic signs can be treated with upfront radiosurgery only, and surgical exploration should be reserved only for patients with rapidly progressing or overt neurologic deficits. For ambulatory patients without neurologic deficit, radiosurgery and DDS appear to be equally effective; 94% of the patients who were able to walk remained ambulatory after surgery (in Patchell et al 's study), and 94% of the patients who were neurologically intact remained intact after radiosurgery (in Ryu et al's study). This suggests a potential use of radiosurgery for ambulatory patients without deficit. For patients with neurologic deficit or nonambulatory, although the end points were different, and direct comparison is impossible, DDS improved ambulation in 62% in Patchell et al's study, and radiosurgery provided 63% neurologic improvement (52% complete recovery and 11% improvement) in Ryu et al's study. It is obvious that immediate surgical decompression will frequently result in a prompt neurological recovery, and thus surgery is preferred in patients

Table 34.2 Results of phase II trial with radiosurgery for metastatic spinal cord compression

Radiographic outcome (at 2 mo after SRS)			
Overall tumor response		80%	
Overall epidural tumor volume reduction		65 ± 14%	
	Pre-SRS	**Post-SRS**	***p* Value**
Epidural tumor size*	0.82 ± 0.08 cm^2	0.41 ± 0.06 cm^2	< 0.001
Thecal sac area*	1.05 ± 0.11 cm^2	1.35 ± 0.11 cm^2	< 0.001
Thecal sac patency*	55 ± 4%	76 ± 3%	< 0.001
Neurologic outcome (median follow-up 11.5 mohs)			
Overall rate of being intact		85% (53/62)	
Remained intact in intact patients		88% (31/35)	
Became intact in deficit patients		59% (16/27)	

* *Measured at the level of most severe spinal cord compression.*
Abbreviation: *SRS, stereotactic radiosurgery.*
Source: *From Ryu S, Rock J, Jain R, et al. Radiosurgical decompression of metastatic epidural compression. Cancer 2010;116(9):2250–2257.*

with neurologic deficit from overt spinal cord compression. The merit of spine radiosurgery is that it is much less invasive treatment than open surgery. Overall, the radiosurgery procedure is convenient, well tolerated, and may be performed on an outpatient basis. In addition, because radiosurgery is administered only to the involved spine and epidural tumor, it offers the additional benefit of sparing the functioning bone marrow of the spine and facilitates continuation of systemic chemotherapy.

Potential Pitfalls and Concerns with Use of Radiosurgery for Metastatic Spinal Cord Compression

During the emergence of spine radiosurgery, patients who presented with impending MSCC have been typically excluded from spine SBRT by most practitioners. The main reason was because of the concern of underdose to the epidural tumor and overdose to the spinal cord, thus leading to the development of frank spinal cord compression and/or neurologic sequelae.

To help understand this issue, it is worthwhile to look at the subset of patients whose epidural tumor progressed after radiosurgery. In Ryu et al's phase II study,[25] 16% overall (9/62 total patients) had neurologic progression; 2 patients were neurologically intact before radiosurgery, and 7 patients had an initial neurologic deficit. Radiographically, these failures were in-field failure in three, immediately adjacent spine in five, and due to a compression fracture in one. These cases of progression are shown in ▶ Fig. 34.2 with potential causes of failure. Upon neurologic progression, five of these patients underwent open surgical resection. In two of the five patients (one with renal cell carcinoma, one with non–small-cell lung carcinoma), surgical specimens showed no evidence of viable tumor. The patient with renal cell carcinoma had a compression fracture with retropulsion without any evidence of tumor. The surgical specimens of three patients (thyroid follicular cancer, melanoma, and breast cancer) showed active tumor. The finding of radiographic and pathologic tumor control provides an argument against potential tumor progression in the small area of underdosing within the epidural target. Indeed, despite being relatively underdosed, the slightly lower dose was still sufficient to reduce the extent of epidural tumor. No correlation could be found with the severity of initial extent of MSCC or the radiosensitivity of the tumor histology. In addition, other studies of patients with radioresistant tumors such as renal cell carcinoma and melanoma have shown that radiosurgery may offer good tumor control.[21,26] The alternative treatment for these tumors can be surgery followed by radiosurgery in the postoperative setting.[27]

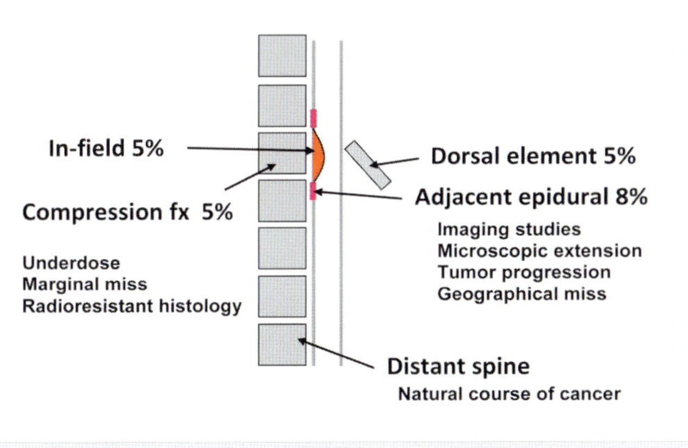

Fig. 34.2 Radiographic pattern of failure after radiosurgery of metastatic spinal cord compression and possible causes ($n = 62$).

There can be microscopic extension outside the grossly visible epidural lesion on MRI. This may be the cause of tumor recurrence in the adjacent spine level or it can be secondary to another separate metastasis to the adjacent bone. The extent of potential microscopic extension is not known at this time. We observed the tumor progression at the immediately adjacent spine in 6% of the patients treated with radiosurgery.[28] In another study, Chang et al reported a similar cause of failure due to the progression of adjacent level disease.[18]

Development of compression fracture of the vertebral bone treated with SRS has been reported. The Sloan-Kettering Memorial Cancer Center experience reported a 39% risk of any degree of vertebral height loss shown on follow-up MRI.[29] On the other hand, MD Anderson Hospital reported a much lower rate of 20%.[30] In terms of bone fracture after high-dose radiation, the incidence of rib fracture has been reported as 21% in a lung radiosurgery series.[31] It is also important to consider that there are many other causes of vertebral compression fractures in this group of mostly elderly patients, including osteoporotic changes from chronic steroid administration. Because not every compression fracture requires any therapeutic intervention, the actual rate of clinically significant compression fracture after radiosurgery may be significantly lower than what has been reported.

In our experience, it appears that symptomatic compression occurs in about 10%. Patients with multiple myelomas have a higher incidence of compression fracture up to 40%, also reflecting the natural behavior of multiple myeloma.[37]

Grading System and Patient Selection

Questions may arise about how patients with MSCC can be selected for the best treatment intervention. This decision requires a reliable grading system of MSCC. The grading system would provide consistency in description and diagnosis of MSCC, in treatment decision making, and in reporting of outcomes by different treatments. Several grading systems have been proposed[32–34] using MRI only to estimate the anatomical extent of spinal cord compression for making decisions regarding surgery and correction of spinal stability. However, there is currently no reliable correlation between the degree of the anatomical spinal cord compression and the actual neurologic status of the patient. MRI and other imaging modalities do not provide any predictive information of the neurologic status of the patient. Therefore, we proposed a dual grading system: radiographic grade (I–V), which evaluates the anatomical extent of MSCC, and neurologic grade (A–E), which provides the functional status. These two are mutually independent.

The radiographic grading system (shown in ▶ Fig. 34.3 and ▶ Table 34.3) is as following. Grade 0 indicates spine bone involvement only, that is, spine bone metastasis. Grade I is involvement of the epidural fat. The thecal sac can be abutted/impinged by the tumor. Grade II is thecal sac compression by the tumor but not to the spinal cord. Grade III is defined as the tumor abutting and impinging on the spinal cord. There is no deformation or displacement of the spinal cord. Grade IV is displacement of the spinal cord. Cerebrospinal fluid (CSF) is still visible on T2-weighted imaging. This denotes a partial block on myelogram. Grade V is frank spinal cord compression. The CSF is no longer visible on T2-weighted images or complete block on myelography. At the level of the cauda, it is defined as grade II when the canal compromise is < 50% and grade IV when the canal compromise is ≥ 50%.

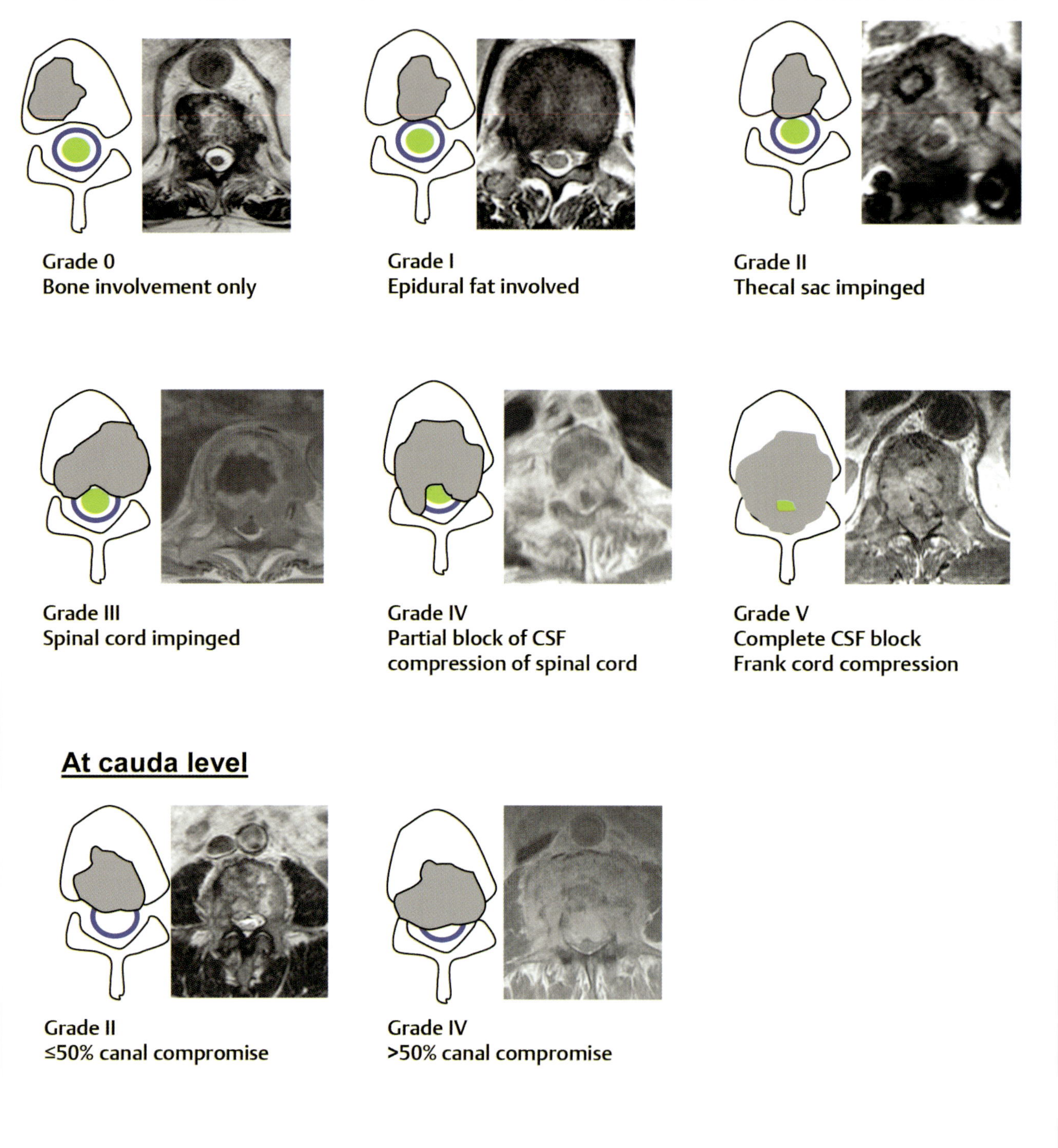

Fig. 34.3 Schematic illustration and magnetic resonance imaging example of radiographic grading.

Table 34.3 Proposed dual grading system of spinal cord compression

Radiographic grade		Neurologic grade	
Grade	Description	Grade	Description
0	Spine bone involved only	A	No abnormality
I	Tumor involves epidural fat and can abut the thecal sac	B	Minor symptoms (e.g., radiculopathy sensory change)
II	Thecal sac compressed, CSF present between tumor and spinal cord	C	Functional paresis with muscle power ≥ 4/5. It can be nerve root sign or spinal cord sign. Involved muscle is functional in the upper extremity and ambulatory in the lower extremity
III	Tumor abuts or impinges spinal cord	D	Functional paresis with muscle power ≤ 3/5. Involved muscle is nonfunctional in the upper extremity and nonambulatory in the lower extremity
IV	Spinal cord displaced, CSF visible within dura	E	Paralysis, incontinence
V	Complete block, spinal cord compressed, no CSF visible within dura		

Abbreviation: *CSF, cerebrospinal fluid.*

The neurologic grading system (▶ Table 34.3) is defined as follows. Grade A is no neurologic abnormality. Grade B is defined as focal minor symptoms, such as radiculopathy or minor sensory change. Grade C is defined as a functional paresis. This includes muscle power 4 or stronger. Either nerve root sign or spinal cord sign can be present. The patient is ambulatory with or without aid. Grade D is defined as nonfunctional paresis. The muscle power is 3 or less. This may involve nerve root sign or spinal cord sign. The involved muscle is no longer functional, and patients are generally nonambulatory. Grade E is defined as paralysis and/or incontinence.

For validation of the dual grading system, the MRI results of pre- and postradiosurgery of the phase II study from MSCC were reviewed by clinicians (neurosurgeon, radiation oncologist, medical oncologist) and five neuroradiologists. Interobserver correlation by Kendall's coefficient for concordance of ordinal response (0.83) was statistically significant ($p < 0.0001$). Correlation between the clinical specialties and neuroradiologists were excellent ($p < 0.0001$), with Kappa coefficient for nominal response of the observers (0.38 ± 0.01). Although there can be many other factors to be considered, this finding supports the usefulness of the proposed dual grading system for clinical use.

Both the surgical and the radiosurgical treatment can provide excellent epidural decompression. Therefore, at our institution, surgical decompression is recommended for patients with neurologic grade C or above regardless of the anatomical extent. Radiosurgery is used for patients with neurologic grade A or B, regardless of the radiographic extent of epidural compression. When there is a high anatomical grade, the patients are closely followed after radiosurgery for any sign of neurologic deterioration.

Future Clinical Trials

The Radiation Therapy Oncology Group (RTOG) 0631 phase II/III study is ongoing with spine radiosurgery for localized spine metastasis, including mild MSCC.[35] The phase II portion of the study has been completed and demonstrates the feasibility and safety of cooperative large-scale clinical trial under vigorous quality assurance. The phase III randomized clinical trial is currently enrolling patients. The study will compare a single dose of external beam radiation (8 Gy) to a single dose of SRS (16 or 18 Gy). The primary end point is pain control measured at 3 months post–study entry. The secondary end points are pain control and quality of life measures and MRI follow-up imaging to assess the radiographic change of vertebral bone, spinal cord, and the tumor response of epidural and paraspinal soft tissue tumors. The study covers any malignant metastatic tumors, including radioresistant tumors such as melanoma, renal cell carcinoma, and soft tissue tumors (▶ Fig. 34.4).

The combined use of radiosurgery with open surgery has been reported. Upfront surgical resection and postoperative radiosurgery to the involved epidural surgical site have been reported by Rock et al.[27] Radiosurgery was performed usually 1 to 2 weeks after open surgery. In this report, 92% of the total 18 patients remained neurologically stable or improved with little or no morbidity. The drawback of postoperative radiosurgery is the difficulty of delineating the tumor and spinal cord due to poor image quality secondary to the interference of hardware used for spine stabilization. This approach may be attractive for patients who have overt spinal cord compression syndrome with neurologic deficit, as these patients need rapid surgical decompression prior to adjuvant radiotherapy or radiosurgery.

The combined treatment of radiosurgery and vertebroplasty or kyphoplasty for spinal cord compression is not well established. The combined treatment of radiosurgery delivered within 1 to 2 weeks after vertebroplasty for spine metastases was well tolerated with excellent results of pain control.[36] However, in the case of the MSCC experience, there is concern that the epidural tumor may be pushed more dorsally into the spinal canal by the injected cement, causing the spinal cord compression to worsen.

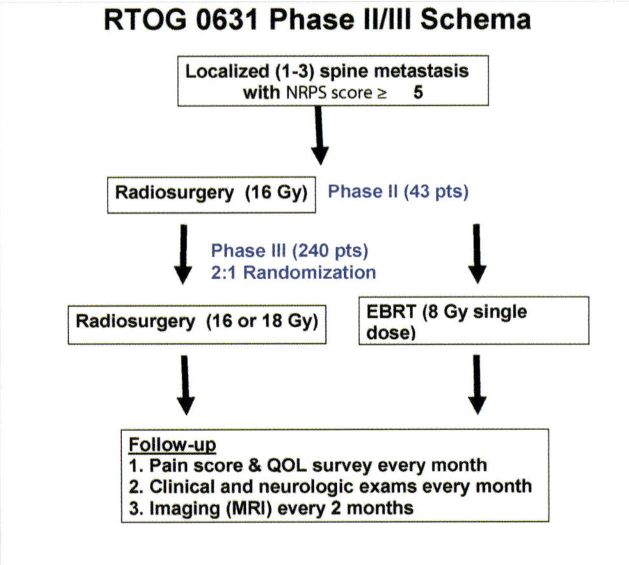

Fig. 34.4 Schema of RTOG 0631 phase II/III spine radiosurgery study for localized spinal metastasis and minimal spinal cord compression. EBRT, external beam radiotherapy; MRI, magnetic resonance imaging; NRPS, Numerical Pain Scale; QOL, quality of life.

There are no supporting data as to whether chemotherapy can be combined with radiosurgery at this time. Because radiosurgery was usually delivered in a single fraction, the concurrent chemotherapy schedule was not altered and not given on the same day. Special caution should be advised because there is the potential for an interaction between some chemotherapy agents and radiation. A more practical advantage of radiosurgery is that functioning red marrow can be preserved in patients who require systemic chemotherapy.

Conclusion

For operable patients who are ambulatory or with minimal neurologic deficit, DDS followed by EBRT remains the standard of care based on the existing evidence. However, emerging data indicate that primary radiosurgery can be as effective as surgery plus radiation in many clinical situations. SRS is noninvasive and does not require any recovery time, whereas DDS is an invasive open surgery that may require instrumentation for spine stabilization. Similar to the treatment of brain metastasis, radiosurgery may ultimately prove to be as efficacious as surgery. If SRS and DDS are proven to be equally successful treatments for similar clinical scenarios, it will provide a wider range of treatment options that will be of great benefit to this already debilitated patient population. Careful patient selection with a pertinent grading system will also help to develop a more individualized treatment strategy.

For the patient with inoperable MSCC, conventional EBRT is currently the de facto standard management strategy. Because these patients are likely to have a suboptimal result with conventional radiotherapy techniques, radiosurgery may offer a much better chance of preserving or improving neurologic function. Likewise, patients with spine metastases that have received prior radiation can still be good candidates for radiosurgery. For patients with overt spinal cord syndrome with neurologic deficit, immediate surgical decompression should be performed whenever possible, particularly when there is a rapid development of symptoms.

Metastatic tumors involving the spinal column are complex. Added to the oncologic problems, symptoms arising from complicating issues, such as intercurrent degenerative changes, osteoporosis and associated bony changes, and spine instability, may directly affect neurologic function and patient quality of life. The management of MSCC therefore requires a multidisciplinary effort to ensure the best comprehensive total care of these spine tumor patients.

References

[1] Byrne TN. Spinal cord compression from epidural metastases. N Engl J Med 1992; 327: 614–619

[2] Quinn JA, DeAngelis LM. Neurologic emergencies in the cancer patient. Semin Oncol 2000; 27: 311–321

[3] Greenberg HS, Kim JH, Posner JB. Epidural spinal cord compression from metastatic tumor: results with a new treatment protocol. Ann Neurol 1980; 8: 361–366

[4] Helweg-Larsen S. Clinical outcome in metastatic spinal cord compression: a prospective study of 153 patients. Acta Neurol Scand 1996; 94: 269–275

[5] Ryu S, Jin JY, Jin R, et al. Partial volume tolerance of the spinal cord and complications of single-dose radiosurgery. Cancer 2007; 109: 628–636

[6] Hirabayashi H, Ebara S, Kinoshita T, et al. Clinical outcome and survival after palliative surgery for spinal metastases: palliative surgery in spinal metastases. Cancer 2003; 97: 476–484

[7] Vecht CJ, Haaxma-Reiche H, van Putten WL, de Visser M, Vries EP, Twijnstra A. Initial bolus of conventional versus high-dose dexamethasone in metastatic spinal cord compression. Neurology 1989; 39: 1255–1257

[8] Loblaw DA, Laperriere NJ. Emergency treatment of malignant extradural spinal cord compression: an evidence-based guideline. J Clin Oncol 1998; 16: 1613–1624

[9] Maranzano E, Latini P. Effectiveness of radiation therapy without surgery in metastatic spinal cord compression: final results from a prospective trial. Int J Radiat Oncol Biol Phys 1995; 32: 959–967

[10] Maranzano E, Latini P, Perrucci E, Beneventi S, Lupattelli M, Corgna E. Short-course radiotherapy (8 Gy 2) in metastatic spinal cord compression: an effective and feasible treatment. Int J Radiat Oncol Biol Phys 1997; 38: 1037–1044

[11] Maranzano E, Trippa F, Casale M, et al. 8 Gy single-dose radiotherapy is effective in metastatic spinal cord compression: results of a phase III randomized multicentre Italian trial. Radiother Oncol 2009; 93: 174–179

[12] Rades D, Stalpers LJ, Hulshof MC, et al. Comparison of 1 8 Gy and 10 3 Gy for functional outcome in patients with metastatic spinal cord compression. Int J Radiat Oncol Biol Phys 2005; 62: 514–518

[13] Rades D, Lange M, Veninga T, et al. Final esults of a prospective study comparing the local control of short-course and long-course adiotherapy for metastatic spinal cord compression. Int J Radiat Oncol Biol Phys 2011; 79: 524–530

[14] Patchell RA, Tibbs PA, Regine WF, et al. Direct decompressive surgical resection in the treatment of spinal cord compression caused by metastatic cancer: a randomised trial. Lancet 2005; 366: 643–648

[15] Rades D, Abrahm JL. The role of radiotherapy for metastatic epidural spinal cord compression. Nat Rev Clin Oncol 2010; 7: 590–598

[16] Rades D, Fehlauer F, Veninga T, et al. Functional outcome and survival after radiotherapy of metastatic spinal cord compression in patients with cancer of unknown primary. Int J Radiat Oncol Biol Phys 2007; 67: 532–537

[17] Ryu S, Fang Yin F, Rock J, et al. Image-guided and intensity-modulated radiosurgery for patients with spinal metastasis. Cancer 2003; 97: 2013–2018

[18] Chang EL, Shiu AS, Mendel E, et al. Phase I/II study of stereotactic body radiotherapy for spinal metastasis and its pattern of failure. J Neurosurg Spine 2007; 7: 151–160

[19] Yamada Y, Bilsky MH, Lovelock DM, et al. High-dose, single-fraction image-guided intensity-modulated radiotherapy for metastatic spinal lesions. Int J Radiat Oncol Biol Phys 2008; 71: 484–490

[20] Gerszten PC, Burton SA, Welch WC, et al. Single-fraction radiosurgery for the treatment of spinal breast metastases. Cancer 2005; 104: 2244–2254

[21] Gerszten PC, Burton SA, Ozhasoglu C, et al. Stereotactic radiosurgery for spinal metastases from renal cell carcinoma. J Neurosurg Spine 2005; 3: 288–295

[22] Degen JW, Gagnon GJ, Voyadzis JM, et al. CyberKnife stereotactic radiosurgical treatment of spinal tumors for pain control and quality of life. J Neurosurg Spine 2005; 2: 540–549

[23] Ryu S, Jin R, Jin JY, et al. Pain control by image-guided radiosurgery for solitary spinal metastasis. J Pain Symptom Manage 2008; 35: 292–298

[24] Sahgal A, Ma L, Gibbs I, et al. Spinal cord tolerance for stereotactic body radiotherapy. Int J Radiat Oncol Biol Phys 2010; 77: 548–553

[25] Ryu S, Rock J, Jain R, et al. Radiosurgical decompression of metastatic epidural compression. Cancer 2010; 116: 2250–2257

[26] Gerszten PC, Burton SA, Quinn AE, Agarwala SS, Kirkwood JM. Radiosurgery for the treatment of spinal melanoma metastases. Stereotact Funct Neurosurg 2005; 83: 213–221

[27] Rock JP, Ryu S, Shukairy MS, et al. Postoperative radiosurgery for malignant spinal tumors. Neurosurgery 2006; 58: 891–898, discussion 891–898

[28] Ryu S, Rock J, Rosenblum M, Kim JH. Patterns of failure after single-dose radiosurgery for spinal metastasis. J Neurosurg 2004; 101 (Suppl 3): 402–405

[29] Rose PS, Laufer I, Boland PJ, et al. Risk of fracture after single fraction image-guided intensity-modulated radiation therapy to spinal metastases. J Clin Oncol 2009; 27: 5075–5079

[30] Boehling NS, Grosshans DR, Allen PK, et al. Vertebral compression fracture risk after stereotactic body radiotherapy for spinal metastases. J Neurosurg Spine 2012; 16: 379–386

[31] Andolino DL, Forquer JA, Henderson MA, et al. Chest wall toxicity after stereotactic body radiotherapy for malignant lesions of the lung and liver. Int J Radiat Oncol Biol Phys 2011; 80: 692–697

[32] Fourney DR, Frangou EM, Ryken TC, et al. Spinal instability neoplastic score: an analysis of reliability and validity from the spine oncology study group. J Clin Oncol 2011; 29: 3072–3077

[33] Tomita K, Kawahara N, Kobayashi T, Yoshida A, Murakami H, Akamaru T. Surgical strategy for spinal metastases. Spine 2001; 26: 298–306

[34] Tokuhashi Y, Matsuzaki H, Oda H, Oshima M, Ryu J. A revised scoring system for preoperative evaluation of metastatic spine tumor prognosis. Spine 2005; 30: 2186–2191

[35] Ryu S, James JL, Gerszten P, Yin FF, Timmerman RD, Hitchcock YJ, Movsas B, Kanner AA, Berk LB, Kachnik LA. RTOG 0631 Phase II/III Study of Image-Guided Stereotactic Radiosurgery for Localized Spine Metastases: Phase II Results. Radiation Oncology Practice 2013 (in print)

[36] Gerszten PC, Germanwala A, Burton SA, Welch WC, Ozhasoglu C, Vogel WJ. Combination kyphoplasty and spinal radiosurgery: a new treatment paradigm for pathological fractures. J Neurosurg Spine 2005; 3: 296–301

[37] Jin R, Anderson J, Jin JY, Chen Q, Rock J, Ajlouni M, Movsas B, Ryu S. Single fraction spine radiosurgery for multiple myeloma epidural spinal cord compression. Journal of Experimental Therapeutics and Oncology 2009; 8: 35–41

35 Spinal Cord Decompression with Surgery

Mari L. Groves, Ryan M. Kretzer, and Daniel M. Sciubba

Introduction

Metastatic disease continues to plague the overall survival as well as quality of life of many patients with cancer, despite improvements in treatment. Of the 1.2 million new patients diagnosed with cancer in the United States each year, 10 to 30% will develop spinal metastases.[1] Postmortem analysis also finds that 30 to 90% of patients have spinal metastases that are not clinically apparent, thus highlighting the number of patients with subclinical disease.[2] These neoplastic lesions occur in the thoracic, lumbosacral, and cervical regions at a distribution of 60, 30, and 10%, respectively.[3] The types of primary tumors that metastasize to the spine are also diverse and include breast (16–7%), lung (12–15%), prostate (9–15%), kidney (3–6%), and thyroid (4%), among others.[1] Metastatic epidural spinal cord compression (MESCC) is defined as an epidural metastatic lesion causing displacement of the spinal cord from its normal position in the vertebral canal on radiological imaging.[4]

The role of surgery has varied over the years. Before radiation was available, simple open decompressive laminectomy was the only treatment available. Early retrospective studies and a small randomized trial did not show any benefit for decompressive laminectomy alone or in combination with radiotherapy[5–13] (▶ Table 35.1). However, most spinal metastases occur in the vertebral body and may not be best decompressed through laminectomy alone. Additionally, laminectomy can result in the destabilization of the spine leading to further compression. With the advent of spinal instrumentation in the 1980s, circumferential decompression followed by instrumented fixation was better able to relieve compression and stabilize the spine. Several uncontrolled surgical series and a meta-analysis showed surgery with or without postoperative radiotherapy is superior to radiation alone[14–42] (▶ Table 35.2). A recent randomized clinical trial also favored surgical decompression for some cases of MESCC.[43]

Presentation

There are 25,000 cases of symptomatic MESCC in the United States each year.[44] Ten percent of patients initially present with symptomatic spinal metastasis with pain as the most common symptom in between 83 and 95% of patients.[45] There are multiple etiologies for pain in this population. Local pain is due to periosteal stretching from tumor growth and the resultant inflammatory process. Mechanical pain results from instability due to bony deterioration and erosion. Radicular pain results from compression or irritation of a nerve root.[46] Patients will often have a combination of both myelopathic and radicular symptoms depending on the level of tumor. Approximately 60 to 80% of patients will have motor weakness at the time of diagnosis.[46] Autonomic dysfunction, including bladder and bowel dysfunction, can also be found. Without intervention these patients progress to complete paralysis.[46] Neurologic status at the time of diagnosis, especially motor function, correlates with prognosis of MESCC;[47] thus, diagnosis prior to neurologic deterioration is important in preservation of function.

Imaging

Magnetic resonance imaging (MRI) and computed tomography (CT) remain dependent adjuncts to diagnosis of spinal metastatic disease. Although MRI is superior in defining the soft tissue anatomy and neural compression, CT is preferred in defining the osseous anatomy and for surgical planning. Patients with MESCC should undergo full body imaging to assess the overall degree of involvement, as this will impact their overall survival when assessing the need for surgery (▶ Fig. 35.1).

Table 35.1 Ambulatory outcome for early cohort studies comparing posterior decompressive laminectomy and radiation therapy

Treatment	No. patients	Ambulatory posttreatment	Mean
Posterior decompressive laminectomy alone			30%
All studies pre-1980 (9 total)	682	32	
Dunn et al[5]	104	33	
Stark et al[6]	32	16	
Findlay[7]	80	24	
Sorensen et al[8]	105	34	
All studies following 1980 (4 total)	321	27	
Radiation alone			48%
All studies pre-1980 (5 total)	386	44	
Greenberg et al[9]	83	57	
Stark et al[6]	32	35	
Constans et al[10]	108	39	
Martenson et al[11]	42	64	
Sorensen et al[8]	149	38	
Ruff & Lanska[12]	41	73	
Posterior decompressive laminectomy + radiation			47%
All studies pre-1980 (4 total)	126	45	
Stark et a[6]	52	37	
Constans et al[10]	465	46	
Martenson et al[11]	21	57	
Sherman & Waddell[13]	111	57	
Sorensen et al[8]	91	53	

Table 35.2 Results in circumferential spinal cord decompression from class III retrospective cohort data

Study	No. patients	Pain improvement	Ambulation	Mortality*	Morbidity*
Harrington[14]	52	N/A	85	12%	17%
Siegal & Siegal[15]	40	92%	80%	8%	20%
Fidler[16]	18	N/A	78%	6%	N/A
Kostiuk et al[17]	100	81%	72% A, 38% P	0%	21%
Harrington[18]	77	N/A	73%	7%	18%
Manabe et al[19]	28	100%	86%	7%	0%
Moore & Uttley[20]	26	71%	77%	31%	8%
Sundaresan et al[21]	54	90%	94%	6%	15%
Hammerberg[22]	56	91%	88%	4%	17%
Cooper et al[23]	33	97%	88%	3%	42%
Sundaresan et al[24]	110	90%	82%	5%	48%
Akeyson et al[25]	25	80%	72%	0	44%
Gokaslan et al[26]	72	92%	93%	3%	43%
Weigel et al[27]	76	89%	93%	7%	24%
Wise et al[28]	80	N/A	89%	3	36
Hatrick et al[29]	42	90%	86%	0	19
Bilsky et al[30]	25	100%	88%	12%	32%
Fourney et al[31]	100	87%	N/A	3%	37%
Jackson et al[32]	79	89%	N/A	3%	37%
Sundaresan et al[33]	80	95%	98%	1.3	29%
Patchell et al[43]	50	N/A	84%	6%	8%
Chen et al[34]	31	N/A	74%	6%	0%
Chaichana et al[35]	78	N/A	89%	3%	12%
Tanaka et al[36]	100	88%	76%	0	3%
Laufer et al[37]	39	N/A	65%	0	5%
Tancioni et al[38]	23	96%	100%	0%	0%
Walcott et al[39]	15	N/A	100%	0%	13%
Kim et al[40]	57	N/A	95%	5%	26%
Tancioni et al[41]	151	91%	63%	0%	N/A
Tancioni et al[42]	25	96%	N/A	0%	0%
Total	1742	86%	80%	4%	21%

Ambulation refers to the percentage of patients who were ambulatory following treatment. Mortality and morbidity are defined as death or complication within 30 days of the operation.
Abbreviations: *A, anterior; P, posterior; N/A, not applicable.*

Scoring System

Several scoring systems for spinal metastases exist using a range of prognostic factors to correlate clinical outcomes and survival. They attempt to categorize these patients into groups that will benefit from surgery versus those who will not. The Weinstein, Boriani, and Biagini (WBB) and Enneking systems of classification also were developed to stage and facilitate treatment planning in patients with primary spine tumors.[2] Tomita and colleagues use the grade of malignancy, presence of visceral metastases, and metastases in bone to predict survival.[2] Tokuhashi et al differentiate the primary site of the neoplasm as well as the patient's neurologic status as markers for survival.[2] The Spinal Oncology Study Group recently released standardized indications for treatment of tumor-related spinal instability.[48] The Spinal Instability Neoplastic Score (SINS) uses location,

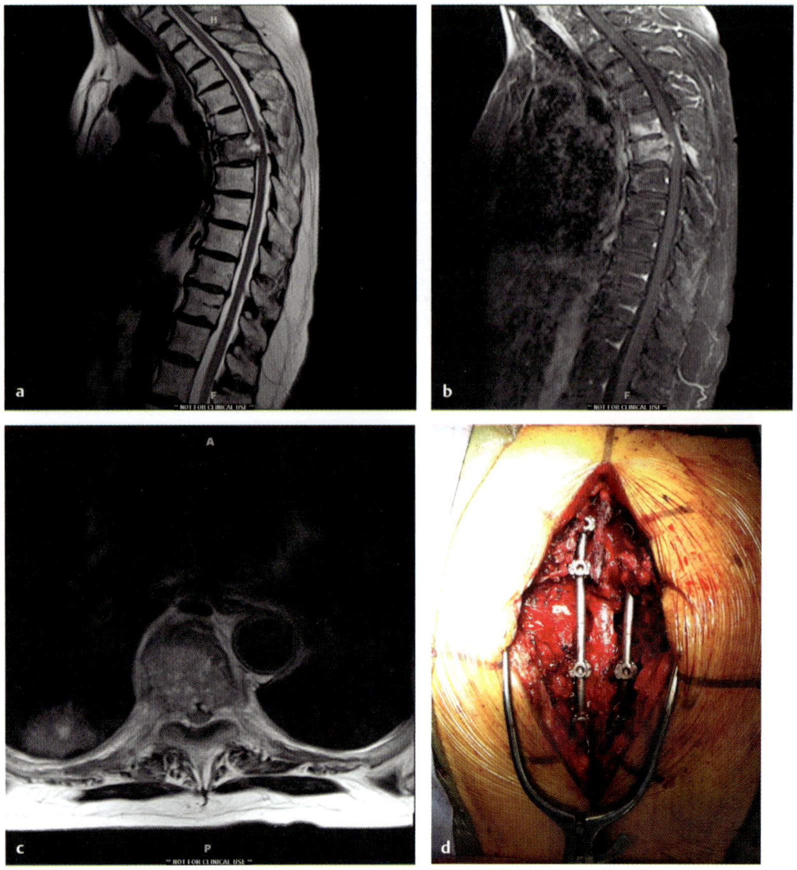

Fig. 35.1 Preoperative magnetic resonance image demonstrating metastatic vertebral body involvement with epidural extension and canal compromise. (a) Sagittal T2- and (b) T1-weighted images with contrast enhancement, as well as (c) axial T2-weighted image showing complete obliteration of the cerebrospinal fluid space. (d) Intraoperative construct demonstrating posterior rod placement as well as anterior tumor resection and cage placement.

pain, type of bone lesion, radiographic alignment, vertebral body collapse, and posterolateral involvement of spinal elements to rate the level of instability. For patients with a SINS score > 7, surgical stabilization was recommended.[48]

Treatment

Surgical indications include spinal instability, epidural compression with spinal cord dysfunction, radioresistant tumors, the need to establish diagnosis, recurrence despite radiotherapy, and neurologic deterioration during radiation treatment. Surgical timing plays an important role in neurologic outcome. If there has been rapid deterioration of the patient's neurologic function then an operation for decompression should be undertaken as soon as possible. Definitive treatment for MESCC should occur within 24 hours, but if the deterioration has been gradual, surgery can proceed at an urgent but not emergent rate.

Tumor type is critical in deciding whether radiation will be efficacious. Indications for radiotherapy in MESCC are for radiosensitive tumors such as lymphoma, myeloma, and small cell carcinoma of the lung. Patients without neurological impairment, spinal instability, or mechanical pain without bony compromise of the spinal canal would also be ideal candidates for radiotherapy as opposed to surgery. The overall tumor burden and life expectancy of the patient should also be considered, as those patients with < 3 months to live may not survive long enough to justify the recovery time following surgery.

Much of the existing literature for MESCC came from early retrospective cohort studies (***level IV***, grade C+) comparing decompressive laminectomy with observation. These studies examined ambulatory status, pain relief, and complications regarding treatment (▶ Table 35.1). These studies show that ambulation following treatment with posterior decompression alone was only 30%. There was no difference found in posttreatment ambulation for patients treated with both laminectomy and radiation versus radiation alone.

Young et al carried out the first randomized control clinical trial and found no statistical difference in outcome or survival between patients treated with radiotherapy and those treated with decompressive laminectomy and radiotherapy.[49] There were no treatment-related complications for either surgery or radiotherapy. However, this study was done with only 29 patients. As a result, laminectomy and surgical interventions fell out of favor. For reasons that are more accepted today, laminectomy alone may worsen a patient's spinal instability causing worsening pain, deformity, and neurological compromise. Additionally, laminectomy alone may be insufficient for decompression if the metastatic lesion is ventral to the spinal cord and inaccessible through a posterior approach.[49]

In subsequent retrospective cohort studies, stabilization procedures in addition to posterior decompression showed some improvement in patient outcome. Patient's functional outcome was improved if posterior stabilization was performed in addition to decompression, with a mean motor improvement of 64%.[50] Over the past 2 decades more aggressive decompression and stabilization methods have been introduced through circumferential decompression. Functional improvement was also noted in those patients who underwent circumferential decompression and stabilization, with a mean neurological improvement of 75% and mean mortality rate of 10% (▶ Table 35.2).

In 2005, Patchell and colleagues published a randomized, prospective clinical trial of direct decompressive surgical resection and stabilization combined with radiotherapy ($n = 50$) versus radiotherapy alone ($n = 51$) for MESCC.[43] They showed that patients who underwent surgery combined with radiation retained the ability to walk for longer and regained the ability to walk more often than patients treated with radiation alone (84% vs 57%, $p = 0.001$).[43] This improvement was also sustained as patients who underwent surgery retained the ability to walk for a median of 122 days compared to 13 days for patients who underwent radiation alone ($p = 0.0003$). For those patients able to walk prior to treatment, 94% in the surgery group were able to do so when compared to only 74% of the radiotherapy group (median 153 days vs 54 days, $p = 0.024$). The median survival was also improved in the surgical cohort at 126 days compared to 100 days in the radiotherapy alone subgroup ($p = 0.033$).[43] There was also a significant improvement in the maintenance of continence, muscle strength, functional ability, and increased survival time when surgery was combined with radiation therapy. The study was closed early due to these findings, and the overall consensus was that in patients without radiosensitive tumors, surgery and radiotherapy led to longer ambulatory status, allowed the recovery of ambulation more frequently, and

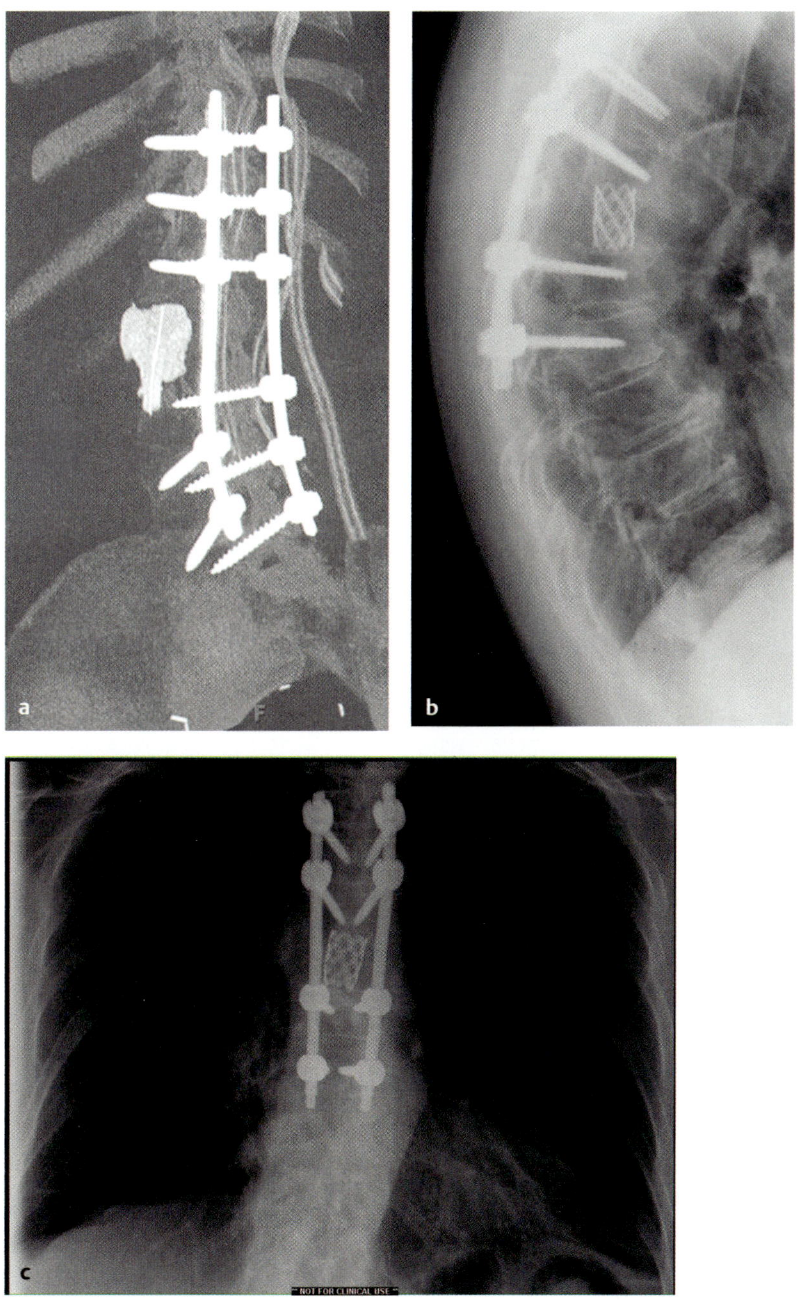

Fig. 35.2 (a) Computed tomographic reconstruction demonstrating intraoperative hardware construct with anterior cage placement at L2–L3 and posterior rod with pedicle screws from T11 to L5. (b) Anteroposterior view of patient in Fig. 35.1 showing anterior cage at T6 and posterior pedicle screw and rod construct from T4 to T8. (c) Lateral view of spine hardware reconstruction.

improved the quality of life for those patients. These improvements in function appeared to be sustained throughout the remainder of the patient's survival time.[43]

Chi and colleagues also conducted a randomized clinical trial that stratified patients according to age. They examined groups of patients receiving surgery versus those receiving only radiation in ages < 65 years and > 65 years.[51] They found that patients < age 65 experienced a greater improvement in ambulation (315 days vs 72 days with radiation alone; $p = 0.0024$). They also showed an improvement in survival with a median time of 126 days with surgery versus 93 days with radiation alone ($p = 0.0048$). This difference was not significant in patients greater than 65 years of age. Their conclusions found that as age increases, the beneficial effect of surgery diminishes and becomes equivalent to radiation therapy alone.[51]

There was some thought that in patients with solitary metastases a total spondylectomy or en bloc resection would improve survival, as has been shown for primary bone tumors of the spine. However, Moulding and colleagues showed that for such patients stereotactic radiosurgery should be the first line of treatment rather than en bloc excision.[52] Additional studies are focusing on tumor types and whether en bloc resection has an impact in overall survival.

Radiation therapy was initially favored and is still considered an important adjunct to surgical resection for relatively radioresistant tumors. With the improvement in targeting, conventional external beam radiation therapy (EBRT) and stereotactic radiosurgery (SRS) help improve local tumor control with minimal patient morbidity.[52] This precise targeting allows a more limited surgical resection of tumor with segmental fixation followed by focused radiation of the residual disease through SRS. Limiting tumor resection may also provide more effective palliation and decreased morbidity for patients who are at high surgical risk.[52]

Surgical Technique

Surgical approach is reliant upon the location of the tumor, site of spinal cord compression, histological type, and the type of reconstruction and stabilization that will be required once the tumor is resected. For vascular metastatic tumors such as renal cell, thyroid, or hepatocellular carcinoma, one should consider preoperative embolization to decrease blood loss. Anterior approaches are commonly thought to provide the best access to the tumor since the vertebral body is commonly involved ▸ Fig. 35.1.

In the upper thoracic spine, the anterior approach is fraught with difficulties as access to this area is limited by the heart and great vessels. For instance, lesions at the cervicothoracic junction may require a combination anterolateral cervical approach and a sternotomy with or without a thoracotomy.[53] As this is clearly complicated by high surgical morbidity, the posterior transpedicular or costotransversectomy approach has been popularized. In the midthoracic spine (T5–T10), a thoracotomy provides direct access to the vertebral body and laterality should be determined by the location of the extravertebral tumor.[53] Alternatively, posterolateral approaches including costotransversectomy can also be utilized in the midthoracic region. Approaches to the thoracolumbar region usually require a combination thoracotomy and retroperitoneal approach for anterior access. Metastasis to the lumbar spine can be reached through a retroperitoneal incision. Given the anterior anatomy at the lumbosacral junction, a posterior approach is favored.

Stabilization of the spine is reliant upon innovations in spinal column reconstruction using titanium cages and plating (▸ Fig. 35.2). Polymethylmethacrylate (PMMA) can also be used by filling a chest tube and securing this to the surrounding bone with screws or pins. Posterior stabilization has been well established with pedicle screw fixation. However, older methods such as hooks and wires can be implemented if the pedicles are unable to be cannulated. To prevent postoperative deformity, lesions requiring more than a single corpectomy should typically be supplemented with posterior instrumentation. Minimally invasive options are possible for some patients and are currently being developed.

Conclusion

There has been a gradual transition in the literature from retrospective cohort studies that showed little difference between laminectomy and radiotherapy to studies that now include well-designed, ***level I evidence*** favoring surgery combined with radiation treatment for the treatment of MESCC. Patchell and colleagues showed that surgery should be considered the primary treatment modality for most patients with isolated MESCC in the setting of reasonable life expectancy and functional status. Overall, surgical decompression and stabilization of the spinal column are more effective at relieving pain, regaining ambulatory status, and preserving bowel/bladder function than conventional radiotherapy.

References

[1] White AP, Kwon BK, Lindskog DM, Friedlaender GE, Grauer JN. Metastatic disease of the spine. J Am Acad Orthop Surg 2006; 14: 587–598

[2] Sciubba DM, Petteys RJ, Dekutoski MB, et al. Diagnosis and management of metastatic spine disease. J Neurosurg Spine 2010; 13: 94–108

[3] Abrahm JL, Banffy MB, Harris MB. Spinal cord compression in patients with advanced metastatic cancer: "all I care about is walking and living my life." JAMA 2008; 299: 937–946

[4] Loblaw DA, Laperriere NJ, Mackillop WJ. A population-based study of malignant spinal cord compression in Ontario. Clin Oncol (R Coll Radiol) 2003; 15: 211–217

[5] Dunn RC, Kelly WA, Wohns RN, Howe JF. Spinal epidural neoplasia: a 15-year review of the results of surgical therapy. J Neurosurg 1980; 52: 47–51

[6] Stark RJ, Henson RA, Evans SJ. Spinal metastases. A retrospective survey from a general hospital. Brain 1982; 105: 189–213

[7] Findlay GF. The role of vertebral body collapse in the management of malignant spinal cord compression. J Neurol Neurosurg Psychiatry 1987; 50: 151–154

[8] Sørensen S, Børgesen SE, Rohde K, et al. Metastatic epidural spinal cord compression: results of treatment and survival. Cancer 1990; 65: 1502–1508

[9] Greenberg HS, Kim JH, Posner JB. Epidural spinal cord compression from metastatic tumor: results with a new treatment protocol. Ann Neurol 1980; 8: 361–366

[10] Constans JP, de Divitiis E, Donzelli R, Spaziante R, Meder JF, Haye C. Spinal metastases with neurological manifestations: review of 600 cases. J Neurosurg 1983; 59: 111–118

[11] Martenson JA, Evans RG, Lie MR, et al. Treatment outcome and complications in patients treated for malignant epidural spinal cord compression (SCC). J Neurooncol 1985; 3: 77–84

[12] Ruff RL, Lanska DJ. Epidural metastases in prospectively evaluated veterans with cancer and back pain. Cancer 1989; 63: 2234–2241

[13] Sherman RM, Waddell JP. Laminectomy for metastatic epidural spinal cord tumors. Posterior stabilization, radiotherapy, and preoperative assessment. Clin Orthop Relat Res 1986 Jun: 55–63

[14] Harrington KD. Anterior cord decompression and spinal stabilization for patients with metastatic lesions of the spine. J Neurosurg 1984; 61: 107–117

[15] Siegal T, Siegal T. Surgical decompression of anterior and posterior malignant epidural tumors compressing the spinal cord: a prospective study. Neurosurgery 1985; 17: 424–432

[16] Fidler MW. Anterior decompression and stabilisation of metastatic spinal fractures. J Bone Joint Surg Br 1986; 68: 83–90

[17] Kostuik JP, Errico TJ, Gleason TF, Errico CC. Spinal stabilization of vertebral column tumors. Spine 1988; 13: 250–256

[18] Harrington KD. Anterior decompression and stabilization of the spine as a treatment for vertebral collapse and spinal cord compression from metastatic malignancy. Clin Orthop Relat Res 1988: 177–197

[19] Manabe S, Tanaka H, Higo Y, Park P, Ohno T, Tateishi A. Experimental analysis of the spinal cord compressed by spinal metastasis. Spine 1989; 14: 1308–1315

[20] Moore AJ, Uttley D. Anterior decompression and stabilization of the spine in malignant disease. Neurosurgery 1989; 24: 713–717

[21] Sundaresan N, Digiacinto GV, Hughes JE, Cafferty M, Vallejo A. Treatment of neoplastic spinal cord compression: results of a prospective study. Neurosurgery 1991; 29: 645–650

[22] Hammerberg KW. Surgical treatment of metastatic spine disease. Spine 1992; 17: 1148–1153

[23] Cooper PR, Errico TJ, Martin R, Crawford B, DiBartolo T. A systematic approach to spinal reconstruction after anterior decompression for neoplastic disease of the thoracic and lumbar spine. Neurosurgery 1993; 32: 1–8

[24] Sundaresan N, Steinberger AA, Moore F, et al. Indications and results of combined anterior-posterior approaches for spine tumor surgery. J Neurosurg 1996; 85: 438–446

[25] Akeyson EW, McCutcheon IE. Single-stage posterior vertebrectomy and replacement combined with posterior instrumentation for spinal metastasis. J Neurosurg 1996; 85: 211–220

[26] Gokaslan ZL, York JE, Walsh GL, et al. Transthoracic vertebrectomy for metastatic spinal tumors. J Neurosurg 1998; 89: 599–609

[27] Weigel B, Maghsudi M, Neumann C, Kretschmer R, Müller FJ, Nerlich M. Surgical management of symptomatic spinal metastases: postoperative outcome and quality of life. Spine 1999; 24: 2240–2246

[28] Wise JJ, Fischgrund JS, Herkowitz HN, Montgomery D, Kurz LT. Complication, survival rates, and risk factors of surgery for metastatic disease of the spine. Spine 1999; 24: 1943–1951

[29] Hatrick NC, Lucas JD, Timothy AR, Smith MA. The surgical treatment of metastatic disease of the spine. Radiother Oncol 2000; 56: 335–339

[30] Bilsky MH, Boland P, Lis E, Raizer JJ, Healey JH. Single-stage posterolateral transpedicle approach for spondylectomy, epidural decompression, and circumferential fusion of spinal metastases. Spine 2000; 25: 2240–2249, discussion 250

[31] Fourney DR, Abi-Said D, Rhines LD, et al. Simultaneous anterior-posterior approach to the thoracic and lumbar spine for the radical resection of tumors followed by reconstruction and stabilization. J Neurosurg 2001; 94 (Suppl): 232–244–;erratum in: J Neurosurg 2001;95(1 Suppl):160

[32] Jackson RJ, Loh SC, Gokaslan ZL. Metastatic renal cell carcinoma of the spine: surgical treatment and results. J Neurosurg 2001; 94 (Suppl): 18–24

[33] Sundaresan N, Rothman A, Manhart K, Kelliher K. Surgery for solitary metastases of the spine: rationale and results of treatment. Spine 2002; 27: 1802–1806

[34] Chen YJ, Chang GC, Chen HT, et al. Surgical results of metastatic spinal cord compression secondary to non-small cell lung cancer. Spine 2007; 32: E413–E418

[35] Chaichana KL, Pendleton C, Sciubba DM, Wolinsky JP, Gokaslan ZL. Outcome following decompressive surgery for different histological types of metastatic tumors causing epidural spinal cord compression: clinical article. J Neurosurg Spine 2009; 11: 56–63

[36] Tanaka M, Nakahara S, Ito Y, et al. Surgical treatment of metastatic vertebral tumors. Acta Med Okayama 2009; 63: 145–150

[37] Laufer I, Hanover A, Lis E, Yamada Y, Bilsky M. Repeat decompression surgery for recurrent spinal metastases. J Neurosurg Spine 2010; 13: 109–115

[38] Tancioni F, Navarria P, Mancosu P, et al. Surgery followed by radiotherapy for the treatment of metastatic epidural spinal cord compression from breast cancer. Spine 2011; 36: E1352–E1359

[39] Walcott BP, Cvetanovich GL, Barnard ZR, Nahed BV, Kahle KT, Curry WT. Surgical treatment and outcomes of metastatic breast cancer to the spine. J Clin Neurosci 2011; 18: 1336–1339

[40] Kim JM, Losina E, Bono CM, et al. Clinical outcome of metastatic spinal cord compression treated with surgical excision ± radiation versus radiation therapy alone: a systematic review of literature.(review) Spine 2012; 37: 78–84

[41] Tancioni F, Navarria P, Pessina F, et al. Assessment of prognostic factors in patients with metastatic epidural spinal cord compression (MESCC) from solid tumor after surgery plus radiotherapy: a single institution experience. Eur Spine J 2012; 21 (Suppl 1): S146–S148

[42] Tancioni F, Navarria P, Pessina F, et al. Early surgical experience with minimally invasive percutaneous approach for patients with metastatic epidural spinal cord compression (MESCC) to poor prognoses. Ann Surg Oncol 2012; 19: 294–300

[43] Patchell RA, Tibbs PA, Regine WF, et al. Direct decompressive surgical resection in the treatment of spinal cord compression caused by metastatic cancer: a randomised trial. Lancet 2005; 366: 643–648

[44] Cobb CA, Leavens ME, Eckles N. Indications for nonoperative treatment of spinal cord compression due to breast cancer. J Neurosurg 1977; 47: 653–658

[45] Helweg-Larsen S, Sørensen PS. Symptoms and signs in metastatic spinal cord compression: a study of progression from first symptom until diagnosis in 153 patients. Eur J Cancer 1994; 30A: 396–398

[46] Sciubba DM, Gokaslan ZL. Diagnosis and management of metastatic spine disease. Surg Oncol 2006; 15: 141–151

[47] Arguello F, Baggs RB, Duerst RE, Johnstone L, McQueen K, Frantz CN. Pathogenesis of vertebral metastasis and epidural spinal cord compression. Cancer 1990; 65: 98–106

[48] Fourney DR, Frangou EM, Ryken TC, et al. Spinal instability neoplastic score: an analysis of reliability and validity from the spine oncology study group. J Clin Oncol 2011; 29: 3072–3077

[49] Young RF, Post EM, King GA. Treatment of spinal epidural metastases: randomized prospective comparison of laminectomy and radiotherapy. J Neurosurg 1980; 53: 741–748

[50] Witham TF, Khavkin YA, Gallia GL, Wolinsky JP, Gokaslan ZL. Surgery insight: current management of epidural spinal cord compression from metastatic spine disease. Nat Clin Pract Neurol 2006; 2: 87–94, quiz 116

[51] Chi JH, Gokaslan Z, McCormick P, Tibbs PA, Kryscio RJ, Patchell RA. Selecting treatment for patients with malignant epidural spinal cord compression—does age matter?: results from a randomized clinical trial. Spine 2009; 34: 431–435

[52] Moulding HD, Elder JB, Lis E, et al. Local disease control after decompressive surgery and adjuvant high-dose single-fraction radiosurgery for spine metastases. J Neurosurg Spine 2010; 13: 87–93

[53] Fourney DR, Gokaslan ZL. Spinal instability and deformity due to neoplastic conditions. Neurosurg Focus 2003; 14: e8

36 Postoperative Spine Radiosurgery

Randa Tao, T. Jonathan Yang, Paul Brown, Laurence D. Rhines, and Stephen H. Settle

Introduction

Given the advances in radiation treatment delivery, stereotactic body radiotherapy (SBRT) is being used in broader scenarios, including in patients who first undergo surgical management of metastatic spinal column tumors.[1] SBRT allows the delivery of a high dose of radiation in one or a few fractions targeted with precision to the tumor and at-risk areas while sparing the adjacent critical structures. It also takes advantage of the greater radiobiological effect afforded by hypofractionation. Prospective studies have demonstrated the safety and efficacy of SBRT to the spine, both in the radiation naive and reirradiation scenarios, with local control rates better than 85 to 90% in some series.[2,3] This technique has proven particularly useful in the treatment of radiation-resistant histologies, such as renal cell carcinoma, which typically respond poorly to conventional fractionated radiation.[4–6] Additionally, this technique allows for the reirradiation of patients who have failed conventional fractionated radiation.

Many of the potential advantages of SBRT to the spine also apply to the postoperative setting and take advantage of the steep dose gradients achievable with SBRT. Ablative doses of radiation can be delivered to postoperative regions that are almost always at risk for harboring residual disease while sparing the adjacent critical structures, most importantly the spinal cord and healing fascial and subcutaneous tissues. Postoperative SBRT can include delivery of high doses of radiation after a variety of surgical procedures ranging from an open surgical vertebrectomy to a minimally invasive percutaneous cement augmentation procedure. When radiosurgery is used in combination with a surgical approach, the potential for achieving durable symptom and tumor control may be possible for appropriately selected patients.

Surgical management of metastatic spinal tumors can immediately relieve neurologic symptoms caused by epidural cord compression. However, this approach is not always undertaken with the goal of complete surgical resection of tumor. Furthermore, when complete resection of tumor is achieved, microscopic disease frequently remains. Adjuvant radiation therapy is indicated to provide local tumor control, and randomized data have shown that surgery followed by conventional radiation results in better outcomes than conventional radiation alone.[7] Patchell et al demonstrated a significant improvement in patients' ability to remain or become ambulatory following surgery plus radiation therapy versus radiation therapy alone.[7] Unfortunately, local tumor control rates are still modest with such an approach[8] and further adjuvant fractionated radiation with the spinal cord within the field is not possible in patients who have received and failed prior conventional radiation. This raises the question of whether more effective radiation treatment can lead to better outcomes. SBRT has the potential of delivering higher biologically effective doses of radiation to achieve this while protecting critical structures such as the spinal cord, hence allowing for reirradiation in some cases.

In addition to the potential of offering durable local control, SBRT in the postoperative setting may have other advantages. Patients who are poor candidates for definitive SBRT due to bulky disease or tumor proximity to normal critical structures can potentially become good candidates for SBRT after open surgery. For example, a patient who has a tumor in a location abutting the spinal cord may undergo upfront surgical resection resulting in anatomy that is subsequently favorable for SBRT. Delivering radiation after surgery can then allow for higher doses of radiation to be given if a tumor abutting the spinal cord is resected. Patients who are in pain and cannot lie still for the period of time required for SBRT may potentially be comfortably treated following surgical stabilization or vertebral body augmentation. Upfront surgical management can also help patients with an impending vertebral body fracture, patients who would be at high risk for fracture following SBRT, or patients with evidence of spinal instability.[9,10] Additionally, anticipating postoperative SBRT can allow for a less extensive surgery to be performed and hence less morbidity for the patient. With planned ablative radiation therapy, the surgeon does not necessarily need to remove an entire involved vertebral body or perform a difficult gross total resection of a large invasive tumor.[11] As such, combining the two treatment approaches can potentially decrease the morbidity of both, which is especially important to consider in the palliative setting of patients with metastatic spine disease.

Radiation doses for postoperative SBRT generally do not differ from doses given with definitive SSRS treatment, though a fractionated approach rather than single-fraction SSRS is sometimes preferred. Dose and fractionation schemes can be delivered at 10 to 24 Gy in one fraction or 18 to 27 Gy in three fractions, resulting in higher biologic equivalent doses than conventional adjuvant fractionated radiation therapy. Whether this technique translates to a higher rate of local tumor control has been evaluated in studies with promising results.

Literature Review

Symptom Control and Local Tumor Control

The literature specific to postoperative spine SBRT is based on retrospective and phase I/II studies representing ***level IIA evidence***. Many of these studies report outcomes on a heterogeneous patient population treated with SBRT, including those treated with definitive SBRT, patients who are treated after previous conventional radiation, or patients treated after a wide range of surgical procedures. The literature on SBRT including 15 patients or more treated postoperatively is summarized in ▸ Table 36.1.

The first study on postoperative spine SBRT (sSBRT) was published from the University of Pittsburgh in 2005, describing 26 patients with spinal compression fractures as a result of their metastatic disease.[12] All of the patients were treated with a percutaneous balloon kyphoplasty procedure followed by single-fraction SBRT. Fiducial markers were placed during the kyphoplasty procedure for use in SBRT image guidance. The

Table 36.1 Summary of literature on postoperative spine stereotactic body radiotherapy

Study	No. postop patients	Total no. tumors/no. patients	Tumor dose/no. fx/Rx isodose	F/u (months) (range)	Local control/criteria
Gerszten et al[12]	26	26/26	Mean 18 Gy/1/80%	Median 16 (range 11–24)	24 of 26 (92%)/clinical
Rock et al[13]	18	18/18	4 of 18: EBRT 25 Gy/10 fx + SBRT boost; median 6 Gy/1/90% 14 of 18: SBRT only; median 14 Gy/1/90%	Median 7 (range 4–36)	17 of 18 (94%)/clinical
Chang et al[14]	29	74/63	32 of 63: 30 Gy/5 fx 31 of 63: 27 Gy/3 fx Rx isodose such that 80–90% target coverage	Median 21.3 (range 1–50)	23 of 29 (79%)/imaging
Moulding et al[19]	21	21/21	Median 24 Gy/1/100%	Median 10.3 (range 1.3–54.8)	17 of 21 (81%)/imaging
Nguyen et al[17]	15	55/48	30 Gy/5 fx 24 Gy/3 fx 24 Gy/1 fx Rx isodose: CTV covered by 80–90%	Median 13.1 (range 3.3–54.5)	10 of 15 (67%)/imaging
Garg et al[3]	16	63/61	18–24 Gy/1 fx Rx isodose: CTV covered by 80–90%	Median 17.8 (range 1.2–52.1)	16 of 16 (100%)/imaging
Laufer et al[11]	186	186/186	24 Gy/1 fx 24–30 Gy/3 fx 18–36/5–6 fx	Median 7.6 (range 1.0–66.4)	156/186 (83.8%)/imaging

Abbreviations: CTV, clinical target volume; EBRT, external beam radiotherapy; f/u follow-up; fx, fraction(s); Rx, prescription; SBRT, stereotactic body radiotherapy.
Source: Adapted from Sahgal A, Bilsky M, Chang EL, et al. Stereotactic body radiotherapy for spinal metastases: current status, with a focus on its application in the postoperative patient: a review. J Neurosurg Spine 2011;14:151, with permission.

patients were treated to a mean dose of 18 Gy (range 16–20 Gy). The median follow-up was 16 months with the focus on the extent of pain relief and side effects associated with treatment. Long-term improvement in pain control was reported in 92% of the patients at 1 year, but there was a limited report of tumor control rates. Follow-up imaging with MRI was used to evaluate for signs of spinal cord injury caused by radiation showing no imaging evidence of toxicity. These results were promising in showing that postkyphoplasty SBRT can achieve symptom control without causing spinal cord injury.

Rock and colleagues at Henry Ford Hospital published a retrospective study on 18 patients who underwent an open surgical procedure such as a laminectomy or corpectomy.[13] This study is often cited as the first initial report of the use of SBRT in the true adjuvant setting as the previous study from University of Pittsburgh only included patients treated after a kyphoplasty procedure. The patients in this study were treated with a single fraction of adjuvant radiosurgery ranging from 6 to 16 Gy with the Novalis Body System (Feldkirchen, Germany). Again, the outcomes from this study were based on symptom control. Of the 13 patients who had preoperative neurologic deficits, 12 patients (92%) remained neurologically stable with 8 patients (62%) experiencing improved symptoms. The authors reported that a follow-up MRI performed for the one patient who had deterioration of symptoms demonstrated disease progression in the local area that was outside the SBRT treated volume. No imaging follow-up on the other patients was reported. Based on this set of patients, the authors concluded that SBRT after an open surgical procedure was safe and offered the chance to improve or at least stabilize neurologic function.

The study with the largest number of postoperative SBRT patients included on a prospective trial was published in 2007.[14] This was a phase I/II study from MD Anderson with 63 patients, including 29 treated with postoperative SBRT, 15 of which underwent surgery followed by SBRT delivered with postoperative intent. In some cases, patients with disease located < 5 mm from the cord underwent surgical resection enabling a more favorable radiation treatment plan, illustrating that surgery offers certain patients an opportunity to receive SBRT. The patients were treated with fractionated SBRT, receiving 30 Gy in six fractions or 27 Gy in three fractions depending on the time of study enrollment. With a median follow-up of 21.3 months, the actuarial local control rate, defined as no tumor progression on MRI, was 84% at 1 year. The radiation dose and fractionation did not significantly affect the local control rates. Interestingly, patients treated with surgery and adjuvant SBRT also did not have a significantly different outcome from those treated with SBRT alone. No grade 3 or 4 neurologic toxicity was observed.

More recently, Laufer et al from Memorial Sloan-Kettering Cancer Center performed a retrospective analysis of 186 patients treated with SBRT after limited surgical decompression and instrumentation of the spine.[11] For these patients, the goal of surgery was to perform decompression with a "separation surgery" to create physical distance between the tumor and the spinal cord. No gross-total or en bloc tumor resection was performed. The patients then received either a single fraction of SRS with 24 Gy, three fractions of SBRT from 24 to 30 Gy, or lower doses of hypofractionation using five or six fractions to deliver 18 to 36 Gy. With a median follow-up of 7.6 months, the 1-year cumulative local control rate was 83.8% for the entire group, 91% for the patients receiving 24 Gy in one fraction, 95.9% for 24 to 30 Gy in three fractions, and 77.4% for patients treated with 18 to 36 Gy in five or six fractions. On univariate analysis, improved local control was found to be significantly associated with a higher hypofractionated dose (HR 1 for low-dose hypofractionation of 18–36 Gy in five or six fractions, HR 0.12 for high-dose 24–30 Gy in three fractions, and HR 0.45 for a single fraction of 24 Gy). This study demonstrated that there may be a dose response for postoperative SBRT in the setting of metastatic spine disease.

The results from these studies have shown promising rates of symptom and/or local tumor control rates for postoperative SBRT, similar to the rates reported for patients treated in the definitive setting. There does not seem to be any indication of increased toxicity with treating to high radiation doses following surgery despite the theoretical concern that disruption of the spinal vasculature during surgery can increase the risk of radiation toxicity. Given the heterogeneity and small size of the postoperative patient population in most of the reported series, it is difficult to compare directly the results of either definitive SBRT or adjuvant SBRT with conventional fractionated radiotherapy. Comparing adjuvant SBRT with adjuvant conventional fractionation is especially difficult, as many patients receiving palliative treatment have very limited long-term follow-up. Symptom control may be followed in these patients, but repeat imaging is infrequently performed.

Additional criticisms of the literature available on postoperative SBRT include the heterogeneity of the patients and treatments. Differences in patient selection, the extent of prior surgery or radiation, multiple dose and fractionation schemes, and the different metrics used to evaluate clinical response limit our ability to make specific conclusions about this technique. More studies are needed in order to evaluate whether the presumed advantages of postoperative SBRT clearly translate into better patient outcomes.

Patterns of Failure

One concern with delivering high doses of radiation to a limited area is the potential for increased marginal failures and subsequent recurrences, as the total target volumes for SBRT are smaller than conventional fields. With conventional radiotherapy fields, the vertebral bodies adjacent to the level with disease are treated, whereas only the involved vertebral bodies are treated with SBRT. Indeed, an entire segment of the spinal cord can be treated with conventional fields as the dose is below cord tolerance, whereas the cord is an avoidance structure with SBRT treatment. This raises the concern for failure at the epidural space where there is a sharp dose falloff, or at the field boundaries, which rarely encompass more than two vertebral body levels in SBRT. There are more data reported on patterns of failure in definitive SBRT. Failure at an adjacent vertebral body was uncommon; the failure rate was 0% in a large series of 500 cases treated with definitive SBRT at the University of Pittsburgh[15] and 5% in a smaller series of 61 cases.[16] However, failure at the epidural space is more commonly reported, representing about half of the total failures in some series.[14,17]

The data on patterns of failure in the postoperative setting are limited, as most reports do not describe the location of the failure. The most extensive data on patterns of failure in the postoperative setting come from the results of the phase I/II trial published from MD Anderson in 2007.[14] Failure rates were obtained based on MRI documentation of tumor progression. There were 6 failures out of the 29 patients treated postoperatively; 3 were in patients who underwent a kyphoplasty or vertebroplasty procedure and occurred in the epidural space or the posterior edge of the vertebral body, where the tumor would be predicted to be under-dosed due to the spinal cord dose constraint. The remaining three failures occurred in patients treated with vertebrectomy or partial resection, and two of the three patients had prior radiation. The failures in these cases included the epidural space, the paravertebral and paraspinal tissues, and the lamina/pedicle.

Technique at MD Anderson Cancer Center

At MD Anderson, postoperative SBRT is generally given to patients who undergo resection for limited spinal metastatic disease. Patients with radioresistant tumor histologies such as renal cell carcinoma, carcinoma of the lung, colon cancer, and melanoma are often considered for SBRT over conventional radiotherapy treatment. Patients with radiosensitive histologies such as breast cancer can be treated with SBRT as well, though conventional radiation is often preferred for radiosensitive histologies, and SBRT is reserved as an option for salvage. Poor candidates for SBRT include those who have had prior SBRT in the vicinity (the same or adjacent vertebral level), close gross tumor proximity to the cord despite open surgery, multilevel spine disease, patients who cannot discontinue cytotoxic chemotherapy, and patients with symptoms that preclude them from lying flat for an extended time (e.g., pain or dyspnea).

All patients are treated with computed tomographic (CT) image guidance using on-board CT imaging integrated with the treating linear accelerator. During simulation, patients are immobilized in a stereotactic body frame system (Bodyfix, Medical Intelligence Elekta, Schwabmuenchen, Germany) with a whole-body vacuum for those with lower spinal disease. For patients with cervical or upper thoracic disease, a large intensity-modulated radiation therapy (IMRT) over-the-shoulders mask is used, along with a whole-body vacuum device. Alignment is achieved with a stereotactic localizer and target positioning frame. The postoperative magnetic resonance imaging (MRI) and often the preoperative MRI is fused with the CT images acquired at simulation. If the instrumentation from surgery is causing significant artifact on the postoperative imaging, preventing adequate visualization of the spinal cord, or is predicted to cause significant artifact on the CT simulation, a CT myelogram can be performed to better delineate the cord–vertebral segment interface. An axial T2-weighted MR image is obtained if it is not possible to obtain a CT myelogram. For patients with disease near the cord, a CT myelogram is preferred.

For target volumes, the gross tumor volume (GTV) is defined as areas of residual disease seen on the postoperative MRI. We define the clinical target volume (CTV) as the GTV plus any residual contiguous bone marrow space and the high-risk postoperative region where there was tumor prior to surgery. Generally, the weight-bearing portion of the bone is targeted with at least one pedicle included. Often the posterior elements of the vertebral body are not included in the field, unless this is the site of disease. The surgical scar is generally not included as part of the CTV. We do not use any additional expansions for a planning treatment volume (PTV) due to the precise stereotactic setup and CT-based image guidance for treatment.[3] The dose and fractionation schemes we use for postoperative SBRT are generally the same as those for definitive SBRT, though fractionated SBRT is often preferred if there is concern for potential decrease in accuracy due to metallic artifacts on the CT and MRI scans or if there is concern that disruption of the vasculature or other potential damage during surgery may put the patient at greater risk for spinal cord injury. Patients who are radiation naïve with a radioresistant tumor histology are usually treated in one fraction to 18 or 24 Gy prescribed to the GTV and 16 Gy prescribed to the CTV. Three fractions are often used for patients who have been previously irradiated or for cervical spine lesions treating the CTV to 27 or 24 Gy. If three fractions are used, it is possible to target the GTV to 27 Gy and the CTV to 24 Gy, though sometimes a separate GTV is not indicated or is not needed in the postoperative setting. Some difficult cases can be treated in five or six fractions to a dose of 30 Gy to the CTV, for example, patients with large-volume disease previously treated with radiation. Inverse-treatment planning is used to create an IMRT plan. The dose constraint goal for the spinal cord as a point dose is set so that no greater than 0.01 cm^3 of the cord receives > 10 to 12 Gy. The anatomical spinal cord with a 2-mm margin is limited to 12 to 14 Gy or less.

Future Studies

Additional studies on postoperative SBRT are needed in order to demonstrate whether this technique is clearly better than surgery followed by conventional radiation treatment. While the data on postoperative SBRT are limited, it is clear that the technique is effective and safe. Additionally, it is important that future studies distinguish between a simple vertebral body augmentation and a more complex open procedure. Vertebral augmentation is only minimally invasive and very effective in relieving pain from a vertebral body compression fracture, a common adverse event associated with spine SBRT.[9,10] The approach of combining vertebral body augmentation with SBRT has been prospectively evaluated by Gerszten et al in 2005 and 2009 and shown to be clinically effective in patients with compression fractures.[12,18] The rate of vertebral body fracture progression at MD Anderson has recently been demonstrated to be 20%[9] and is as high as 39% in some series.[10] Given the high risk of vertebral body fracture in this patient population, the treatment paradigm of minimally invasive surgery for vertebral body augmentation (e.g., vertebroplasty or kyphoplasty) followed by SBRT for patients who are at risk for vertebral body compression fracture should be explored prospectively.

Additionally, a prospective trial comparing postoperative SBRT with conventional radiation could provide robust evidence as to whether SBRT translates into better clinical outcomes, especially if detailed clinical and radiographic response are compared. Additional studies on how to use surgical techniques to better separate the radiation target and the cord may potentially demonstrate the ability to further escalate the radiation dose. More studies are also needed to determine the true radiation dose tolerances of the spinal cord and other critical structures in the hypofractionated setting. This may help improve the amount of tissue that can be covered and potentially reduce the rate of failure at the epidural space. As more patients are living longer with metastatic cancer, innovations in both surgery and radiation techniques may allow us to take full advantage of the therapeutic window to balance effective treatment with limited morbidity.

Conclusion

The rationale for treating patients with spine metastases with SBRT in the postoperative setting is multifold. To date, the evidence supporting this treatment paradigm is based on retrospective data and phase I/II trials. Although it is difficult to compare directly the outcomes with conventional treatment, the literature on postoperative SBRT consistently demonstrates that the treatment is safe and effective. Future studies may show that the combination of surgery with SBRT results in even better outcomes and can offer patients with limited metastatic disease the chance of effective long-term palliation along with durable tumor control.

References

[1] Sahgal A, Bilsky M, Chang EL, et al. Stereotactic body radiotherapy for spinal metastases: current status, with a focus on its application in the postoperative patient. J Neurosurg Spine 2011; 14: 151–166

[2] Garg AK, Wang XS, Shiu AS, et al. Prospective evaluation of spinal reirradiation by using stereotactic body radiation therapy: The University of Texas MD Anderson Cancer Center experience. Cancer 2011; 117: 3509–3516

[3] Garg AK, Shiu AS, Yang J, et al. Phase 1/2 trial of single-session stereotactic body radiotherapy for previously unirradiated spinal metastases. Cancer 2012; 118: 5069–5077

[4] Cannady SB, Cavanaugh KA, Lee SY, et al. Results of whole brain radiotherapy and recursive partitioning analysis in patients with brain metastases from renal cell carcinoma: a retrospective study. Int J Radiat Oncol Biol Phys 2004; 58: 253–258

[5] Sundaresan N, Scher H, DiGiacinto GV, Yagoda A, Whitmore W, Choi IS. Surgical treatment of spinal cord compression in kidney cancer. J Clin Oncol 1986; 4: 1851–1856

[6] Maranzano E, Latini P. Effectiveness of radiation therapy without surgery in metastatic spinal cord compression: final results from a prospective trial. Int J Radiat Oncol Biol Phys 1995; 32: 959–967

[7] Patchell RA, Tibbs PA, Regine WF, et al. Direct decompressive surgical resection in the treatment of spinal cord compression caused by metastatic cancer: a randomised trial Lancet 2005; 366: 643–648

[8] Klekamp J, Samii H. Surgical results for spinal metastases. Acta Neurochir (Wien) 1998; 140: 957–967

[9] Boehling NS, Grosshans DR, Allen PK, et al. Vertebral compression fracture risk after stereotactic body radiotherapy for spinal metastases. J Neurosurg Spine 2012; 16: 379–386

[10] R , ose PS, Laufer I, Boland PJ, et al. Risk of fracture after single fraction image-guided intensity-modulated radiation therapy to spinal metastases. J Clin Oncol 2009; 27: 5075–5079

[11] Laufer I, Iorgulescu JB, Chapman T, et al. Local disease control for spinal metastases following "separation surgery" and adjuvant hypofractionated or high-dose single-fraction stereotactic radiosurgery: outcome analysis in 186 patients. J Neurosurg Spine 2013; 18: 207–214

[12] Gerszten PC, Germanwala A, Burton SA, Welch WC, Ozhasoglu C, Vogel WJ. Combination kyphoplasty and spinal radiosurgery: a new treatment paradigm for pathological fractures. J Neurosurg Spine 2005; 3: 296–301

[13] Rock JP, Ryu S, Shukairy MS, et al. Postoperative radiosurgery for malignant spinal tumors. Neurosurgery 2006; 58: 891–898, discussion 891–898

[14] Chang EL, Shiu AS, Mendel E, et al. Phase I/II study of stereotactic body radiotherapy for spinal metastasis and its pattern of failure. J Neurosurg Spine 2007; 7: 151–160

[15] Gerszten PC, Burton SA, Ozhasoglu C, Welch WC. Radiosurgery for spinal metastases: clinical experience in 500 cases from a single Institution Spine 2007; 32: 193–199

[16] Ryu S, Rock J, Rosenblum M, Kim JH. Patterns of failure after single-dose radiosurgery for spinal metastasis. J Neurosurg 2004; 101 (Suppl 3): 402–405

[17] Nguyen QN, Shiu AS, Rhines LD, et al. Management of spinal metastases from renal cell carcinoma using stereotactic body radiotherapy. Int J Radiat Oncol Biol Phys 2010; 76: 1185–1192

[18] Gerszten PC, Monaco EA. Complete percutaneous treatment of vertebral body tumors causing spinal canal compromise using a transpedicular cavitation, cement augmentation, and radiosurgical technique. Neurosurg Focus 2009; 27: E9

[19] Moulding HD, Elder JB, Lis E, et al. Local disease control after decompressive surgery and adjuvant high-dose single-fraction radiosurgery for spine metastases. J Neurosurg Spine 2010; 13: 87–93

37 Neoadjuvant Spinal Radiosurgery

Kevin C. Yao and Seth Blacksburg

Introduction

Stereotactic radiosurgery has emerged as a promising and exciting field in the management of primary and metastatic spinal malignancy. Much as intracranial radiosurgery redefined the roles of both surgery and conventional fractionated external beam radiotherapy for the treatment of intracranial pathology, spine radiosurgery is an evolving technique that is redefining the treatment paradigm of spinal neoplasms. The first application of spinal radiosurgery was to metastatic tumors wholly contained within the confines of the vertebral cortex, thereby providing a margin for radiation dose falloff between the tumor and the spinal cord. Results have been impressive, with excellent local control rates independent of radiosurgical treatment device, radiation delivery schedule, primary tumor histology, and history of prior radiation.[1–3] More recently, spine radiosurgery has also proven to be an effective adjuvant treatment following the surgical tumor debulking of spinal metastases causing spinal cord compression.[4] Despite its rise in popularity and use, the optimal timing and sequence of radiosurgery and surgery in the treatment of spinal neoplasms remain unknown.

As the field of spine radiosurgery progresses, not only will optimal radiosurgery doses and planning techniques be determined, but optimal timing and sequence of radiosurgery with surgery will also be elucidated. There is a slowly emerging body of research founded on the use of neoadjuvant radiosurgery for brain metastases.[5,6] By extension of principle, neoadjuvant radiosurgery, otherwise known as "planned preoperative" radiosurgery, may also provide significant benefit in the treatment of spinal neoplasms. In this chapter, we aim to highlight the potential advantages of neoadjuvant radiosurgery, particularly in comparison to the currently evolving paradigm of postoperative adjuvant spine radiosurgery. For the reasons discussed below, it is reasonable to forecast that future data concerning neoadjuvant spine radiosurgery may validate its approach, particularly when applied to metastatic epidural spinal cord compression and primary spinal tumors.

Rationale for Neoadjuvant Radiosurgery for Spinal Neoplasms

Neoadjuvant Radiosurgery Provides More Accurate Tumor Volume Contouring

A clear advantage to the neoadjuvant approach involves the ability to carefully delineate tumor volumes in unviolated tissue planes. Tumor volume delineation in the unoperated patient is generally straightforward. Using a combination of computed tomography (CT), magnetic resonance imaging (MRI), and occasionally CT myelography, excellent differentiation between spinal cord, thecal sac, and tumor is usually possible.[7] In contrast, the postoperative determination of tumor volumes may be quite difficult. Postoperative fibrosis and fluid often contrast enhance like unresected tumor on imaging. Furthermore, radiographic scatter and streak artifact from implanted instrumentation obscure the MR and CT imaging of residual tumor.[8,9] Consequently, postoperative treatment volumes are often contoured larger than necessary, incurring higher dose to surrounding organs and, therefore, increasing the potential for greater radiation toxicity.

To minimize the volume of irradiated uninvolved adjacent normal tissue, clinical judgment must be employed to discriminate between areas at high risk of harboring microscopic disease from normal postoperative radiographic signal change that does not contain malignant potential. This is, by nature, a subjective process. Preoperative and postoperative contoured tumor volumes are typically fused and compared. Whereas gross treatment volume (GTV) (the volume containing gross residual disease) is often apparent, differentiating normal postoperative radiographic signal change from clinical treatment volume (CTV) (the volume containing both GTV and areas of microscopic tumor within the tumor bed or vertebra that may contain malignant potential), can be very difficult. While the image fusion of preoperative and postoperative tumor volumes can be helpful, spine image fusion by itself is often fraught with imprecision. This is largely due to differences in patient positioning that can be further compounded by the postoperative radiographic change and surgical instrumentation that obscure anatomical landmarks used for image fusion. Furthermore, changes in spinal alignment brought about by surgery can also make spinal image fusion over several vertebral levels nearly impossible.

Ultimately, the treating physicians utilize fused preoperative and postoperative images while incorporating intraoperative surgical observations to identify GTV, CTV, and organs at risk, most notably spinal cord. The final result of this rigorous, but often multilayered subjective process, are postoperative treatment volumes that tend to be larger than necessary. These volumes are frequently larger than the preoperative tumor volume due to radiographic ambiguity and the natural tendency of treating physicians to over-, rather than under-, compensate for areas likely to harbor residual tumor. The existing small body of literature regarding postoperative radiosurgery has not demonstrated an increased risk of radiation myelopathy. However, as radiosurgery delivery devices become more precise and radiation doses escalate, more precise and accurate tumor volume delineation as provided by the neoadjuvant approach will ultimately make spine radiosurgery safer.

Upfront Radiosurgery May Obviate Surgery in the Setting of Epidural Compression

Patients with spinal cord compression are often symptomatic with signs of myelopathy that may include paresis, bladder dysfunction, or inability to ambulate. This unfortunate but not uncommon scenario traditionally has been deemed an emergency.[10–17] The customary position has been that every minute from the time of diagnosis until spinal cord decompression is achieved diminishes the likelihood that return of neurologic function will occur. Because the therapeutic tumor-shrinking effects of conventional external beam radiation have traditionally been considered minimal and delayed, this treatment modality has not been typically utilized in the setting of symptomatic neoplastic epidural compression except for exquisitely radiosensitive tumors such as lymphoma and multiple myeloma. In this limited setting, conventional external beam radiation has afforded only moderate success. For most other clinical scenarios involving neoplastic epidural compression, direct open surgical decompression of the spinal cord has been the traditional initial treatment of choice.[18,19]

Upfront spine radiosurgery has only been used sparingly in the setting of spinal cord compression.[1,20] Providing ablative doses of radiation to tumor while simultaneously minimizing spinal cord radiation dose is currently very difficult to achieve in the setting of spinal cord compression where the tumor directly abuts and compresses the spinal cord. Combined with the significant time required to adequately image, simulate, volume contour, and deliver radiation with current treatment planning systems, radiosurgery has not typically been used in the setting of clinical spinal cord compression.

Ryu et al published the only data (***level IV evidence***) to date regarding upfront radiosurgical treatment for metastatic epidural spinal cord compression.[21] In this cohort series, 62 patients harboring 85 tumors causing epidural compression, ranging from minimal canal compromise and thecal indentation to actual displacement of the spinal cord, were treated with radiosurgery. Radiosensitive tumors (e.g., lymphoma, multiple myeloma, small cell carcinoma, and germ cell tumors) were excluded, as were patients who demonstrated weakness graded 3 out of 5 or worse on the Medical Research Council scale. Patients were treated with both steroids and radiosurgery within 24 to 48 hours of the initial diagnosis. Linear accelerator (LINAC)–based radiosurgery dose ranged from 14 to 20 Gy prescribed to the 90% isodose line, delivered in a single fraction. The spinal cord dose constraint was 10 Gy delivered to no more than 10% of the contoured spinal cord volume. With a mean follow-up of 11.5 months following radiosurgery, the overall volumetric tumor response rate was 80%, including complete response in 27% (complete volumetric resolution of epidural tumor) and partial response in 30% (defined as more than 50% epidural tumor volume reduction). Fourteen percent of patients demonstrated no tumor volume reduction, whereas 6% of patients experienced tumor progression. Of the 35 patients who were neurologically intact at presentation, 33 patients (94%) remained neurologically intact at last follow-up. Among the 27 patients who presented with a neurologic deficit, 14 patients (52%) had complete recovery to normal, 3 patients (11%) improved, and another 3 (11%) remained unchanged or stable. Sixteen percent (9 of 62 patients) of patients deteriorated neurologically following treatment: 2 of these patients were neurologically intact at the time of presentation, whereas 7 patients had a pretreatment neurologic deficit. In no case was neurologic deterioration attributable to radiation myelopathy.

These class IV data demonstrate that a significant percentage, if not the majority, of patients with metastatic epidural compression can effectively be treated with spinal radiosurgery as upfront treatment. Following this treatment, only a minority of patients with metastatic epidural compression will deteriorate neurologically and/or demonstrate tumor growth. With more experience, stratification for predicting risk of failure following upfront radiosurgery for spinal neoplasms, both primary and metastatic, with or without epidural compression will likely be possible. This stratification would allow for the determination of the likelihood of tumor control based on tumor histology and several radiosurgical parameters determined prior to treatment. These parameters would likely include maximum achievable radiosurgical dose to epidural tumor and remaining GTV, and extent of dose distribution to the CTV and involved vertebral level. These parameters would be determinable after radiosurgery planning prior to treatment. The treating physician could therefore identify patients at a high risk of further tumor growth due to underdosing of tumor from spinal cord constraints. Parameters predictive of eventual pathologic collapse could also identify patients at risk for pathologic collapse after radiosurgery treatment. These patients, as well as those patients who demonstrate overt spinal instability at the time of presentation, would then require planned postradiosurgery surgical decompression and stabilization following upfront radiosurgery. This approach would effectively select for those patients who would best be served by sequencing both modalities for optimal treatment benefit.

One traditional rationale for not employing planned preoperative radiation is poor wound healing and associated wound complications.[4,22] In several series, preoperative conventional fractionated external beam radiotherapy for spinal metastatic disease resulted in wound complication rates of up to 30%. However, conformal stereotactic therapy effectively minimizes dose to the skin and subcutaneous tissues, thus theoretically minimizing these wound-related complications. As described above, radiosurgery treatment volumes tend to be larger in the postoperative setting as opposed to the preoperative setting. Consequently, dose to the subcutaneous tissues and skin is minimized with neoadjuvant radiosurgery. Soft tissue injury and vascular damage, both precursors to wound complications, are less likely to occur in the setting of neoadjuvant radiosurgery. Thus far, there is evidence to suggest that wound healing is not negatively affected in the setting of neoadjuvant radiosurgery for spinal tumors.

Preoperative Radiosurgery is Provided in a More Timely Manner than Postoperative Radiosurgery

There are several factors that theoretically render the timing of radiosurgery and surgery more predictable when radiosurgery is employed preoperatively rather than postoperatively. A schedule of neoadjuvant radiosurgery followed by surgery is more likely to be accelerated rather than delayed. Neurological deterioration following neoadjuvant radiosurgery prior to planned surgery would be the primary scenario that would affect the timing of planned surgical tumor resection. In this situation, such deterioration would most likely hasten the time to surgery.

In contrast, there are several factors that may potentially delay radiosurgery and allow tumor repopulation in the postoperative setting. Reestablishment of thecal sac patency does not always occur immediately following surgery. Despite adequate surgical thecal sac decompression and tumor resection, postoperative blood, seroma, or soft tissue edema may reconstitute the surgical void, thereby obliterating the surgically created margin around the thecal sac. Consequently, postoperative radiosurgery may be delayed up to several weeks or even months until thecal sac patency is restored. This clinical scenario might result in pressure to deliver the radiosurgery dose closer to the spinal cord than originally planned to avoid a delay in postoperative radiosurgery.

Successful patient immobilization for the safe application of radiosurgery may also be difficult to achieve in the immediate postoperative setting. Including patient setup and dose delivery, radiosurgery treatment can take 60 to 90 minutes, during which time the patient is expected to remain motionless, typically in a supine position. Patients recovering from recent surgery often cannot accomplish this due to incisional pain and muscular deconditioning. Consequently, postoperative radiosurgery may need to either be delayed or performed under anesthesia. Any delay to postoperative radiosurgery may allow tumor repopulation, which is particularly relevant in the metastatic population where tumor growth can occur rapidly when effective systemic therapy is not available or is once again withheld from the patient in the immediate postoperative setting. Therefore, neoadjuvant radiosurgery offers the optimal treatment delivery schedule to minimize the likelihood of tumor growth and maximize long-term tumor control.

Neoadjuvant Radiosurgery Increases Radiosensitivity and Makes Dose Delivery More Predictable

Another potential advantage to neoadjuvant radiosurgery is enhanced oxygenation of nearby tissues, a unique advantage to irradiating tissues prior to surgery. One of the main principles of radiation biology involves the relative biological advantage of treating a tumor in an oxygen-rich environment. The oxygen enhancement ratio (OER) is a formalized attempt to measure the difference in sensitivity of tumor cells to hypoxic and oxygen-rich environments. From numerous biological studies conducted during the mid- to late 20th century, it is known that hypoxic cells are resistant to low linear energy transfer (LET) radiation, such as X-rays and protons. Poorly vascularized regions, including postoperative tissue with small vessel destruction and vascular distortion, likely have lower concentrations of oxygen with the potential for suboptimal tumor kill as compared to tissues not violated by surgery.[23]

Dose deflection from surgical instrumentation can also make dose delivery less reliable. Studies regarding this potential uncertainty have unfortunately been limited in scope. The general premise is that both contouring and treatment planning are based on diagnostic kilovoltage CT imaging. The difficulty in outlining postoperative residual tumor due to scatter artifact has previously been described. However, commercially available treatment planning software uses the same CT imaging. Treatment software calculates dose based on tissue density and, hence, attenuation of dose deposited in tissues, which in the case of metallic artifact, can be erroneous. The algorithm used by such software effectively lacks the ability to take into account the actual density and atomic number (Z) of the particular metal instrumentation. Thus, titanium, steel, and cobalt alloy-based implants are all treated equally. From principles involving the interaction of photons with metals, areas close to metal have higher doses deposited related to Compton (back) scatter; the degree of this is related, in turn, to the energy of photons and the type of metal. The actual result of this uncertainty is the potential for areas of increased dose abutting metal, with decreased dose downstream. It is important to note that these effects are likely diminished with the utilization of multiple beam arrangements. However, especially as the treatment planning software does not take these actual changes in real dose deposition into account, it remains a real theoretical disadvantage to a modality that relies on steep dose gradients to maximally spare dose-sensitive structures such as the spinal cord. Although similar dosimetric issues might be more popularized for cases of hip prostheses in the definitive radiation treatment for prostate cancer, it is relatively unique from a stereotactic treatment perspective in the setting of adjacent critical radiation-sensitive tissues.[24–26]

Neoadjuvant Radiosurgery and Conventional Radiation: Proof of Principle

The utilization of neoadjuvant radiation—often concurrent with chemotherapy—to sterilize presurgical fields and enhance the ability for gross total tumor resection is well characterized in various malignancies. Similarly, an advantage of radiosurgery for spinal lesions is the theoretical ability to facilitate negative margins with oncologic resections as well as to decrease spillage of viable tumor from intralesional surgery. Even with the sharp delineation of tumor and prescription of full dose to a planning treatment volume (PTV), a significant portion of low dose radiation is received by adjacent regions that might harbor microscopic disease. Theoretically, this surrounding lower dose might sterilize subclinical disease and enhance surgical outcomes.

Neoadjuvant radiosurgery is particularly attractive in the treatment of primary spinal tumors such as chordoma, chondrosarcoma, and sarcoma. In these tumors, en bloc tumor resection has been reported to offer the most durable long-term local control. However, en bloc surgery remains a highly technical and morbid surgical procedure that is often not applicable to a large percentage of patients due to proximity of the tumor to critical structures. Preliminary results of neoadjuvant radiotherapy for primary spine tumors have been promising. DeLaney et al employed a conventional fractionation approach for 50 patients with chordomas or primary spine sarcomas; 37 patients went on to receive surgical resection, with 5-year local control and disease-free survival rates of 78 and 63%, respectively.[27] Wu et al reported the outcome for a 72-year-old patient treated with a single fraction of 24 Gy to an L3 vertebral body chordoma. At 4 months after treatment, the tumor was resected due to symptoms of mechanical instability. Pathology at that time showed 99% tumor necrosis.[28] These anecdotal reports provide only ***level IV*** data. Nevertheless, it is reasonable to conclude that the neoadjuvant radiosurgery approach for the treatment of primary spinal tumors is a paradigm that warrants further investigation.

Conclusion

Neoadjuvant radiosurgery is a promising treatment that may prove to be the most rational means of applying radiosurgery to spinal neoplasms. Due to the lack of ***level I, II,*** or ***III*** data, this approach can currently only be recommended weakly. However, in the foreseeable future, the evolution of radiation treatment planning devices and radiosurgery delivery techniques will dovetail with the development of a sophisticated understanding of hypofractionated radiobiology. These advances will likely result in upfront radiosurgery emerging as the initial treatment modality of choice for most spinal neoplasms. Preliminary data being accrued at institutions performing the first trials of neoadjuvant radiosurgery for spine tumors will help define the potential efficacy of this neoadjuvant approach. Eventually clinical trials comparing outcomes of neoadjuvant radiosurgery to postoperative radiosurgery will be necessary.

References

[1] Yamada Y, Bilsky MH, Lovelock DM, et al. High-dose, single-fraction image-guided intensity-modulated radiotherapy for metastatic spinal lesions. Int J Radiat Oncol Biol Phys 2008; 71: 484–490

[2] Ryu S, Rock J, Rosenblum M, Kim JH. Patterns of failure after single-dose radiosurgery for spinal metastasis. J Neurosurg 2004; 101 (Suppl 3): 402–405

[3] Ryu S, Fang Yin F, Rock J, et al. Image-guided and intensity-modulated radiosurgery for patients with spinal metastasis. Cancer 2003; 97: 2013–2018

[4] Itshayek E, Yamada J, Bilsky M, et al. Timing of surgery and radiotherapy in the management of metastatic spine disease: a systematic review. Int J Oncol 2010; 36: 533–544

[5] Yamamoto MKT, Kawabe T, Barfod B, et al. Can pre-operative GKRS prevent meningeal dissemination in brain met patients? A case-matched study. Paper presented at: the 10th Biennial Congress and Exhibition of the International Stereotactic Radiosurgery Society; May 2011; Paris, France

[6] Chang JH. The comparative results of neoadjuvant radiosurgery, adjuvant radiosurgery, and adjuvant WBRT for treatment of large metastatic brain tumors. Paper presented at: the 10th Biennial Congress and Exhibition of the International Stereotactic Radiosurgery Society; May 2011; Paris, France

[7] Dahele M, Zindler JD, Sanchez E, et al. Imaging for stereotactic spine radiotherapy: clinical considerations. Int J Radiat Oncol Biol Phys 2011; 81: 321–330

[8] Thariat J, Castelli J, Chanalet S, Marcie S, Mammar H, Bondiau PY. CyberKnife stereotactic radiotherapy for spinal tumors: value of computed tomographic myelography in spinal cord delineation. Neurosurgery 2009; 64 (Suppl): A60–A66

[9] Sahgal A, Bilsky M, Chang EL, et al. Stereotactic body radiotherapy for spinal metastases: current status, with a focus on its application in the postoperative patient. J Neurosurg Spine 2011; 14: 151–166

[10] Siegal T. Spinal cord compression: from laboratory to clinic. Eur J Cancer 1995; 31A: 1748–1753

[11] Maranzano E, Latini P. Effectiveness of radiation therapy without surgery in metastatic spinal cord compression: final results from a prospective trial. Int J Radiat Oncol Biol Phys 1995; 32: 959–967

[12] Bach F, Larsen BH, Rohde K, et al. Metastatic spinal cord compression: occurrence, symptoms, clinical presentations and prognosis in 398 patients with spinal cord compression. Acta Neurochir (Wien) 1990; 107: 37–43

[13] Helweg-Larsen S, Johnsen A, Boesen J, Sørensen PS. Radiologic features compared to clinical findings in a prospective study of 153 patients with metastatic spinal cord compression treated by radiotherapy. Acta Neurochir (Wien) 1997; 139: 105–111

[14] Maranzano E, Latini P, Beneventi S, et al. Comparison of two different radiotherapy schedules for spinal cord compression in prostate cancer. Tumori 1998; 84: 472–477

[15] Kim RY, Spencer SA, Meredith RF, et al. Extradural spinal cord compression: analysis of factors determining functional prognosis—prospective study. Radiology 1990; 176: 279–282

[16] Greenberg HS, Kim JH, Posner JB. Epidural spinal cord compression from metastatic tumor: results with a new treatment protocol. Ann Neurol 1980; 8: 361–366

[17] Martenson JA, Evans RG, Lie MR, et al. Treatment outcome and complications in patients treated for malignant epidural spinal cord compression (SCC). J Neurooncol 1985; 3: 77–84

[18] van den Bent MJ. Surgical resection improves outcome in metastatic epidural spinal cord compression. Lancet 2005; 366: 609–610

[19] Patchell RA, Tibbs PA, Regine WF, et al. Direct decompressive surgical resection in the treatment of spinal cord compression caused by metastatic cancer: a randomised trial. Lancet 2005; 366: 643–648

[20] Gerszten PC, Burton SA, Ozhasoglu C, Welch WC. Radiosurgery for spinal metastases: clinical experience in 500 cases from a single institution. Spine 2007; 32: 193–199

[21] Ryu S, Rock J, Jain R, et al. Radiosurgical decompression of metastatic epidural compression. Cancer 2010; 116: 2250–2257

[22] Ghogawala Z, Mansfield FL, Borges LF. Spinal radiation before surgical decompression adversely affects outcomes of surgery for symptomatic metastatic spinal cord compression. Spine 2001; 26: 818–824

[23] Hall EJ. Radiobiology for the Radiologist. Hagerstown, MD: Harper & Row; 1973

[24] Su A, Reft C, Rash C, Price J, Jani AB. A case study of radiotherapy planning for a bilateral metal hip prosthesis prostate cancer patient. Med Dosim 2005; 30: 169–175

[25] Reft C, Alecu R, Das IJ, et al. AAPM Radiation Therapy Committee Task Group 63. Dosimetric considerations for patients with HIP prostheses undergoing pelvic irradiation: report of the AAPM Radiation Therapy Committee Task Group 63. Med Phys 2003; 30: 1162–1182

[26] Lin SY, Chu TC, Lin JP, Liu MT. The effect of a metal hip prosthesis on the radiation dose in therapeutic photon beam irradiations. Appl Radiat Isot 2002; 57: 17–23

[27] DeLaney TF, Liebsch NJ, Pedlow FX, et al. Phase II study of high-dose photon/proton radiotherapy in the management of spine sarcomas. Int J Radiat Oncol Biol Phys 2009; 74: 732–739

[28] Wu AJ, Bilsky MH, Edgar MA, et al. Near-complete pathological response of chordoma to high-dose single-fraction radiotherapy: case report. Neurosurgery. 2009; 64: E389–E390, discussion E390

Benign Spine Tumors

38 Treatment of Benign Spinal Tumors with Surgery

Lee Hwang, Jason Liauw, Sheng-fu Larry Lo, and Timothy Witham

Extramedullary spinal tumors represent the majority of intradural spinal tumors in both adults and in children. The most common primary intradural extramedullary lesions are derived from meningeal cells (meningiomas) or nerve sheath cells (schwannomas and neurofibromas). The majority of spinal meningiomas, schwannomas, and neurofibromas are noninfiltrative, histologically benign, and amenable to complete open surgical resection. On the other hand, certain patients are less than ideal candidates for the standard surgical resection due to their age and medical comorbidities, the recurrent nature of a tumor type, or the presence of multiple lesions in the setting of familial phakomatoses. In these cases, additional therapeutic modalities, including stereotactic radiosurgery, are available as an alternative to surgical resection. Microsurgical resection remains the treatment of choice for benign spinal tumors that cause myeloradiculopathy and/or spinal cord compression.

In this chapter, we assess the clinical and radiological outcomes of the surgical management for the most frequently encountered benign extramedullary spinal tumors. At the same time, we hope to emphasize the pivotal role of surgery as a safe and effective therapeutic option for patients with these benign spinal tumors.

■ Spinal Meningiomas

Representing 25 to 45% of spinal tumors, spinal meningiomas occur less frequently than intracranial meningiomas. The majority of spinal meningiomas are meningoepithelial (29–59%) or psammomatous (21–57%). Anaplastic meningiomas of the spine are less common. Approximately 80% of cases involve the thoracic spine; low cervical and lumbar meningiomas are rare. In the younger population, cervical meningiomas are more common and account for 14.0 to 18.5% of spinal meningiomas.[1] Cervical meningiomas are frequently located anterior to the spinal cord, which may complicate the open surgical management. Most spinal meningiomas are entirely intradural, but up to 10% may be both intradural and extradural or entirely extradural. Unlike intracranial meningiomas, spinal meningiomas do not penetrate the pia and usually manifest signs of spinal cord compression relatively early. Meningiomas with extradural extension have been described as more aggressive variants. Additionally, their resection is often complicated by epidural bleeding and indistinct tumor planes. En plaque meningiomas are rarer and may be difficult to remove, often requiring multiple surgical resections. Favorable features include an absence of ventral location and lack of bone or major blood vessel involvement. Genetic predisposition, neurofibromatosis type 2 (NF2), and prior exposure to ionizing radiation are all well-established risk factors.[2]

Asymptomatic patients with spinal meningiomas can be followed clinically with serial imaging studies. Treatment is indicated in the presence of severe pain, significant neurologic deficits, aggressive growth, or spinal cord compression on imaging. Surgical resection is usually recommended, given that meningiomas tend to be extramedullary with a distinct plane of surgical dissection (▶ Fig. 38.1), and complete surgical removal can be achieved in > 90% of cases.

After gross total resection of spinal meningiomas, the tumor recurrence rate ranges from 1.3[3] to 13%.[4] In general, complete resection is achievable with an identifiable tumor–spinal cord plane of dissection as long as the dural involvement is not too extensive or ventral. The intraoperative decision to pursue subtotal resection is usually based on the size of the tumor, histological features that indicate a high grade lesion, location relative to the spinal cord, and involvement of adjacent vasculature.

▶ Table 38.1 summarizes the surgical series describing outcomes with resection of spinal meningiomas. King et al[3] conducted a prospective study between 1974 and 1994, and 77 out of 78 patients underwent a gross total resection of spinal meningiomas. Ninety-five percent of their patients showed improvement and were independently mobile upon follow-up evaluations. Three of the four patients who were paraplegic prior to surgery were asymptomatic after long-term recovery. One of these patients died postoperatively secondary to a pulmonary embolism. The tumor recurrence rate was 1.3%, the lowest reported in the literature. Solero et al[5] also performed a prospective study with a mean follow-up period of 15 years. One hundred fifty out of 156 patients underwent gross total resection, and 6% of these patients experienced tumor recurrence, compared to 17% of patients who underwent subtotal tumor resection; 92% of the total patient population reported absent or mild neurologic impairment postoperatively. The mortality rate was 1.4%; however, 16 patients were lost to follow-up evaluation. In another prospective study, Setzer et al[6] performed gross total resection of spinal meningiomas in 75 out of 80 patients with a mean follow-up period of 43.5 months. The recurrence rate of 10% was associated only with high-grade and atypical low-grade lesions. Postoperative neurologic function improved in 71% of patients and remained unchanged in 23%. The mortality rate was 1.25%, whereas the complication rate was 5%. The most common complications were cerebrospinal fluid (CSF) leak or fistula, spinal instability, wound infection, and deep venous thrombosis or pulmonary embolism.

More recent retrospective studies report similar findings. Sandalcioglu et al[7] operated on 131 patients with a mean follow-up period of 61 months. The tumor recurred in four patients, three of whom were initially treated with gross total resection. All recurrent tumors required repeat surgical resection. Thirty-nine percent of patients were unable to ambulate independently preoperatively, but 69% of these patients regained the ability to ambulate postoperatively. Overall, 96% of patients experienced improvement or no change in neurologic function postoperatively. One patient died, and three patients experienced postoperative complications with full recovery. Similarly, Postalci et al[8] treated 38 out of 46 patients with gross total resection. There was no case of tumor recurrence after gross total resection, but all eight patients who underwent subtotal resection experienced tumor recurrence. Seven out of these eight patients underwent a repeat operation; one elderly patient was treated nonsurgically due to medical comorbidities. At the latest follow-up evaluation, 61% of patients demonstrated

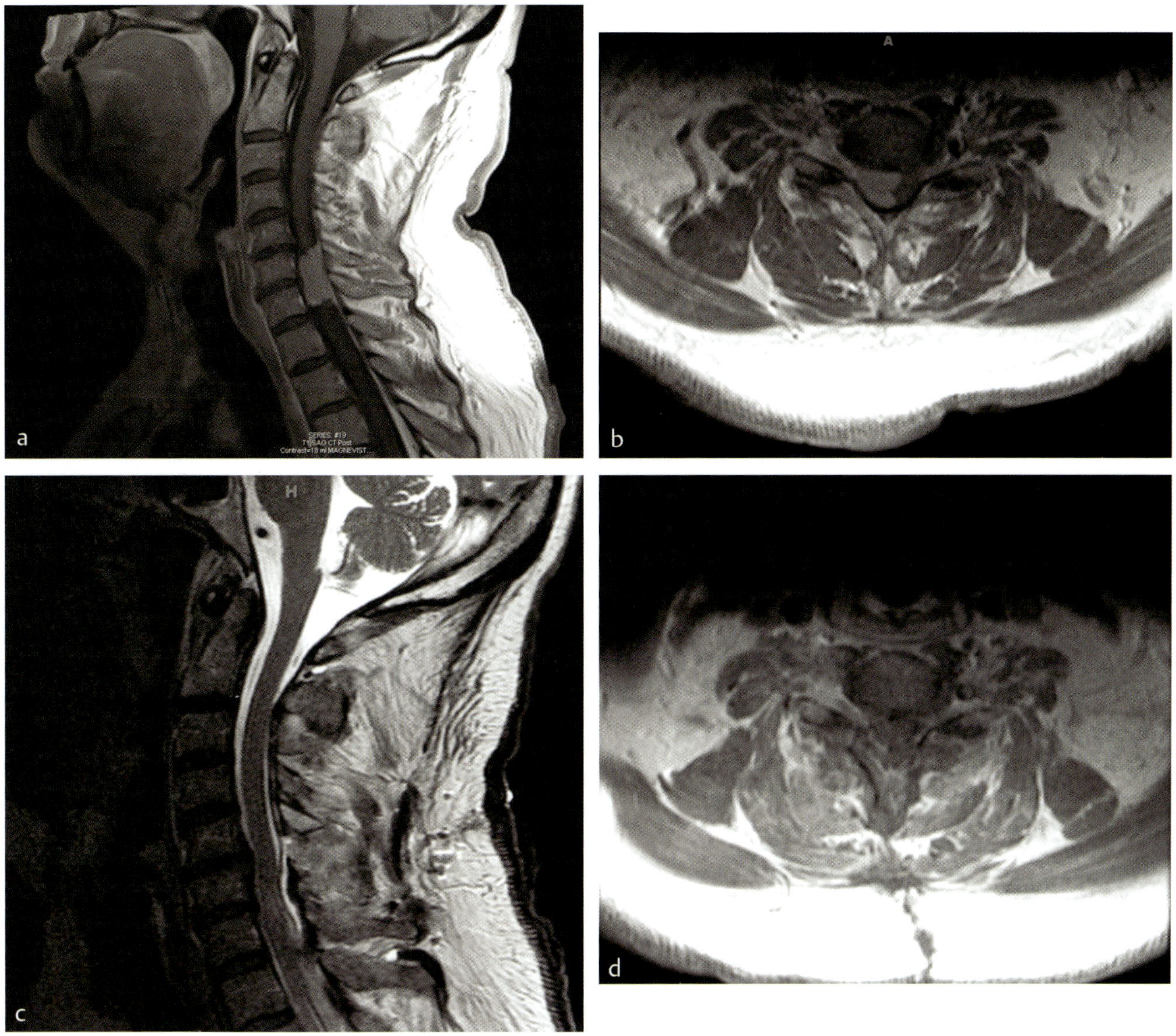

Fig. 38.1 The patient is a 61-year-old man who presented with progressive neck pain, right upper extremity pain, right lower extremity weakness, paresthesias, and gait dysfunction. He underwent C6 and C7 laminoplasty and microscope-assisted resection of this dural-based intradural extramedullary tumor that proved to be a typical meningioma. He was discharged without any complications on postoperative day 3. Preoperative imaging): Contrast-enhanced T1-weighted magnetic resonance imaging (MRI), (a) sagittal and (b) axial views, showing dural-based mass causing severe spinal cord compression and significant motor deficit. In this case, surgical resection is preferable over radiosurgery, which would not adequately, rapidly, and reliably decompress the spinal cord. In addition, the potential risk of radiation-induced myelopathy must be considered given the extent of spinal cord compression. Postoperative imaging: T2-weighted MRI sagittal view (c) and contrast enhanced T1-weighted MRI axial view (d) showing decompression of the spinal cord and complete resection of the spinal meningioma

improved neurologic function, whereas 30% remained unchanged. Fifteen percent of patients experienced postoperative complications, which were transient or nondebilitating. In the most recent retrospective study by Nakamura et al,[9] 62 out of 68 patients underwent gross total resection, and ~ 10% of these patients experienced tumor recurrence. However, all six patients who initially underwent subtotal resection experienced tumor recurrence. The authors surmise that the higher tumor recurrence rate may be due to the lower mean patient age at the time of surgery (56 y) and the longer mean postoperative follow-up period (12 y).

Several other studies have reported tumor recurrence rates higher than the range usually encountered in the literature. Klekamp and Samii[10] treated 115 out of 117 patients with gross total resection of spinal meningiomas. For these patients, the tumor recurrence rate was 14.6% at 1 year and 29.5% at 5 years. The two patients who underwent subtotal resection both experienced tumor recurrence at 5 years. 80% of the 31 patients who were nonambulatory preoperatively became independently mobile after surgery. The mortality rate was 5.1%, and the overall complication rate was 11.2%. Similarly, Cohen-Gadol et al[1,1] reported a higher than expected tumor recurrence rate.

Table 38.1 Surgical series for spinal meningioma resection

Study	Level of evidence	Treatment (surgery or surgery + radiotherapy [RT])	No. patients	Tumor recurrence	Neurologic outcome	Complications
Solero et al[5]	II-1 Mean f/u 15 y	S	156 (150 GTR + 6 STR)	6 (GTR) 17 (STR)	92% mild impairment, 8% severe impairment (*n* = 126)	1.4% mortality (2 died immediately postop; 29 unrelated deaths)
Roux et al[14]	III-2 Mean f/u 28 mo	S + RT (RT for 2 patients w/recurrence after 2–3 y)	54 (50 GTR)	3.7 (STR)	85% very good (walk normally), 13% stable 2% worse (Nurick's grade)	No mortality
King et al[3]	II-1	S	78 (77 GTR)	1.3	95% improved (independently mobile)	1.3% mortality (1 died 2/2 PE), 1 paraplegia, 3 CSF leak
Klekamp & Samii[10]	II-1	S	117 (115 GTR)	14.6 at 1 y, 29.5 at 5 y (GTR); 52 at 1 y, 100 at 5 y (STR)	80% of 31 patients independently mobile (not walk preop)	6 died 2/2 cardiopulmonary causes; 11.2% complication rate (infection, meningitis, CSF leak, hemorrhage, instability, UTI)
Gezen et al[13]	III-2 f/u 2–15 y	S + RT	36 (35 GTR; 2 surgery + radiotherapy)	5.6 (2 patients: 5 y s/p STR and 8 y s/p GTR)	83% improved, 14% unchanged (Cooper-Epstein grade of UE/LE)	3 unrelated deaths: 1 CSF leak, 2 wound infection
Gottfried et al[15]	IV	S + RT	25 (23 GTR; 1 surgery + radiotherapy)	4	75–97% ambulatory (33–74% preop)	No M/M
Cohen-Gadol et al[11]	III-2 (age < 50 y)	S	40	22.5 (20% in 10 patients age < 21 y)	Almost all with ataxia improved; 10/16 w/preop weakness complete resolution and 5/16 unchanged; 12/16 normal bladder control; 27/32 sensory improved postop	4 died (1 prolonged intubation, 2 NF2 progression, 1 incompletely resected malignant meningioma); 20% complication rate (spine instability, CSF leaks)
Setzer et al[6]	II-1 Mean f/u 43.5 mo	S (RT for 2 high-grade and 1 progressive atypical low-grade)	80 (75 GTR)	10 (high-grade or atypical)	25% symptom free; 38.8% mild deficits; 17.5% sensorimotor deficits but ambulating; 10% more severe deficits requiring orthotics; 3.75% major deficits and fully dependent (71.3% improved, 22.5% stable, 5% deteriorated/died)	1.25% mortality; 5% complication rate (CSF leak, wound infection, PE)
Sandalcioglu et al[7]	III-2 Mean f/u 61 mo	S	131	3 (4 patients) 3 s/p GTR and 1 s/p STR	39% unable to walk independently preop; 96.2% improved or unchanged; 3% worse	0.8% mortality (1 died 2/2 MI), 1 DVT, 1 CSF fistula, 1 prolonged wound healing (all recovered completely w/conservative tx)
Zada[37]	III-2 Mean f/u 75 mo	S + RT	116 (72 surgery + radiotherapy)	6 (7 patients) Mean progression time 90 mo	unavailable	1 pediatric patient died after 7 y; 8% complication rate (CN III deficit, cerebral edema or necrosis, hydrocephalus)
Postalci et al[8]	III-2	S	46 (38 GTR)	17 (8 patients all s/p STR), 7/8 reoperate (not 1 elderly w/comorbidities)	61% improved; 30% unchanged; 9% deterioration	15% complication rate (transient neuro deficits and CSF fistula)

Table 38.1 continued

Study	Level of evidence	Treatment (surgery or surgery + radiotherapy [RT])	No. patients	Tumor recurrence	Neurologic outcome	Complications
Nakamura et al[9]	III-2	S	68 (62 GTR)	9.7% (GTR); all 6 STR recurred, reoperate in 5 y average	unavailable	unavailable

Abbreviations: *CN III, third cranial nerve; CSF, cerebrospinal fluid; DVT, deep venous thrombosis; f/u, follow-up; GTR, gross total resection; LE, lower extremity; MI, myocardial infarction; M/M, TK; NF2, neurofibromatosis type 2; PE, pulmonary embolis; s/p, status post; STR, subtotal resection; UE, TK; UTI, urinary tract infection.*

Their retrospective study assessed 40 patients, all under the age of 50. Nine patients experienced tumor recurrence, and only one of these patients initially underwent gross total resection. This unusually high recurrence rate of 22.5% is similar to the 20% reported by Deen et al[12] in 10 patients under the age of 21. The mortality rate and complication rate were also unusually high at 10% and 20%, respectively. On the other hand, the number of patients included in these two studies was lower than the others. Overall, outcomes from surgical resection of spinal meningiomas are favorable and often lead to acceptable functional status. However, it appears that spinal meningiomas affecting younger aged patients tend to present more aggressively, have a higher incidence of epidural extension, and often require repeat resection.

The literature supports the fact that the optimal treatment for primary spinal meningioma is gross total microsurgical resection. Some authors advocate adjunctive radiotherapy in the setting of tumor recurrence. Additionally, stereotactic radiosurgery may be a treatment option even after gross total resection in order to irradiate the adjacent dura that may contain infiltrative neoplastic cells (▶ Fig. 38.2). In a retrospective analysis with a follow-up period of 2 to 15 years, Gezen et al[13] assessed 36 patients, 35 of whom underwent gross total resection of spinal meningiomas. One patient who initially underwent subtotal resection experienced tumor recurrence after 5 years, whereas one patient who initially underwent gross total resection experienced tumor recurrence after 8 years. Both of these patients were treated with repeat operations along with adjuvant radiotherapy. Neither experienced recurrence after combination therapy. Roux et al[14] also performed radiosurgery for two patients with recurrent tumors after subtotal resection. They were both stable at follow-up evaluation after 5 years. Gottfried et al[15] performed gross total resection for 23 out of 25 patients. One patient experienced tumor recurrence 2 years after a subtotal resection. After a second operation, this patient received adjuvant radiotherapy which resulted in decreased tumor size as well as long-term stabilization of neurologic function.

As radiosurgery for spinal tumors is increasingly becoming a popular option in patients with medical comorbidities or multiple spinal lesions, the long-term benefit of radiosurgery still remains to be determined. When treating spinal meningiomas, an approach incorporating both surgical and radiosurgical options may be preferable as they are not mutually exclusive. Such combination therapy can often be implemented after subtotal resection to reduce tumor growth and recurrence.

It is the authors' experience that limitations to radiosurgery include tumor size relative to the compressed spinal cord and patients presenting with a motor deficit. Although radiosurgery has shown to halt the growth of spinal meningiomas in some circumstances,[16,17] individuals presenting with a motor deficit may not benefit due to the lack of timely decompression. In fact, many tumors will become more edematous following radiosurgery, which may be devastating in the setting of severe spinal cord compression.

Spinal Schwannomas

Nerve sheath tumors, schwannomas, and neurofibromas, account for up to one third of intradural spinal tumors in adults, and most are solitary schwannomas that develop proportionally throughout the spinal column. Anatomically, schwannomas tend to arise from the dorsal nerve roots. Most lesions are entirely intradural but 30% extend through the dural root sleeve, resulting in a dumbbell shape with both intradural and extradural components.[18]

Both neurofibromatosis type 1 (NF1) and type 2 (NF2) are associated with nerve sheath tumors. Schwannomas are more common in NF2 and tend to be more aggressive than those not associated with NF2. Multiple schwannomas can develop without neurofibromatosis in a syndrome referred to as schwannomatosis.[19]

▶ Table 38.2 and 38.3 provide a summary of surgical outcomes for the resection of spinal nerve sheath tumors with levels of evidence. Due to the well-documented benign nature of sporadic spinal schwannomas, gross total surgical removal is usually attempted and successfully achieved. In a retrospective study by Kim et al,[20] 31 complete resections were performed with less than 23% of patients experiencing postoperative neurologic deficits, none of which were functionally debilitating. Tumor recurrence rate and postoperative complications were not reported. Seppälä et al[18] retrospectively assessed 187 patients, 167 of whom underwent gross total resection of spinal schwannomas over a mean follow-up period of 12.9 years. The 11 patients who experienced tumor recurrence all initially underwent subtotal resection. Seventy-eight percent of patients improved clinically, and 81% of patients who were unable to walk independently before surgery became ambulatory postoperatively. The most common early complications included local and radiating pain, and late complications included cystic myelopathy (2%), spinal arachnoiditis (6%), and spinal deformity (6%), as well as severe pain (7%).

More recent retrospective studies report similar findings. Conti et al[21] operated on 152 patients with a mean follow-up period of 17.5 years. The tumor recurrence rate was 4.5% and was noted only in cases of subtotal resection. The 1.4% mortality rate was due to unrelated causes. Safavi-Abbasi et al[22]

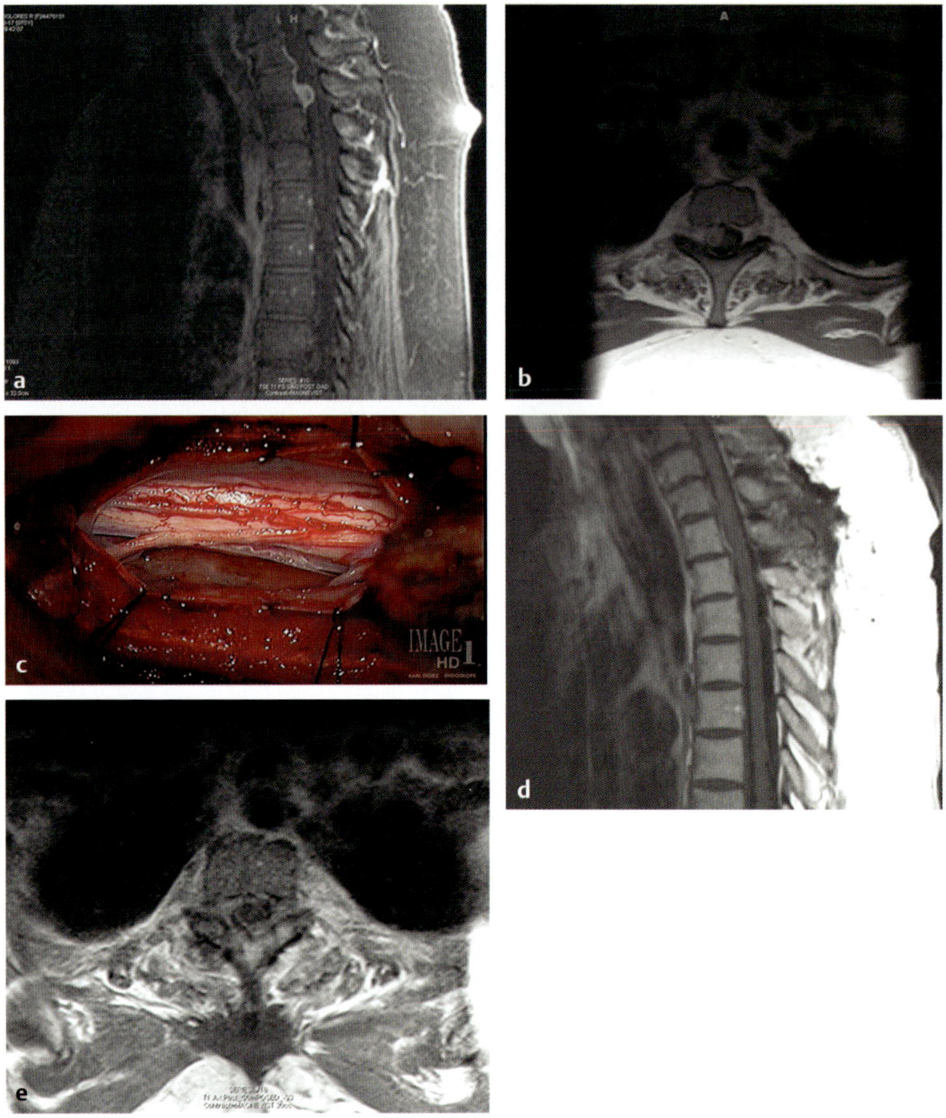

Fig. 38.2 The patient is a 71-year-old woman who presented with what was thought to be cervical myelopathy and gait dysfunction. However, cervical spine imaging did not demonstrate significant stenosis, and a lesion was identified at the T2–T3 level with spinal cord compression. She underwent a T2 laminoplasty with resection of this intradural extramedullary lesion that proved to be a typical meningioma. There were no immediate postoperative complications, but she returned to the clinic with swelling and discomfort at the base of her neck. Imaging revealed a pseudomeningocele that was successfully treated with 5 days of lumbar drainage with complete resolution of her symptoms. Preoperative imaging: contrast-enhanced T1-weighted MRI, (a) sagittal and (b) axial views, showing a lesion at T2–T3 with spinal cord compression. (c) Intraoperative imaging after complete tumor resection. Postoperative imaging: contrast enhanced T1-weighted MRI (d) sagittal and (e) axial views showing complete tumor resection and decompression of the spinal cord. The dural enhancement was sagittal, imaging was closely followed. In this case, recurrence after serial imaging would be optimally treated with radiosurgery given that the diagnosis was well-established and that radiosurgery would effectively prevent further growth of such a lesion.

performed gross total resection in 127 out of 131 patients with a mean follow-up period of 4.25 years. The 2.3% mortality rate was due to unrelated causes. Surprisingly, the 3.9% tumor recurrence rate was associated with only gross total resection. The lack of tumor recurrence after subtotal resection may be due to the short-term follow-up period; in addition, eight patients were lost to follow-up evaluation.

In summary, the tumor recurrence rate for spinal schwannomas ranges between 3.9 and 5.9%, predominantly associated with subtotal resection. The mortality rates as well as perioperative complication rates are low, though late complications have been reported.[15]

The role of adjuvant radiotherapy remains controversial due to the lack of large-scale studies with long-term follow-up evaluations. Murovic et al[23] reported that out of eight patients with spinal schwannomas who underwent a single operation, symptoms improved in seven patients. The two patients who were treated with surgery followed by radiosurgery both experienced symptom improvement. One patient who underwent surgery clinically improved, received radiosurgery, and then worsened after 48 months. The authors concluded that any patient with signs and symptoms of myeloradiculopathy and with MRI evidence of spinal cord compression should undergo surgical tumor debulking prior to radiosurgery for optimal outcome.

Spinal Neurofibromas

The spinal nerve root tumors in NF1 are typically neurofibromas. Unlike schwannomas, neurofibromas more frequently involve the ventral root. Other than this anatomical difference, schwannomas and neurofibromas can be indistinguishable on MRI.[24] Multiple neurofibromas help to establish the diagnosis of NF1, but this syndrome should be considered even in patients with solitary lesions.

Complete surgical excision is the treatment of choice for these benign nerve sheath tumors, especially for patients with

Table 38.2 Surgical outcomes for resection of spinal schwannomas

Study	Level of evidence	Treatment (surgery [S] or surgery + radiotherapy [RT])	No. patients	Tumor recurrence (%)
Kim et al[20]	III-2	S	31 (all GTR)	unavailable
Seppälä et al[18]	III-2 Mean f/u 12.9 y	S	187 (167 GTR)	5.9 (11/20 all s/p STR); only two repeat operations (others conservative tx due to medical comorbidities)
Conti et al[21]	III-2 Mean f/u 17.5 y	S	152	4.46% all s/p STR
Safavi-Abbasi et al[22]	III-2 Mean f/u 4.25 y	S	131 (127 GTR)	3.9% all s/p GTR
Murovic et al[23]	III-2 f/u 2–24 mo	S + RT	11 (4 surgery + radiotherapy)	unavailable

Abbreviations: *f/u, follow-up; GTR, gross total resection; s/p, status post; STR, subtotal resection; tx, treatment*

Table 38.3 Surgical outcomes for resection of spinal neurofibromas

Study	Level of evidence	Treatment (surgery [S] or surgery + radiotherapy [RT])	No. patients	Tumor recurrence (%)	Neurologic outcome	Complications
Seppälä et al[18]	III-2	S	32 (26 GTR; 22 w/NF1)	12.5% (4/32: 3 with NF1); 7 second new tumor; 4 multiple new tumors	Out of 15 alive: 69% improved; 12% unchanged; 16% deteriorated; 2 remained paraplegic; 1 symptom free; 8 local neck/back pain; 6 radicular pain; 1 severe dysesthetic pain; 6 sensory deficit (preoperative deficit in 2); 5 mild motor weakness; 9 walked normally (6 with NF1); 2 bladder dysfunction (1 with NF1)	53% mortality (17/32: 11 NF1) Late complications: Spinal deformity in 2 NF1 patients, severe dysesthesia in 2 patients (1 NF1 and 1 non-NF1)
Murovic 2010	III-2 f/u 2–24 mo	S + RT	4 (3 w/NF1; 1 patient 2 surgeries + radiotherapy)	25%	2/3 improved and 1/3 unchanged with surgery alone; 1 patient unchanged or improved after 2 surgeries + CyberKnife	unavailable

symptomatic or enlarging lesions. Seppälä et al[25] retrospectively assessed 32 patients, 26 of whom underwent gross total resection of spinal neurofibromas. Four patients experienced tumor recurrence (12.5%), and three of these patients were previously diagnosed with NF1. Seven patients developed a second tumor, and four patients developed multiple new tumors. Eleven out of the 17 patients who died (53% mortality rate) were previously diagnosed with NF1. Of the 15 patients alive, 69% experienced improved neurologic function, 12% remained unchanged, and 16% clinically deteriorated. Only one patient was reported to be free of symptoms. Late complications included spinal deformities in two NF1 patients and severe dysesthesias in two (one NF1 and one non-NF1) patients.

The overall poor outlook associated with spinal neurofibromas is most likely related to the younger age at presentation compared with spinal schwannomas. Levi et al[26] reported that the average age at presentation for spinal neurofibromas was 39.8 years, which was significantly lower than the average age at presentation for schwannomas (52.2 y). Furthermore, neurofibroma excision tends to be more difficult and complicates the decision between attempting gross total resection and preserving neurologic function.

Murovic et al[23] treated four patients with spinal neurofibromas. Three patients had NF1, and one of these patients underwent radiosurgery 5 years after surgical resection. This patient showed clinical improvement over time but initially experienced upper extremity weakness and hyperesthesia, proximal lower extremity weakness, as well as spastic gait. No tumor was evident after 6 years of follow-up evaluation. The other three patients with spinal neurofibromas underwent surgery only. One patient reported no symptoms and was neurologically intact after 24 months of follow-up evaluation. Another patient reported improved symptoms and was neurologically intact at 17 months, with no evidence of tumor at 12 months. The last patient showed symptomatic as well as clinical improvement at 1 month, with no evidence of tumor after 18 months of follow-up evaluation.

Spinal Hemangioblastomas

Spinal hemangioblastomas are relatively rare, representing between 2 and 15% of intramedullary tumors.[27] Despite being histologically benign, these lesions can cause significant neurological morbidity secondary to the frequently associated edema, cyst, or syrinx formation. They most commonly involve the thoracic spine and occasionally extend to multiple noncontiguous levels. They must be differentiated from spinal ependymomas, which also demonstrate feeding arteries and draining veins on angiography.

They may develop sporadically (two thirds of cases) or in association with von Hippel-Lindau (VHL) disease (one third of cases). Hemangioblastomas associated with this disease typically present at an earlier age of onset than sporadic cases.[27] The indications for surgical resection differ between sporadic lesions and those associated with VHL disease. For sporadic lesions, resection is often required for diagnosis and strongly recommended before symptom development. Because of the typically long quiescent period of growth and the usual need for multiple surgeries in a lifetime, patients with VHL disease are advised to undergo surgical removal only when the lesion becomes symptomatic.[28] ▶ Table 38.4 summarizes the surgical series documenting treatment of spinal hemangioblastomas.

Several retrospective studies have reported favorable outcome after surgical management of spinal hemangioblastomas, with and without concurrent VHL disease. Lonser et al[29] assessed 44 patients with VHL disease who underwent surgical resection with a mean follow-up period of 44 months. Eighty-four percent of patients remained neurologically stable postoperatively. The overall mortality rate was 2%. Nine percent of cases were complicated by CSF leaks, and 4% were affected by superficial wound infections. The tumor recurrence rate was not reported presumably due to the short-term follow-up period. Na et al[30] also conducted a retrospective study of nine patients, five of whom were diagnosed with VHL disease. Gross total resection was achieved in six cases, and the mean follow-up period was 22 months. Most patients, with and without VHL disease, experienced an improvement or no change in neurologic function. There was no perioperative mortality, and the tumor recurrence rate was not reported. The most recent retrospective study by Mandigo et al[31] reported gross total resection in all 15 of their patients, four of whom were diagnosed with VHL disease. There was no clinical or radiological evidence of residual or recurrent tumor in any patient at follow-up ranging from 15 months to 6 years. Eighty-seven percent of patients were neurologically stable postoperatively. There was no perioperative mortality; however, three cases were complicated by neuropathic pain, CSF leak, and infection, respectively. No adjuvant therapy was indicated or implemented in any of these studies.

Moss et al[32] assessed 31 patients with spinal hemangioblastomas after radiosurgery, 25 patients with VHL disease and 26 patients who were previously treated with one or more operations. Nearly all patients with VHL disease had disease-associated tumors outside of the central nervous system. Most of these patients had recurrent tumors after prior operations,

Table 38.4 Surgical series for spinal hemangioblastoma resection

Study	Level of evidence	Treatment (surgery [S] or surgery + radiotherapy [RT])	No. patients	Tumor recurrence (%)	Neurologic outcome	Complications
Lonser et al[29]	III-2 Mean f/u 44 mo	S	44 with VHL	unavailable	7% improved; 84% unchanged; 9% worsened	2% mortality rate 9% CSF leaks 4% superficial wound infection
Na et al[30]	III-2 Mean f/u 22 mo	S	9 (5 with VHL; 6 GTR)	unavailable	Most improved or stable	No mortality
Mandigo et al[31]	III-2 Mean f/u 35 mo	S	15 (4 with VHL; GTR in all)	0	87% unchanged; 1 patient improved and 1 patient unchanged	No mortality; 20% complication rate (3/15 with neuropathic pain, CSF leak, infection)
Moss et al[32]	III-2 f/u 5–164 mo	S + RT	31 (25 with VHL; 26 surgery + radiotherapy)	Out of 10 lesions with > 2 y f/u: 50% decreased size, and 50% unchanged size	Out of 41 tumors p/w pain or neurologic deficit: 88% improved or resolved	22.5% mortality rate, 16% radiation necrosis

Abbreviations: *CSF, cerebrospinal fluid; f/u, follow-up; GTR, gross total resection; P/W, tk; VHL, von-Hippel-Lindau syndrome.*

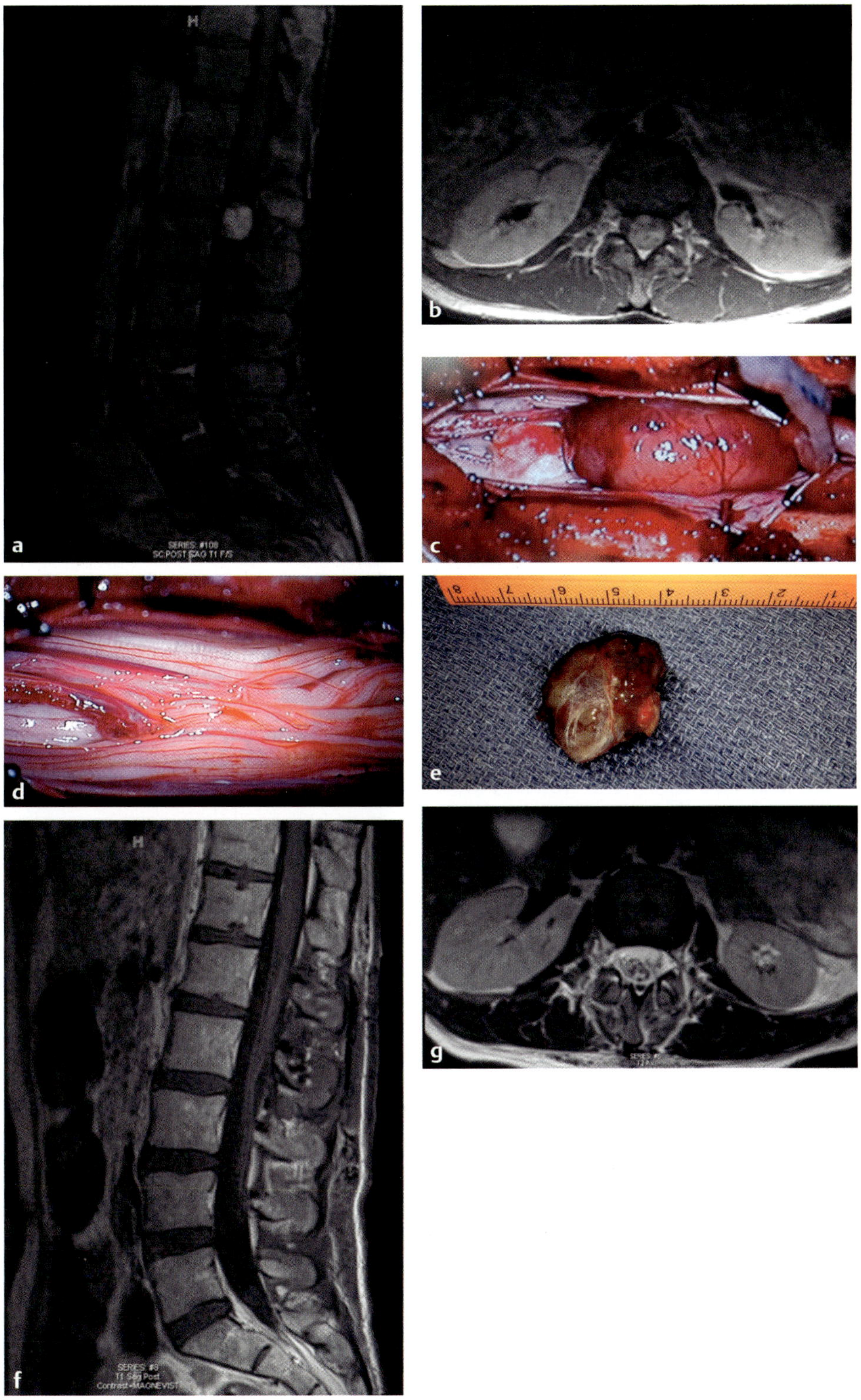

Fig. 38.3 The patient is a 38-year-old female who presented with a 2.5 year history of progressive low back pain and a 2.5 month history of bilateral lower extremity sciatic pain. Preoperative imaging (A-B): Contrast enhanced T1-weighted MRI sagittal (A) and axial (B) views showing a contrast-enhancing lesion involving the distal conus medullaris and proximal cauda equina and occupying the majority of the spinal canal. The differential diagnosis for a lesion in this location includes benign lesions, such as a schwannoma, and also potentially more aggressive lesions, such as a myxopapillary ependymoma. Open surgery is preferred initially to establish the diagnosis.Intraoperative imaging (C-D) and specimen for pathology (E): Intraoperative imaging shows the lesion at the distal conus medullaris and filum terminale before (C) and after (D) gross total resection. Pathology proved to be a myxopapillary ependymoma, which is associated with variable biological behavior and occasionally requires adjuvant therapies. Radiosurgery as an initial therapeutic approach would not have clarified the diagnosis. Postoperative imaging (F-G): Contrast enhanced T1-weighted MRI sagittal view (F) and T2-weighted MRI axial view (G) showing complete tumor resection

experienced postoperative neurological impairment, and opted to avoid further surgical resection. Among the 10 spinal hemangioblastomas followed for more than 2 years, 5 lesions decreased in size, and the remaining 5 lesions were unchanged in size. 88% of tumors associated with pain and/or neurologic deficits at initial presentation showed significant clinical improvement or complete resolution of symptoms. Six lesions considered local failures were treated with surgical drainage and resection less than 3 months after radiosurgery due to the development of symptomatic cysts. Furthermore, radiation necrosis occurred in five patients with associated symptoms of numbness, extremity weakness, and new-onset headaches.

Complete surgical resection is the definitive treatment of choice for patients with spinal cord hemangioblastomas because incomplete resection may result in significant morbidity and mortality in patients. Patients with VHL disease impose special considerations in the therapeutic approach. These patients tend to present with multiple hemangioblastomas, many of which are asymptomatic and/or relatively small. For symptomatic lesions, open resection is often required to promptly relieve the associated mass effect on the spinal cord. When to treat asymptomatic lesions remains controversial. Although many exhibit slow growth, some hemangioblastomas can suddenly increase in size and cause devastating neurological deficits. Moss et al[32] recommend radiosurgery for VHL patients with asymptomatic hemangioblastomas > 5 mm in size if they are cystic or enlarging on serial imaging studies. The goal is to prevent neurologic deterioration and potential morbidity resulting from repeat operations for these lesions with a greater risk of becoming symptomatic.

Conclusion

Advances in spinal microsurgical techniques have allowed for safer and more aggressive resection of spinal tumors. The postoperative functional outcome is closely correlated to the severity of preoperative deficits; therefore, an early diagnosis markedly influences the functional prognosis, and surgical candidates must be carefully selected. Minimally symptomatic patients tend to experience the greatest benefit and the least risk from surgery. Surgical outcome is also related to the presence of spinal cord atrophy and arachnoid scarring, both indicating chronic spinal cord compression.[33] Furthermore, predictors of long-term morbidity and mortality include tumor type, identification of a tumor–spinal cord plane of dissection (POD), and extent of surgical resection, which are all closely interrelated. Patients with tumors that can be totally removed due to a more identifiable POD are more likely to lead a normal life after surgery with a higher rate of progression-free survival than patients with tumors less amenable to complete resection.

Although the safety and effectiveness of microsurgical resection of most benign spinal tumors are well-documented in the literature, some patients are not ideal surgical candidates due to other risk factors or the characteristics of their tumor. In such clinical circumstances, the optimal treatment may become somewhat controversial. One potential therapeutic modality that is currently being extensively investigated is stereotactic radiosurgery. An obvious benefit of radiosurgery over microsurgery includes the noninvasive nature of this treatment modality. Numerous studies have recently demonstrated long-term control of spinal meningiomas,[16,17] nerve sheath tumors,[16,17,34,35] and hemangioblastomas[32] using stereotactic radiosurgery. However, with radiosurgery, a diagnosis is assumed based only upon imaging studies alone and no histopathological correlation. In this situation, the prognosis can only be predicted based on the assumed imaging diagnosis. Furthermore, when preoperative spinal imaging is indeterminate and the differential diagnosis includes benign as well as malignant lesions, surgery is indicated for histopathological diagnosis and appropriate management (▶ Fig. 38.3). Stereotactic radiosurgery is a useful adjunct to an initial operation with any suspicion of residual tumor and with evidence of tumor recurrence during follow-up evaluations. This therapeutic modality should also be considered for patients with multiple lesions associated with phakomatoses, patients with significant medical comorbidities, as well as younger patients. On the other hand, patients who present with significant signs of myeloradiculopathy and marked spinal cord compression on MRI typically do not benefit from stereotactic radiosurgery.

As experience with stereotactic radiosurgery continues to grow, the risk for radiation-induced myelopathy has become increasingly apparent. Gibbs et al[36] reported six patients who were previously irradiated for primary (three patients) and metastatic (three patients) spinal lesions and then developed signs of myelopathy more than 6 months later. The authors assert that hypofractionated radiosurgery is safe but recommend using caution when exposing > 1 cm^3 of spinal cord to more than 8 Gy of radiation. Although there are numerous reports of radiation-induced malignancy after treatment of intracranial tumors, there is currently limited data on such a risk with spinal tumors after radiotherapy. Because secondary tumors can significantly impact the patient's quality of life and complicate further treatment, it is important to consider this potential morbidity and continuously monitor the patient with long-term follow-up evaluations.

The field of stereotactic radiosurgery is rapidly expanding and gaining favor as an adjuvant or alternative therapy for some benign extramedullary spinal tumors. However, gross total resection must always be considered initially because it significantly impacts recurrence rates. When treatment is indicated, early microsurgical intervention remains the recommendation for all intradural extramedullary spinal cord tumors to confirm histology as well as to prevent growth and neurologic deterioration.

References

[1] Helseth A, Mørk SJ. Primary intraspinal neoplasms in Norway, 1955 to 1986. A population-based survey of 467 patients. J Neurosurg 1989; 71: 842–845

[2] Chamberlain MC, Tredway TL. Adult primary intradural spinal cord tumors: a review. Curr Neurol Neurosci Rep 2011; 11: 320–328

[3] King AT, Sharr MM, Gullan RW, Bartlett JR. Spinal meningiomas: a 20-year review. Br J Neurosurg 1998; 12: 521–526

[4] Mirimanoff RO, Dosoretz DE, Linggood RM, Ojemann RG, Martuza RL. Meningioma: analysis of recurrence and progression following neurosurgical resection. J Neurosurg 1985; 62: 18–24

[5] Solero CL, Fornari M, Giombini S, et al. Spinal meningiomas: review of 174 operated cases. Neurosurgery 1989; 25: 153–160

[6] Setzer M, Vatter H, Marquardt G, Seifert V, Vrionis FD. Management of spinal meningiomas: surgical results and a review of the literature. Neurosurg Focus 2007; 23: E14

[7] Sandalcioglu IE, Hunold A, Müller O, Bassiouni H, Stolke D, Asgari S. Spinal meningiomas: critical review of 131 surgically treated patients. Eur Spine J 2008; 17: 1035–1041

[8] Postalci L, Tugcu B, Gungor A, Guclu G. Spinal meningiomas: recurrence in ventrally located individuals on long-term follow-up; a review of 46 operated cases. Turk Neurosurg 2011; 21: 449–453

[9] Nakamura M, Tsuji O, Fujiyoshi K, et al. Long-term surgical outcomes of spinal meningiomas. Spine 2012; 37: E617–E623

[10] Klekamp J, Samii M. Surgical results for spinal meningiomas. Surg Neurol 1999; 52: 552–562

[11] Cohen-Gadol AA, Zikel OM, Koch CA, Scheithauer BW, Krauss WE. Spinal meningiomas in patients younger than 50 years of age: a 21-year experience. J Neurosurg 2003; 98 (Suppl): 258–263

[12] Deen HG, Scheithauer BW, Ebersold MJ. Clinical and pathological study of meningiomas of the first two decades of life. J Neurosurg 1982; 56: 317–322

[13] Gezen F, Kahraman S, Canakci Z, Bedük A. Review of 36 cases of spinal cord meningioma. Spine 2000; 25: 727–731

[14] Roux FX, Nataf F, Pinaudeau M, Borne G, Devaux B, Meder JF. Intraspinal meningiomas: review of 54 cases with discussion of poor prognosis factors and modern therapeutic management. Surg Neurol 1996; 46: 458–463, discussion 463–464

[15] Gottfried ON, Gluf W, Quinones-Hinojosa A, Kan P, Schmidt MH. Spinal meningiomas: surgical management and outcome. Neurosurg Focus 2003; 14: e2

[16] Gerszten PC, Quader M, Novotny J, Flickinger JC. Radiosurgery for benign tumors of the spine: clinical experience and current trends. Technol Cancer Res Treat 2012; 11: 133–139

[17] Sachdev S, Dodd RL, Chang SD, et al. Stereotactic radiosurgery yields long-term control for benign intradural, extramedullary spinal tumors. Neurosurgery 2011; 69: 533–539, discussion 539

[18] Seppälä MT, Haltia MJ, Sankila RJ, Jääskeläinen JE, Heiskanen O. Long-term outcome after removal of spinal schwannoma: a clinicopathological study of 187 cases. J Neurosurg 1995; 83: 621–626

[19] Halliday AL, Sobel RA, Martuza RL. Benign spinal nerve sheath tumors: their occurrence sporadically and in neurofibromatosis types 1 and 2. J Neurosurg 1991; 74: 248–253

[20] Kim P, Ebersold MJ, Onofrio BM, Quast LM. Surgery of spinal nerve schwannoma. Risk of neurological deficit after resection of involved root. J Neurosurg 1989; 71: 810–814

[21] Conti P, Pansini G, Mouchaty H, Capuano C, Conti R. Spinal neurinomas: retrospective analysis and long-term outcome of 179 consecutively operated cases and review of the literature. Surg Neurol 2004; 61: 34–43, discussion 44

[22] Safavi-Abbasi S, Senoglu M, Theodore N, et al. Microsurgical management of spinal schwannomas: evaluation of 128 cases. J Neurosurg Spine 2008; 9: 40–47

[23] Murovic JA, Charles Cho S, Park J. Surgical strategies for managing foraminal nerve sheath tumors: the emerging role of CyberKnife ablation. Eur Spine J 2010; 19: 242–256

[24] Levy WJ, Latchaw J, Hahn JF, Sawhny B, Bay J, Dohn DF. Spinal neurofibromas: a report of 66 cases and a comparison with meningiomas. Neurosurgery 1986; 18: 331–334

[25] Seppälä MT, Haltia MJ, Sankila RJ, Jääskeläinen JE, Heiskanen O. Long-term outcome after removal of spinal neurofibroma. J Neurosurg 1995; 82: 572–577Erratum in: J Neurosurg 1995 Jul;83(1):186

[26] Levi AD, Ross AL, Cuartas E, Qadir R, Temple HT. The surgical management of symptomatic peripheral nerve sheath tumors. Neurosurgery 2010; 66: 833–840

[27] Neumann HP, Eggert HR, Scheremet R, et al. Central nervous system lesions in von Hippel-Lindau syndrome. J Neurol Neurosurg Psychiatry 1992; 55: 898–901

[28] Lonser RR, Oldfield EH. Spinal cord hemangioblastomas. Neurosurg Clin N Am 2006; 17: 37–44

[29] Lonser RR, Weil RJ, Wanebo JE, DeVroom HL, Oldfield EH. Surgical management of spinal cord hemangioblastomas in patients with von Hippel-Lindau disease. J Neurosurg 2003; 98: 106–116

[30] Na JH, Kim HS, Eoh W, Kim JH, Kim JS, Kim ES. Spinal cord hemangioblastoma : diagnosis and clinical outcome after surgical treatment. J Korean Neurosurg Soc 2007; 42: 436–440

[31] Mandigo CE, Ogden AT, Angevine PD, McCormick PC. Operative management of spinal hemangioblastoma. Neurosurgery 2009; 65: 1166–1177

[32] Moss JM, Choi CY, Adler JR, Soltys SG, Gibbs IC, Chang SD. Stereotactic radiosurgical treatment of cranial and spinal hemangioblastomas. Neurosurgery 2009; 65: 79–85, discussion 85

[33] Cristante L, Herrmann HD. Surgical management of intramedullary spinal cord tumors: functional outcome and sources of morbidity. Neurosurgery 1994; 35: 69–74, discussion 74–76

[34] Dodd RL, Ryu MR, Kamnerdsupaphon P, Gibbs IC, Chang SD, Adler JR. Cyber-Knife radiosurgery for benign intradural extramedullary spinal tumors. Neurosurgery 2006; 58: 674–685, discussion 674–685

[35] Murovic JA, Gibbs IC, Chang SD, Mobley BC, Park J, Adler JR. Foraminal nerve sheath tumors: intermediate follow-up after cyberknife radiosurgery. Neurosurgery 2009; 64 (Suppl): A33–A43

[36] Gibbs IC, Patil C, Gerszten PC, Adler JR, Burton SA. Delayed radiation-induced myelopathy after spinal radiosurgery. Neurosurgery 2009; 64 (Suppl): A67–A72

[37] Zada G, Pagnini PG, Yu C, Erickson KT, Hirschbein J, Zelman V, Apuzzo MLJ. Long-term outcomes and patterns of tumor progression after gamma knife radiosurgery for benign meningiomas. Neurosurgery 2010; 67: 322–328, discussion 328–329

39 Treatment of Benign Spinal Tumors with Radiosurgery

Judith A. Murovic and Steven D. Chang

Introduction

The Horsley–Clarke stereotactic apparatus was invented in 1908 by British neurosurgeon Sir Victor Horsley and his colleague Robert Clarke, a mathematician. Their Cartesian coordinate stereotactic device was fixed to a monkey's skull via a head frame and allowed for the stereotactic electrocoagulation of a target in deep-seated brain structures.[1] In 1947 an American neurologist, Ernest Spiegel, and Henry Wycis, then a medical student who became a neurosurgeon, designed a stereotactic device using polar coordinates for use in humans based on the Horsley–Clarke apparatus.

In 1951 the Swedish neurosurgeon Lars Leksell developed the concept of radiosurgery.[2] Using a cyclotron, Leksell and the physicist Borje Larsson employed proton beams originating from several directions, which allowed for the destruction of brain lesions, first in animals and then in humans. This device was thus a new, noninvasive method for destroying discrete anatomical regions within the brain while minimizing the effect on the surrounding normal tissues.

The first CyberKnife radiosurgery system (Accuray, Inc. Sunnyvale, CA) was developed at Stanford University Medical Center (SUMC) by John Adler and was used to treat its first patient in 1994. The CyberKnife radiosurgery device had two new features that set it apart from other stereotactic therapy methods—robotic mounting and image guidance. Thus, the CyberKnife device has a maneuverable robotic manipulator with an attached lightweight, 285-lb, 6-MV linear accelerator (LINAC) X-ray energy source. The robot positions and aims the LINAC toward a patient on a remotely repositional treatment couch. Real-time digital X-ray imaging is used via two cameras that acquire fluoroscopic X-rays of treatment site –associated skeletal features. Image registration techniques are then used to determine and then relay the treatment site's coordinates to the manipulator, which in turn directs the beams to the treatment site within the patient. When the target moves, the process detects this change and corrects the beam pointing in near real time. This real-time image guidance eliminates the need for skeletal fixation in positioning. The system delivers multiple cross-fired beams to a designated lesion via six degrees of freedom with a 0.3-mm precision.[2]

Rationale for Radiosurgery of Benign Spinal Tumors

Radiosurgery has been used in the past to treat benign skull-based meningiomas, such as benign tumors within the cavernous sinus. When standard open surgical techniques are employed to remove these tumors, they have been shown to be difficult to access and the open surgical approach has the associated potential for brainstem and adjacent cranial nerve injury. In a recent review, Kondziolka et al[3] presented a long-term control rate of 93% after the use of the Gamma Knife (Elekta AB, Stockholm, Sweden) to treat 1,045 intracranial benign (World Health Organization [WHO] grade I) meningiomas. In a subset of 488 patients for which serial imaging was obtained, 215 tumors regressed and 256 were unchanged for a control rate of 97%. Only 19 tumors enlarged. Likewise, in a study from SUMC, using the CyberKnife radiosurgery system, 13 trigeminal schwannomas had a 100% control rate, with 2 tumors remaining stable and the remainder reducing in size.[4] Thus, similar spine tumors would be expected to respond to radiosurgery in a like manner.[5]

Radiosurgery has been used extensively to treat malignant spinal metastases. The controversy has been raised, however, that patients with benign spinal tumors have longer life expectancies than those with malignant spinal tumors; thus the potential of experiencing a delayed myelopathy is of more concern. This controversy of the possibility of spinal cord injury after treatment of benign spine tumors with radiosurgery will be addressed throughout the chapter by quoting the various complication percentages for such management.

The first patient with a benign spinal tumor, a hemangioblastoma, was treated at SUMC using CyberKnife radiosurgery in 1997.[5] The outcomes of the treatment of two such lesions were summarized by Chang et al. in 1998.[6] These two tumors decreased in size by 33 and 70%, respectively, after an 18-month follow-up.

Dodd et al.[5] presented the SUMC CyberKnife radiosurgery treatment outcomes of 51 patients with 55 benign spinal tumors including 30 schwannomas, 9 neurofibromas, and 16 meningiomas managed between 1999 and 2005. Murovic et al[7] presented a longer follow-up on a subset of Dodd et al's patients with schwannomas and neurofibromas. A summary of the latter subset will be included in this chapter further, focusing on the tumors' clinical and imaging responses after radiosurgery as a rational for such treatment. Moss et al[8] evaluated the outcomes of 16 spinal hemangioblastomas treated from 1991 to 2007, and these also will be analyzed. The review by Sachdev et al[9] of outcomes of spinal meningiomas treated with CyberKnife radiosurgery will be presented as well.

Literature Supporting Radiosurgery Treatment of Benign Spinal Tumors

A literature review covering 2005 to 2010 that searched for publications using CyberKnife radiosurgery to treat benign spinal tumors elicited 10 publications, four of which were from our institution. A critical evaluation of all six outside studies was carried out. Studies having documentation of the same parameters used in this chapter's SUMC CyberKnife radiosurgery analysis of outcomes in various benign spinal tumors yielded two outside institution papers that met the requisite rigorous criteria (▶ Table 39.1).

Table 39.1 Literature review of imaging outcomes after CyberKnife radiosurgery of benign spinal tumors

Study	Study type, level of evidence	Tumor type, No. patients	Mean age (range yrs.)	Asscted. genetic disorder, pt. no.	Mean tumor volumes (range) (cm^3)	Mean SRS Maximum Tumor doses (range) (Gy)*	Mean f/u times, (range) (mos.)	Pain outcomes (Pt. No)	N.E. outcomes (Pt. No)	Imaging results (Pt. No)
Gerszten et al[10]	Prospective, cohort study, II**	Schwannomas, 35	50 (21–85)	NF2, 9	11.0 (1.0–47.7)	22.03 (17.5-25)	Not included****	Improved (14), stabilized (2), worse (1)	Improved (3), stabilized(1), worse (1)	Improved (1), stabilized (11); worse (1) ****
		Neurofibromas, 25	30 (33–57)	NF2, 20	12.6 (0.3-93.4)	21.3 (15–25)	Not included***	Improved (8); stabilized(4)†; worse (1)	Improved (2); stable (2)	Stable (8)
		Meningiomas, 13	41 (18–77)	N/A	4.9 (0.8–16.0)	21.25 (17.5–25.0)††	Not included	N/A	N/A	Stabilized (13)
Chang et al[13]	Prospective cohort study, II	Hemangioblastomas, 5 (8 tumors)	26 (22–33)	VHL, 3	0.3 0.04–0.71)	25.8 (13–33)	50 (23–72)	N/A	Improved (1); stable (7)	Improved. (6); stabilized (1); worse (1)

* *One fraction was used in all cases in both authors' patients, except for one meningioma, in the Gerszten et al series, which caused cord compression and received three fractions.*

** *Fisher CG, Wood KB. Introduction to and techniques of evidence-based medicine. Spine 2007;32:S66–S72.*

*** *Follow-up time for neurofibromas, schwannomas, and meningiomas combined was 37 months with a range of 8 to 71 months.*

**** *The one patient who was described as worse developed S1 Numbness and had open surgery.*

† *Two patients temporarily improved.*

†† *One patient received 45 Gy.*

Abbreviations: *N/A, not applicable; NF2 neurofibromatosis type 2; Pt. No., patient number; SRS, stereotactic radiosurgery; VHL, von Hippel-Lindau disease.*

Source: *Data from Gerszten PC, Burton SA, Ozhasoglu C, McCue KJ, Quinn AE. Radiosurgery for benign intradural spinal tumors. Neurosurgery 2008;62(4):687–896; and Chang UK, Rhee CH, Youn SM, Lee DH, Park SQ. Radiosurgery using the CyberKnife for benign spinal tumors: Korea Cancer Center Hospital experience. J Neurooncol 2011;101(1):91–99.*

A Critical Review of "Radiosurgery for Benign Intradural Spinal Tumors" by Gerszten et al

In the first literature review publication, Gerszten et al[10] analyzed 73 patients with benign intradural-extramedullary spinal tumors, which were treated with CyberKnife radiosurgery. The authors used a prospective cohort study approach (i.e. level II evaluation per the Fisher and Wood classification regarding levels of evidence for a primary research question).[11] The outcomes of three intradural-extramedullary types of benign spinal tumors were evaluated including 35 schwannomas, 25 neurofibromas, and 13 meningiomas. The authors carefully outlined the mean patients' ages with ranges, associated genetic disorders, mean tumor volumes and ranges, mean stereotactic radiosurgery (SRS) maximum tumor dosages and imaging results. The mean follow-up for all three types of tumors was 37 months, with a range of 8 to 71 months; this follow-up information was not available, however, for each individual tumor type.

Schwannomas

Nine (36%) of 35 patients with schwannomas, who were treated with CyberKnife radiosurgery had associated neurofibromatosis type 2 (NF2). The mean tumor volume for schwannomas was 11.0 cm^3 (1.0–47.7 cm^3), and the mean SRS maximum tumor dose was 22.03 Gy. The patient outcomes were delineated using changes in three parameters including pain, neurologic deficits, and imaging pre- and post-treatment with radiosurgery.

A subgroup of 17 patients had pre- and post–CyberKnife radiosurgery pain levels evaluated. The levels of pain improved in 14 (82%) patients, 2 (12%) had stable pain levels, and 1 (6%) had a new numbness. A second subgroup of five patients had neurological deficit progression following pre- and post–CyberKnife radiosurgery. Of this subgroup, three (60%) patients improved, one (20%) was stable, and one (20%) became worse.

Radiosurgery was used as the primary treatment in seven asymptomatic patients, and imaging was used as the outcome modality for this subgroup: five lesions (71%) were stable at the time of the last follow-up imaging, and one (14%) was smaller. One (14%) of these seven patients required surgery for the development of S1 numbness. An additional six patients had been treated for imaging progression after primary resection and all six (100%) had stable imaging at the time of follow-up. Thus, of a total of 13 patients for whom imaging was involved in the outcome determination, 11 (85%) lesions were stable, one (8%) improved, and one (8%) "progressed without quotes" per the article, though the indication for operation was the described S1 numbness.

Neurofibromas

Evaluating 25 neurofibromas, 20 (80%) were associated with NF2. A mean maximum tumor dosage of 21.3 Gy was used to treat these 25 tumors using radiosurgery. The mean tumor volume was 12.6 cm^3 and the range was 0.3 to 93.4 cm^3.

Parameters used for evaluating outcomes were pain in 13 patients, of whom 8 (62%) improved and 2 (15%) remained stable and 3 (23%) regressed (2 of these 3 had temporarily improved, however).

Four patients with neurofibromas underwent radiosurgery for progressive neurologic deficits. Of these four patients, two (50%) patients improved and two (50%) stabilized. Of three patients who underwent radiosurgery for imaging progression after open resection, three (100%) patients had stable imaging. Five (100%) of five asymptomatic patients also remained stable with regard to their imaging after radiosurgery.

Meningiomas

Thirteen patients with meningiomas, who were treated with an SRS tumor maximum dose of radiosurgery had an average tumor volume of 4.9 cm^3 (0.8–16.0 cm^3) and were treated with 21. 3 Gy. For this group, of 11 patients who had open surgical resection and underwent SRS for tumor progression on imaging, all (100%) remained stable with regard to their imaging after treatment of their tumors. Two patients underwent radiosurgery as a primary treatment and both had imaging that showed tumor control during follow-up.

Complications

Of the total of 73 benign tumors, two schwannoma patients and one meningioma patient developed SRS-related cord injury manifesting as a Brown-Séquard syndrome, 5 to 13 months posttreatment. These three patients were treated with a combination of steroids, vitamin E, and gabapentin; one patient underwent hyperbaric oxygen therapy. The authors stated that a commonality to two of three cases was prior open surgical resections of the tumors, which, they postulated, may have caused a predisposition of the spinal cord to radiation injury.[10]

A Critical Review of "Radiosurgery Using the CyberKnife for Benign Spinal Tumors: Korea Cancer Center Hospital Experience" by Chang et al

Hemangioblastomas

Hemangioblastomas are vascular tumors that are intramedullary in location and situated near the pial surface.[12] Chang et al[13] in an outside institution review evaluated 30 benign spinal tumors in 20 patients of which 8 tumors were hemangioblastomas. The subgroup of hemangioblastomas from this paper was chosen for its rigorous specification of treatment data and to enable a comparison to the SUMC experience to be presented later in this chapter.

In this publication by Chang et al, three tumors were associated with von Hippel-Lindau (VHL) disease. All tumors were treated with 13-23 Gy as the single equivalent SRS dosage, which was given in one fraction. These authors indicated that the follow-up period was 50 months with a range of 23 to 72 months.

Of six patients who were asymptomatic prior to radiosurgery treatment, all (100%) remained asymptomatic after radiosurgery. In one patient who had gait difficulties, the gait improved. In another patient with unspecified neurologic deficits, the

Table 39.2 Imaging outcomes after SUMC CyberKnife radiosurgery of schwannomas and neurofibromas

Pt no.	Tumor types and location	Gender, ages (y)	Asscted. genetic disorders	Prior ORs	CK RS dates	Tumor volumes (cm³)†	SRS doses (Gy), fxs	F/u times (mos.)	Sx. outcomes	NE outcomes	Imaging results
	Schwannomas										
1	R C1–C2	F, 38	N/A	None	8/03	16.86	21, 3	48	Improved	Improved	Improved
2	R C1–C2	M, 71	N/A	None	11/04	5.65	20, 2	30	Improved	Progressed then improved post-OR	Improved
3	L C2–C3	M, 38	FS	None	9/04	1.60	18, 1	12	Improved	Stabilized	Improved
4	R C3–C4	M, 42	N/A	None	4/03	1.36	18, 1	36	Improved	Stabilized	Improved
5	L C4–C5	M, 55	N/A	None	5/03	2.18	18,1	24	Stabilized	Improved	Improved
6	L C4-–C5	M, 47	N/A	STR, 3/02	10/03	6.61	21, 3	48	Improved then progressed post-AA, then improved post-shunt	Improved, then progressed post-AA, then improved post-shunt	Improved
7	L C4–C5	F, 53	N/A	None	12/04	1.70	18, 1	24	Improved.	Improved	Improved
8	L C5–C6	F, 61	N/A	GTR, 1993	5/00	1.70	18, 1	72	Progressed	Improved post-OR	Progressed
9	R L4–L5	M, 61	N/A	STR, 2003	3/04	8.56	20, 1	48	Improved	Improved	Improved
10	R L4–L5	F, 63	N/A	None	5/06	5.80	16, 1	6	Improved	Improved	Stabilized
	Neurofibromas										
1	R, L C1–C2**	M, 25	NF1	None	9/03	14.50*	20, 2*	12	Progressed	Progressed then improved post-OR	R Progressed L Progressed
2	LC5–C6	F, 47	NF1	STRs, 2000, 2003	9/05	2. 6	20,2	12	Improved	Improved	Stabilized
3	R, L C7–T1	M, 25	NF1	None	9/03	10.04*	20, 2*	12	Progressed then improved post-OR	Improved	R Improved L Progressed
4	R L5–S1	F, 28	NF2	None	9/04	3.08	20, 2	20	Improved	Progressed but due to distal nerve per EMG/ NCVs	Improved
5	R L5–S1	F, 63	N/A	None	6/03	5.83	18, 1	36	Improved	Stabilized	Improved

† *The formula for an idealized ellipsoid, volume = 0.5 × width × length × height, was used to estimate the tumor volume on a contrast magnetic resonance imaging scan*
* *Both tumors were treated as a single volume in two fractions*
** *Patients 1 and 3 were the same patient who underwent treatment of four tumors, two each treated at separate times.*
Abbreviations: *Asscted., associated; CK RS, CyberKnife radiosurgery; EMG/NCVs, electromyography and nerve conduction velocities; FS, familial schwannomatosis; F/u, follow-up; GTR, gross total resection; L, left; NE, neurologic examination; NF1, neurofibromatosis type 1; R, right; N/A, not applicable; NF2, neurofibromatosis type 2; ORs, surgeries; SRS, stereotactic radiosurgery; Sx., symptom; STR, subtotal resection.*
Source: *Adapted from Murovic J et al. Foraminal nerve sheath tumors: intermediate follow-up after CyberKnife radiosurgery. Neurosurgery 2009; 64(2): A33–A43, with permission.*

neurologic examination remained stable. Using imaging evaluation, six tumors regressed, and one each stabilized and progressed, respectively. No complications were mentioned to have occurred in any patients in this publication.

The SUMC CyberKnife Radiosurgery Experience with Schwannomas and Neurofibromas

Intradural-extramedullary tumors represent 40% of all spinal tumors.[12] The majority of tumors in this location that have been treated with radiosurgery at our institution consisted of schwannomas, neurofibromas, and meningiomas. The data from our experience between 1999 and 2006 with schwannomas and neurofibromas were reviewed in a publication by Murovic et al.[7] and are summarized here. For schwannomas and neurofibromas the range for prescribed doses was 16 to 20 Gy, and they were delivered in one to three fractions of 6 to 20 Gy. Target volumes ranged from 1.36 to 16.9 mL.

A nonrigid immobilization device, either an Aquaplast face mask (WFR/Aquaplast Corp, Wyckoff, NJ) or a vacuum foam body cradle was used for simulation, treatment planning, and delivery of the CK RS. Digital reconstruction radiographs were generated from 1.25-mm computed tomographic (CT) slices, and contrast magnetic resonance imaging (MRI) was fused with the CT for treatment planning. Critical structures were contoured per Sachdev et al,[9] and the inverse treatment planning is also described there. The information there is representative of the methods followed for each SUMC article summarized hereafter.

Schwannomas

Schwannomas and neurofibromas represent 25% of intradural-extramedullary lesions in the spine.[14] While these tumors have traditionally been treated with open surgery, detailed data regarding the CyberKnife radiosurgery treatment of 10 patients with 10 schwannomas and 4 patients with 7 neurofibromas, who underwent SRS between 1999 and 2005 at our institution are presented here.[7]

Schwannoma patients' outcomes after radiosurgery treatment are summarized in ▶ Table 39.2. Eight (89%) of nine patients with schwannomas, who were symptomatic upon presentation had significant improvement in either pain or dysesthesias after radiosurgery treatment. Seven (88%) of eight schwannoma patients' symptoms improved by 6 months post-radiosurgery treatment and the remaining one case (patient 1) experienced symptom improvement after 24 months. One (11%) patient (patient 8) had symptoms increase in severity at 72 months after treatment. Neurologically, 9 (90%) of 10 schwannomas improved (6 did so within 2 d–24 mo) or remained stable (3). Patient 6 worsened after an automobile accident but improved to baseline after a ventriculoperitoneal shunt was placed. Patient 6 became worse at 72 months after radiosurgery treatment but improved after surgical intervention.

The imaging characteristics are also summarized, since this was an effective objective way to determine radiosurgery response. After a mean follow-up period of 34.8 months (range 6–72 months), 8 (80%) of 10 patients with schwannomas were found to have radiographic improvement (i.e., their tumors regressed in size on serial MRIs). The MRIs were carried out every 6 months for 2 years and then yearly thereafter. Patient 1's tumor increased in size on MRI at 60 months, and patient 10's tumor remained the same size (i.e., stabilized at 6 mo follow-up).

Neurofibromas

Among four neurofibroma patients with seven tumors, three patients improved, while the other with four tumors had increased pain. The requisite time to symptom improvement ranged from 12 to 36 months. The neurological examination after radiosurgery treatment worsened in the one patient with bilateral C1–C2 and C7–T1 tumors. The examination did improve after open surgical resection.

Three (43%) of seven neurofibromas (the right C7-T1 tumor of patient 3, and patients 4 and 5)) decreased in size after radiosurgery treatment. Three tumors increased in size: the right and left C1–C2 tumors in patient 2 and the left C7–T1 tumor also from patient 2. Patient 2's tumor remained radiographically stable during the 12-month observation period.

Thus, patients with schwannomas had a better result from radiosurgery than did those patients with neurofibromas. This may be due to the schwannoma tumor tissue being unobstructed by nerve tissue, since the tumor displaces the nerve fibers. The neurofibroma tumor tissue, in contrast, is intertwined between the nerve fibers, and thus the radiation is less effective against the tumor tissue.

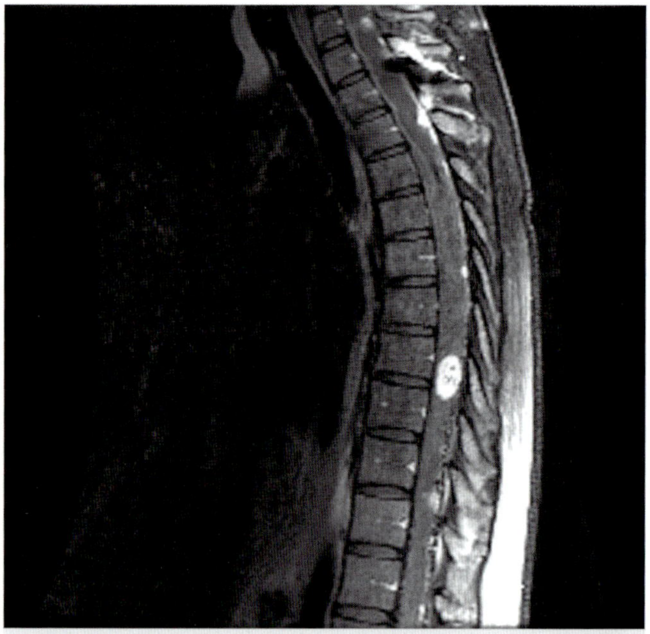

Fig. 39.1 An example of a T2-weighted postcontrast magnetic resonance image of a predominantly T7 hemangioblastoma in a patient with von Hippel-Lindau disease (patient 12 in Table 39.3). The tumor is intramedullary in location and avidly enhances. Other smaller hemangioblastomas were present in the spine but had remained stable and thus were not treated at this time.

The majority of patients who did not benefit from radiosurgery in this series presented with significant signs of radiculomyelopathy and marked spinal cord compression on MRI. There were no delayed radiation-induced myelopathies in this group of spine radiosurgery-treated patients.

The SUMC CyberKnife Radiosurgery Experience with Hemangioblastomas

Intramedullary spinal cord tumors are less common than intradural-extramedullary tumors and represent 5% of all spinal cord tumors. In the intramedullary location, astrocytomas occur 30% of the time, ependymomas have an incidence of 30%, and hemangioblastomas, 3 to 8%.[12,14] Sixteen spinal hemangioblastomas treated at SUMC with radiosurgery between 1991 and 2007 are summarized here. The locations, radiosurgery dosages, and outcomes using imaging sizes on serial MRIs are also presented.[8]

Hemangioblastomas

Hemangioblastomas are the most common tumors associated with VHL (▶ Fig. 39.1). However, these tumors can also occur sporadically.

Moss et al[8] evaluated 92 cranial and spinal hemangioblastomas in 31 patients who were treated with radiosurgery at our institution (▶ Table 39.3). Of these patients, 16 tumors were located in the spinal cord.

The median follow-up time for the spinal hemangioblastoma patients was 33,5 months with a mean of 37.2 months. The tumor dosages ranged from 20 to 25 Gy and were delivered in one to three fractions. Target volumes ranged from 0.06 to 2.65 cm^3. Fifteen of the 16 hemangioblastomas either remained stable (9) or improved (6). Only one patient's tumor increased in size during the follow-up period. Importantly, in this series of 16

Table 39.3 Summary of SUMC CyberKnife radiosurgery of hemangioblastomas

Pt. no.	Tumor types and locations	Gender, age (y)	Asscted. genetic disorders	Prior ORs	Prior SRS†	CK RS dates	Tumor volumes (cm^3)	SRS Doses (Gy), fxs	F/u times (mo)	Imaging results	ORs post-CK RS
	Hemangioblastomas										
1	C2	M,43	VHL	2001	2002	2004	2.36	21, 3	24	Improved	None
2	C2–C3	F, 39	VHL	None	None	1/96	1.1	21, 3	26	Improved	1/97
3	C3	F, 19	VHL	2001	None	2/02	0.36	21, 3	73	Stabilized	None
4	C4	F, 19	VHL	None	None	2/02	0.625	21, 3	73	Stabilized	None
5	C5	F, 26	VHL	None	None	2/04	0.10	22, 2	57	Improved	None
6	C6–C7	F, 28	VHL	None	None	6/04	0.11	20, 1	22	Progressed	None
7	C7	M, 53	VHL	None	None	6/01	0.46	21, 3	55	Improved	None
8	C7–T1	F, 19	VHL	None	None	2//02	0.81	21, 3	73	Improved	None
9	T1	M, 40	VHL	1975, 1984	None	7/95	0.06	21, 3	32	Improved	None
10	T2–T3	M, 39	N/A	STR, 10/03	None	12/03	0.09	25,1	36	Stabilized	None
11	T7	M, 37	VHL	STR, 7/05, STR, 8/05	None	5/06	0.41	20,1	12	Stabilized	None†††
12	T7	F, 28	VHL	None	None	6/04	0.07	20, 1	22	Stabilized	None
13	T11–T12	M, 50	VHL	6/00	None	10/03	0.22	20, 2	35	Stabilized	None
14	T11–T12	F, 29	VHL	95	None	10/05	0.06	22,1	6	Stabilized	None
15	T11	F, 51	N/A††	STR,10/05, GTR,12/05	None	5/06	0.24	20, 1	12	Stabilized	None
16	L2-L3	M, 60	N/A	STR,11/01, STR, 11/01	None	12/02	2.5	25, 1	37	Stabilized	None

† Refers to lesion only.
†† Negative genetic testing for VHL, but presented with a history of having had a cervical hemangioblastoma removed in the past, so she may have an indolent form of VHL.
††† Died of renal failure 5/98.
Abbreviations: *Asscted., associated; CK RS, CyberKnife radiosurgery; F, female; fx, fraction(s); f/u follow-up; GTR, gross total resection; M, male; N/A, not applicable; ORs, surgeries; SRS, stereotactic radiosurgery; STR, subtotal resection; VHL, von Hippel-Lindau disease.*
Source: *Adapted from Moss JM, Choi CYH, Adler JR Jr, Soltys SG, Gibbs IC, Chang SD. Stereotactic radiosurgical treatment of cranial and spinal hemangioblastomas. Neurosurgery 2009;65(1):79–85, with permission.*

hemangioblastomas managed as shown in ▶ Table 39.3, no patients developed spinal cord radiation toxicity.

The SUMC Radiosurgery Experience with Meningiomas

From 1999 to 2008, 32 spinal meningiomas were treated with radiosurgery at SUMC. The follow-up of these patients is being updated at this time; thus a summary of the results of the analysis of Sachdev et al[9] from our institution will be presented.

Meningiomas

Thirty-two spinal meningiomas were managed using radiosurgery between 1999 and 2008 at SUMC. Seventeen (53%) of 32 tumors had undergone prior resection, and these patients were being treated for residual or recurrent tumor. Histology was confirmed for 17 (53%) of 32 meningiomas.

The average tumor volume was 3.03 cm^3 with a range of 0.14 to 11.05 cm^3. The average prescribed dose was 20.6 Gy with a range of 16 to 30 Gy. The median treatment fractions were two with a range from one to five.

Considering tumor volume response, 47% of meningiomas remained stable, while 53% had a documented decrease in volume. Of those that decreased in volume, 56% decreased by more than half of the original pretreatment.

Complications

One patient developed the only incidence of transient radiation myelitis in this group of meningiomas, postradiosurgery treatment. This patient with a C7–T2 recurrent meningioma had previously undergone a subtotal tumor resection. The treated tumor volume was 7.6 cm^3 with a treatment dose of 24 Gy that was delivered in three fractions; the intratumorial maximal dose was 34.3 Gy. The volume of spinal cord irradiation included 4.7 cm^3 receiving over 8 Gy and 0.1 cm^3, over 27 Gy. The maximum spinal cord dosage was 29.9 Gy. The patient's posterior column dysfunction stabilized with corticosteroid administration. The spinal cord edema seen on MRI in the involved region resolved over time and was replaced by a small degree of myelomalacia in the region.

A study by Gibbs et al[15] from our institution described this complication in six patients out of more than 1,075 treated cases. Gibbs et al suggested that potential predisposing genetic factors may be present that could be responsible for this complication. Germ line alterations in genes such as transforming growth factor beta 1 and ataxia telangiectasia may be associated with radiation-induced late effects.[16]

Conclusion

Radiosurgery has been shown to be an effective treatment for a variety of benign spinal tumors that include foraminal schwannomas and neurofibromas, hemangioblastomas, and meningiomas. This was documented by both the literature review publications as well as publications from our own institution. The data presented in this chapter from both sources were comparable. These data show that for these benign spine tumors, pain relief and neurological improvement, as well as a decrease in tumor size by serial imaging, are all important outcomes that will need to be further evaluated for each tumor type. The improvement in all three of these parameters using radiosurgery shows promise in this management strategy for these tumors. Furthermore, the paucity of cases of radiation-induced myelopathy bodes well for the more widespread use of radiosurgery in the future for benign spinal tumors.

References

[1] Lasak JM, Gorecki JP. The history of stereotactic radiosurgery and radiotherapy. Otolaryngol Clin North Am 2009; 42: 593–599

[2] Adler JR Jr, Chang SD. CyberKnife image-guided radiosurgery. Neurosurgery 2009; 64 (Suppl): A1

[3] Kondziolka D, Mathieu D, Lunsford LD, et al. Radiosurgery as definitive management of intracranial meningiomas. Neurosurgery 2008; 62: 53–58, discussion 58–60

[4] Sakamoto GT, Borchers DJ, Xiao F, et al. Cyberknife radiosurgery for trigeminal schwannomas. Neurosurgery 2009; 64 (Suppl): A14–A18

[5] Dodd RL, Ryu MR, Kamnerdsupaphon P, et al. CyberKnife radiosurgery for benign intradural extramedullary spinal tumors. Neurosurgery 2006; 58: 675–684, discussion 684–685

[6] Chang SD, Murphy M, Geis P, et al. Clinical experience with image-guided robotic radiosurgery (the Cyberknife) in the treatment of brain and spinal cord tumors. Neurol Med Chir (Tokyo) 1998; 38: 780–783

[7] Murovic JA, Gibbs IC, Chang SD, et al. Foraminal nerve sheath tumors: intermediate follow-up after cyberknife radiosurgery. Neurosurgery 2009; 64 (Suppl): A33–A43

[8] Moss JM, Choi CY, Adler JR Jr, et al. Stereotactic radiosurgical treatment of cranial and spinal hemangioblastomas. Neurosurgery 2009; 65: 79–85, discussion 85

[9] Sachdev S, Dodd RL, Chang SD, et al. Stereotactic radiosurgery yields long-term control for benign intradural, extramedullary spinal tumors. Neurosurgery 2011; 69: 533–539

[10] Gerszten PC, Burton SA, Ozhasoglu C, et al. Radiosurgery for benign intradural spinal tumors. Neurosurgery 2008; 62: 887–895

[11] Fisher CG, Wood KB. Introduction to and techniques of evidence-based medicine. Spine (Phila Pa 1976) 2007; 32: S66–72

[12] Greenberg M. Handbook of Neurosurgery. New York, NY: Thieme; 2006

[13] Chang UK, Rhee CH, Youn SM, et al. Radiosurgery using the CyberKnife for benign spinal tumors: Korea Cancer Center Hospital experience. J Neurooncol 2011; 101: 91–99

[14] Parsa AT, Lee J, Parney IF, et al. Spinal cord and intradural-extraparenchymal spinal tumors: current best care practices and strategies. J Neurooncol 2004; 69: 291–318

[15] Gibbs IC, Patil C, Gerszten PC, et al. Delayed radiation-induced myelopathy after spinal radiosurgery. Neurosurgery 2009; 64 (Suppl): A67–A72

[16] Travis EL. Genetic susceptibility to late normal tissue injury. Semin Radiat Oncol 2007; 17: 149–155

Index

A

B

T

U

V